Cancer Diagnostics

Current and Future Trends

Edited by

Robert M. Nakamura, MD
Scripps Clinic, La Jolla, CA

Wayne W. Grody, MD, PhD
UCLA School of Medicine, Los Angeles, CA

James T. Wu, PhD
ARUP Labs, Salt Lake City, UT

Raymond B. Nagle, MD, PhD
Arizona Cancer Center, Tucson, AZ

HUMANA PRESS ✳ TOTOWA, NEW JERSEY

© 2004 Humana Press Inc.
999 Riverview Drive, Suite 208
Totowa, New Jersey 07512

www.humanapress.com

Due diligence has been taken by the publishers, editors, and authors of this book to assure the accuracy of the information published and to describe generally accepted practices. The contributors herein have carefully checked to ensure that the drug selections and dosages set forth in this text are accurate and in accord with the standards accepted at the time of publication. Notwithstanding, since new research, changes in government regulations, and knowledge from clinical experience relating to drug therapy and drug reactions constantly occur, the reader is advised to check the product information provided by the manufacturer of each drug for any change in dosages or for additional warnings and contraindications. This is of utmost importance when the recommended drug herein is a new or infrequently used drug. It is the responsibility of the treating physician to determine dosages and treatment strategies for individual patients. Further, it is the responsibility of the health care provider to ascertain the Food and Drug Administration status of each drug or device used in their clinical practice. The publishers, editors, and authors are not responsible for errors or omissions or for any consequences from the application of the information presented in this book and make no warranty, express or implied, with respect to the contents in this publication.

This publication is printed on acid-free paper. ∞
ANSI Z39.48-1984 (American Standards Institute) Permanence of Paper for Printed Library Materials.

Production Editor: Wendy S. Kopf.
Cover design by Patricia F. Cleary.
Cover illustration: Figure 3 from Chapter 11, "New Applications of Flow Cytometry in Caner Diagnosis and Therapy," by Sophie Song and Faramarz Naeim.

For additional copies, pricing for bulk purchases, and/or information about other Humana titles, contact Humana at the above address or at any of the following numbers: Tel: 973-256-1699; Fax: 973-256-8341; E-mail: humana@humanapr.com, or visit our Website: http://humanapress.com

Printed in the United States of America. 10 9 8 7 6 5 4 3 2 1
e-ISBN: 1-59259-791-2
Library of Congress Cataloging in Publication Data
Cancer diagnostics : current and future trends / edited by Robert M.
Nakamura ... [et al.].
     p. ; cm. -- (Contemporary cancer research)
Includes bibliographical references and index.
 ISBN 1-58829-167-7 (alk. paper)
 1. Cancer--Diagnosis. 2. Cancer--Molecular diagnosis.
 [DNLM: 1. Neoplasms--diagnosis. 2. Laboratory Techniques and
Procedures. 3. Tumor Markers, Biological--diagnostic use. QZ 241 C2152
2004] I. Nakamura, Robert M., 1927- II. Series.
 RC270.C345 2004
 616.99'4075--dc22
                              2003026932

Preface

In the past, many tumor marker laboratory tests have not been sensitive enough for the very early detection of cancer. However, many of them have nonetheless proved useful in monitoring therapy, following the course of the tumor, and predicting prognosis. Today, cancer may be viewed as a genetic disease with various specific chromosomal and nucleotide aberrations, such as mutations, deletions, gene amplification, gene rearrangements, and translocations occurring during the transformation of a normal cell into a malignant cell.

The considerable advances in technology during the past several years have greatly enhanced our ability to detect human cancers in the very early stages of tumor formation. These technologies include: (1) nucleotide molecular assays (genomics); (2) proteomics (multiplex protein measurements); (3) DNA microarrays; and (4) bioinformatics. Many of these technologies are already helping in the integration and use of multiple biomarkers for tumors. Although the individual biomarkers may reveal only limited information, the use of multiple biomarkers can help markedly elevate the diagnostic capabilities for early detection of tumors.

Nucleic acid molecular tests are unusual in that the tests do not measure any physiological state and can be performed on fresh, frozen, or archival biological tissue specimens. Many of the molecular tests may be specific to one disease. The modern approach to the diagnosis and understanding of cancer has been characterized by the use of molecular and protein profiling. With the help of bioinformatics, artificial intelligence, and neural networks, even more accurate and sensitive diagnostic tests for cancer will surely be developed.

Cancer Diagnostics: Current and Future Trends is concerned primarily with those clinical laboratory tests that may already, or in the near future, help in the early detection, evaluation, and prediction of human tumors for specific therapeutic decisions. It should be of high interest and value to physicians who diagnose and treat cancer patients, and to clinical laboratory scientists and pathologists who are interested in diagnostic clinical laboratory tests for cancer and their future evaluation.

Robert M. Nakamura, MD
Wayne W. Grody, MD, PhD
James T. Wu, PhD
Raymond B. Nagle, MD, PhD

Contents

Contributors

DANIEL A. ARBER, MD • *Departmen of Pathology, Stanford University Medical Center, Stanford, CA*

KENNETH J. BLOOM, MD • *Senior Medical Director, US Labs, Irvine, CA*

JENNIE C. C. CHANG, PhD • *Beckman Coulter Inc., San Diego, CA*

HELEN H. CHUN, PhD • *Division of Molecular Pathology, Department of Pathology and Laboratory Medicine, The David Geffen School of Medicine at UCLA, Los Angeles, CA*

ALISTAIR J. COCHRAN, MD, FRCP • *Departments of Pathology and Laboratory Medicine and Surgery, The David Geffen School of Medicine at UCLA, Los Angeles, CA*

JUDITH A. FINLAY, PhD • *Hybritech Inc., A Subsidiary of Beckman Coulter Inc. San Diego, CA*

PATRICIA A. GANZ, MD • *Department of Hematology and Oncology and School of Public Health, Department of Health Services and Medicine and The David Geffen School of Medicine at UCLA, Los Angeles, CA*

RICHARD A. GATTI, MD • *Division of Molecular Pathology, Department of Pathology and Laboratory Medicine, The David Geffen School of Medicine at UCLA, Los Angeles, CA*

ARMAND B. GLASSMAN, MD • *Department of Pathology and Laboratory Medicine, The University of Texas MD Anderson Cancer Center, Houston, TX*

KAREN GRAY, PhD • *Millennium Pharmaceuticals Inc., Cambridge, MA*

WAYNE W. GRODY, MD, PhD • *Divisions of Medical Genetics and Molecular Pathology, Departments of Pathology and Laboratory Medicine, Pediatrics, and Human Genetics, The David Geffen School of Medicine at UCLA, Los Angeles, CA*

DAVE S. B. HOON, PhD • *Department of Molecular Oncology, John Wayne Cancer Institute, Santa Monica, CA*

VICKI L. HOPWOOD, MS • *Cytogenetic Technology Program, MD Anderson Cancer Center, The University of Texas, Houston, TX*

PETER C. HU, MS • *Cytogenetic and Medical Technology Programs, MD Anderson Cancer Center, The University of Texas, Houston, TX*

YASUSHI KASAHARA, PhD, DMSc • *Department of Clinical Pathology, School of Medicine, Showa University, Tokyo, Japan*

FERDYNAND KOS, PhD • *Beckman Coulter Inc., San Diego, CA*

KRISTINE KUUS-REICHEL, PhD • *Beckman Coulter Inc., San Diego, CA*

FRANK J. LIU, MD • *F. J. Medical Consultation Services, Sugar Land, TX*

KEVIN S. LIU, MD • *Department of Family Medicine, Scott & White Clinics (Waco Clinic), Texas A&M University College of Medicine, Waco, TX*

ALFREDO MARTÍNEZ, PhD • *Cell and Cancer Biology Branch, National Cancer Institute, Bethesda, MD*

STEPHEN D. MIKOLAJCZYK, MS • *Hybritech Inc., A Subsidiary of Beckman Coulter Inc. San Diego, CA*

MIDORI MITSUI, PhD • *Division of Molecular Pathlogy, Department of Pathology and Laboratory Medicine, The David Geffen School of Medicine at UCLA, Los Angeles, CA*

REBECCA MOSHER, MD • *Millennium Pharmaceuticals Inc., Cambridge, MA*

JAMES L. MULSHINE, MD • *Cell and Cancer Biology Branch, National Cancer Institute, Bethesda, MD*

FARAMARZ NAEIM, MD • *Department of Pathology and Laboratory Medicine, UCLA Medical Center, Los Angeles, CA*

RAYMOND B. NAGLE, MD, PhD • *Department of Pathology, Arizona Cancer Center, Tucson, AZ*

SHAREEF A. NAHAS, MS • *Division of Molecular Pathology, Department of Pathology and Laboratory Medicine, The David Geffen School of Medicine at UCLA, Los Angeles, CA*

ROBERT M. NAKAMURA, MD • *Department of Pathology, Scripps Clinic, La Jolla, CA*

CHARLES T. NUGENT, PhD • *Beckman Coulter Inc., San Diego, CA*

THOMAS M. PRIBYL, PhD • *Hybritech Inc., A Subsidiary of Beckman Coulter, Inc., San Diego, CA*

ASIF RASHID, MD, PhD • *Department of Pathology, The University of Texas MD Anderson Cancer Center, Houston, TX*

RAMUNE RELIENE, PhD • *Department of Pathology and Laboratory Medicine, The David Geffen School of Medicine at UCLA, Los Angeles, CA*

HARRY G. RITTENHOUSE, PhD • *Hybritech Inc., A Subsidiary of Beckman Coulter, Inc., San Diego, CA*

ALICE A. ROBERTS, MD, PhD • *Department of Pathology and Laboratory Medicine, The David Geffen School of Medicine at UCLA, Los Angeles, CA*

JEFFREY S. ROSS, MD • *Department of Pathology and Laboratory Medicine, Albany Medical College, Albany, NY and Millennium Pharmaceuticals Inc., Cambridge, MA*

ROBERT H. SCHIESTL, PhD • *Departments of Pathology, Environmental Health, and Radiation Oncology, UCLA Schools of Medicine and Public Health, Los Angeles, CA*

JOYCE L. SELDON, MS CGc • *Jonsson Comprehensive Cancer Center, University of California, Los Angeles, CA*

SOPHIE SONG, MD, PhD • *Department of Pathology and Laboratory Medicine, The David Geffen School of Medicine at UCLA, Los Angeles, CA*

JAMES STEC • *Millennium Pharmaceuticals Inc., Cambridge, MA*

BRET TABACK, MD • *Department of Molecular Oncology, John Wayne Cancer Institute, Santa Monica, CA*

ENG M. TAN, MD • *W. M. Keck Autoimmune Disease Center, Department of Molecular and Experimental Medicine, The Scripps Research Institute, La Jolla, CA*

JORDI TAULER, PhD • *Cell and Cancer Biology Branch, National Cancer Institute, Bethesda, MD*

C. HOWARD TSENG, MD, PhD • *College of Medicine, Chung Shan Medical University, Taichung, Taiwan*

YUTAKA TSUKADA, MD, PhD • *Hachioji Main Labs, SRL Inc., Tokyo, Japan*

R. BRUCE WALLACE, PhD • *Hybritech Inc., A Subsidiary of Beckman Coulter, Inc., San Diego, CA*

JAMES T. WU, MD • *ARUP Labs, University of Utah, Salt Lake City, UT*

TSUNG-TEH WU, MD, PhD • *Department of Pathology, The University of Texas MD Anderson Cancer Center, Houston, TX*

I
INTRODUCTION

General Considerations in the Use and Application of Laboratory Tests for the Evaluation of Cancer

Robert M. Nakamura and Wayne W. Grody

1. INTRODUCTION

Cancer Diagnostics is concerned with diagnostic tests for the detection and evaluation of human tumors. A cancer cell is the result of malignant transformation of a normal cell *(1)*. Cancer cells are associated with significant growth dysregulation. The identification of a universal tumor-specific epitope or marker has remained elusive. In the past, many types of tumor markers have been characterized The serological and serum tumor markers have included enzymes, proteins, hormones, mucin, and blood group substances *(1)*. Many current tumor marker tests are useful primarily for prediction of prognosis and monitoring therapy of previously diagnosed cancers. However, significant research efforts have been directed to finding laboratory tests that may be useful for screening or early detection of tumors. One useful organ-specific marker has been the prostate specific antigen (PSA) test which has been useful for helping the clinician in the decision to proceed to prostatic biopsy for the diagnosis of cancer vs prostatic hyperplasia *(2)*.

Within recent years, there has been a revolutionary development of molecular pathology tests for the diagnosis and evaluation of cancer. Many of these molecular tests can specifically characterize the type of tumor. Many have demonstrated that they can be useful for the early diagnosis of certain cancers and even the prediction of those that are hereditary *(3–5)*.

Following completion of the sequencing phase of the human genome project, there has been an emphasis on the study of human proteins as drug targets, combining the newer efforts of proteomics and pharmacogenomics. The study of proteins will undoubtedly become a central component in diagnostics *(6)*. Currently, several comprehensive approaches to the identification of protein markers in cancer are being developed *(7,8)*, building on advances in two-dimensional electrophoresis, mass spectrometry, and chip-based technologies, including tissue and antibody arrays. Through the use of serum proteomic patterns, Petricoin et al. *(8)* identified 50 ovarian cancers in a masked set that included 18 stage I cases. The 50 cases were compared to 66 cases of nonmalignant disease, of which 63 were noncancer patients. The results yielded a sensitivity of 100%, specificity of 95% and a positive predictive value of 94%, far exceeding any other existent general screening test for malignancy.

From: *Cancer Diagnostics: Current and Future Trends*
Edited by: R. M. Nakamura, W. W. Grody, J. T. Wu, and R. B. Nagle © Humana Press Inc., Totowa, NJ

In this chapter, to set the stage for the remaining contributors in this volume, there will be a brief discussion of the modern concepts of cancer and general discussion of the characteristics of various clinical laboratory tests.

2. MODERN CONCEPTS OF CANCER

Most cancers are caused by the combined interaction of genetic factors, lifestyle, and environmental exposures *(9,10)*. Over the past several years, cancer research efforts have made extensive progress in the definition of the molecular basis for malignant transformation and proliferation of cells.

Today, cancer may be viewed as a genetic disease with its various specific chromosomal and nucleotide aberrations *(1,4,11)*. The multiple genetic changes include mutations, deletions, gene amplifications, gene rearrangements, and translocations during the transformation of a normal cell into a malignant one.

Researchers have made significant advances in the study of mutations in DNA sequences that lead to amplification or suppression of oncogenes or to the deletion of tumor suppressor genes encoding regulatory proteins that normally suppress cellular proliferation *(1,4)*. The mutations in cancer can be either germline mutations—which are inherited and associated with specific familial cancer syndromes—or somatic acquired mutations. The somatic mutations are sporadic and are the most frequent abnormalities associated with tumor formation and progression *(12,13)*.

Environmental influences that cause oncogenic mutations include radiation, ultraviolet light exposure, and chemical carcinogens. Also, infectious agents, such as the human papilloma virus (HPV) or the Epstein-Barr virus (EBV), can promote malignancy through interaction with the host genome *(9,10,14,15)*. A genetic susceptibility to cancer can result from mutations that alter the normal cellular regulatory or DNA repair mechanisms.

Most cancers are the result of multiple events involving multiple genes. Certain genetic mutations precede tumor formation, and other mutations evolve during tumor progression *(16–20)*. Fearon and Vogelstein *(21)* document evidence that the pathogenesis of colon cancer is a multi-step process. Colorectal carcinomas may arise from a pre-existing benign adenoma. The colorectal tumors have mutational events that result in activation of oncogenes and inactivation of tumor suppressor genes. Thus, many carcinomas require at least five genetic alterations in a multi-step process. The nature and progression of the tumor is influenced by the total accumulation of changes rather than the sequence of events.

3. REASONS FOR REQUESTING CLINICAL LABORATORY TESTS

There are several indications for physicians requesting a clinical laboratory test *(22,23)*. These indicators are listed in Table 1.

In general, clinical laboratory tests are commonly ordered for diagnosis of diseases, monitoring therapy, and predictions of prognosis. The most frequent and important tests requested are those used to influence therapeutic decisions and to monitor the course of therapy.

A laboratory test that may not be useful and necessary for medical care today may nevertheless be important in the future when a new therapeutic drug or modality is discovered. For example, tests for a variety of oncogenes and anti-oncogenes (i.e., tumor suppressor genes, such as *p53*) will probably be very important tests in the future much as testing for HER-2/neu oncogene amplification has become *(23,24)*. A mutation in the *ras* oncogene or a dele-

Table 1
Uses and Reasons for Requesting a Laboratory Test Diagnosis

1. Assessment of prognosis and severity
2. Monitoring course of disease or response to therapy
3. Genetic classification
4. Screening of defined populations, i.e., high risk
5. Establishment of baseline values for assessment of future change
6. Risk assessment
7. Clinical research studies

tion of *p53* is often involved in tumor formation. Investigators are developing anticancer agents which can block the induction of tumors by mutated *ras* genes *(24,25)*. When such agents become generally available, many laboratories will need to institute assays to detect *ras* oncogene mutations in order to determine which patients would be candidates for these specific gene-targeted therapies.

The value of a laboratory test depends on its ability to answer a specific clinical question for patient management *(26)*. The clinical value of a new test should be determined by how well it outperforms currently available tests and whether this performance can be economically justified. The cost effectiveness of the new laboratory test in clinical practice should be determined *(27,28)*.

The predictive value of a test result is not a real measure of its clinical value, especially when it is used in the later stages of a diagnostic workup *(29)*. The clinical value can be determined by the amount of useful information for patient management provided by the test result. Thus, a useful laboratory test ordered by the physician will be needed for and applied to a medical and therapeutic decision based upon the results. Many clinicians today are aware of an aphorism which states, "Before ordering a laboratory test, decide what you will do if the results are normal or abnormal. If both answers are the same, the test is not necessary" *(22)*.

4. SENSITIVITY, SPECIFICITY, AND PREDICTIVE VALUE OF LABORATORY TESTS

There are several characteristics used to describe laboratory tests. It is critical for the clinician to have some information on the sensitivity and specificity of the laboratory test being ordered *(30–34)*. Sensitivity can be defined as "positivity in disease" or the probability of a test being positive in patients who actually have the disease. Specificity concerns the ability of the test to distinguish the patients who have the disease from the patients who do not have the disease.

Positive predictive value (PPV) is the likelihood that the patient has the disease if the test is positive. Negative predictive value (NPV) is the likelihood that the patient does not have the disease if the test result is negative. There are important issues that should be emphasized *(31)*:

1. Positive and negative results must be well defined so they can be compared.
2. The disease in question must be defined clearly and have relevance to decisions made in practice.
3. The calculation of specificity should be done using well-defined reference groups:

Table 2
Immunological and Serologic Methods

Methods	Use
Immunofluorescence	Sensitive assay for screening
Enzyme immunoassay (EIA)	Sensitive assay for screening
Double immunodiffusion (ID)	Requires precipitin reaction; high specificity but not very sensitive procedure
Counterimmunoelectrophoresis (CIE)	Increased sensitivity and speed as compared with ID
Particle agglutination	More sensitive than ID
Immunoblotting (IB)	Very sensitive and allows detection of antibodies to soluble and insoluble antigens.

    a. A group that has been carefully selected to exclude the specific disease in question, or
    b. A "healthy" group defined by the absence of any major illness.
4. If the test is used to screen a population for the specific disease, then the prevalence of the disease must be considered.
5. If the test is used to distinguish options on the differential diagnosis of two different diseases, then the relative prevalence of these two conditions is more important than the prevalence of either condition in the population as a whole.

None of the current immunological or serologic tumor marker assays approach the 100% specificity and sensitivity of an ideal assay *(1)*. Table 2 lists commonly used immunochemical and serologic testing methods.

Immunofluorescence assays, enzyme immunoassays, immunoblotting assays, and chemiluminescence assays involve a primary antibody-antigen reaction and are sensitive. Such primary antigen-antibody assays are 1000 times more sensitive than secondary antigen-antibody assays, such as immunodiffusion, counterimmunoelectrophoresis (CIE), and particle agglutination assays *(35)*. As a general rule, highly sensitive tests useful for exclusion of disease have low diagnostic specificity, whereas the less sensitive assays may offer greater diagnostic specificity. Sensitivity and specificity are inversely related and have much to do with the cutoff level or upper limit of the normal reference range. In many assays for a particular tumor marker, the cutoff level is commonly set at the 95th percentile of the so-called "normal population" that is not known to have the cancer. However, there is often an overlap between the cancer patients and normal population, patients with benign tumors, and patients with diseases other than cancer.

Often there are reports of new tumor markers stating that the difference between the mean of the tumor population and that of the normal population is significant. However, if the difference in the mean of the two populations is five- to ten-fold, the marker may be useful and show promise. If the mean of the population of normal and cancer patients shows only 2 -to 2.5-fold difference, then when patients with other diseases are examined, there usually will be considerable overlap and the test will not demonstrate good sensitivity and specificity.

5. DIAGNOSTIC TESTING VS EVALUATIVE TESTING

Ward *(36,37)* has emphasized that clinical laboratory tests may be categorized as diagnostic or evaluative. The usefulness of a new diagnostic test is determined by how the test categorizes diseased persons as diseased and unaffected persons as unaffected based on comparison with a gold standard indicator of disease. For a diagnostic test to be useful it must be able to demonstrate high sensitivity and specificity on the differences between individual patients. Good diagnostic tests should give reproducible results over time. Evaluative tests are used to measure and assess changes in disease activity over time and to determine indexes of change *(38)*. The evaluative tests are used to compare the current status of a patient with his or her status at a previous point in time to determine if there is improvement or disease progression. The value and accuracy of an evaluative test is determined by how it monitors changes in disease activity. The test should be compared with changes in an accepted gold standard measurement of disease activity. An example of a useful evaluative test would be to determine the serum level of the acute phase inflammatory C-reactive protein in rheumatic fever or rheumatoid arthritis. The C-reactive protein levels parallel the inflammatory activity during the course of the disease *(39,40)*.

6. ASSESSING NEW EVALUATIVE LABORATORY TESTS

Before a new laboratory test is recommended to be incorporated in clinical practice, the following points should be considered *(36)*:

1. The test should be standardized so that findings of the test in clinical research studies can be reproduced and applied in a nonresearch setting.
2. Test results should available in a timely manner for good patient care and clinical decision-making.
3. The new test should be more valid or sensitive to change when compared to evaluative tests already in use.
4. The new test should be compared with existing tests by randomized trials to determine cost effectiveness *(41)*.

7. CUTOFF VALUES (REFERENCE RANGES) AND MULTIPLICITY OF LABORATORY TESTS

Each clinical laboratory must define and establish cutoff values between a normal and abnormal result. The assignment of the cutoff values will determine the proportion of false-positive and false-negative results *(42)*. For example, does the "normal reference range" include 95, 97.5, or 99% of the so-called normal population? Are age-related reference ranges assigned?

For many clinical laboratory tests, the cutoff is set to include only 95% of the normal population, therefore allowing a 5% false-positive rate. Thus, if someone without the specific disease has one test performed, there is a 5% chance the result will be outside of the reference range. When multiple tests are performed, with a cutoff to include 95% of the normal population, then the likelihood of obtaining a false-positive result rises dramatically with the number of tests performed. The likelihood of one abnormal result with five tests is 22% *(34,43)*. Therefore, abnormal results must be interpreted with caution if multiple tests have been performed.

8. NUCLEIC ACID MOLECULAR MARKERS FOR CANCER

Nucleic acid-based molecular tests are unusual as the tests do not measure any physiological state and can be performed on fresh, frozen, or archival biologic tissue specimens. Many of the molecular tests may be specific to one disease. The modern approach to diagnosis and understanding of cancer has been with the use of molecular profiling *(45–47)*. Under this technology, an additional category of testing exists besides the usual diagnostic, evaluative, and prognostic tests for cancer. The molecular tests are used to determine the risk of future disease in an individual who is healthy at the time of testing. In the cancer field, such tests have become prominent in the setting of familial cancer syndromes.

Most of the heritable familial cancer syndrome genes have multiple possible mutations, many of which are quite rare or even unique to one family.Thorough laboratory testing may require direct sequencing of the gene to attain the highest accuracy and sensitivity of mutation detection and allow individuals to make critical diagnostic and therapeutic decisions *(3,4)*.

Molecular techniques have provided many basic tools that will allow successful detection, specific diagnoses, and rapid treatment of cancers. Through the use of molecular tests, it will also be possible to reliably differentiate similar cancers from one another.

DNA microassay techniques are now used for a comprehensive detection of many cancer-associated mutations, or for gene expression in an effort to fingerprint various cancers for diagnosis and therapeutic evaluation *(7,48,49)*.

9. EXAMPLES OF MOLECULAR MARKERS FOR EARLY DETECTION OF CANCERS

Several researchers have reported on the use of a new generation of panels of molecular tests for the early detection of tumors of the pancreas and lung, colorectal tumors, liver carcinoma, and head and neck tumors. These molecular techniques may provide a new approach to cancer screening, diagnosis and therapy in the future. The molecular assays have been applied to DNA extracted from stool, serum, and body fluids for detecting various types of cancer.

9.1. Circulating Serum/Plasma Tumor DNA

Small amounts of free DNA circulate in both normal and diseased human plasma *(50–52)*. However, increased concentrations of DNA are present in plasma of cancer patients. In cancer patients, mutations of oncogenes (i.e., *ras* gene) and tumor suppressor genes (*p53*), and microsatellite alterations have been detected. Plasma DNA analysis may become a useful noninvasive diagnostic approach for detection and evaluation of many different types of cancer *(53,54)*.

9.2. Colorectal Carcinoma

Molecular assays on DNA extracted from stool specimens have been reported for detection of colorectal cancers *(55–57)*. The reported incidence of *k-ras* mutations is between 7 and 80% *(58)*, and 40% *(58,59)*. The mutations in *k-ras* codons12 and 13 were present in 53 and 89% of colon cancers, respectively *(60,59)*. The application of *k-ras* and *p53* mutation gene analyses in the feces was only able to detect 57.7% of patients with colorectal cancer *(61)*.Therefore, the study of other genes involved in colorectal carcinogenesis was found to be necessary.

Gocke et al. *(62)* have reported that *p53* and APC (adenomatous polyposis coli) mutations are detectable in the plasma and serum of patients with colorectal cancer or adenomas.

The following panel of molecular markers detecting gene mutations in DNA extracted from stool specimens was reported to be useful for early detection of colorectal carcinoma *(56)*. These panels included assays for APC, *k-ras*, *p53*, and *Bat 26* as described below.

Adenomatous polyposis coli gene (APC) plays a role in cell adhesion and migration. In a mutated form, the protein β-catenin accumulates in high levels and stimulates cell growth. *k-ras* is involved in signal transduction from activated transmembrane receptors to protein kinases. Wildtype *p53* genes will initiate cell cycle arrest and DNA repair. Mutated forms lead to decrease or absence of *p53* function. Thus, the damaged cells do not repair their DNA properly and produce more damaged cells. *Bat-26* is a marker of microsatellite instability (MSI). In the normal genome, tandem repeats of 1 to 6 nucleotide (microsatellites), are scattered and fixed in number. With errors in the DNA mismatch repair mechanism, the microsatellites are expanded in repeat number. Ten to 15% of colon cancers have MSI *(62,63)*.

9.3. Pancreatic Carcinoma

Pancreatic cancers are difficult to detect early. The serological tumor markers, such as CEA and CA-19-9, have not been sensitive enough to screen patients for pancreatic cancers at an early stage *(1)*. Molecular markers have been reported to show promise of early detection of pancreatic cancers by serum and stool analysis. Pancreatic cancers are known to have a high incidence (over 90%) of *k-ras* gene mutations *(64,65)*.

A potential noninvasive source of DNA in pancreatic cancer patients is the serum *(64–66)*. Also, *k-ras* mutations have been detected in stool, in pancreatic duct secretions, and pancreatic cytology smears *(67)*. Mulcahy et al. *(66)* found *k-ras* mutations in the DNA from plasma of 17 of 24 patients with pancreatic cancer. They also noted that plasma DNA alterations were found 5 to 14 mo before clinical diagnosis of pancreatic cancer in four patients.

9.4. Cervical Carcinoma

Recently, the FDA's Microbiology Device Panel made recommendations to the FDA *(68)* that HPV molecular testing should be added to the Pap smear for primary screening of high-grade cervical disease or cancer in women over 30 yr of age. The current primary screening tool for cervical cancer is the Pap smear and is not performed on approximately one-third of the eligible women. The sensitivity of the Pap has been estimated to be 35–81% *(68)*. If both the Pap smear and HPV test are negative, the negative predictive value of the combined test is virtually 100%. HPV tests can be used as a follow-up of ASCUS Pap (abnormal squamous cells of undetermined origin). A negative HPV test on an ASCUS follow-up would indicate that the patient does not have a carcinoma or a significant dysplasia *(69,70)*.

The oncogenic proteins E6 and E7 of HPV types 16, 18, 31, and 33 bind to tumor suppressor genes *p53* and RB, respectively *(71,72)*. The process results in impaired tumor-suppressor gene function, involving DNA repair, decreased apoptosis, mutations, and eventual virus-induced cervical carcinogenesis.

10. QUALITY CONTROL AND QUALITY ASSURANCE ISSUES WITH MOLECULAR TESTS

Molecular genetic and oncology tests can provide unique information not available by any other clinical method. However, many of the tests are often "home brew" and the performance and quality assurance issues are mainly the responsibilities of the individual clinical laboratory *(5,73,74)*.

The recommendations and guidelines regarding quality control and assurance issues have been defined for all clinical laboratories performing DNA testing. The procedures are described in detail in the laboratory inspection checklists and guidelines for molecular pathology and molecular genetics, published by the College of American Pathologists, American College of Medical Genetics and the National Committee on Clinical Laboratory Standards (NCCLS) *(5)*.

Each laboratory should conduct the various quality control and quality assurance procedures recommended. In addition, for each molecular assay, the clinical laboratory should perform a clinical validation study or literature review and determine the medical utility and usefulness. The guidelines as recommended by CLIA-88 (Clinical Laboratory Improvement Ammendments) should be followed. Proficiency testing procedures as defined by CLIA-88 must be implemented *(75)*.

11. ETHICAL ISSUES IN MOLECULAR TESTS

There are certain unique ethical issues raised by molecular tests, especially those pertaining to testing for genetic diseases by virtue of their predictive nature and the implications of positive findings for insurability, employment, and other family members. Although not widespread, there have been instances of adverse effects and discrimination as a result of genetic testing, even for recessive mutations *(4,76–78)*. Information in the medical record is legally recognized as private and confidential *(3,76)*. Pathologists, clinicians, and health care workers should not disclose confidential information to others without the patient's consent, actual or implied. With current information technology and the numerous personnel with legitimate access to medical records in electronic form, there has been a perceived need for new regulations and technology to provide greater security of the data and maintain confidentiality. Laboratories performing molecular testing have a heightened role to play in ensuring their appropriate use, confidentiality, and meaningful reporting. Because this area of clinical laboratory testing is so new and complex, many primary care physicians are not comfortable with result interpretation, and inaccurate, potentially harmful, misinformation may be conveyed to patients even when the analytic portion of the test was performed impeccably *(79)*. Molecular testing laboratories must therefore be highly cognizant of the pre- and post-analytic aspects of these tests, to ensure their proper use and enhance their clinical utility.

12. SUMMARY

The clinical laboratory should clearly state the immunochemical or immunological test procedure performed, along with the definition of reference range to include the cutoff value and what percent of the normal population is included in the reference range.

The clinical interpretation of the specific laboratory test can be influenced by many factors, including the sensitivity and specificity of the test, the clinical setting in which the test was requested, the reason the test was requested, and the number of tests performed. The clinician should order the test on the basis of "what question does he or she want answered?" and, what he will do or recommend when the results of the clinical laboratory are normal or definitely abnormal. The test request is not necessary or definitely necessary for patient care if the physician will not change his clinical care or recommendation if the results are either normal or definitely abnormal.

The newer approach for laboratory tests in the diagnosis and management of cancer will likely be panel testing at the genetic and protein levels, since cancer is now known to result from multiple genetic abnormalities accumulating over a long period of time. Data will be accumulated on specific types of tumor panel assays, which will become available for "fingerprint analysis" of specific types of tumors.

The assay panels may include specific gene loci and sequences, oncogenes and suppressor gene products, mini-satellite instability analysis, chromosome analysis, etc. Such panels or "microassays" will be analyzed by a sophisticated software program with access to a large database for early detection and diagnosis, evaluation and therapeutic management of the cancer patients.

REFERENCES

1. Wu JT. 1997. Types of tumor markers, in Human Circulating Tumor Markers: Current Concepts and Clinical Applications. Nakamura RM and Wu JT, eds., American Society of Clinical Pathology Press: Chicago, Illinois pp. 37–75.
2. Catalona WJ, Smith DS, Wolfert RL, et al. 1995. Evaluation of Percentage of Free Serum Prostate-Specific Antigen to Improve Specificity of Prostate Cancer Screening. JAMA 274:1214–1220.
3. Nakamura RM. 1997. Laboratory diagnosis and evaluation of human tumors: Future perspectives, in Human Circulating Tumor Markers: Current Concepts and Clinical Applications. Nakamura RM and Wu JT, eds., American Society of Clinical Pathology Press: Chicago, Illinois, pp. 225–248.
4. Gregg JP and Grody WW. 1997. Diagnostic Molecular Genetics: Current Applications and Future Technologies. Pediatric. Ann. 9:553–561.
5. Grody WW. 1998. Molecular assays for genetic diseases, in Clinical Diagnostic Immunology: Protocols in Quality Assurance and Standardization. Burek CL, Cook L, Folds JD, Nakamura RM and Sever JL, eds. Blackwell Sciences: Boston, MA, pp. 471–480.
6. Srimivas PR, Verma M, Zhao Y, Srivatava S. 2002. Proteomics for Cancer Biomarker Discovery Clin. Chem. 48:1160–1169.
7. Liotta L and Petricoin E. 2000. Molecular Profiling of Human Cancer. Nat. Rev. Genetic 1:48–56.
8. Srinvas PR, Srivastava S, Hanash S, Wright GL. 2001. Proteomics in Early Detection of Cancer. Clin. Chem. 47:1901–1911.
9. McPhee SJ. 1995. Screening for Cancer: Useful Despite its Limitations. West. J. Med. 163:169–172.
10. Ames B, Willett WC, Swirsky-Gold L. 1995. The Causes and Prevention of Cancer. Proc. Natl. Acad. Sci. USA 92:5258–5265.
11. Wilman CL and Fenoglio-Preiser CM. 1987. Oncogenes, Suppressor Genes, and Carcinogenesis. 1987. Hum. Pathol. 18:895–902.
12. Cordon-Cardo C. 1995. Mutation of Cell Cycle Regulators: Biological and Clinical Implications for Human Neoplasia. Am. J. Pathol. 147:545–560.
13. Malkin D. 1994. Germline *p53* Mutations and Heritable Cancer. Annu Rev Genet. 28:443–465.
14. Mutirangura A. 2001. Serum/plasma Viral DNA: Mechanisms and Diagnostic Applications to Nasopharyngeal and Cervical Carcinoma. Ann. NY Acad. Sci 945:59–67.
15. Ferenczy A and Franco E. 2002. Persistent Human Papillomavirus Infection and Cervical Neoplasia. Lancet Oncol. 3:11–16.
16. Goldberg D and Diamandis EP. 1993. Models of Neoplasia and their Diagnostic Implications: A historical Perspective. Clin. Chem. 39:2360–2374.
17. Burck KB, Lieu ET, Larrick JW. 1998. Oncogenes: An Introduction to the Concept of Cancer Genes. Springer-Verlag: New York, NY.

18. Bishop JM. 1987. Molecular Genetics of Cancer. Science 235:305–311.

19. Diamandis EP. 1992. Oncogenes and Tumor Suppressor Genes: New Biochemical Tests. Crit. Rev. Clin. Lab. Sci. 29:269–305.

20. Weinberg RA. 1989. Oncogenes, Antioncogenes, and the Molecular Bases of Multistep Carcinogenesis. Cancer Res. 49:3717–3721.

21. Fearon ER and Vogelstein B. 1990. A Genetic Model for Colorectal Tumorigenesis. Cell 61:759–767.

22. Nakamura RM and Bylund DJ. 1992. New Developments in Clinical Laboratory Molecular Assays. J. Clin. Lab. Analysis 6:73–83.

23. Nakamura RM and Bylund DJ. 1994. Factors Influencing Changes in the Clinical Immunology Laboratory. Clin. Chem. 40:2193–2204.

24. Travis J. 1993. Novel Anti-cancer Agents Move Closer to Reality. Science 260:1877–1878.

25. James EL, Goldstein JL, Brown MS, et al. 1993. Benzodiazepine Peptidomimetrics: Potent Inhibitors of Ras Fanesylation in Animal Cells. Science 260:1937–1942.

26. Robertson EA, Zweig MH, Van Steirteghem AC. 1983. Evaluating the Clinical Efficiency of Laboratory Test. Am. J. Clin Path. 79:78–86.

27. Pannal P, Marshall W, Jabor A, Magid E. 1996. A Strategy to Promote the Rational Use of Laboratory Tests. J. Int. Fed. Clin. Chem. 8:16–19.

28. Johnson HA. 1995. Diagnostic Information as a Commodity. Clin. Chem. 41:781–784.

29. Johnson HA. 1993. Predictive Value and Informational Value of a Diagnostic Test. Annals Clin. Lab. Sci. 23:159–164.

30. Galen RS and Gambino SR. 1975. Beyond Normality: The Predictive Value and Efficiency of Medical Diagnosis. Wiley: New York, NY.

31. Dawkins RL. 1985. Sensitivity and specificity of autoantibody testing, in The Autoimmune Diseases. Mackay IR and Rose NR, eds. Academic Press: San Diego, CA, pp. 669–706.

32. Vecchio TJ. 1985. Predictive Value of a Single Diagnostic Test in Unselected Populations. NEJM 274:1171–1173.

33. Ransohoff DF and Feinstein AR. 1978. Problems of Spectrum and Bias in Evaluating the Efficacy of Diagnostic Tests. NEJM 299:926–930.

34. Sibley J. 1995. Laboratory Tests. Rheum. Dis. Clin. NA 21:407–428.

35. Hang L and Nakamura RM. 1997. Current Concepts and Advances in Clinical Laboratory Testing for Autoimmune Diseases. Crit. Rev. Clin Lab Sci. 343:275–311.

36. Ward MM. 1995. Evaluative Laboratory Testing. Assessing Tests that Assess Disease Activity. Arthritis Rheum. 38:1555–1563.

37. Ward MM. 1993. Clinical Measurer in Rheumatoid Arthritis: Which are Most Useful in Assessing Patients? J. Rheum. 21:17–21.

38. Kirshner B and Guyatt G. A 1985. Methodological Framework for Assessing Health Indices. J. Chronic Dis. 38:27–36.

39. Otterness IG. 1994. The Value of C-reactive Protein Measurement in Rheumatoid Arthritis. Semin. Arthritis Rheum. 24:91–104.

40. Sox HC. 1996. The Evaluation of Diagnostic Tests: Principles, Problems and New Developments. Ann. Rev. Med. 47:463–471.

41. Guyatt GH, Tugwell PX, Feeny DH, et al. 1986. A Framework for Clinical Evaluation of Diagnostic Technologies. Can. Med. Assoc. J. 134:587–594.

42. Einstein AJ and Bodian CA. 1997. The Relationship Among Performance Measures in the Selection of Diagnostic Tests. Arch. Path. Lab. Med. 121:110–117.

43. Cupples LA, Heeren T, Schatzkin A, et al. 1984. Multiple Testing of Hypothesis in Comparing Two Groups. Ann. Int. Med. 100:122–219.

44. Heim RA and Silverman LM. 1994. Molecular Pathology: Approaches to Diagnostic Human Disease in the Clinical Laboratory. Caroline Academic. Durham, NC. p. 104.

45. Mao L and Sidransky D. 1994. Cancer Screening in Genetic Alterations in Human Tumors. Cancer Res. 54:1939S–1940S.

46. Ahrendt SA and Sidransky, D. 1999. The Potential of Molecular Screening. Surgical Oncol.Clin. N.A. 8:641–656.

47. Mao L. 2000. Microsatellite Analysis, Applications and Pitfalls. Ann. NY Acad. Sci. 906:55–62.

48. Marx J. 2000. Medicine. DNA Assays Reveal Cancer in its Many Forms. Science. 289:1670–1672.

49. Bertucci, F, Houlgatte R, Nguyen C, Urens P, Jordan BR, Birnbaum D. 2001. Gene Expression Profiling of Cancer by Use of DNA Assays: How Far from the Clinic? Lancet Oncol. 2:647–82.

50. Anker P and Stroun M. 2000. Circulating Nucleic Acids in Plasma or Serum. Ann. NY Acad. Sci. 906:1–169.

51. Sidransky D. 2000. Circulating DNA: What We Know and What We Need to Learn. Ann. NY Acad. Sci. 906:1–4.

52. Jen J, Wu L, Sidransky D. 2000. An Overview on the Isolation and Analysis of Circulating Tumor DNA in Plasma and Serum. Ann. NY Acad. Sci. 906:8–12.

53. Kopreski MS and Gocke CD. 2000. Cellular-versus Extracellular-based Assays: Comparing Utility in DNA and RNA Molecular Marker Assessment. Ann. NY Acad. Sci. 906:124–128.

54. Anker P, Mulcahy H, Chen XQ, Stroum M. 1999. Detection of Circulating Tumor DNA in the Blood (plasma/serum) of Cancer Patients. Cancer Metastasis Rev. 18:65–73.

55. Ahlquist DA, Skoletsky JE, Boynton KA, et al. 2000. Colorectal Cancer Screening by Detection of Altered Human DNA in Stool: Feasibility of a Multitarget Assay Panel. Gastroenterology 119:1219–1227.

56. Willis MS, Freda FS, Chenault CB. 2002. Current Methods of Colorectal Cancer Screening. Medical Lab. Observer 34:12–14.

57. Sidransky D, Tokino T, Hamilton SR, et al. 1992. Identification of Ras Oncogene Mutations in the Stool of Patients with Curable Colorectal Tumors. Science 256:1102–105.

58. Minamoto T, Mai M, Ronai Z. 2000. K-*ras* Mutation: Early detection in Molecular Diagnosis and Risk Assessment of Colorectal, Pancreas, and Lung Cancers-A Review. Cancer Detect. Prev. 1:1–12.

59. Lev Z, Kislitsin D, Rennert G, Lerner A. 2000. Utilization of K-*ras* Mutations Identified in Stool DNA for the Early Detection of Colorectal Cancer. J. Cell. Biochem. Suppl. 34:35–39.

60. Martinez-Garza SG, Nunez-Salazar A, Calderon-Garciduenas AL, et al. 1999. Frequency and Clinicopathology Associations of K-ras Mutations in Colorectal Cancer in a Northeast Mexican Population. Dig. Dis. 17:225–229.

61. Notarnicola M, Cavallini A, Cardone R, Pezzolla F, Demma I, Di Leo A. 2000. K-ras and *p53* Mutations in DNA Extracted from Colonic Epithelial Cells Exfoliated in Faeces of Patients with Colorectal Cancer. Dig. Liver Dis. 32:131–136.

62. Gocke CD, Benko FA, Kopreski MS, McGarrity TJ. 2000. *p53* and APC Mutations are Detectable in the Plasma and Serum of Patients with Colorectal Cancer (CRC) or Adenomas. Ann. NY Acad. Sci. 906:44–50.

63. Samowitz WS, Slattery ML, Potter JD, Leppert MF. 1999. Bat-26, and BAT-40 Instability in Colorectal Adenomas and Carcinomas and Germline Polymorphisms. Am. J. Path. 154:1637–1641.

64. Theodur L, Melzer E, Sologov M, Bar-Meir S. 2000. Diagnostic Value of K-*ras* Mutations in Serum of Pancreatic Cancer Patients. Ann. NY Acad. Sci. 906:19–24.

65. Mulcahy H and Farthing MJ. 1999. Diagnosis of Pancreatico-biliary Malignancy: Detection of Gene Mutations in Plasma and Stool. Ann. Oncol. 10 Suppl 4:114–117.

66. Mulcahy,HE, Lyautey J, Lederrey C. 1998. A Prospective Study of K-*ras* Mutations in the Plasma of Pancreatic Cancer Patients. Clin. Cancer. Res. 4:271–275.

67. Apple SK, Hecht JR, Novak JM, Nieberg RK, Rosenthal DL, Grody WW. 1996. Polymerase Chain Reaction-based K-ras Mutation Detection of Pancreatic Adenocarcinoma in Routine Cytology Smears. Am. J. Clin. Pathol. 105:321–326.

68. Sainato D. 2002. A Role for HPV in Cervical Cancer Screening? Clin. Lab. news. 28:4–10.

69. Vassilakos P, Petignat P, Boulvain M, Campana A. 2002. Primary Screening for Cervical Cancer

Precursors by the Combined Use of Liquid-based Cytology, Computer-assisted Cytology and HPV DNA Testing. Br. J. Cancer 3:382–388.

70. Wright TC Jr, Cox JT, Massad, LS, Twiggs LB, Wilkinson EJ. 2002. ASCCP-Sponsored Consensus Conference. 2001 Consensus Guidelines for the Management of Women with Cervical Cytological Abnormalities. JAMA 16:2120–2129.

71. Brooks LA, Sullivan,A, O'Nions J, et al. 2002. E7 Proteins from Oncogenic Human Papillomavirius Types Transactivate p73: Role in Cervical Intraepithelial Neoplasia. Br. J. Cancer 86:263–268.

72. Ferenczy A and Franco E. 2002. Persistent Human Papillomavirus Infection and Cervical Neoplasia. Lancet Oncol. 3:11–16.

73. Dequeker E, Ramsden S, Grody WW, Stenzel TT, Barton DE. 2001. Quality Control in Molecular Genetic Testing. Nat. Rev. Genet. 2:717–23.

74. McGovern MM, Benach MO, Wallenstein S, Desnick RJ, Keenlyside R. 1999. Quality Assurance in Molecular Genetic Testing Laboratories. JAMA 281:835–841.

75. Grody WW. 1994. Proficiency Testing in Diagnostic Molecular Pathology. Diagn. Mol. Pathol. 3:211–213.

76. Grody WW and Pyeritz RE. 1999. Report Card on Molecular Genetic Testing. Room for Improvement? JAMA 9:845–847.

77. Grody WW. 1999. Cystic Fibrosis: Molecular Diagnosis, Population Screening, and Public Policy. Arch. Pathol. Lab. Med. 123:1041–6.

78. Billings, PR, Kahn MA, de Cuevas M, Beckwith J, Alper JS, Natowicz MR. 1992. Discrimination as a Consequence of Genetic Testing. Am. J. Hum. Genet. 50:476–482.

79. Giardiello FM, Brensinger JD, Petersen GM. et al. 1997. The Use and Interpretation of Commercial APC Gene Testing for Familial Adenomatous Polyposis. N. Engl. J. Med. 336:823–827.

2

New Insights and Future Advances in Cancer Diagnostics

Limitations of Conventional Tumor Markers

Yasushi Kasahara and Yutaka Tsukada

1. INTRODUCTION

Tumor markers for malignant diseases can be divided into various stages, namely screening, diagnostic, monitoring and prognosis, and in the foreseeable future, preventive testing. Neither conventional serological tumor markers, spanning from carcinoembryonic antigen (CEA) *(1)* to prostate-specific antigen (PSA) *(2)*, nor the genomic markers *(3)* reported in the past 20 yr, have risen to our expectations with regard to early diagnostic or early disease detection.

There are currently about 50 serological tumor makers available *(4)*, some are used for diagnostic purposes in European countries and in Japan. In the United States, however, the application of tumor markers is restricted to monitoring or prognosis rather than diagnosis, except for PSA and nuclear matrix protein (NMP) *(5)*, owing to insufficient sensitivity for early stage detection. Even CA19–9 *(6)* and CA125 *(7)* were just approved as diagnostic markers in 2002 for the Medicare reimbursement system.

Relentless efforts have been exerted to find better ways to diagnose cancer. The logistic regression model using multiple makers has been used to improve the sensitivity and accuracy of diagnosis, with only limited success. The proteomics assay *(8)* especially matrix-assisted laser desorption/ ionization (MALDI) *(9)* is expected to serve as a new tool for the enhancement of multiple m arker assays and for the discovery of new markers.

The simultaneous detection of large numbers of targets such as in proteomics *(10)* on micro chips *(11)* as well as in DNA/RNA array will help shed light on the disease process of cancer, but the advantages and efficacies of this technique for diagnostic application will need to be assessed.

Malignant transformations are associated with the mutation or genetic alternation of oncogenes *(3)* or suppressor genes *(12)*. Suppressor gene alternation is detected in a broader spectrum of cancers than oncogene alternation. More than one gene alternation is required to transform a cell into a cancer cell regardless of whether it is a germ line cell or a somatic cell. In cancer cells, oncogenes mostly involved in growth signal transaction are upregulated from transcriptional stage to phenotypic activity, while suppressor genes involved in DNA repair and genomic integrity are downregulated. Oncogenes are known to be tumor associated rather than tumor specific, in the same way that tumor markers are known to be tumor-associated antigens. From the point of view of clinical application, genomic markers may not be as attractive as anticipated.

From: *Cancer Diagnostics: Current and Future Trends*
Edited by: R. M. Nakamura, W. W. Grody, J. T. Wu, and R. B. Nagle © Humana Press Inc., Totowa, NJ

Table 1
Tissue Specificity and Overall Sensitivity/Specificity
of Typical Serological Markers

Serological markers	Primary type tumor	Other tumors	Overall sensitivity/ specificity
CEA[a]	Colorectal	Pancreatic, kidney, stomach	65%/65%
α-Fetoprotein[a]	Hepatic Cell	Testicular, ovarian	80%/70%
SCC	Cervical	SCC (Head & Neck, Lung)	50%/85%
PSA	Prostate	85%/80%	
CA 19-9[b]	Pancreatic	Gastric, colorectal	80%/70%
CA 125	Ovarian	Cervical75%/75%	
CA 15-3[b]	Breast	Renal Cell, Cervical	45%/90%
CA 72-4[b]	Gastric	Ovarian, Colorectal	50%/90%

[a]Carcinoembryonic protein.
[b]Carbohydrate antigens defined by monoclonal antibody.

On the other hand, through molecular research findings, it has been possible to gain some insight on the molecular pathways that allow malignant growth for some types of cancer. Numerous target cancer drugs are currently under development *(13)*. In pharmacogenomics, a diagnosis is required to identify the cause of cancer for each patient, and new molecular markers are selected for more accurate treatment with fewer side effects when using target cancer drugs instead of conventional cancer drugs. Because each targeting drug requires a specific assay, this field offers interesting prospects of expansion.

Through the advancement of PC-aided graphic imaging technology for cancer diagnostics, it is now possible to detect tumors of less than 10 mm in diameter and determine the exact location of the cancer *(14)*. Medical imaging technology is the most feasible method for the screening or diagnosis of the early stage of cancer and it will likely soon replace serological markers on solid tumors.

It is worth considering imaging technology not only with conventional tracer reagent but also with new tumor markers *(15)*. In the near future, imaging technology is likely to become more cost effective and sensitive, and to detect disease at the earliest stage possible. Cancer diagnosis for prevention or possible risk prediction is the ultimate goal.

2. ADVANTAGES AND LIMITATIONS OF CONVENTIONAL TUMOR MAKERS IN SERUM

The development of tumor specific epitopes or molecules has been elusive in spite of research efforts in science and medicine. Table 1 shows the overall characteristics of popular tumor markers in serum *(16–25)*, selected among over 100 markers reported in the past 50 yr *(4)*. CEA *(1)* was identified from tumor tissue of colorectal cancer patients through serological adsorption using adjacent normal tissue, a technique similar to the subtraction method using gene cloning.

In terms of sensitivity and specificity at the cutoff point of each marker, CEA is not adequate for diagnostic purposes *(16)*. The α-fetoprotein has a higher sensitivity than CEA with 80%, but its specificity is lower because of the positivity of benign diseases *(18)*.

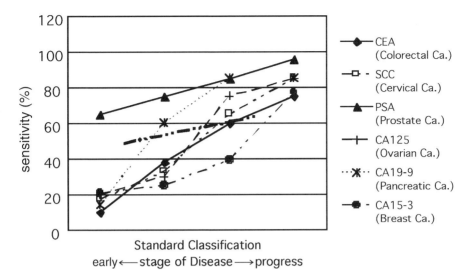

Fig. 1. Relation between sensitivity and disease progression for typical tumor markers.

CA 19–9, the first tumor marker to be defined by monoclonal antibody, recognizes the sugar chain as specific epitope, not as a whole molecule *(6)*. This specific epitope is present on a wider variety of molecules. It shows about 85% sensitivity and 70% specificity for pancreatic cancer *(22)*. PSA has the highest detection sensitivity with 85% and 85% specificity, and is currently the best serum marker for prostatic cancer *(21)*. CA 15–3 and CA 72–4 both have low sensitivity and high specificity *(24,25)*.

Even typical markers shown here are not sensitive or specific enough for diagnostic and screening purposes. PSA, the most sensitive marker, is highly organ specific, squamous cell carcinoma (SCC) is rather tissue specific *(20)*, and all other markers are less organ specific.

Figure 1 shows the brief relation between detection sensitivity and the stage of diseases at standard classifications for various markers. Most markers increase in serum concentration with the size of the tumor, and the detection sensitivity percent is proportional to the advancement of the tumor. If specific tumor markers without the cutoff value were developed in the near future, more sensitive detection methodology would be required to detect the earliest stage of disease.

Only PSA shows a relatively better sensitivity at the early stage *(26,27)*. PSA is elevated in serum even in tumors of less than 1 cm in diameter *(21)*. NMP bladder cancer marker using urine as specimen has the same sensitivity as PSA at the early stage *(28,29)*.

To improve diagnostic sensitivity and accuracy, an algorithm based on a combination of multiple markers has been applied to various tumors, some achieved improvement on detection sensitivity; however, decisive results have not been obtained *(30)*.

The search for a more sensitive and reliable method is now turning to proteomics analysis *(10,31)*, which allows for the simultaneous measurement of hundreds of test parameters in serum on a chip. However, only two reports have shown proteomic assays as a promising tool for cancer diagnostics.

An assay based on mass spectrometry, surface-enhanced laser desorption/ionization (SELDI), was able to detect ovarian cancer at 100% sensitivity with 95% specificity, including all 18 cases of stage I patients as shown by cluster pattern analysis *(32)*. SELDI assay showed 93% sensitivity for all breast cancer cases at 91% specificity using 3 makers selected from among 147 markers *(10)*. SELDI is a promising method for the discovery of new biological markers. However, further data using serum as specimen must be collected to assess the value of this technology for practical applications in the future. The sensitivity of existing markers at the early stage of diseases is inadequate for diagnostic or screening, but acceptable for monitoring of cancer or prognosis. Following the discovery of PSA 15 yr ago, no other adequate marker has been reported, and therefore we need to look into new genomic related markers as suitable tumor marker candidates. Only in vitro diagnostics using biomarkers can predict the risk of cancer prior to its onset, not imaging diagnostics.

3. NUCLEIC ACID MOLECULE DETERMINATION AS TUMOR MARKERS

Molecular science and gene analysis have contributed to the understanding of cancer biology *(33)*. A single gene defect, developing several hereditary tumors has been reported, and more than hundreds of oncogenes and suppressor genes have been identified *(3)*.

Thus, too much has been expected of gene markers for cancer diagnostics; the development of most cancers involves a complex series of steps *(34)*, and the genes themselves do not reflect any physiological state in the body. A recent study on identical twins has revealed that cancer is weakly influenced by genetic makeup. That means nurture is more important than nature's encoding *(35)*. The possible targets of nucleic acid determination with regards to cancer so far are as follows:

- Oncogenes/suppressor genes mutation.
- Inactivation of suppressor genes through methylation on CpG island or instability of promoter region.
- mRNA profile of somatic cell.
- Microsatellite mutation (instability).
- Telomere stability and telomerase activity.

Most oncogenes related with intracellular signal-transduction pathways cause cancer by overexpression as a result of mutation, especially in the case of *ras*-related genes. However, oncogenes or oncogene profiles for cancer diagnostics have proven inadequate for clinical application in spite of intensive investigation.

The mutation of *MIC, KRAS/KRAF, Her2/EGFR, BCL-2* and other genes is found in a certain percentage of various malignancies *(36,37)*. The combination of oncogenes with conventional tumor markers, such as K-*ras* mutation with CA19-9 for colorectal and pancreatic cancer improves detection sensitivity and prognostic value *(38)*. The mutation of suppressor genes such as *p53* and *BR* is more common in overall cancers than that of oncogenes.

Table 2 shows the suppressor genes that might be important for possible application on cancer testing *(3,39–45)*. These can be divided into categories according to function of transcription related activity *(40)*, cell-cycle controller, and DNA repair *(45,46)*. Those functions require normal cells to prevent disturbing factors such as mismatch accumulation, abnormal cell growth, and cell transformation.

The loss-of-function of single suppressor genes in germline mutations such as *p53, RB, BLM* causes hereditary cancer. Mutations of *BLM (44)* and *BRCA1/BRCA2* cause colon *(42)*, breast, and ovarian cancer respectively resulting from a defect in DNA repair. *PETEN* mutation *(46)*, a lack of activity reducing the amount of kinase Akt product, is found in various cancers. *KLF6* gene *(41)* of transcription factor is mutated in 77% of primary prostate cancers.

Table 2
Important Tumor Suppressor Genes Causing Cancer

Genes	Function	Type of cancer
p53	Cell-cycle response	Colon, various
p27	Cell-cycle inhibitor	Breast
RB	Cell-cycle inhibitor	Lung, AML
BRCA	DNA stability	Breast, ovarian
PTEN	Signal transduction	Various, systemic
RARb2	Retinoic acid receptor	Colon, APL
KLF6	Transcription factor	Gastric
RUNX3	Transcription related	Gastric
EZH2	Transcription repressor	Prostate
Blm	DNA repair	Bowel, colon

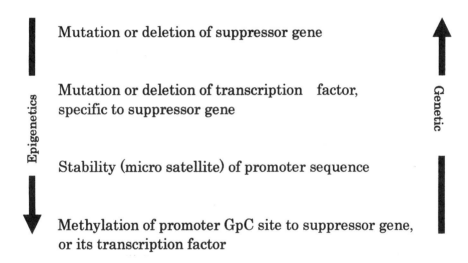

Fig. 2. Impact of inactivation or silencing of suppressor gene on tumor.

Various factors trigger the inactivation of suppresser genes. Figure 2 shows various factors for the inactivation of suppressor genes that are sleeping or switched off with methylation on the CpG island within the promoter region *(47)*, other than the existing concepts of deletion or mutation of suppressor genes. Current research reveals the importance of the silencing of suppressor gene by promoter methylation on tumors.

DNMT1/DNMT3b encoded methyltransferase is a key molecule responsible for the methylation of suppressor genes *(43)*. *RERb2*, retinoic acid receptor gene silenced by methylation *(48)*, which causes acute promyelocytic leukemia (APL) or acute myeloid leukemia (AML), has been confirmed in experimental models. In addition, cases of colon, lung, lym-phoma,, and breast cancer with a high percentage of methylation have been reported. Tumor suppressor genes play a crucial role in anticancer defense. Suppressor gene somatic cells have, in principle, the same potential to inform on risk of cancer onset and early stages of cancer than oncogenes.

However, whether methylation for genes silenced by the methyletransferase expression product of DNMT1/DNMT2 is specific to the suppressor gene locus or to global genes remains to be solved, and how many genes are involved in the methylation of suppressor genes in cancer in addition to DNMT1/ DNMT3b also remains unclear *(43)*.

Microarray applied on gene expression profile uses tissue or cell as specimen. To improve prognosis and classification of prostate cancer, Saravana et al., analyzed thousands of genes using transcription profile, from normal adjacent prostate to metastatic cancer for over 700 clinical specimens.

The expression of hepsin and pim-1 transcript screen showed the correlation with clinical outcome reflecting the progression of the disease *(49)*. In a subsequent study, they identified enhancer of zeste homolog 2 (EZH2) as a candidate of most specific markers for prostatic cancer with regard to the metastatic and lethal progression of the disease *(50,51)*. In addition, gene-expression analysis of solid tumors between primary tumors and metastases showed a set of genes associated with metastasis and metastatic cells being present in primary tumors.

Prostasin, a potential serum marker for ovarian cancer was also identified through microarray technology *(51)*. The transcription profile-method using microarray is a useful tool for the discovery of new markers. This technology, although more complicated than routine diagnostic application, provides more precise data and should be used in conjunction with pathological diagnosis.

The somatic mutation of microsatelllite instability is comparable to a molecular clock showing tumor cell divisions through changes in diversity *(53)*. Current reports show that microsatellite diversity is detected even in the serum of cancer patients using PCR amplification of DNA.

Microsatellite mutation in serum is detected in 71% of patients with small cell lung cancer *(53)* as well as colon, head, and neck cancers *(54)*, among others. DNA analysis of microsatellite instability in serum, detected 71% of hepatocellular carcinoma in cancer patients with an α-fetoprotein serum concentration of less than cutoff level, and overall hepatocellular carcinoma at 100% sensitivity and 81% specificity when using the profile of 19 marker DNAs *(55)*. Thus, microsatellite instability is a unique potential marker in serum for nonorgan specific cancer, offering the possibility of detecting the early stage of events in cancer. Telomerase activity has been detected in over 90% of human cancers from tissue specimen *(56,57)* and normal germ cells but not in normal adjacent tumor tissues and is associated with more aggressive tumor behavior.

Telomerase activity measured by telomeric repeat amplification protocol was positive in 81% of colocectal cancers and in 70% of gastric cancers *(58,59)*; another study detected positive telomerase activity in 93% of overall breast cancers *(60)*, including 68% of primary tumors and 95% of advanced stage tumors, among surgically resected samples.

Telomerase detection in body fluids, such as ascites, bronchial washings, and urine has also been demonstrated in various cancers *(61)*. Telomerase enzyme activity was detected in 94.7% of bladder cancers using bladder washes as specimen. Telomerase activity in cancer has no organ specificity, but detection sensitivity and specificity is high compared with other tumor markers in serum.

4. PHARMACOGENOMIC TESTING OF CANCER FOR TARGETING DRUGS

Current advancements in pharmacogenomics are anticipated to lead toward a tailored cancer therapy targeting specific molecules that cause particular tumors *(12)*. Target drugs pro-

Table 3
Target Drugs to Specific Genes for Cancer Therapy

Drug	Target Gene	Function	Cancer
Herceptin	*HER-2*	Monoclonal antibody to HER-2 protein TK inactivation	Breast
Gleevec	*bcr/abl*	Tyrosinekinase Inhibitor	Leukemia
Iressa	*EGFR*	Tyrosinekinase Inhibitor	Lung
bevacizumab	*VEGF*	Monoclonal antibody to VEGF for anti-angiogenesis	Breast, Colorectal
CC1-779	*PETN/mTOR-S6*	mTOR/S6 kinase Inhibitor in PTEN-deficient tumor	Prostate, Brain

vide for accurate treatment, offering a judicious, and cost-effective alternative to conventional drugs; they ensure that the optimum dose of the right drug is given to the right patient with fewer adverse effects. Each new target drug needs a specific test to identify the pharmacogenomic background of the patient prior to dose administration. For instance, Herceptin, a breast cancer drug already on the market, is restricted to patients with an overexpression of HER-2/neu. Patients who carry an overexpressed HER-2/neu receptor protein, about 20% of all cancer patients, must be differentiated from others for therapy *(62)*.

Table 3 shows a number of target drugs and their brief characteristics. Gleevec is an Food amd Drug Administration (FDA)-approved drug *(63,64)*. Bcr-Abl tyrosine kinase inhibitor is about 90% effective in the early stage of chronic myelogenous leukemia (CML) caused by Bcr-Abl tyrosine kinase abnormality. Iressa *(65,66)*, EGFR tyrosine kinese inhibitor, has only been approved for nonsmall lung cell cancer in Japan.

Both avastin *(67)*, a monoclonal antibody to VEGF protein, and CCI-779 *(68,69)*, an inhibitor to mTOR-S6 kinase signal transaction in PTEN-deficient tumors, are in clinical trial stage. The next target drug should focus on the genes associated with the invasion or metastasis of cancer. Pharmacogenomics might thus provide the chance to develop new molecular marker testing methods that will provide detailed information on the functioning mechanism of targeting drugs. All targeting drugs listed in the table require a new cancer testing approach that characterizes the tumor of each patient with molecular markers, thereby reducing side effects and avoiding the unnecessary use of expensive drugs *(70)*.

5. IMPACT OF IMAGING DIAGNOSTICS ON CANCER IN RELATION WITH TUMOR MARKERS

Tumor biomarkers have improved with time for prognosis and monitoring purposes mainly, but for earlier detection and risk assessment their development have not yet reached a level adequate for clinical applications. In the past two decades, noninvasive imaging technology based on various platforms for cancer diagnostics has made significant advances with the surrounding computer-aided technologies, not only for clinical applications but also for basic research *(13)*.

In the case of lung cancer, early detection is needed to improve prognosis because most cancers are metastasized when first detected by biomarkers or by cytological assessment of sputum. Mass screening for lung cancer with low-dose X-ray spiral computerized tomography (CT) in mobile units was performed on 5483 individuals from the general population in Japan *(13)*. The detection rate with CT was 0.48%, including cancers of less then 10 mm in diameter, whereas that of standard mass screenings done previously in the same area were 0.03–0.05%, 10 times less sensitive. This high-resolution CT also constitutes an excellent tool for confirmatory discrimination of subtypes of small peripheral lung peripheral adenocarcinomas *(71)*. Magnetic resonance imaging (MRI) on preoperative local staging of patients with pancreatic cancer was applied to discriminate resectability. MRI results showed 98% sensitivity, 92% specificity, and 96% accuracy in patients with suspected pancreatic tumor *(72)*. MRI-guided intervention is now expanding to diagnosis and treatment of prostate cancer, as in the case of fiber-guided endoscopy for colorectal or gastric cancer.

A recently developed method, optical coherence tomography (OCT) combined with optical fiber may differentiate flat malignant from inflammatory lesions, without requiring biopsy. Ultrasonography with improved resolution is now a common screening tool for the physical check-up of healthy individuals.

Ultrasonography used as a second-line test to serum CA125 shows an increased detection sensitivity in ovarian cancer *(73)*, similar to the combination of occult blood testing with fiber endoscope in colorectal cancer.

Positron emission tomography (PET), which produces images by detecting the radiation given off by tracer molecules, has improved in terms of sensitivity; its applications have also been expanded through the development of new tracers responding to specific targets. PET using tracers responding to target genes are being adapted to gene expression study in experimental animals *(14)*. PET imaging of *HSV1-tk* expression using thymidine analog called FIAU labeled with radioisotope was used in a clinical gene-therapy trial.

Imaging technologies in diagnostics of cancer have acquired a strong position in relation to molecular and biomarkers in serum or tissue. Advancements in imaging technology will soon lead to the development of a downsized and more cost-effective system with higher resolution that will be easier to use. Without additional improvement, most tumor markers could serve as supplemental tools to imaging diagnosis in the near future. The development of tumor markers as possible tracers with the intervention of imaging analysis, a form of functional molecular imaging analysis, and the development of new primary test markers prior to the application of imaging diagnostics, are promising paths to explore for cancer testing. However, imaging technologies are limited in the sense that they cannot predict cancer risk or provide information on the aggravation of the disease *(74)*.

6. SUMMARY

New biomarkers in serum that make up for the limitations of conventional tumor markers need to be improved both in terms of organ specificity and detection sensitivity at the early stage of disease. The proteomics assay, especially that based on SELDI, and the gene expression assay are considered promising tools for the discovery of new biomarkers. The development of new biomarkers that reflect both aggravation and metastasis of tumors is highly desirable.

Compared with phenotypic biomarkers, oncogenes/suppressor genes are not very specific in cancer somatic cells, in spite of initial expectations, and they are not likely to become mainstream in routine cancer diagnostics. Further studies on suppressor gene silencing as a result of methylation of the promoter region and microsatellite instability need to be evaluated as possible markers to a broad spectrum of cancers.

Telomerase activity expressed in somatic cancer cells and associated with aggressive tumor behavior, is the most specific marker. Telomerase activity measured by telomeric repeat has been detected in over 90% of tissue specimen in solid tumors and body fluids. If greater detection sensitivity for telomerase activity is achieved, serum rather than tissue will be used as specimen. The early stage detection of solid tumors in routine screening is thus foreseeable with telomerase activity combined with imaging analysis.

Pharmacogenomic testing for targeting cancer drugs is the most promising emerging routine diagnostics tool. In contrast to conventional cancer drugs, new targeting drugs require corresponding molecular testing to select the right dose for the right patient with fewer adverse effects and effective cost containment.

Imaging technologies based on various platforms have progressed significantly with the aid of computer-aided technologies. Imaging diagnostics can detect as little as 10 mm in diameter of solid tumor in addition to showing localization. Most conventional tumor markers for diagnostics are likely to disappear in the future. The development of new biomarkers either for primary testing prior to imaging diagnostics or for specific tracers of imaging analysis is one option worth investigating for early cancer diagnostics. Only in vitro diagnostics using biomarkers can predict the risk of cancer prior to its onset, not imaging diagnostics.

REFERENCES

1. Gold P and Freedman SO. 1965. Specific carcinoembryonic antigens of the human digestive system. J. Exp. Med. 122(3):3:467–481.
2. Ban Y, Wang MC, Chu TM. 1984. Immunologic markers and the diagnosis of prostatic cancer. Urol Clin North Am. 11(2):269–276.
3. Blume-Jensen P and Hunter T. 2001. Oncogenic Kinase Signalling. Nature 411:355–365.
4. Wu JT. 2001. Diagnosis and management of cancer using serolgic tumor, in: Diagnosis and Management by Laboratory Method Markers. vol. 20, Henry JB, ed., S. Saunders Co., Philadelphia, pp. 1028–1042.
5. Landman J, ChangY, Kavaler E, Droller MJ, Liu, BC. 1998. Sensitivity and specificity of NMP-22, telomerase, and BTA in the detection of human bladder cancer. Urology 52(3):398–402.
6. Koprowski H, Steplewski Z, Mitchell K, Herlyn M, Herlyn D. 1979. Colorectal carcinoma antigens detected by hybridoma antibodies. Somatic Cell Genet. 5(6):957–971.
7. Bast RC Jr, Feeney M, Lazarus H, Nadler LM, Colvin RB, Knapp RC. 1981. Reactivity of a monoclonal antibody with human ovarian carcinoma. J. Clin. Invest. 68(5):1331–1337.
8. Hanash, S. 2003. Disease Proteomics. Nature 422:226–232.
9. Aebersold R and Mann M. 2003. Mass spectrometry-based Proteomics. Nature 422:198–207.
10. Li J, Zhang Z, Rosenzweig J, Wang YY, Chan DW. 2002. Proteomics and bioinformatics approaches for indentification of serum biomarkers to detect breast cancer. Clin. Chem. 48(8):1296–1304.
11. Robin LS, Martinsky T, Schena M. 2003. Trends in microarray analysis. Nature Med. 9(1)1: 140–145.
12. Balmain A. 2002. New-age tumour suppressors. Nature 417:235–237.
13. Couzin J. 2002. Smart weapons prove tough to design. Science 298:522–525.
14. Sone S, Takashima S, Li F, Yang , et al. 1998. Mass screening for lung cancer with mobile spiral computed tomography scanner. Lancet 351(9111):1242–1245.
15. Lok C. 2001. Picture perfect. Nature 412:372–374.

16. Bel Hadj Hmida Y, Tahri N, Sellami A, Yangui N, Jlidi R, Beyrouti MI, et al. 2001. Sensitivity, specificity and prognostic value of CEA in colorectal cancer: results of a Tunisian series and literature review. Tunis. Med. 79(8–9):434–440.

17. Pezzilli R, Billi P, Plate, L, Laudadio Ma, Sprovieri G. 1995. Serum CA 242 in pancreatic cancer. Comparison with CA 19-9 and CEA. Ital. J. Gastroenterol. 27(6):296–299.

18. Johnson PJ. 2001. The role of serum alpha-fetoprotein estimation in the diagnosis and management of hepatoceller carinoma. Clin. Liver Dis. 5(1):145–159.

19. Aoyagi U. 2001. [Japanese]Alpha fetoprotein and I'ts fucocylation index in early Diagnostic diagnostic of Hepatocarcinomahepatocarcinoma. Nippon Rinsho. 59(6):42–348.

20. Takeda M, Sakuragi N, Okamoto K, et al. 2002. Preoperative serum SCC, CA125, and CA19-9 levels and lymph node status in squamous cell carcinoma of the uterine cervix. Acta. Obstet. Gynecol. Scand. 81(5):451–457.

21. Krumholtz JS, Carvalhal GF, Ramos CG, et al. 2002. Porstate-specific antigen cutoff of 2.6 ng/mL for prostate cancer screening is associated with favorable pathologic tumor features. Urology 60(3):469–474.

22. Kokhanenko NIU, Ignashov AM, Varga EV, et al. 2001. Role of the tumor markers CA 19-9 and carcinoembryonic antigen (CEA) in diagnosis, treatment and prognosis of pancreatic cancer. Vopr. Onkol. 47(3):294–297.

23. Gemer O, Segal S, Kopmar A. 2001. Preoperative CA-125 level as a predictor of non optimal cytoreduction of advanced epithelial ovarian cancer. Acta. Obstet. Gynecol. Scand. 80(6): 583–585.

24. Tampellini M, Berruti A, Gorzegno G, et al. 2001. Independent factors predict supranormal CA 15-3 serum levels in advanced breast cancer patients at first disease relapse. Tumour Biol. 22(6):367–373.

25. Ychou M, Duffour J, Kramar A, Gourgou S, Grenier J. 2000. Clinical significance and prognostic value of CA72-4 compared with CEA and CA19-9 in patients with gastric cancer. Dis. Markers. 16(3–4):105–110.

26. Yamamoto T, Ito K, Ohi M, et al. 2001. Diagnostic significance of digtal rectal examination and transrectal ultrasonography in men with prostate-specific antigen levels of 4 ng/mL or less. Urology 58:994–998.

27. D'amico AV, Whittington R, Malkowicz SB, et al. 1999. Pretreatment nomgram for prostate-specific antigen recurrence after radical prostatectomy or external-beam radiation therapy for clinically localized prostate cancer. J. Clin. Oncol. 17:168–172.

28. Gutierrez Banos JL, Rebollo Rodrigo MH, Antolin Juarez FM, Martin Garcia, B. 2001. NMP 22, BTA stat test and cytology in the diagnosis of bladder cancer: a comparative study. Urol Int. 66(4):185–190.

29. Saad A, Hanbury DC, McNicholas TA, Boustead GB, Morgan, S, Woodman AC. 2002. A study comparing various noninvasive methods of detecting bladder cancer in urine. BJU Int. 89(4): 369–373.

30. Ali SM, Leitzel K, Chinchilli VM,et al. 2002. Relationship of serum HER-2/neu and serum CA 15-3 in patients with metastatic breast cancer. Clin. Chem. 48(8):1314–1320.

31. Festsch PA, Simone NL, Bryant-Greewood PK, et al. 2002. Protemic evaluation of archival cytologic material using SELDI affinity mass spectrometry: potential for diagnostic applications. Am. J. Clin. Pathol. 118(6):870–876.

32. Petricoin EF, Ardekani AM, Hitt BA, et al. 2002. Use of proteomic patterns in serum to identify ovarian cancer. Lancet 359(9306):572–577.

33. Ponder BA. 2001. Cancer genetics. Nature 411:336–341.

34. Evan IG and Vousden KH. 2001. Proliferation, cell cycle and apoptosis in cancer. Nature 411:342–348.

35. Chakravarti A and Little P. 2003. Nature, nurture and human disease. Nature 421:412–414.

36. Salgia R and Skarin AT. 1998. Molecular abnormalities in lung cancer. J. Clin. Oncol. 16(3):1207–1217.

37. Rajagopalan H, Bardelli A, Lengauer C, et al. 2002. NATURE. RAF/RAS oncogenes and mismatch-repair status. Nature 418:934.

38. Dinxu F, Shengdao Z, Tianquan H, Yu J, Ruoging L, Zurong Y, Xuezhi W. 2002. A prospective study of detection of pancreatic carcinoma by combind plasma K-ras mutation and serum CA 19-9 analysis. Pancreas 25(4):336–341.

39. Kovar H, Jug G, Aryee DN, et al. 1997. Among genes involved in the RB dependent cell cycle regulatory cascade, the p16 tumor suppressor gene is frequently lost in the Ewing family of tumors. Oncogene 15(18):2225–2232.

40. Zetter BZ and Banyard J. 2002. The silence of the genes. Nature 419:572–573.

41. Narla G, Heath KE, Reeves HL, et al. 2001. KLF6, a candidate tumor suppressor gene mutated in prostate cancer. Science

42. Yang H, Jaffrey PD, Miller J, et al. 2002. BRCA2 Function function in DNA Binding binding and Recombination recombination from a BRCA2-DSS1-ssDNA Structurestructure. Science 297:1837–1848.

43. Rhee I, Backman KE, Park BH, et al. 2002. DNMT1 and DNMT3b cooperate to silence genes in human cancer cells. Nature 416:552–556.

44. Gruber SB, Ellis NA, Rennert G, Offit K. 2002. BLM heterozygosity and the risk of colorectal cancer. Science 297:2013.

45. Pellegrini L, Yu DS, Lo T, et al. 2002. Insights into DNA recombination from the structure of a RAD51-BRCA2 complex. Nature 420:287–290.

46. Penninger JM and Woodgett J. 2001. PTEN-Coupling Tumor Suppression to Stem Cells? Science 294:2116–2118.

47. Robert MF, Morin S, Beaulieu N, et al. 2003. DNMT1 is required to maintain CpG methylation and aberrant gene silencing in human cancer cell. Nat. Gemet. 33:61–65.

48. Esteller M, Fraga M, Paz MF, et al. 2002. Cancer epigenetics and methylation. Science 297:1807–180.9

49. Varambally S, Dhanasekaran SM, Zhou M, et al. 2002. The polycomb group protein EZH2 is involved in progression of prostate cancer. Nature 419:624–628.

50. Dhanasekaran SM, Barrette TR, Ghosh D, et al. 2001. Delineation of prognostic biomarkers in prostate cancer. Nature 412:822–826.

51. Mok SC, Chao J, Skates S, et al. 2001. Prostasin, a potential serum marker for ovarian cancer: indentification through microarray technology. J. Natl. Cancer Ins. 93(19):1458–1464.

52. Shibata D, Navidi W, Salovaara R, Li Z, Aaltonen LA. 1996. Somatic microsatellite mutations as molecular tumor clocks. Nat. Med. 2(6):676–681.

53. Chen XQ, Stroun M, Magnenat JL, et al. 1996. Microsatllite alterations in plasma DNA of small cell lung cancer patients. Nat. Med. 2(9):1033–1035.

54. Gebert J, Sun M, Ridder R, et al. 2000. Molecular profiling of sporadic colorectal tumors by microsatellite analysis. Int. J .Oncol. 16(1):169–179.

55. Chang YC, Ho CL, Chen HH, et al. 2002. Molecular diagnosis of primary liver cancer by microsatellite DNA analysis in the serum. Br. J. Cancer. 87(12):1449–1453.

56. Elemore LW, Forsythe HL, Ferreira-Gonzalez A, Garrett CT, Clark GM, Holt SE. 2002. Real-time quantitative analysis of telomerase activity in breast tumor specimens using a highly specific and sensitive fluorescent-based assay. Diagn. Mol. Pathol. 11(3):177–185.

57. Marx J. 2002. Tackling Cancer at the telemeres. Science 295:2350–2351.

58. Tang SJ, Dumot JA, Wang L, et al. 2002. Telomerase activity in pancreatic endocrine tumors. Am. J. Gastroenterol. 97(4):1022–1030.

59. Katayama S, Shiota G, Oshimura M, Kawasaki H. 1999. Clinical usefulness of telomerase activity and telomere length in the preoperative diagnosis of gastric and colorectal cancer. J. Cancer Res. Clin. Oncol. 125(7):405–410.

60. Hiyama E, Gollahon L, Kataoka T, et al. 1996. Telomerase activity in human breast tumors. J. Natl. Cancer Inst. 88(2):116–122.

61. Hess JL and Highsmith WE Jr. 2002. Telomerase detection in body fluids. Clin. Chem. 48(1):18–24.

62. Bilous M. 2001. HER2 Testing Advisory Board. HER2 testing recommendations in Australia. Pathology 33(4):425–427.
63. Hung M, Dorsey JF, Epling-Burnette PK, et al. 2002. Inhibition of Bcr-Abl kinase activity by PD 180970 blocks constitutive activation of Stat5 and growth of CML cells. Oncogene 21(57): 8804–8816.
64. Marx J. 2001. Why some leukemia cells resist STI-571. Science 292:2231–2232.
65. Natele RB and Zaretsky SL. 2002. ZD1839 (Iressa): What's in it for the patient? Oncologist 7(4):25–30.
66. Herbest RS. 2002. Targeted therapy in non-small-cell lung cancer. Oncology 9(9):19–24.
67. Whang YE, Wu X, Suzuki H, et al. 1998. Inactivation of the tumor suppressor PTEN/MMAC1 in advanced human prostate cancer through loss of expression. Proc. Natl. Acad. Sci. USA 95(9):5246–5250.
68. Neshat MS, Mellinghoff IK, Tran C, et al. 2001. Enhanced sensitivity of PTEN-deficient tumors to inhibition of FRAP/mTOR. Proc. Natl. Acad. Sci. USA 98(18):10,314–10,319.
69. Watanabe T, Katsumata N, Ando M, et al. 2002. [Japanese] Genetic testing for effective Herceptin therapy. Nippon Rinsho. 60(3):603–611.
70. Schubert CM. 2003. Microarray to be used as routine clinical screen. Nat. Med. 9(1):9.
71. Yang ZG, Sone S, Takashima S, Li F, Honda T, Maruyama Y, Hasegawa M, Kawakami S. et al. 2001. High-resolution CT analysis of small peripheral lung adenocarcinomas revealed on screening helical CT. AJR Am. J. Roentgenol. 176(6):1399–1407.
72. Fischer U, Vosshenrich R, Horstmann O, et al. 2002. Preoperative local MRI-staging of patients with a suspected pancreatic mass. Eur. Radiol. 12(12):296–303.
73. Menon U, Talaat A, Rosenthal AN. et al. 2000. Performance of ultrasound as a second line test to serum CA125 in ovarian cancer screening. BJOG 107(2):165–169.
74. Ramaswamy S, Ross K, Lander E, Golub,T. 2003. A molecular signature of metastasis in primary solid tumors. Nat. Genet. 33:49–53.

3

The Changing Role of the Pathologist in the Management of the Cancer Patient

Raymond B. Nagle

1. INTRODUCTION

1.1. The Difficult Diagnosis

The experienced surgical pathologist routinely uses paraffin embedded tissue stained with hematoxylin and eosin (H&E) to establish the correct cancer diagnosis. A number of circumstances arise, however, in which the H&E slide is insufficient to establish the correct diagnosis. This occurs in approx 4–10% of all tumors and is usually owing to the fact that the tumors are undifferentiated and the cell of origin remains elusive. These undifferentiated tumors tend to fall into three categories:

1. The large cell undifferentiated tumor.
2. The small cell undifferentiated tumor.
3. The spindle cell undifferentiated tumor.

A second circumstance is the tumor presents as a metastasis with an uncertain origin. Often these tumors are poorly differentiated adenocarcinomas in which the organ of origin cannot be ascertained from the histological pattern of the metastasis. Approximately 20% of all cancer patients present with metastasis. Studies have revealed that in as many as 4% of these patients the primary cancer is never found, even with complete autopsy examination.

2. CURRENT USE OF IMMUNOHISTOCHEMICAL MARKERS OF CELL LINEAGE

Beginning in the 1980s, antibodies specific to various cell linage proteins that could be used in immunohistochemical applications became available to the pathologist. It was found that all epithelial neoplasms expressed cytoskeleton proteins of the cytokeratin family. It was discovered that there were 20 such proteins, and exact combinations of these proteins were expressed with great fidelity in various cell lines *(1)*. These findings were adapted for diagnostic use, allowing many undifferentiated tumors to be clearly diagnosed as carcinomas after demonstrating that they expressed cytokeratins. Shortly thereafter, other proteins were discovered that also were cell lineage specific. Over the years this has evolved and now there are a great number of antibodies that are useful in classifying undifferentiated neoplasms or in defining the site of origin of metastatic neoplasms.

Examples of the use of such antibodies for identifying large cell undifferentiated neoplasms *(2–4)* or neoplasms of uncertain origin is shown in Fig. 1. Antibodies useful in the

From: *Cancer Diagnostics: Current and Future Trends*
Edited by: R. M. Nakamura, W. W. Grody, J. T. Wu, and R. B. Nagle © Humana Press Inc., Totowa, NJ

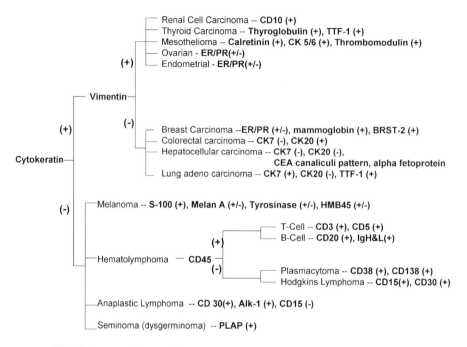

Fig. 1. Large cell undifferentiated or neoplasms of unknown origin.

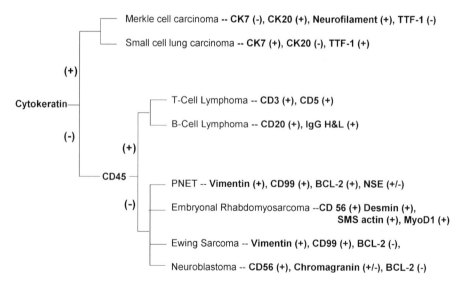

Fig. 2. Small cell undifferentiated neoplasm.

differential diagnosis of small cell undifferentiated neoplasms *(5–8)* are shown in Fig. 2 and those used for poorly differentiated spindle cell neoplasms *(9–11)* are shown in Fig. 3. Using an algorithm approach to tumor diagnosis, which utilizes a few relatively inexpensive immunohistochemical tests, has resulted in better patient care and reduced cost. Use of these markers has also better categorized tumors so that clinical drug trials and other studies are on a firmer basis in terms of the tumor classification.

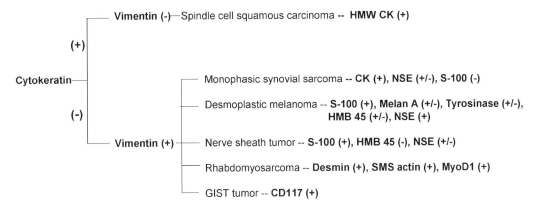

Fig. 3. Poorly differentiated spindle cell neoplasms.

3. TECHNOLOGICAL ADVANCES

This effort to establish cell lineage specific marker reagents was enhanced by two technological developments: First, the discovery by Kohler and Milstein that monoclonal antibodies could be made by fusing specifically immunized murine spleen cells with murine myeloma cells resulting in a cell line producing a specific antibody that could be grown in tissue culture. This resulted in the production of specific monoclonal antibodies that were easily made in great quantity and could be sent around the world to various laboratories enabling the establishment of standardized immunohistochemical testing. Unfortunately, the majority of these antibodies were made against conformational epitopes, which were often denatured during standard formalin fixation of clinical specimens. A second major technologic advancement was the discovery of heat antigen retrieval in which cross-linking by formalin was reversed by exposing the tissue to various protocols of steam or boiling. This enabled many monoclonal antibodies that were previously only used on fresh frozen tissue to be used in archival, formalin fixed, paraffin-embedded tissue.

The impact of cloning the human genome has resulted in the ability to predict amino acid sequences for any human protein. Peptides can be synthesized or constructed and recombinant proteins can be made in bacterial plasmids that can be used as immuogens. This has resulted in monoclonal antibodies (MAbs) specific for every human gene product now being possible. With the advent of microarray analysis, gene expression for a variety of human tumors is being determined. These studies will undoubtedly result in a new set of targets and generation of MAbs with greater specificity and clinical relevance.

4. PREDICTIVE MARKERS

In general, antibody markers have been used to confirm or rule out a diagnosis in the context of comparing immunohistochemical results with morphology and clinical information. They were used, therefore, as adjuncts to conventional pathologic diagnosis. The new challenge presented to pathologists is the use of immunohistochemistry to detect therapeutic protein targets. The current thinking in medical oncology is to move away from general cytotoxic agents to customized therapy, where certain target proteins expressed in the individual patient are being treated with protein-specific agents. These target proteins have been shown to function in strategic signaling pathways or other fundamentally important biochemical pathways in various cancers and have been chosen as targets for therapy. Drugs specifically interacting with targeted proteins would block these pathways and lead to the selective killing of tumor cells. The quantification of the amount of target present in the tumor is therefore used to predict therapeutic response.

The great advantage of detecting these targets by immunohistochemistry rests in the ability to directly associate the target with the malignant cells. A sample of current protein target molecules for which there are already drugs available is shown in Table 1. The drug development industry is moving very rapidly and has presented the field with a great challenge in developing tests for these targets. Only one of these target detection reagents, HER-2/neu, has Premarket Approval (PMA) status as a diagnostic reagent (Table 1).

Currently, there are a few approved as In Vitro Diagnostic (IVD) status but most of these are being currently used as Analytic Specific Reagents (ASR). The need for standardization of these tests is great, because unlike the previous diagnostic immunohistochemical tests that were correlated with morphology and clinical histories, these tests are "stand alone" tests. For example, the level of HER-2/neu growth factor receptor expression in a breast cancer predicts whether the patient might respond to HerceptinR, independent of the morphology or other pathologic features. Detection of HER-2/neu expression is an independent test and therefore test standardization needs to be rigidly controlled.

Currently, there is a great deal of confusion as to how one measures these protein levels, and whether or not this can be quantitated using digital imaging and image analysis. One of the technological developments that may be important in this regard is the widespread use of immunohistochemical automation that better ensures run to run consistency *(12)*. There is increasing pressure on pathology labs to quantitate these results so that the therapeutic trials and testing of the new reagents are on a more sound basis. The College of American Pathology is currently proposing a plan for testing and qualifying laboratories performing these predictive tests.

5. CHALLENGES FOR PREDICTIVE TESTS

The "stand alone " predictive test raises a number of new challenges for pathologists. The first challenge is to have proper positive controls. The use of a series of cell lines with known levels of protein expression is an attractive solution. Cell lines however, are not equivalent to tissue sections and their use requires stringent control of their culture, fixation, and method used for their attachment to glass slides.

Perhaps the most important barrier to the study of predictive protein markers is the effect of cross-linking or precipitating fixatives routinely applied by pathology laboratories. The conformation of certain protein epitopes is adversely affected by formalin fixation and is dependant on time, temperature, and the buffering system used in the original processing of the tissue. These procedures are not standardized and until this problem is addressed the full potential of protein target detection by immunohistochemical assays will not be realized.

Even if these test procedures can be standardized there is still the question of whether the results can be quantified. Predictive markers such as the estrogen and progesterone receptors and Her-2/neu are currently being investigated to determine whether modern optical methods can be used to obtain clinically relevant quantification. It is likely that as neoplasms progress or respond to a given therapeutic regimen they will evolve into cell clones using different survival strategies and therefore change their phenotype. This will require resampling and rephenotyping the neoplasm to enable the therapist to adjust customized

Table 1
Drug Targets Now in Use and the Statues of Their Detection Tests[a]

Target	ASR Class 1	IVD Class 2	PMA Class 3
Estrogen Receptor		X	
HER-2/neu		X	X
EGFR	X		
CD20	X	X	
CD52	X		
Progesterone Receptors	X		
Androgen receptor	X		
Asparagine synthase (low levels cause sensitivity)	X		
Thymidylate synthase (low levels cause sensitivity)	X		
Dihydrofolate reductase (low levels cause sensitivity)	X		
GAR transformylase	X		
Mismatch repair abnormal cells	X		
Thymidine phosphorylase (high levels casues activation of the agent)			
CD117	X		
Adenosine deaminase	X		
Somatostatin Receptor	X		
Topoisomerase I	X		
Topoisomerase II	X		
RAR	X		
COX-2	X		
DNA polymerase	X		
RXR	X		
IL2 receptor	X		
Ribonucleotide reductase	X		

[a]Protein targets for which there are therapeutic drugs currently in use or in clinical trial.
Notes: The table indicates the current levels at which existing reagents are approved.
Class 1-Analytic specific reagent (ASR).
Class 2-In vitro diagnostic (IVD).
Class 3-Premarket approval (PMA).

therapy that would be the most appropriate for the patient. Resampling most likely will be restricted to small samples such as needle aspirates or perhaps even circulating tumor cells. The analysis of this type if specimen again will present new challenges to the pathologist and may require the use of more sensitive methods of individual cell analysis including the use of the new fluorescent probes and laser microscopy. Undoubtedly, these developments will improve cancer patient care. On the other hand, they will create technological challenges for pathology laboratories and health care providers who will demand that these new tests are accurate and cost effective.

REFERENCES

1. Moll R, Franke WW, Schiller DL. 1982. The catalog of human cytokeratins: Patterns of expression in normal epithelium, tumors, and cultured cells. Cell 31:11–24.
2. Linder J. 1990. Immunohistochemistry in surgical pathology: the case of the undifferentiated malignant neoplasm. Clin. Lab. Med. 10:59–76.
3. Jaramillo M, Rangel C, Grogan T. 2000. Immunohistochemistry in leukemias and lymphomas, in: Methods in Molecular Medicine, vol 55, Hematologic Malignancies: Methods and Techniques. Humana Press: Totowa, NJ, pp. 301–319.
4. Orchard GE. 2000. Comparison of immunohistochemical labeling of melanocyte differentiation antibodies melan-A, tyrosinase and HMB-45 with NKIC3 and S100 protein in the evaluation of benign naevi and malignant melanoma. Histochem. J. 32:475–481.
5. Hasegawa T, Hirose T, Ayala AG, et al. 2001. Adult neuroblastoma of the retroperitoneum and abdomen Am. J. Surg. Path. 25:918–925.
6. Stevenson A, Chatten J, Bertoni F, et al. 1994. CD99 (p30/32MIC2) neuroectodermal/Ewing's sarcoma antigen as an immunohistochemical marker: review of more than 600 tumors and the literature experience. Appl. Immunohistochem. 2:231–240.
7. Folpe AL, Patterson K, Gown AM. 1997. Antineuroblastoma Antibody NB-84 Also Identifies a Significant Subset of Other Small Blue Round Cell Tumors. Immunohistochem. 4:239–245.
8. Hess E, Cohen C, DeRose PB, Yost BA, Costa MJ. 1997. Nonspecificity of p30/32MIC2 Immunolocalization with the 013 Monoclonal Antibody in the Diagnosis of Ewing's Sarcoma: Application of an Algorithmic Immunohistochemical Analysis. Immunohistochem. 5:94–103.
9. Shipley WR, Hammer RD, Lennington WF, Macon WR. 1997. Paraffin Immunohistochemical Detection of CD56, a Useful Marker for Neural Cell Adhesion Molecule (NCAM), in Normal and Neoplastic Fixed Tissues. Immunohistochem. 5:87–93.
10. Thompson LDR, Wieneke JA, Miettinen M and Heffner DK. 2002. Spindle Cell (Sarcomatoid) Carcinomas of the Larynx. Am. J. Surg. Pathol. 2:153–170.
11. Boyle JL, Haupt HM, Stern J, Multhaupt HAB. 2002. Tyrosinase Expression in Malignant Melanoma, Desmoplastic Melanoma, and Peripheral Nerve Tumors. Arch. Pathol. Lab. Med. 126:153–170.
12. Grogan TM, Rangel C, Rimsza L, et al. 1995. Automated Double-Labeled Immunohistochemistry and in situ Hybridization in Diagnostic Pathology. Advances in Pathol and Lab Med. vol. 8. Mosby: Year Book, Inc. 79–99.

II
SEROLOGICAL TUMOR MARKERS

4

Types of Circulating Tumor Markers and Their Clinical Applications

1. INTRODUCTION

1.1. Enzymes, Serum Proteins, and Hormones

It was during the 1950s and 1960s when we began to realize that the concentration of many molecules circulating in the blood reflected tumor cell activity. Because blood could be sampled repeatedly, these circulating molecules were used to monitor the success of cancer treatment in patients, which allowed for the adjustment of therapeutic regiment from time to time. These molecules included enzymes, isoenzymes, serum proteins, and hormones that could be found in normal blood circulation *(1)*.

During this time there were only a limited number of circulating molecules used as tumor markers for the management of cancer patients. These markers included norepinephrine for pheochromocytoma, tryptophan hyroxyindole acetic acid for carcinoid tumors, serum proteins for multiple myeloma, hormones for various endocrine tumors and several glycolytic enzymes *(2)*. All these molecules were also detectable in normal blood circulation. The blood concentration of these molecules was sufficiently high that it could be detected without the use of a sensitive immunoassay. Although it was realized that these ubiquitous serum molecules were not specific to cancer, their levels often reflected tumor progression and paralleled the clinical status of the patient. They were therefore clinically useful for monitoring the success of therapy but not for diagnosis. Among these circulating molecules, several enzymes had been frequently used (Table 1) *(3)*. Many of these enzymes may complement currently used tumor markers in terms of improved sensitivity and specificity when used together in a multiple marker panel.

Although total enzyme activity was being used for monitoring cancer therapy, isoenzymes were also found useful as circulating tumor markers (Table 2). Because many isoenzymes are tissue specific, their detection at elevated levels may be useful to suggest the tissue site of the tumor, such as elevated bone alkaline phosphatase isoenzyme for bone cancer.

Unfortunately, most serum proteins and enzymes exhibited low sensitivity and specificity when used as tumor markers. As illustrated in the study of breast cancer by Coombes et al. *(3)*, most serum proteins and enzymes were elevated only in patients with advanced metastatic disease. Most of these molecules could not detect cancer at an early stage. Even at the advanced stage, only 8 of the 21 markers were elevated in slightly over half the patients. In

From: *Cancer Diagnostics: Current and Future Trends*
Edited by: R. M. Nakamura, W. W. Grody, J. T. Wu, and R. B. Nagle © Humana Press Inc., Totowa, NJ

Table 1
Enzyme as Tumor Marker

Enzyme	Associated malignant disease
Prostatic acid phosphatase	Prostate carcinoma at a late stage
Lactate dehydrogenase	Acute leukemia; malignant lymphoma; germ cell tumors; metastatic colon, breast, and lung cancers
5'-Nucleotide phosphodiesterase	Lung cancer; liver metastases
Sialyltransferase	Nonspecific
Fucosyltransferase	Multiple malignant tumors
Urinary arylsulfatase	Myeloid leukemia
Thymidine kinase	Hodgkins lymphoma, certain leukemias, and small cell carcinoma of the lung
Terminal deoxynucleotidyl transferase	Lymphoblastic cancer

Table 2
Most Frequently Used Serum Isoenzyme as Tumor Marker

Isoenzyme	Associated malignant diseases
CK-BB	Adenocarcinoma of the prostate, lung, and stomach, not very specific
Type-2 Macro-CK (oligomeric mitochondrial CK	Metastatic liver cancer and various carcinomas
Type I macro CK (complex between CK-BB and IgG	Various neoplastic diseases
Mitochondrial CK-IgA complex	Detected in various carcinomas. Appears to be a prognosticator for patients with advanced tumors
Galactosyltransferase II[2]	Ovarian, liver, and esophageal cancers
Placental ALP (PLAP)[a] (Regan isoenzyme)	Advanced colorectal cancer, not very specific placental-like ALP
	The highest frequency was found in germ-cell tumors (e.g. seminomas) and ovarian cancers, not very specific
Bone ALP	Osteosarcoma, bone metastases
LD-1	Testicular germ cell tumors (seminomas, yolk sac tumor)
LD-4 and LD-5 isoenzymes	Elevated in most cancers at advanced stage

[a]The placental-like isozyme has different biochemical and immunochemical properties compared to the placental ALP. However, there is 98% homology in amino acid sequence between these two enzymes.

Table 3
Some Commonly-Known Carcinoembryonic Proteins

Carcinoembryonic proteins	Comments
CEA	For cancers of the gastrointestinal tract
AFP	Hepatoma and yoc sac tumors
ALP	Multiple isoenzymes of ALP can be detected in cancer tissue
IgGT	It is the hepatoma-specific γ-glutamyltranspeptidase migrating in the a_1-globulin region that can be found in cancer and fetal liver cells
5'NDPase-V	The specificity and sensitivity of 5'-nucleiotide phosphodiesterase isoenzyme-V makes it better than CEA for metastatic breast cancer
POA	Pancreatic oncofetal antigen measurement is useful both as a diagnostic test and for monitoring the clinical course of pancreatic cancer

all probability, the low sensitivity and specificity of these enzymes and protein markers limited their clinical usefulness for cancer management. The types of tumor markers used in the early days differ dramatically in terms of specificity and sensitivity from tumor markers used in recent years. These enzymes, serum proteins, and hormones were known from their normal physiologic functions. They all play specific roles in normal metabolism and therefore can be detected under normal conditions. However, monitoring these molecules in cancer patients may still allow us to relate their elevated concentrations to the molecular basis of malignant growth. Their measurement may also provide clues to the location of tumors such as elevated 5'-nuclotidase is usually associated to the tumor in the liver.

The measurement of enzyme concentration in physiological fluid may also aid in the prognosis of specific types of cancer. For example, lactate dehydrogenase (LDH) in peritoneal fluid was found to be a reliable biochemical marker related to prognosis in patients with ovarian carcinoma. Peritoneal fluid LDH appeared to have prognostic value owing to its correlation with advanced stage, poor histologic type, higher grade, and positive abdominal cytology of serous ovarian cancer *(4)*.

2. CARCINOEMBRYONIC PROTEINS

Carcinoembryonic proteins are proteins that can be detected in high concentration in the fetal tissue, are absent in the normal adult tissue but reappear in an elevated concentration in tumor tissue. Originally, they were called fetal tumor antigens and were latter changed to carcinoembrionic proteins because they are not necessarily immunogenic. A list of carcinoembryonic proteins is shown in Table 3. Placental alkaline phosphatase (the Regan isoenzyme) could be one of the earliest, if not the first, carcinoembryonic protein identified *(6)*. This is an enzyme normally produced by the syncytiotrophoblasts in the placenta after the 12th wk of pregnancy but is also found elevated in advanced colorectal cancer. In the late 1970s, it was the discovery of carcinoembrionic antigen (CEA) in colorectal carcinoma and the development of a sensitive radioimmunoassay for quantifying plasma CEA by Thomson et al. *(7)* that provoked the beginning of a new era of tumor marker investigations and applications. The discovery of CEA also initiated an intensive search for additional carcinoembryonic proteins and tumor-specific markers. Even though the results were disappointing we learn many valuable lessons about how to utilize tumor markers in the management of cancer patients.

The expression of carcinoembryonic protein associated with tumorigensis suggests that these proteins may be related specifically to the events of cancer development. Unfortunately, none of these carcinoembryonic proteins were later found to be tumor specific, although their specificity and sensitivity were improved over the enzymes and serum proteins used as tumor marker. The serum concentration of these carcinoembryonic proteins correlates well with tumor activity. Because of their insufficient sensitivity and specificity, they are not recommended for cancer screening, or for diagnosis. They are most frequently used to monitor the success of treatment for cancer patients. However, their appearance in blood circulation is usually several months before any clinical symptom. They are also useful for detecting recurrence for cancer patients postoperatively.

Unlike enzymes and hormones, many of these carcinoembryonic proteins, such as CEA and α-fetoprotein (AFP), do not have clearly defined physiological functions. Most of these molecules are present in nano- and picogram concentrations in the blood circulation. Quantification of their concentrations circulating in the blood for patient management requires the sensitivity of a radioimmunoassay or enzyme immunoassays. Again, unlike enzymes, these newly discovered tumor markers are usually associated with cancers of higher incidence, such as with epithelial cell-derived carcinomas.

3. MONOCLONAL-DEFINED TUMOR MARKERS

Monoclonal-defined tumor markers are related to epitopes defined by monoclonal antibodies. Note that these monoclonal kits recognize only the epitope, not the entire molecule and that the same epitope may appear in different molecules. Currently, they are frequently used in the management of cancer patients. The development of monoclonal-defined tumor markers was originally an attempt to improve the specificity and sensitivity of tumor marker of carcinoembryonic proteins such as CEA. It was thought that replacing polyclonal with monoclonal antibody in the assay eliminated the cross-reaction between various tumor markers because of the sharing of some epitopes between tumor markers. It was hoped that the use of monoclonal antibodies (MAbs) would lead us to the identification of tumor-specific markers (or tumor-specific epitopes). Although none of the epitopes identified turned out to be tumor-specific, the overall specificity and sensitivity of the monoclonal kits have been improved when compared to polyclonal kits.

Several monoclonal tumor marker kits have become available commercially in recent years (Table 4). These monoclonal antibodies have provided a greater degree of specificity and sensitivity than the polyclonal CEA assay in the management of patients with breast, ovarian, and pancreatic carcinomas. However, they are still limited in their clinical utilities. The major functions of these monoclonal tumor markers are still limited in the monitoring of treatment and detection of recurrence. They are not recommended for screening or for diagnosis. As a result, when a malignant disease is associated with a monoclonal kit, it is understood that the monoclonal tumor marker is only the major marker associated with the malignancy and is not necessarily specific for the malignant disease. In fact, almost all monoclonal tumor markers can be found in all carcinomas though in varying concentrations.

Table 4
Monoclonal Antibody Defined Tumor Markers

Monoclonal kit	Associated major malignant disease
CA 125	Ovarian carcinoma
Hybri-BREScan (CA 549)[a] or CA 15-3	Breast carcinoma
Hybri-CMark (CA 195)[a] or CA 19-9	Pancreatic carcinoma
CA 72-4	Gastric carcinoma
CEA	MAbs are used, specificity has been changed

[a]From Hybritech (San Diego, CA)

Because the monoclonal antibody recognizes only the epitope, not the entire molecule, monoclonal tumor marker assays may react with different molecules as long as they both express the same epitope. For example, the antigen purified from the cell membrane for CA 19-9 is a ganglioside, whereas the molecule circulating in the patients' sera is a glycoprotein, However, because both molecules express the CA 19-9 epitope, consequently, these two different molecules are both CA 19-9 positive. Listed below are some more detail descriptions of these monoclonal-defined tumor markers

3.1. CA 15-3

The CA 15-3 monoclonal tumor marker is best for monitoring patients with breast carcinoma during treatment and for the detection of recurrence. Elevated CA 15-3 is usually not detectable in benign breast tumors. Elevated CA 15-3 appears in blood circulation most frequently after metastases. The epitope associated with the tumor marker CA 15-3 is found on the polymorphic epithelial mucin (PEM) antigen and also in the milk fat globule membrane. Two MAbs, MAb 115D8 and MAb DF3, measure the tumor marker CA 15-3 in a sandwich format. However, only MAb DF3 is specific for the CA 15-3 epitope, whereas MAb 115D8 is only used to catch the tumor marker in the serum. The epitope recognized by DF3 MAb appears as tandem repeats in the serum tumor-marker molecule. CA 549, CA M26, and CA M29 are all epitopes present on the circulating molecule.

3.2. CA 125

CA 125 is the best monoclonal tumor marker for serous ovarian carcinoma and is not elevated in mucinous ovarian tumor. Although not specific for ovarian cancer, elevated CA 125 appears early at benign stages and has the potential for screening ovarian cancer at early stages. The epitope corresponding to tumor marker CA 125 is present in a large molecular weight, mucin-like glycoprotein complex that can be found in sera from patients with ovarian cancer. This epitope recognized by MAb OC 125 is considered a peptide in nature because of its sensitivity to protease and its relative stability to glycosidases.

3.3. CA 19-9

CA 19-9 is the best monoclonal tumor marker for monitoring patients with pancreatic carcinoma. This epitope, identified by MAb 19-9, was produced by a hybridoma prepared from spleen cells of a mouse immunized with a human colon carcinoma cell line, designed to replace polyclonal CEA to improve both specificity and sensitivity of polyclonal CEA.

However, it turned out that the resultant CA 19-9 was better for pancreatic cancer, although it was still reactive with colon cancer. The mucin glycoprotein, expressing CA 19-9 in the serum, has a MW of $= 5 \times 10^6$. The epitope is also shared by glycolipids in the cell membrane *(8)*. CA 19-9 is one of the gastrointestinal cancer-associated antigens defined by MAbs, which includes CA 50 and sialyl-Lewis^x (CSLEX-1). Patients with Lewis negative antigens (Le^a-Le^b-) will not express elevated CA 19-9 regardless of how advanced their pancreatic cancer is.

3.4. CA 19-5

This epitope identified by MAb CC3C-195 is very similar to CA 19-9 *(9)*. CA 195 also reacts with both Le^a and sialyl-Le^a epitopes *(10)*. MAb CC3C-195 binds with higher affinity with the sialylated Le^a blood group antigen than the nonsialylated counterpart.

3.5. CA 50

The epitope defined by the CA 50 assay is similar to the epitope of CA 19-9 and CA 195 but lacks a fucose residue, the same epitope found in Lewis negative (Le $^{a-b-}$) individuals *(11)*. Assays for CA 19-9, CA 195, and CA 50 all produce elevated levels of activity in sera from many patients with colon and pancreatic cancers.

4. BLOOD GROUP SUBSTANCES

It is interesting to note that many blood group substances are closely related to many tumor markers currently used for cancer patient management. For example, an integral part of the CEA molecule is its blood group substance. CEA from entodermally derived adenocarcinoma is found to be an incomplete blood group substance of the ABO system. The deficient antigens have tumor-specific activity resulting from the unmasking of a structural sequence that is cryptic in normal situations. Holburn et al. and Ball JP et al. *(12–14)* have demonstrated that the A, B, Le^a, and Le^b and H detected in CEA preparations were consistent with the patients' blood group and not the result of contaminations. In addition, glycolipid extracts from various human cancer tissues and cell lines show various blood group antigenicities and represent a tumor-associated epitope (carbohydrate epitope) owing to aberrant glycosylation *(13)*. IgM antibodies to T antigen, an immediate precursor of blood groups M and N expressed in about 90% of carcinomas, are present in severely depressed levels in patients with breast, lung, or gastrointestinal (GI) cancers.

Many of the tumor-associated antigens are carbohydrate in nature. It appears that the accumulation of sugar chains, such as sialyl-Le^a and sialyl-Le^x, is the major carbohydrate alteration associated with malignant transformation. The first monoclonal antibody made against such cancer altered blood group antigens with gastrointestinal cancer specificity is CA 19-9. CA 19-9 is a carbohydrate moiety with the sugar sequence containing a sialylated Le^a-active pentasaccharide directed against epitopes on a monosialoganglioside from colorectal cancer cell lines and against mucin molecules in the serum of gastrointestinal carcinoma patients *(15)*. Most of these carbohydrate antigens in epithelial tumors are derived from the Lewis blood group-related antigens. Lewis blood group antigen (Le) specificities have been found to reside in glycosphingolipids and glycoprotein molecules on the surface of erythrocytes, epithelial and endothelial cells, as well as in bound or free glycoprotein oligosaccharides secreted into various body fluids, such as saliva, ovarian-cyst fluid, urine, and milk. Co-expression and an increase in Lewis blood group-antigen-active glycolipids have been found in human adenocarcinoma. Le^a and Le^b carbohydrate determinants coexist in both glycolipid

Table 5
Glycosyl Transferases as Tumor Markers

Glycosyltransferase*	Donor substrate	Associated diseases malignant
Galactosyl-transferases	UDP-Gal	Isoenzyme II is sensitive for pancreatic cancer
Sialyl-transferase	CMP-NeuAc	Elevated in various carcinomas
Fucosyl-transferases	GDP-Fuc	Early stage of gastric cancer, malignant endometrial tissue and various metastatic carcinomas *(44)*

and glycoprotein forms in the same cells. The distribution of the Le^a and Le^b activities in the glycoprotein fraction corresponded well with that in glycolipids (Table 5).

Altered blood group antigens (or their carbohydrate epitopes) are frequently overexpressed in malignant tissues. Overexpression of altered blood group antigens is usually related to the process of tumor progression and is associated with poor prognosis. This overexpression is nonspecific and can be found in most carcinomas of varying degrees of advancement. During neoplastic transformation and neoplastic growth, blood group antigen expression in the glycoprotein and glycolipid antigens of tissues changes profoundly. Neoplastic cells may "lose" or "acquire" new antigens expressed or not expressed, respectively, by their normal counterparts.

Many of these malignancy associated blood group antigens relating to blood groups A, B, H, and Lewis antigens and their precursors are results of incomplete biosynthesis of the major blood group antigens. These precursor-like substances accumulated frequently in tumor cells *(16)*. For example, blood group A, B, and H antigens are deficient in many human adenocarcinomas. Loss of antigen expression has been found in bladder cancer, correlating with invasiveness. Modifications of these glycoproteins were also found through fucosylation and sialylation, affecting expression of blood group antigens and resulting in the production of most of the known tumor-associated carbohydrate antigens. Typical examples of tumor-associated antigens in gastrointestinal and colorectal lesions are fucosylated mono- and multimeric Le^x, Le^y, and sialylated Le^x and Le^a structures. The expression of blood group ABH antigen of the oncodevelopmental type was discovered in colonic epithelia and tumors *(17)*. Conceivably, monoclonal antibodies against these altered carbohydrate epitopes may prove useful for identification and establishment of tumor marker immunoassays. Many MAbs directed to individual types of structures have been used as probes for the detection of these antigens as tumor-associated markers. An increased synthesis of one type of antigen and decreased formation of another type seems to be frequently associated with carcinogenesis in breast, lung, and ovarian cancer *(18)*.

4.1. Glycosyltransferases

Because of the association of blood group substances with tumor markers, the enzymes that catalyze the addition of specific sugar residues from an activated donor substrate to glycoproteins, namely glycosyltransferases, also reflect tumor cell activity and could be used as tumor marker *(18)*. Past observations suggest that cell-type specific glycosylation

Table 6
Nmps Found in Various Human Tumors*

Tumor Type	Name/Designation of Altered NMP
Prostate	PC-1
Colon	CC 1-6, NC 1-4
Breast	NM200.4;NMBc 1-6; NMBC W-Z
Head and neck	C 1-11; N 12-15
Cervix	p69; p186; p200
Bladder	NMP 22 (NuMA)
Osteosarcoma	No formal designation

*Modified from ref. *19.*

sequences can result from the regulated expression of glycosyltransferase genes. The specificity of the enzymes for their donor and acceptor substrates constitutes the primary basis for determining the structures of the sugar chains produced by a cell. Changes in terminal glycosylation during development, differentiation, and oncogenic transformation are determined by these enzyme activities. Therefore, the activity of glycosyltransferases, which appear in the tumor tissue, determine the type of carbohydrate tumor markers eventually detected in cancer patients. In other words, the changes in glycolipid or glycoprotein glycosylation in transformed cells correspond to quantitative or qualitative changes in the expression of the relevant glycosyltransferases. It has been estimated that 100 or more glycosyltransferases are required for the synthesis of known carbohydrate structures on glycoproteins and glycolipids, and most of these are involved in elaborating the highly diverse terminal sequences found in mucinous glycoproteins. These enzymes are grouped into families based on the type of sugar they transfer. Several of the glycosyltransferases appear to associate specifically with certain tumor activity and have been used as tumor markers (Table 5). Serum fucosyltransferase has been found to respond to therapy designed for colon cancer patients with metastases. Galactosyltransferase has been determined useful for differentiating between benign and malignant pancreatic carcinoma.

5. NUCLEAR MATRIX PROTEINS

Nuclear matrix proteins (NMPs) were originally thought to be primarily an architectural protein network responsible for maintaining nuclear shape but now are known as a dynamic family of proteins that has a vital role in such fundamental cell processes as steroid hormone binding, gene transcription, and protein translation (Table 6). In the past, NMP was not expected to be released from the nucleus of tumor cells in quantities sufficient to be measured by conventional immunological techniques. Initially NMPs did not receive much attention as tumor markers. It was thought that only through the shedding of cell surface antigens or active secretion of cellular products would they be detectable in the extracellular space and blood circulation. Because these views have been revised, one would expect to see increasing reports of new NMPs for tumor diagnosis.

NMPs have been viewed as a potential target for diagnostic tests in cancer patients and for anticancer therapies. NMPs have been suggested as biomarkers of neoplastic disease in serum, body fluids, and tissue *(19)*. It is interesting to note that many NMPs found in the tumor were not detectable in normal tissue *(20)* NMPs can be released to the blood circulation upon cell death. NMP was also detectable in urine, and the NMP22 urine assay has been used as a screening test for recurrent disease in patients with a history of transitional cell carcinoma (TCC) of the bladder. The sensitivity of the test was almost 100% in patients with invasive TCC. The NMP22 assay may represent a useful alternative or adjunct to cystoscopy and cytology for disease surveillance in patients with TCC *(21)*. A new NMP, namely BLCA-4, was found to be sensitive (96.4%) and specific (100%) marker for bladder cancer. A urine-based immunoassay has been developed and can be used for bladder cancer diagnosis *(22)*. A cervical tumor-associated nuclear matrix antigen, NMP179, was found useful for early detection of high and low-grade cervical intraepithelial neoplasia. The NMP179 assay detected squamous-intraepithelial lesions with high accuracy (96.7%). The assay was 79.3% sensitive for the detection of low and high-grade cervical intraepithelial neoplasia (grades 1–3), with a specificity of 70.4%. NMP179 may be an effective marker for the early detection of preneoplastic-squamous intraepithelial lesions of the cervix and may be useful as an adjunctive tool for better management of cervical intraepithelial neoplasia *(23)*.

The NMP22 test kit is marketed by Matritech (Newton, Mass). Several new NMPs have been developed by Matritech for colon, breast (NMP66), and prostate cancer. Although the initial results are promising, further studies are needed to confirm the clinical utilities of the NMPs. Recently urinary NMP22 levels were found to be useful in the diagnosis of upper urinary tract cancer in patients with a tubeless cutaneous ureterostomy but had no diagnostic value in patients with urinary diversion using a bowel segment *(24)*.

6. CELL-SPECIFIC MARKERS

Currently, the most popular monoclonal-defined tumor markers, such as CA 15-3, CA 125, and CA 199 are used for monitoring of therapy and detection of recurrence of epithelial cell-derived carcinomas. However, tumors are heterogeneous in their cell composition. Many solid tumors may contain malignant cells other than epithelial cell. In these cases, tumors may not be detected if only tumor markers specific for epithelial cell are used. Measuring these tumor markers of different cell-specificity is not only important in increasing the sensitivity of tumor detection but also provide information leading for the design of appropriate therapeutic strategy.

6.1. SCC

Squamous cell has been found in tumors such as cervical cancer, lung cancer, head and neck cancer, and esophageal carcinoma. The tumor marker specifically associated with squamous cell is squamous carcinoma antigen (SCC antigen), which is a subfraction of TA-4. TA-4 was purified from squamous cell carcinoma tissue of the uterine cervix, which is also a glycoprotein with a molecular weight of approx 48 kDa. Elevated serum SCC has been detected in patients with cervical, lung, head and neck, and esophageal cancer. However, elevated serum SCC can also be detected in benign diseases, including pulmonary benign diseases, ovarian cystoma, uterine myoma, endometriosis, hepatitis, and cirrhosis. The frequency and the serum levels of SCC in these benign diseases were low *(24,25)*, with few cases exceeding 5 ng/mL. In cervical squamous cell carcinoma (CSCC) SCC appears to increase with the advance of clinical stages of the cancer. SCC was highest in patients with recurrence malignant diseases. A decline of serum SCC was observed in patients responding to chemotherapy. SCC complements CEA in the detection of CSCC: a combination of SCC and CEA raised the sensitivity for CSCC compared to the single antigen test *(26)*.

6.2. CgA

Two cell-specific tumor markers can be found in tumors containing neuroendocrine cells: chromogranin A (CgA) and neuron-specific enlonase (NSE). CgA is an acidic glycoprotein with a molecular weight of 68 kDa. CgA is present in a variety of polypeptide secreting endocrine cells that possess secretory granules, such as neuroendocrine cells. Although serum CgA is a well-known marker for the neuroendocrine cell, it is rarely used. Resulting from the lack of commercial assay kits in the United States in the past, serum CgA rarely has been measured for the diagnosis and management of patients with neuroendocrine tumors such as neuroblastoma, pheochromocytoma, small cell lung carcinoma, and carcinoid-like tumors. CgA has been found to be more stable and thus more easily manageable marker than plasma and urinary catecholamines, which were traditionally used, for the diagnosis and management of pheochromocytoma *(27)*.

Neuroendocrine cells, in general, have not been found in nonendocrine carcinomas, nor has serum CgA been detected in carcinomas except in those tumors whose normal counterparts contain neuroendocrine cells, such as the prostate tumors *(28)*. However, elevated serum CgA can frequently be detected in carcinomas at more advanced stages *(27)*.

6.3. NSE

Neuron specific enolase is a glycolytic enzyme normally present in neurons, peripheral nerve tissues, and neuroendocrine tissues, especially in the cells of the amine precursor uptake decarboxylation (APUD) system. NSE is a dimer and possesses either αG or γG two monomers with a molecular weight of approx 95 kDa, which are expressed preferentially in neurons and neuroendocrine cells and APUD cells. NSE is found at high levels in tumors of neuroendocrine origin such as small cell carcinoma of the lung and neuroblastoma *(29)*. Highly elevated serum NSE is also associated with advanced cancer. Repeated measurements of NSE during treatment can help with the evaluation of its effectiveness and the prediction of a possible relapse. Most importantly, elevated serum NSE has been found in 78% of patients with SCLC but only 17% of patients with other solid malignant tumors *(29)*. Importantly, moderately increased serum levels of NSE have also been found in a small percentage of patients with pneumonia *(30)*.

7. ASSOCIATION WITH METASTASIS

It is recognized that tumor metastasis is associated with an unfavorable outcome, and is the major cause of death in cancer patients. Because the entire process of metastasis is known, markers associated with individual events of metastasis can be identified. These markers are then used to identify patients at high risk and predict prognosis *(31)*.

The process of metastases can be roughly divided into several major stages *(32)*. In order for tumor cells at the primary site to metastasize, the process involves the digestion of the basement membrane, expression of specific receptors, expression of adhesion molecules, cellular adhesion, and cell migration. The cell components and products associated with these processes, such as proteolytic enzymes and their receptors, cell adhesion molecules, and various polypeptide growth factors, are all candidates for markers of metastasis. Moreover, a family of tumor cell-derived motility-inducing cytokines, fibronectin, collagen *(33)*, and laminin in the extracellular matrix are also potentially useful markers. When tumor cells are ready to spread, there may also be a release of type IV collagen, glycoproteins, and proteoglycans from the basement membranes when they are hydrolyzed by proteolytic enzymes derived from tumor cells *(34)*.

7.1. Protease

Among all markers identified with metastasis, the most clinically useful tumor marker is probably the protease. Following transformation by oncogenes, proteases may be found in cells that are not present in normal parental cells. For example, a single major extracellular matrix metalloprotease was secreted by human bronchial epithelial cells after being transformed by *H-ras* oncogene *(34)*.These secreted extracellular matrix metalloproteases represent a group of type IV collagenase, coded by a newly recognized gene family, associated with their metastatic potential. In addition, elevated levels of cathepsin D and urokinase-type plasminogen activator (uPA) found in the tumor tissue of a breast cancer patient was related to a higher risk for the development of metastasis and a reduced prospect of overall-survival. Studies with tumor tissues or tumor cell lines also suggested that tumor invasion and metastasis were associated with elevated levels of proteases.

Four different classes of proteases are known to be correlated with malignancy:

1. Serine proteases (e.g., uPA and plasmin).
2. Cysteinyl proteases (e.g., cathepsin B and L).
3. Aspartyl proteinases (e.g., cathepsin D).
4. Metalloproteases (e.g., gelatinases, collagenases, stromelysins).

The ability of tumor cell derived proteases to dissolve structures in the immediate vicinity of the cell is the first step of metastasis. Degradation of the surrounding extracellular matrix is necessary to allow the migration of tumor cells away from their primary site. These proteases assist active tumor cells in the penetration of basement membranes and interstitial stroma during the transition from *in situ* to invasive carcinoma. Proteases may also act directly and indirectly in the role of plasminogen activators in tissue degradation in neoplasia. The plasmin can activate proenzyme forms of other proteases or may directly degrade the extracellular matrix including the basement membrane *(35)* Increasing evidence has suggested that proteases may serve as prognostic factors in solid tumors, especially in breast cancer, to predict the outcome of the disease. Both uPA and cathepsin D, measured in extracts of breast cancer tissues, have a major impact on the prediction of relapse and overall survival time for the cancer patient. Wolf et al. *(36)* reported that the stromelysin 3 gene, which encodes a putative matrix metalloproteinase, is expressed in all invasive breast carcinomas.

8. NONSPECIFIC TUMOR MARKERS

Two criteria, namely specificity and sensitivity, are often employed to evaluate the clinical utility of a tumor marker. Few tumor markers discovered today have a desirable specificity and sensitivity. On the other hand, there are several nonspecific markers that are clinically useful for monitoring disease during treatment and for detecting recurrence. Although these tumor markers are detectable nonspecifically in a large variety of cancers, their concentrations are nevertheless sensitive to changes of the tumor activity. Many of these nonspecific tumor markers are inexpensive and simple to measure, and are therefore useful for monitoring therapy and detecting recurrence for patients with a known diagnosis. For example, Lipid associated sialic acid in the plasma (LASA-P) can be quantified with a simple, rapid, and inexpensive calorimetric procedure and its serum concentration closely parallels the serum concentrations of many tumor markers of higher specificity. Nonspecific tumor markers could also be useful in multiple marker formats to improve both the sensitivity and specificity of individual tumor marker assays.

Serum tissue polypeptide specific antigen (TPS), despite its nonspecificity, has been shown to be complementary to CA 15-3 in the management of breast cancer. The addition of TPS to CA 15-3 not only increases the sensitivity of CA 15-3 from 28.6% up to 44.4% in the overall population, and from 71.9% to 87.6% in patients with metastases but also increased the overall sensitivity by 12.7% during postsurgical follow-up *(37)*. Changes in the TPS level showed the strongest association with clinical response after the first course of chemotherapy. TPA and TPS were better indicators of disease progression than CA 15-3 in breast cancer patients treated with chemotherapy *(38)*.

8.1. Proliferation Marker

Despite its nonspecificity, proliferation markers have been widely used clinically in cancer patient management because the deregulated cell proliferation is one of the major factors contributing to tumor growth. The overall rate of proliferation may be indirectly related to the clinical outcome of many types of tumors. Because the cell cycle is the major mechanism controlling cell proliferation, expression of these proliferation markers is usually related to various phases of cell cycle progression. There are several proliferation markers that have demonstrated clinical utility.

8.2. Ki-67

Ki-67 is identified by MIB-1 MAb utilizing immunohistochemistry. MIB-1, recognizes proliferating cells in all phases of the cell cycle except G_o. Ki-67 works well in formalin-fixed paraffin-embedded sections with appropriate antigen retrieval. Ki-67 antigen expression generally correlates well with mitotic activity. The Ki-67 antigen was expressed in S phase cells although not in G_1 cells in human mitogen-stimulated peripheral blood lymphocytes entering the first cell cycle. The monoclonal antibody (mAb) Ki-67 has been used for about 10 yr, mainly to monitor proliferating cells in tissue sections, but to date little is known about the proteins it recognizes. The new monoclonal Ki-S3 and Ki-S5 antibodies detect proliferating cells in frozen and paraffin-embedded tissues. They recognize proteins with the same molecular mass as Ki-67 in Western blot. In immunoprecipitation experiments, the measurement of Ki-67 (as MIB-1 proliferation index) has proven useful in predicting the clinical outcome of the neuroendocrine tumors of the pancreas. The index also appeared useful for determining the prognosis for the survival of an individual *(39)*. Soluble Ki-67 was not detectable in blood circulation. The failure of Ki-67 detection is likely to the result of its instability in blood circulation.

8.3. PCNA

Proliferating cell nuclear antigen (PCNA) is a 36-kD nuclear protein present in highest amounts during the S phase. PC10, a MAb against PCNA, is used to stain PCNA in paraffin-fixed tissue *(40)*.

8.4. CYFRA 21-1

CYFRA 21-1 is the serum fragments of cytokeratin 19, which has been widely assessed as a serum marker of several malignancies. Assay for CYFRA 21-1 is commercially available. Cytokeratins are proteins of the intermediate filament family and a main component of the cell cytoskeleton. Cytokeraton is composed of different types of filaments with different sizes; actin, intermediate filaments, myosine, and microtubules. At present, 20 cytokeratins have been described, and all are proteins restricted only to epithelial cells.

CYFRA 21-1 appears to be a useful marker for non-small cell lung cancer (NSCLC), especially the squamous type with a sensitivity of 55%. Increased levels correlate with the severity of the disease *(41)*. In a group of squamous-cell lung cancer patients at different stages of disease, measurement of CYFRA 21-1 and SCC have showed significant prognostic value for clinical stages. A significant relationship between marker level and survival was observed for CYFRA 21-1 as well as SCC levels. In a multivariate analysis, CYFRA 21-1 and/or TPS remained significant predictors of survival *(42)*. The Combination of proliferation markers with other tumor markers appears most effective. Combination of CYFRA 21-1 and NMP22 help determine the need for cystoscopy in patients with bladder cancer *(43)*.

8.5. TK1

Cytosolic thymidine kinase 1 (TK1) is one of the enzymes involved in DNA replication. TK1 is activated at late G_1 of cell cycle, and its activity correlates with cell proliferation. A polyclonal anti-TK1 antibody against a synthetic peptide from the C-terminus of human TK1 is available. TK1 is located in the cytoplasm of cells, and is strongly expressed in the cells in S+G_2 period, raised at late G_1 and decreased during mitosis *(44)*.

8.6. Mitosin

Mitosin is a 350 kD nuclear phosphoprotein involved in cell division. It is expressed in the late G_1, S, G_2, and M phases of the cell cycle but is absent in G_0. Presently, only the immunohistochemical method has been used for its detection in formalin-fixed, paraffin-embedded tumors. Mitosin has been determined useful in node-negative breast cancer *(45)*.

8.7. LASA-P

Sialic acids (*N*-acetylneuraminic acids) are the acylated derivatives of neuraminic acid and are the terminal residues at the nonreducing end of the carbohydrate chains in many glycoproteins, glycolipids, and proteoglycans. Sialoglycoproteins on the tumor cell surface have a long history of being associated with invasiveness and metastases *(46)*. LASA-P is found elevated in a variety of malignant diseases, such as in the breast, or in those diseases associated with the gastrointestinal tract and the lung—leukemia, lymphoma, Hodgkin's disease, and melanoma—but also in nonmalignant inflammatory diseases. Apparently LASA-P is not specific to any specific type of tumor and is used in conjunction with other tumor markers for increased levels of sensitivity and specificity *(47,48)*. This lack of tumor specificity substantially limits its use as a tumor marker for diagnosis; however, it compares favorably with the most widely used tumor markers for following a patient's response to therapy and for the early detection of recurrent disease *(49)*. The sensitivity of LASA-P assay for various cancers was reported to range from 77 to 97%.

9. ECTOPIC TUMOR MARKER

It is important to note that most ectopic tumor markers are related to metastasis. The term "ectopic tumor marker" is used to describe markers that are unexpectedly or ectopically produced by certain tumors and that have no apparent association with the parent tissue of these tumors. Their appearance may also be related to the genetic control of protein

Table 7
Some Known Ectopic Tumor Markers

Ectopic marker	Ectopic appearance
AFP (>1000 ng/mL)	GI tumor and gallbladder carcinoma, renal, breast, ovarian carcinomas *(50)*
Calcitonin	Carcinoma of lung, islet cell, carcinoid, breast and medullary carcinoma of the lung and ovary, pheochromocytoma
Chromogranin A	Endocrine tumors (medullary thyroid Ca. anterior pituitary adenoma, pancreatic islet-cell Ca.)
ACTH	Pancreatic and oat-cell carcinoma
Free α-HCG subunit	Colorectal, pancreatic, and brochogenic carcinoma
β_1 subunit of HCG	Nontrophblstic cancers (For endocrine tumors (medullary thyroid Ca., anterior pituitary adenoma, pancreatic islet-cell ca
A subunit of the glycoprotein tropic hormones	Metastatic gastric carcinoid
Thyroglobulin	Differentiated thyroid carcinoma

expression; the same theory explains why carcinoembryonic proteins appear in tumors. Both carcinoembryonic proteins and ectopic markers have identical features in common; both are expressed at fetal tissues, and both expressions are suppressed during normal growth or cell differentiation and re-expressed after the transformation of normal cells into tumor cells. Similar to carcinoembryonic proteins, ectopic markers are detectable in malignant tumors because the malignant tumor contains the same genetic composition as its parent fetal tissue. It is the result of de-repression or loss of genetic control in the tumor that accounts for the re-appearance of carcinoembryonic proteins and ectopic markers. We believe that the appearance of ectopic markers may occur further on in the passage of tumor progression (at a later stage, after multiple mutations). In other words, the re-expression of the ectopic markers in the tumor cell requires a greater loss of genetic control, a loss that occurs, for example, during advanced malignant disease or metastasis. Because of the close association of ectopic tumor markers with metastasis, the detection of ectopic makers would suggest a poor prognosis.

The elevation of serum concentrations of AFP found in neoplasms, such as colon, ovarian, pancreatic, and breast carcinomas, is a typical example of an ectopic marker (Table 7). The serum concentration of the ectopic AFP may be highly elevated at the thousandth nanogram range. As expected, the fetal cells of these AFP-producing, nonhepatic tumors are also capable of producing AFP. Note that in most cases, these nonhepatic tumors do not synthesize AFP. Ectopic AFP production usually occurs in rapidly growing and poorly differentiated tumors, such as tumors having regional or distant metastases, although liver function tests may be normal. Ectopic markers are frequently found in polypeptide hormones. In fact, many of these ectopic hormones in the serum even precede clinical recognition of the tumor. Their quantification may also be useful in monitoring responses to therapy. Detection of ectopic AFP has been found to be a useful preoperative tumor marker for differentiating between the patient with primary gallbladder carcinoma and the patient with gallbladder hydrops. Gallbladder carcinoma is rarely diagnosed before surgery, which sometimes inhibits operative planning.

10. SUMMARY

All molecules appearing in the blood circulation can be used as tumor markers providing their concentrations correlate with certain aspects of tumor activity. The serum or plasma concentration of any molecule that correlates with malignant transformation, tumor cell proliferation, tumor size, and metastasis can be used as a tumor marker for cancer management. Circulating tumor markers can be divided into various groups based on their differences in clinical application.

REFERENCES

1. Bodansky O. 1974. Reflections on biochemical aspects of human cancer. Cancer 33:364–371.
2. Warburg O. 1956. On the origin of cancer cells. Science 123:309–314.
3. Coombes RC, Powles TJ, Gazet JC, et al. 1977. Biochemical markers in human breast cancer. Lancet 1:132–137.
4. Yuce K, Baykal C, Genc C, Al A, Ayhan A. 2001. Diagnostic and prognostic value of serum and peritoneal fluid lactate dehydrogenase in epithelial ovarian cancer. Eur. J. Gynaecol. Oncol. 22:228–232.
5. Fishman WH, Inglis NI, Stolbach LL, et al. 1968. A serum alkaline phosphatase isoenzyme of human neoplastic cell origin. Cancer Res. 28:150–154.
6. Gold P and Freedman SO. 1963. Demonstration of tumour specific antigens in human colonic carcinomata by immunological tolerance and absorption techniques. J. Exptl. Med. 121:439–61.
7. Thomson DMP, Krupey J, Freedman SO, et al. 1969. The radioimmunoaasy of circulating carcinoembryonic antigen of the human digestive system. Proc. Natl. Acad. Sci. USA 64:161–167.
8. Takasaki H, Uchida E, Tempero MA, et al. 1988. Correlative study on expression of CA 19-9 and DU-PAN-2 in tumor tissue and in serum of pancreatic cancer patients. Cancer Res. 48: 1435–1438.
9. Fukuta S, Magnani JL, Gaur PK, et al. 1987. Monoclonal antibody CC3C 195, which detects cancer-associated antigens in serum, binds to human Lea blood group antigen and to its sialylated derivative. Arch. Biochem. Biophys. 255:214–2146.
10. Blaszczyk M, Pak KY, Herlyn M, et al. 1985. Characterization of Lewis antigens in normal colon and gastrointestinal adenocarcinomas. Proc. Natl. Acad. Sci. USA 82:3552–3556.
11. Stroud MR, Levery SB, Nudelman ED, et al. 1991. Extended type 1 chain glycosphingolipids: dimeric $Le^a(III^4V^4Fuc_2Lc_6)$ as human tumor-associated antigen. J. Biol. Chem. 266:8439–8446.
12. Dimmons DA and Rand Perlmann P. 1973. Carcinoembryonic antigen and blood group substances. Cancer Res. 33:313–322.
13. Holburn AM, Mach JP, Mac Donald D, et al. 1974. Studies of the association of the A, B, and Lewis blood group antigens with carcinoembryonic antigen (CEA). Immunology 26:831–843.
14. Ball JP, Magous R, Lecou C, et al. 1976. Presence of blood group H antigen on a carcinoembryonic antien, and its enzymatic modification into blood group A and B specificities. Cancer Res. 36:2124–2129.
15. Magnani JL, Steplewski Z, Koprowski H, et al. 1983. Identification of the gastrointestinal and pancreatic cancer-associated antigen detected by monoclonal antibody 19-9 in the sera of patients as a mucin. Cancer Res. 43:5489–5492.
16. Feizi T, Turberville C, Westwood JH. 1975. Blood-group precursors and cancer-related antigens. Lancet 2:391–393.
17. Dabelsteen E, Graem N, Clausen H, et al. 1988. Structural variations of blood group A antigens in human normal colon and carcinomas. Cancer Res. 48:181–187.

18. Narita T, Funahashi, Satoh Y, et al. 1993. Association of expression of blood group-related carbohydrate antigens with prognosis in breast cancer. Cancer 71:3044–3053.
19. Hughes JH and Cohen MB. 1999. Nuclear matrix proteins and their potential applications to diagnostic pathology. Am. J. Clin. Pathol. 111:267–274.
20. Davis F, Gyorkey F, Busch RK, Busch H. 1979. Nucleolar antigen found in several human tumors but not in the nontumor tissues studied. Proc. Natl. Acad. Sci. USA 76:892–896.
21. Ishii T, Okadome A, Takeuchi F, Hiratsuka Y. 2001. Urinary levels of nuclear matrix protein 22 in patients with urinary diversion. Urology 58:940–942.
22. Konety BR, Nguyen TS, Dhir R, et al. 2000. Detection of bladder cancer using a novel nuclear matrix protein, BLCA-4. Clin. Cancer Res. 6:2618–2625.
23. Keesee SK, Meyer JL, Hutchinson ML, et al. 1999. Preclinical feasibility study of NMP179, a nuclear matrix protein marker for cervical dysplasia. Acta. Cytol. 43:1015–1022.
24. Collazos J and Rodriguez J. 1993. Squamous cell carcinoma antigen in patients with cirrhosis. Clin. Chem. 39:548–553.
25. Molina R, Filelia Z, Torres MD, et al. 1990. SCC antigen measured in maliganat and nonmalignant diseases. Clin. Chem. 36:251–254.
26. Sarandakou A, Phocas I, Botsis D, et al. 1998. Tumour-associated antigens CEA, CA125, SCC and TPS in gynaecological cancer. Eur. J. Gynaecol. Oncol. 19:73–77.
27. Wu T-L, Chang CP-Y, Tsao K-C, Sun C-F, Wu JT. 1999. Development of a microplate assay for serum chromogranin A (CgA): establishment of normal reference values and the detection of elevated CgA in carcinomas. J. Clin. Lab. Anal. 13:312–319.
28. Tsao KC and Wu JT. 2001. Development of an ELISA for the detection of serum chromogranin A (CgA) in prostate and non-neuroendocrine carcinomas Clin. Chim. Acta. 313:21–29.
29. Burghuber OC, Worofka B, Schernthaner G, et al. 1990. Serum neuron-specific enolase is a useful tumor marker for small cell lung cancer. Cancer 65:1386–1390.
30. Collazos J and Rodriguez J. 1993. Squamous cell carcinoma antigen in patients with cirrhosis. Clin. Chem. 39:548–553.
31. Graeff H, Harbeck N, Pache L, et al. 1992. Prognostic impact and clinical relevance of tumor-associated proteases in breast cancer. Fibrinolysis 6(Suppl 4):45–53.
32. Fidler IJ and Hart IR. 1982. Biological diversity in metastatic neoplasms:origins and implications. Science 217:998–1003.
33. Miyamoto KK, Mcsherry SA, Robins SP, et al. 1994. Collagen cross-link metabolites in urine as markers of bone metastases in prostatic carcinoma. J. Urol. 151:909–913.
34. Collier IE, Wilhelm SM, Eisen AZ, et al. 1988. H-ras oncogene-transformed human bronchial epithelial cells (TBE-1) secrete a single metalloprotease capable of degrading basement membrane collagen. J. Biol. Chem. 263:6579–6587.
35. Graeff H, Harbeck N, Pache L, et al. 1992. Prognostic impact and clinical relevance of tumor-associated proteases in breast.
36. Wolf C, Rouyer N, Lutz Y, et al. 1993. Stromelysin 3 belongs to a subgroup of proteinases expressed in breast carcinoma fibroblastic cells and possibly implicated in tumor progression. Proc. Natl. Acad. Sci. USA 90:1843–1847.
37. D'Alessandro R, Roselli M, Ferroni P, et al. 2001. Serum tissue polypeptide specific antigen (TPS): a complementary tumor marker to CA 15-3 in the management of breast cancer. Breast Cancer Res. Treat. 68:9–19.
38. Sjostrom J, Alfthan H, Joensuu H, Stenman UH, Lundin J, Blomqvist C. 2001. Serum tumour markers CA 15-3, TPA, TPS, hCGbeta and TATI in the monitoring of chemotherapy response in metastatic breast cancer. Scand. J. Clin. Lab. Invest. 61:431–441.
39. Perret AG, Mosnier JF, Buono JP, et al. 1998. The relationship between MIB-1 proliferation index and outcome in pancreatic neuroendocrine tumors. Am. J. Clin. Pathol. 109:286–293.
40. Ogala K, Kurki P, Celis JE, et al. 1987. Monoclonal antibodies to nuclear protein (PCNA/clclin) associated with DNA replication. Exp. Cell. Res. 168:475–486.

41. Rastel D, Ramaioli A, Cornillie F, Thirion B. 1994. CYFRA 21-1, a sensitive and specific new tumour marker for squamous cell lung cancer. Report of the first European multicentre evaluation. European J. Cancer 30A:601–606.

42. Kulpa J, Wojcik E, Radkowski A, Kolodziejski L, Stasik Z. 2000. CYFRA 21-1, TPA-M, TPS, SCC-Ag and CEA in patients with squamous cell lung cancer and in chemical industry workers as a reference group. Anticancer Res. 20:5035–5040.

43. Sanchez-Carbayo M, Herrero E, Megias J, Mira A, Soria F. 1999. Comparative sensitivity of urinary CYFRA 21-1, urinary bladder cancer antigen, tissue polypeptide antigen, tissue polypeptide antigen. J. Urol. 6:1951–1956.

44. Wang N, He Q, Skog S, Eriksson S, Tribukait B. 2001.Investigation on cell proliferation with a new antibody against thymidine kinase 1. Anal. Cell. Pathol. 23:11–19.

45. Clark GM, Allred DC, Hilsenbeck SG, et al. 1997. Mitosin (a new proliferation marker) correlates with clinical outcome in node-negative breast cancer. Cancer Res. 57:5505–5508.

46. Yogeeswaran G and Salk PL. 1981. Metastatic potential is positively correlated. Science 212:1514–1516.

47. Dnistrian AM, Smith C, and Schwartz MK. 1986. Sialic acid as a tumor marker. Clin. Invest. 27:156–159.

48. Dwivedi C, Dixit M, Hardy REK. 1990. Plasma lipid-bound sialic acid alterations in neoplastic diseases. Acta. Diabetol. Lat. 27:357–364.

49. Petru E, Sevin BU, Averette HE, et al. 1990. Comparison of three tumor markers-CA-125, lipd-associated sialic acid (LSA), and NB/70k-in monitoring ovarian cancer. Gynecol. Oncol. 38: 181–186.

50. Brown JA and Roberts CS. 1992. Elevated serum a-fetoprotein levels in primary gallbladder carcinoma without hepatic involvement. Cancer 70:1838–1840.

5

Identification of Risk Factors for Early Neoplasm

James T. Wu

1. INFLAMMATION MARKER

Inflammation, especially chronic inflammation, is a significant factor in the development of solid tumor malignancies *(2)*. Several inflammation markers, including interleukin 6 (IL-6), C-reactive protein (CRP), and amyloid protein, can be detected in the blood circulation and serve as risk factors for early neoplasm. CRP is nonspecific but is the most sensitive marker of inflammation. IL-6, IL-1, and tumor necrosis factor alpha induce the synthesis of CRP in hepatocytes. Its role as a predictor of survival has been shown in multiple myeloma, melanoma, lymphoma, ovarian, renal, pancreatic, and gastrointestinal tumors *(3)*. Chronic infection by viruses, bacteria, parasites, chemical irritants, nondigestible particles, or noninfectious sources all may result in chronic inflammation, a major risk factor for cancer. The longer inflammation persists, the higher the risk of associated carcinogenesis. It is well known that during the phagocytosis of bacteria or virus-infected cells, a powerful mixture of oxidants such as nitric oxide (NO), O_2 and H_2O_2 are released. These oxidants from infection may cause oxidative damage to DNA, leading to mutations and eventually carcinogenesis *(4)*.

In addition to reactive oxygen species, inflammatory cells and cytokines are also found in tumors, which mediate the inflammatory pathway (e.g., NF-κB and COX-2) and are likely to contribute to tumor growth and progression. They increase cell cycling, cause the loss of tumor suppressor function, and stimulate oncogene expression, all of which may lead to malignancy. For example, both hereditary and sporadic forms of chronic pancreatitis are associated with an increased risk of developing pancreatic cancer. The combined increase in genomic damage and cellular proliferation, both of which are seen with inflammation, strongly favors the malignant transformation of pancreatic cells *(4,5)*. Ulcerative colitis and colonic Crohn's disease (known collectively as inflammatory bowel disease [IBD]) are both associated with increased risk for colorectal cancer *(6)*. The genetic alterations found in ulcerative colitis associated colorectal cancer involve many of the same targets found in sporadic colorectal tumors and include multiple sites of allelic deletion, microsatellite instabilities, and mutations of APC, *p53*, *k-ras* as well as *msh2* and other genes. The progression of dysplasia to carcinoma is generally accompanied by an accumulation of these mutations and the similarities in the biology of colorectal cancer associated with ulcerative colitis and sporadic colorectal cancer appear to outweigh their differences *(7)*.

From: *Cancer Diagnostics: Current and Future Trends*
Edited by: R. M. Nakamura, W. W. Grody, J. T. Wu, and R. B. Nagle © Humana Press Inc., Totowa, NJ

Table 1
Associations of Various Known Pathogens With Cancer

Pathogen	Malignancy
Helicobacter pylori (bacteria)	Gastric carcinoma
Helicobacter pylori	Mucosal-associated lymphoid tissue
Schistosoma haematobium (parasite)	Bladder cancer
HTLV-1 (virus)	Adult T-cell leukemia/lymphoma
HTLV-II	Hairy cell leukemia
HBV	Hepatoma
HHV-8	Kaposi's sarcoma
EBV	Lymphoproliferative disorders
EBV	Nasopharyngeal carcinoma
EBV	Burkitt's lymphoma
HPV	Anogenital carcinoma, cervical cancer, head and neck carcinoma
HIV	

Abbr: HIV, human immunodeficiency virus; HTLV, human T-cell leukemia/lymphoma virus; HHV, human herpes virus; EBV, Epstein-Bar virus; HBV, hepatitis B virus; HPV, human papilloma virus.

2. BACTERIAL AND VIRUS INFECTION

There is a well-known link between bacterial or virus infection and cancer risk (Table 1). The key determinants of this risk are bacterial and virus infection-induced inflammation. This risk, however can be identified by direct detection of bacteria or virus in the blood circulation, which may also serve as an early marker for early neoplasm. It has been recently recognized that viruses and other pathogens play an important role in the etiology of human cancers *(8)*. In other words, the bacterial and virus infections themselves are considered to be risk factors for cancer. Table 1 lists the associations of various know pathogens with cancer.

The most well known link between virus and cancer is the link between human papillomavirus (HPV) and cervical cancer. DNA of specific HPV types has been found in almost all cervical cancer biopsies *(9)*. Current screening protocols are based on the use of Pap smears. In fact, high-risk HPV genotypes are also found to be responsible for other anogenital cancers, and squamous-cell carcinoma of the head and neck *(10)*. The screening of high-risk HPV can be performed by the detection of viral DNA and cellular proteins (viral onocoproteins) by cytological and coloscopic analysis. The identification of specific types of HPV as causative agents for cancer of the cervix and its precursor lesions led to the development of a new method for cancer screening and early diagnosis. HPV genomes and viral oncoproteins should present convenient markers for a transient of persistent infection. The detection of high-risk HPV markers should be followed by a careful clinical investigation and repeated testing for HPV persistence. Because HPV is the cause of essentially all cervical cancers, testing for HPV is the most effective screening method with inconclusive Pap tests (high sensitivity and high negative predictive value) and a negative predictive value approaching 100% for Pap smear plus HPV testing *(9)*.

The association of *Helicobacter pylori* infection with the development of gastric cancer is well recognized as well *(11)*. The key pathophysiologic event in *H. pylori* infection is the initiation and continuance of an inflammatory response. Oxidative and nitrosative stress associated with *H. pylori*-caused inflammation plays an important role in gastric carcinogenesis as a mediator of carcinogenic compound formation, DNA damage, and cell proliferation *(12)*. *H. pylori* infection is identified by histologic examination, the rapid urease test, and serologic evaluation. Stool cultures for *H. pylori* or a direct detection of *H. pylori* antigen in stools by PCR are expensive, tedious, and exhibit low sensitivity. A more sensitive enzyme immunoassay (EIA) has been developed to detect *H. pylori* antigen *(13)*.

Cancer remains a significant burden for human immunodeficiency virus-infected individuals. The discovery of a high incidence of Kaposi's sarcoma in patients with acquired immune deficiency syndrome (AIDS) is now believed to be caused by Kaposi's-sarcoma-associated herpesvirus/human herpesvirus 8. AIDS-lymphoma is known to be associated with Epstein-Barr virus (EBV) and/or KSHV infection. AIDS-related malignancies also include HPV-related cancer. The FDA considers human papillomavirus (HPV) to be a primary screening tool for cervical cancer *(14)*.

It has been reported that hepatocellular carcinoma (HCC), a major type of primary liver cancer, is etiologically linked to viral factors such as chronic infections with the hepatitis B virus (HBV). In addition, about 5% of HCC patients have the hepatitis C virus (HCV) infection *(15)*. Recently, associations between infection with HPV-16 and 18, anal and perianal skin cancer *(16)*, as well as between EBV and oral squamous cell carcinoma (OSCC) have been reported *(17)*.

In addition to the detection of viral or bacterial genomes by PCR, the detection of antipathogen antibodies in the blood by serologic tests such as enzyme-linked immunosorbent assay (ELISA) has also been proposed. The presence of these antibodies in the blood indicates an infection eradicated long before the cancer began to evolve. The staging of the disease, as well as follow up of therapy can be monitored by differentially determining the concentrations of IgM and IgG antibodies.

3. 8OH DG

DNA lesions caused by oxidative stress appear to be early risk factors for cancer. Oxidative stress is a potential mutagen leading to the accumulation of frameshift mutations and may contribute to microsatellite instability in human DNA in the setting of chronic inflammation *(18)*. Oxidants generated during normal metabolism can react with DNA and cause damage. The body continuously repairs its own DNA, but any oxidative lesion that is not repaired can lead to mutations, increasing the risk of cancer *(19)*. Human 8-Oxoguanine-DNA-glycosylase (hOGG1) is a major enzyme for repair of 8-OH-G lesion in human cells and 8-hydroxyguanine (8-OH-G), the most abundant product of oxidative damage, is the site of frequent mutagenic lesions of DNA produced by oxidative damage. As a result, 8-hydroxy deoxyguanine (8-OHdG) became a biomarker of generalized, cellular oxidative stress. The measurement of 8-OHdG in the urine appears to be an indicator of generalized, cellular oxidative stress. Musarrat et al., *(20)* also found a statistically significant 9.76-fold higher level of 8-OHdG in malignant breast tissue with invasive ductal carcinoma compared with normal breast tissue. They believed that the accumulation of 8-OHdG in DNA has a predictive significance for breast cancer risk assessment and is conceivably a major contributor in the development of breast neoplasia.

4. HOMOCYSTEINE

It was found recently that homocysteine, a well-known risk factor for cardiovascular diseases, is also a risk factor for malignant diseases *(21,22)*. Elevated serum or plasma homocysteine can be found in most cancer patients. Several biochemical changes, including folate deficiency, oxidative stress, aberrant DNA methylation, and production of homocysteine thiolactone have been identified in association with hyperhomocysteinemia. All of the events mentioned above may lead to carcinogensis and eventually cancer. Conceivably plasma or serum homocysteine can be treated as a risk factor for early neoplasm.

As suggested by Ziegler et al. *(23)*, circulating homocysteine may be an especially accurate indicator of inadequate folate, an integratory measurement of insufficient folate in tissues, or a biomarker of disruption of one carbon metabolism. Higher levels of plasma homocysteine were also detected in head and neck squamous cell carcinoma *(24)*. There was also a report concerning the association of methylenetetrahydrofolate reductase polymorphism C677T and dietary folate; both have an impact on homocystene level, with the risk of cervical dysplasia. A polymorphic variant (TT) has been linked to reduced levels of plasma folate, aberrant DNA methylation in leucocytes, and increased risk of colorectal cancer (CRC) under conditions of low folate intake. Serum homocysteine has been strongly and significantly predictive of invasive cervical cancer risk *(25)*. As a result, maintaining adequate folate and pyridoxine status and lower levels of homocysteine will reduce the risk of pancreatic cancer.

5. PSA, CA 125, CA 19-9, AND CEA

The use of serum tumor markers for the early detection of cancer is not suggested because of their low sensitivity and low positive predictive value. It has been the experience of investigators that most circulating tumor markers currently being used are elevated only when tumors begin to metastasize. However, when a panel of three serum tumor markers was used, such as OVX1, CA-125-II, and macrophage-colony stimulating factor (M-CSF) the sensitivity was significantly greater than that of the CA-125-II assay alone in patients with primary ovarian epithelial tumors of different histotypes including early-stage, potentially curable diseases *(26)*. When a single marker, CA-125-II, was used, it could only distinguish invasive Stage I tumors from apparently healthy women.

Multiple serum markers have been analyzed in women with early stage epithelial, interleukin-6 (IL-6), IL-10, lipid-associated sialic acid (LSA), M-CSF, OVX1, TAG72 (CA 72-4), tumor necrosis factor (TNF), and tissue polypeptide antigen (TPA). The serial measurement of complementary serum markers can improve the use of marker screening for epithelial ovarian cancer. This approach improves the sensitivity, specificity, and positive predictive value of serum markers CA 125 and OVX1. A procedure that measures complementary serum markers over time can be used as a primary screening technique followed by transvaginal ultrasonography. This procedure can provide a cost-effective means of early detection and can significantly decrease the probability of surgical intervention for false-positive test results *(27)*.

In Taiwan, a study screened a total of 41,495 asymptomatic individuals for cancer by measuring multiple tumor markers *(28)*. The purpose of the screening was to find cancer among asymptomatic individuals. Included in the panel of tumor markers for screening were α-fetoprotein (AFP), CA 125, CA 15-3, CA 19-9, CEA, and prostate-specific antigen (PSA).

We detected elevated tumor markers in 3070 of asymptomatic individuals. However, only 384 of the 3070 individuals with elevated levels of tumor markers returned for a more detail examination by oncologists. Among these 384 individuals, 131 of them (34.1%) were found to have a tumor. The good news was that some of the tumors detected were discovered at the benign stage. In particular, for individuals having elevated CA 125, 16 had benign ovarian tumors and only five individuals were found to have malignant ovarian cancer (9%). Apparently, the sensitivity of tumor detection was increased when multiple tumor markers were monitored. Many tumors would have gone undetected had we not measured multiple tumor markers. Therefore, we believe that screening with multiple tumor markers not only helps detect tumors but also may detect tumors at an early stage.

6. COX 2

Cyclooxygenase (COX) enzymes catalyze the first step in the conversion of arachidonic acid to prostaglandins. There are two isoforms, COX-1 and COX-2; both are glycoproteins and sit on the nuclear membrane. Both COX isoforms are normally absent in most cells but can be transiently up-regulated in response to growth factors and cytokines. Recently it was found that COX-2 appears to play an emerging role in inflammation and carcinogenesis.

Overexpression of COX-2 inhibits apoptosis, which could predispose to cancer *(29)*. Moreover, prostaglandins are believed to be important in the promotional phase of tumorigensis. As a key regulatory enzyme in the synthesis of prostaglandins, COX-2 conceivably plays an important role in the early development of tumorigenesis and may serve as an early tumor marker.

Although the COX-2 reactivity was higher in transitional and adenocarcinomas as well as in squamous cell carcinoma, COX-2 reactivity can also be detected in the nonmalignant urothelium, mainly in areas of regenerative atypical, dysplasia or squamous metaplasia *(30)*. COX-2 mRNA is highly elevated in most human colorectal cancers but is also found in a subset of adenomas. Non-neoplastic mucosa adjacent to the colon tumor also expresses COX-2 *(31)*. COX-2 can be found expressed in polyps 2 mm and larger, suggesting an early role for the enzyme in the development of the polyp. Expression of COX-2 may occur earlier than *K-ras* following the mutation of the tumor suppressor adenomatouys polyposis coli (APC) in the development of familial adenomatous polyposis and the majority of sporadic colorectal cancers.

COX-2, also a marker of inflammation and can be induced by *H. pylori* infection through the activation of nuclear factor-κB (NF-κB). NF-κB is an oxidant-sensitive transcription regulator. In gastric cancer cells, expression of mRNA and protein for COX-2 was inhibited by antioxidants glutathione (GSH), *N*-acetylcysteine (NAC), and NF-κB inhibitor, pyrrolidine dithiocarbamate (PDTC) *(32)*.

7. TGF-α AND TGF-α1

Cytokines, growth factors, and hormones are the primary driving force for most biological reactions. The elevation of cytokines is likely an early event in tumorigensis *(33)*. The measurement of cytokines such as TGF-α and TGF-α1 can be potentially useful for the early detection of tumors. TGF-α/EGFR autocrine signaling plays an important role in squamous cell carcinoma of the head and neck (SCCHN), and upregulation of TGF-α and EGFR have been suggested to be an early event in SCCHN carcinogenesis *(34)*. Expression of

Table 2
Circulating Oncoproteins That Could be Used as Early Markers

Cancer	Corresponding Genes
Colorectal	APC, *ras*, DCC
Stomach	tpr-met, *ras*
Breast	*ras*, c-*erb*B-2
Endometrial	*ras*
Pancreatic cancer in melanoma-prone families	p16^{INK4}

Adapted from ref. *69.*

TGF-α1 levels was found higher in low grade and early stage of bladder transitional cell carcinoma than in high grade and advanced stage tumors. It is suggested that TGF-α1 expression might be specific to early stage human bladder cancer *(35).*

8. C-ERBB-2, RAS (P21), AND IGF-1

The linear path from cytokine and growth factor to membrane receptor and eventually DNA replication is the most important cascade in growth regulation. A large number of extracellular signals are transmitted through signaling transduction pathways via G proteins (RAS protein), leading to diverse biological consequences (Table 2). G protein behaves as a sorting point, capable of interacting with different effectors and connects to distinct signaling pathways *(33).* Consequently, receptors such as c-erbB-2 and RAS protein are crucial regulators of cell growth in eukaryotic cells. There are several *ras* genes, including *k-ras*, *H-ras* and *N-ras*. The *ras* genes give rise to a family of related proteins with a molecular weight of 21 kDa (hence p21) that have strong transforming potential. The *ras* gene family is one of the most commonly mutated genes in both solid tumors and hematological neoplasm. Among them, the *k-ras* gene is most prone to mutation *(33).*

8.1. C-erbB-2

C-erbB-2 gene alterations have been detected in mammary tumors as early as stage I or II and in ductal carcinomas *in situ (36)*, suggesting that overexpression of c-erbB-2 oncoprotein (p185) and the appearance of the serum ectodomain of the c-erbB-2 oncoprotein may also be an early event in carcinogenesis. Expression of p185 has been found to be significantly higher in preneoplastic lesions (95.8% of cases) than in colorectal cancer; therefore, it was also suggested that p185 overexpression might be associated with the early stages of colorectal cancer.

8.2. Ras Protein

As we know now, one of the best characterized tumor-related genes is *k-ras,* which somatically mutates in several types of sporadic human cancers. Because mutations of this gene occur exclusively in three hot spots (codons 12, 13, and 61), and are frequently detected and well characterized in colorectal, pancreas, and lung cancers, molecular diagnosis and susceptibility (risk) assessment targeting *k-ras* mutations are being developed. Clinical samples used for molecular diagnosis and risk assessment include stool and lavage fluid, pancreatic and duodenal juices for colorectal cancers, and pancreas and sputum for lung cancers. Molecular analysis has begun to show promise in assessing susceptibility to, or risk of developing sporadic cancers *(37)*.

Several studies have suggested that the activation of p21 could also be an early event of carcinogenesis. The early mutation of *ras* gene and early expression of p21 have been observed in mucinous ovarian tumors, gastric carcinomas and in endometrial carcinomas *(38–40)*.

8.3. IGF-1

The insulin-like growth factors (IGFs) are a ubiquitous family of growth factors involved in normal cell growth and development. They are also implicated in numerous pathological states, including malignancy. IGF-I receptor (IGF-IR), a cell-surface tyrosine kinase receptor with a 70% homology to the insulin receptor, may be overexpressed owing to mutations in tumor suppression gene products (such as *p53*) and WT-1 or growth factors (such as bFGF and PDGF). This family of growth factors, especially the IGF-I, may present an excellent target for new therapeutic agents in the treatment of cancer and other disorders of excessive cellular proliferation *(41)*. Stattin et al. *(42)* in their study of prostate cancer found a strong association between the increase of prostate cancer and men with elevated plasma IGF-I. This association was particularly strong in younger men, suggesting that circulating IGF-I may be specifically involved in the early pathogenesis of prostate cancer.

Measurement of serum levels of IGF-1 and the calculation of IGF-1/PSA ratios were also found by Djavan et al. *(43)* to significantly improve the detection of prostate cancer over the use of PSA alone. They suggested that the increase in IGF-1 levels (i.e., the IGF-1/PSA ratio) not only was associated with an increased risk of prostate cancer but might also be a useful tool for its early detection.

9. P53 AND P53 AB

9.1. p53 Mutant Protein

p53 is a suppressor gene. Wild type *p53* protein suppresses cell growth and plays a crucial role in maintaining genomic stability in both normal and tumor cells. A mutation of the *p53* gene and the appearance of mutated p53 proteins seem to play an important role in early tumorigenesis. Several reports have indicated that p53 protein can be used as an early marker. CagA(+) *H. pylori* infection, for example, is associated with an early, higher prevalence of *p53* mutations in gastric adenocarcinoma *(44)*. The p53 protein has been detected in esophageal precancerous lesions. Wang et al. *(45)* suggested that accumulation of p53 protein might be an early biomarker for identifying high-risk subjects for esophageal cancer. The p53 protein was found in patients with early stage laryngeal carcinoma by Narayana et al. *(46)* and in patients with early gastric cancer *(47)*.

In colorectal tumors, the mutation of the *p53* suppressor gene appears earlier in the adenoma-carcinoma sequence than the *k-ras* mutation. The *p53* gene seems to play a more important role than the *k-ras* mutation in the early stages of colorectal tumorigenesis *(48)*. The detection of *p53* gene alterations is also possible in sputum samples by PCR-SSCP-silver stain for early diagnosis of lung cancer *(49)*. Additionally, overexpression of the *p53* mutant protein was found in early stage diseases of squamous cell carcinoma of the cervix and in HPV 16/18 positive tumors *(50)*. Detection of micrometastasis of the regional lymph nodes of ovarian cancer by immunohistochemical staining of *p53* protein is also possible in predicting the prognosis of patients with stage I or II epithelial ovarian cancer *(51)*.

9.2. *p53 Ab*

Mutated *p53* protein induced anti-p53 antibodies (p53 Ab) in sera of patients with various types of malignant neoplastic disease. Measureming (p53 Ab) in blood circulation appears to be another marker of potential use for early cancer detection. The finding of antibody against p53 in the sera of individuals who are at high risk of cancer, such as asbestos exposed workers or heavy smokers, indicates that measuring antibody against p53 has promising potential in the early detection of cancer *(52)*. Similar findings have also been reported for esophageal cancer *(53)*. The detection of serum p53 Ab is also useful in the early diagnosis of superficial colorectal cancer *(54)*.

9.3. *VEGF*

Vascular endothelial growth factor (VEGF) is an endothelial-cell-specific mitogen; a potent angiogenic factor specific for vascular endothelial cells. Detection of VEGF in serum is usually related to tumor metastasis, in which new blood vessels are formed to obtain nutrients for tumor growth. However, Giatromanolaki et al. *(55)* found that VEGF could be an early marker that may appear at the early-stage of NSCL cancer (including squamous cell carcinomas and adenocarcinomas). They found that the expression of VEGF occurred before the appearance of other markers, such as *p53, bcl-2*, epidermal growth factor receptor, and c-erbB-2 oncoprotein in NSCL cancer. It was suggested by Kuroi et al. *(56)* that VEGF could be used to determine the risk of carcinogenesis, screen for early cancer, distinguish benign from malignant disease, and distinguish between different types of malignancies. VEGF expression may stimulate tumor cell proliferation in the early stages of cervical cancer, and may be responsible for cervical tumorigenesis *(57)*.

10. CELL-FREE DNA

"Cell-free DNA" or circulating plasma DNA is not a marker by itself. However, it carries identical mutations as the DNA from the tumor of the same patient. In other words, cell-free DNA is the perfect specimen to be used for early detection of tumorigenesis. It is important that the procedure for obtaining cell-free DNA is noninvasive. The sampling of plasma or serum can be performed in asymptomatic individuals and can be performed as frequently as required. The detection of microsatelite instability, DNA hypermethylation, and *k-ras* mutations has been performed successfully with cell-free DNA obtained from cancer patients. The study of plasma DNA with the detection of genetic abnormalities associated with specific cancers has produced promising results. Taback et al. *(58)* have discovered the presence of circulating microsatellite alterations in the serum from patients with early stage breast cancer.

Blood tests for circulating tumor genetic markers are likely to provide valuable prognostic information. Assays of genetic alterations in circulating plasma DNA may be developed as a useful addition to conventional techniques for the diagnosis of lung cancer *(59)*.

Circulating tumor DNA appears to shed early on in the disease process. Consequently, the detection of genetic alteration in cell-free DNA holds significant promise for early detection of breast cancer *(60)*. The possibility that cell-free plasma or serum DNA may become a useful diagnostic tool for early and potentially curable cancers has also been suggested by Chen and colleagues *(61)*. The possibility of early diagnosis was also proposed by Nunes et al. *(62)* for head and neck squamous cell carcinomas. It is important to note that the detection of specific losses of heterozygosity (LOH), microsatellite instability (MI), and promoter hyper-methylation was made possible using circulating, cell-free DNA in breast cancer patients with small or even *in situ* lesions. Genetic alterations were found in plasma or serum DNA from patients with various cancers. Early tumor detection by noninvasive screening proce-dures appears feasible by measuring microsatellite instability (allele shifts) and loss of het-erozygosity in plasma DNA *(63)*. Detection of *p53* mutations in plasma DNA have been reported as a likely prognostic factor and an early marker to indicate recurrence or distant metastasis *(64)*.

11. DNA AND PROTEIN ARRAY (ANTIBODY ARRAY)

As discussed above, the advantages of measuring multiple tumor markers for improving both the sensitivity and specificity for early risk detection of cancer are apparent. Through the development of high-throughput technology, such as genomics and proteomics in recent years, the simultaneous measurement of multiple genes and proteins in a single sample is now possible. The new technology will certainly aid in the screening of high-risk individu-als. In particular, the protein array (or antibody array), a branch of proteomics, is useful for the measurement of several known markers at the same time.

Using a high-throughput proteomic classification system, Adam et al. *(65)* provided an accurate and innovative approach for the early detection/diagnosis of prostate cancer. A protein biochip surface enhanced laser desorption/ionization mass spectrometry approach coupled with an artificial intelligence learning algorithm was used to generate protein profil-ing with proteomic patterns that differentiate prostate cancer from noncancer cohorts. Feroze-Merzoug et al. *(66)* also has measured the gene expression patterns (both mRNA and protein expression profiling) to differentiate between normal prostate and prostate tumor, and between tumors at different stages.

Petricoin et al. *(67)* detected proteomic patterns in serum to distinguish neoplastic from nonneoplastic diseases within the ovary and for the detection of early-stage ovarian cancer. They generated proteomic spectra by mass spectroscopy (surface-enhanced laser desorption and ionisation that completely discriminated cancer from noncancer). Their result yielded a sensitivity of 100%, specificity of 95%, and positive predictive value of 94%. This proves that it is possible to use a prospective population-based assessment of proteomic pattern technology in serum as a screening tool for all stages of ovarian cancer in high-risk and general populations.

12. SUMMARY

Cancer is a complex genetic disease. It is generally believed that the accumulation of multiple gene mutations leads to the development of cancer *(1)*. In addition to inherited mutations, additional mutations have to be acquired for the development of a cancer. At early stages of tumorigenesis, there may be only a few mutations present. The detection of phenotypes corresponding to these early mutations in the circulation makes the detection of early neoplasm possible at a curable stage. Recently it was found that several risk factors might also lead to tumorigensis, which can be eliminated with diet adjustment and life style changes. Most of these risk factors related to inflammation and oxidative stress may also be detected in the blood circulation or urine. The measurement of all of these mutant pheno-types and risk factors in the circulation may help to identify individuals at risk for cancer, or to detect early tumors at benign stage. In this chapter, we identify risk markers and biomarkers during the preclinical stage in order to offer opportunities for early intervention.

REFERENCES

1. Vogelstein B, Fearon ER, Hamilton SE, et al. 1988. Genetic alterations during colorectal-tumor development. N. Engl. J. Med. 319:525–532.
2. Balkwill F and Mantovani A. 2001. Inflammation and cancer: back to Virchow? Lancet 357: 539–545.
3. Mahmoud FA and Rivera NI. 2002. The role of C-reactive protein as a prognostic indicator in advanced cancer. Curr. Oncol. Rep. 4:250–255.
4. Shacter E, Beecham EJ, Covey JM, Koha KW, Potter M. 1988. Activated neutrophils induce prolonged DNA damage in neighboring cells. Carcinogenesis 9:2297–2304.
5. Farrow B and Evers BM. 2002. Inflammation and the development of pancreatic cancer. Surg. Oncol. 10:153–169.
6. Ullman TA. 2002. Cancer in Inflammatory Bowel Disease. Curr. Treat. Options Gastroenterol. 5:163–171.
7. PohlC, Hombach A, Kruis, W. 2000. Chronic inflammatory bowel disease and cancer. Hepatogastroenterology 47:57–70.
8. Julie Parsonnet, ed. 1999. Microbes and malignancy. Infection as a cause of human cancers, Oxford University Press, New York.
9. zur Hausen H. 2002. Papillomaviruses and cancer: from basic studies to clinical application. Nat. Rev. 2:342–350.
10. Mork J, Lie AK, Glattre E, et al. 2001. Human papillomavirus infection as a risk factor for squamous-cell carcinoma of the head and neck N. Engl. J. Med. 344:1125–1131.
11. Uemura N, Okamoto S, Yamamoto S, et al. 2001. *Helicobacter pylori* infection and the development of gastric cancer. N. Engl. J. Med. 345:784–789.
12. Naito Y and Yoshikawa T. 2002. Molecular and cellular mechanisms involved in Helicobacter pylori-induced inflammation and oxidative stress. Free Radic. Biol. Med. 33:323–336.
13. Kim PS, Lee JW, Pai SH, et al. 2002. Detection of Helicobacter pylori Antigen in Stool by Enzyme Immunoassay. Yonsei Med. J. 43:7–13.
14. Boshoff C and Weiss R. 2002. AIDS-related malignancies. Nat. Rev. 2:373–382.
15. Levy L, Renard CA, Wei Y, Buendia MA. 2002. Genetic alterations and oncogenic pathways in hepatocellular carcinoma. Ann. NY Acad. Sci. 963:21–36.
16. Bjorge T, Engeland A, Luostarinen T, et al. 2002. Human papillomavirus infection as a risk factor for anal and perianal skin cancer in a prospective study. Br. J. Cancer 87:61–64.
17. Sand LP, Jalouli J, Larsson PA, Hirsch JM. 2002. Prevalence of Epstein-Barr virus in oral squamous cell carcinoma, oral lichen planus, and normal oral mucosa. Oral Surg. Oral Med. Oral Pathol. Oral Radiol. Endod. 93:586–592.
18. Gasche C, Chang C, Rhees J, Goel A, Boland CR. 2001. Oxidative stress increases frameshift mutations in human colorectal cancer cells. Cancer Res. 61:7444–7448.
19. Poulsen HE, Prieme H, Loft S. 1998. Role of oxidative DNA damage in cancer initiation and promotion. Eur. J. Cancer Prev. 7:9–16.
20. Musarrat J, Arezina-Wilson J, Wani AA. 1996. Prognostic and aetiological relevance of 8-hydroxyguanosine in human breast carcinognesis. Eur. J. Cancer. 32A:1209–1214.
21. Sun C-F, Thomas R, Haven TR, Wu T-L, Tsao K-C, Wu JT. 2002. Serum homocysteine increases with the rapid proliferation rate of tumor cells and decline upon cell death: a potential new tumor marker. Clin. Chim. Acta. 321:55–62.
22. Wu LL and Wu JT. 2002. Hyperhomocysteinemia is a risk factor for cardiovascular disease and a marker for cancer risk: biochemical bases. Clin. Chim. Acta. 322:21–28.
23. Ziegler RG, Weinstein SJ, Fears TR. 2002. Nutritional and genetic inefficiencies in one-carbon metabolism and cervical cancer risk. J. Nutr. 132(8 Suppl):2345S–2349S.

24. Almadori G, Bussu F, Galli J,et al. 2002. Serum folate and homocysteine levels in head and neck squamous cell carcinoma. Cancer 94:1006–1011.
25. Weinstein SJ, Ziegler RG, Selhub J, et al. 2001. Elevated serum homocysteine levels and increased risk of invasive cervical cancer in US women. Cancer Causes Control. 12:317–324.
26. van Haaften-Day C, Shen Y, Xu F,etal. 2001. OVX1, macrophage-colony stimulating factor, and CA-125-II as tumor markers for epithelial ovarian carcinoma: a critical appraisal. Cancer 92:2837–2844.
27. Berek JS and Bast RC Jr. 1995. Ovarian cancer screening. The use of serial complementary tumor markers to improve sensitivity and specificity for early detection. Cancer 76(Suppl): 2092–2096.
28. Tsao K-C, Wu TL, Sun C-F, Chang C, Wu JT. Screening Asymptomatic Individuals for Cancer with Multiple Tumor Markers: Taiwan Experience. Submitted.
29. Buttar NS and Wang KK. 2000. The "aspirin" of the new millennium: cyclooxygenase-2 inhibitors. Mayo Clin. Proc.Oct. 75(10):1027–38.
30. El-sheikh SS, Madaan S, Alhasso A, Abel P, Stamp G, Lalani E-N. 2001. Cyclooxygenase-2: a possible target in schistosoma-associated bladder cancer. B.J.U. International 88:921–927.
31. Peleg II and Wilcox CM. 2002. The role of eicosanoids, cyclooxygenases, and nonsteroidal anti-inflammatory drugs in colorectal tumorigenesis and chemoprevention. J. Clin. Gastroenterol. 34:117–125.
32. Kim H, Lim JW, Seo JY, Kim KH. 2002. Oxidant-sensitive transcription factor and cyclooxygenase-2 by Helicobacter pylori stimulation in human gastric cancer cells. J. Environ. Pathol. Toxicol. Oncol. 21:121–129.
33. Wu JT. 2002. Circulating tumor markers of the new millennium. AACC Press: Washington, DC.
34. Song JI and Grandis JR. 2000. STAT signaling in head and neck cancer. Oncogene 19: 2489–2495.
35. Miyamoto H, Kubota Y, Shuin T, et al. 1995. Expression of transforming growth factor-beta 1 in human bladder cancer. Cancer 75:2565–2570.
36. McCann AH, Dervan PA, O'Regan M, et al. 1991. Prognostic significance of c-erbB-2 and estrogen receptor status in human breast cancer. Cancer Res. 51:3296–3303.
37. Minamoto T, Mai M, Ronai Z. 2000. K-ras mutation: early detection in molecular diagnosis and risk assessment of colorectal, pancreas, and lung cancers—a review. Cancer Detect. Prev. 24:1–12.
38. Duggan BD, Felix JC, Muderspach LI, Tsao J-L, Shibata K. 1994. Early mutational activation of the c-Ki-ras in endometrial carcinoma. Cancer Res. 54:1604–1607.
39. Duggan BD, Rodenhuis S, van de Wetering ML, Moor WJ, Evers SG, van Zandwijk N, et al. 1987. Mutational activation of the k-ras oncogene. A possible pathogenetic factor in adenocarcinoma of the lung. N. Engl. J. Med. 317:929–935.
40. Cuatrecasas M, Villanueva A, Matias-Guiu,X, Prat J. 1997. K-ras mutations in mucinous ovarian tumors. Cancer 79:1581–1586.
41. Czerniak S, Herz F, Gorczyca W, Koss LG. 1989. Expression of ras oncogene p21 protein in early gastric carcinoma and adjacent gastric epithelia. Cancer 64:1467–1473.
42. Werner H and Le Roith D. 2000. New concepts in regulation and function of the insulin-like growth factors: implications for understanding normal growth and neoplasia. Cell. Mol. Life Sci. 57:932–942.
43. Stattin P, Bylund A, Rinaldi S, et al. 2000. Plasma insulin-like growth factor-I, insulin-like growth factor-binding proteins, and prostate cancer risk: a prospective study. J. Natl. Cancer Inst. 92:1910–1917.
44. Djavan B, Bursa B, Seitz C,et al. 1999. Insulin-like growth factor 1 (IGF-1), IGF-1 density, and IGF-1/PSA ratio for prostate cancer detection. Urology 54:603–606.
45. Shibata A, Parsonnet J, Longacre TA, et al. 2002. CagA status of Helicobacter pylori infection and p53 gene mutations in gastric adenocarcinoma. Carcinogenesis 23:419–424.
46. Wang L-D, Hong J-Y, Qiu,S-L, Gao H, Yang CS. 1991. Accumulation of p53 protein in human esophageal precancerous lesions: a possible early biomarker for carcinogenesis. Cancer Res. 53:1783–1787.

47. Narayana A, Vaughan ATM, Gunaratne A. 1998. Is p53 an independent prognostic factor in patients with laryngeal carcinoma. Cancer 82:286–291.

48. Oiwa H, Maehara Y, Ohno S, et al. 1995. Gowth pattern and p53 overexpression in patients with early gastric cancer. Cancer 75:1454–1459.

49. Hosaka S, Aoki Y, Akamatsu T, Nakamura N, Hosaka N, Kiyosawa K. 2002. Detection of genetic alterations in the p53 suppressor gene and the K-ras oncogene among different grades of dysplasia in patients with colorectal adenomas. Cancer 94:219–227.

50. Wang B, Li L, Yao L, et al. 2001. Detection of p53 gene alteration in sputum sample and its implications in early diagnosis of lung cancer Zhonghua Nei Ke Za Zhi. 40:101–104.

51. Ngan HY, Cheung AN, Liu,SS, Cheng DK, Ng TY, Wong LC. 2001. Abnormal expression of pan-ras, c-myc and tp53 in squamous cell carcinoma of cervix: correlation with HPV and prognosis. Oncol. Rep. 8:557–561.

52. Suzuki M, Ohwada M, Saga Y, Kohno T, Takei Y, Sato I. 2001. Micrometastatic p53-positive cells in the lymph nodes of early stage epithelial ovarian cancer: prognostic significance. Oncology 60:170–175.

53. Soussi T. 2000. p53 Antibodies in the sera of patients with various types of cancer: a review. Cancer Res. 60:1777–1788.

54. Hagiwara N, Onda M, Miyashita M, Sasajima K. 2000. Detection of circulating anti-p53 antibodies in esophageal cancer patients. J. Nippon Med. Sch. 67:110–117.

55. Takeda A, Shimada H, Nakajima K, et al. 2001. Serum p53 antibody as a useful marker for monitoring of treatment of superficial colorectal adenocarcinoma after endoscopic resection. Int. J. Clin. Oncol. 6:45–49.

56. Giatromanolaki A, Koukourakis MI, Kakolyris S, et al. 1998. Vascular endothelial growth factor, wild-type p53, and angiogenesis in early operable non-small cell lung cancer. Clin. Cancer Res. 4:3017–3024.

57. Kuroi K and Toi M. 2001. Circulating angiogenesis regulators in cancer patients. Int. J. Biol. Markers 16:5–26.

58. Fujiwaki R, Hata K, Iida K, Maede Y, Miyazaki K. 2000. Vascular endothelial growth factor expression in progression of cervical cancer: correlation with thymidine phosphorylase expression, angiogenesis, tumor cell proliferation, and apoptosis. Anticancer Res. 20:1317–1322.

59. Taback B, Giuliano AE, Hansen NM, Hoon DS. 2001. Microsatellite alterations detected in the serum of early stage breast cancer patients. Ann. NY Acad. Sci. 945:22–30.

60. Allan JM, Hardie LJ, Briggs JA, et al. 2001. Genetic alterations in bronchial mucosa and plasma DNA from individuals at high risk of lung cancer. Int. J. Cancer 91:359–365.

61. Shao ZM and Nguyen M. 2002. Tumor-specific DNA in plasma of breast cancer patients. Anticancer Drugs 13:353–357.

62. Chen X, Bonnefoi H, Diebold-Berger S, et al. 1999. Detecting tumor-related alterations in plasma or serum DNA of patients diagnosed with breast cancer. Clin. Cancer Res. 5:2297–2303.

63. Nunes DN, Kowalski LP, Simpson,AJ. 2001. Circulating tumor-derived DNA may permit the early diagnosis of head and neck squamous cell carcinomas. Int. J. Cancer 92:214–219.

64. Sozzi G, Musso K, Ratcliffe C, Goldstraw P, Pierotti MA, Pastorino U. 1999. Detection of microsatellite alterations in plasma DNA of non-small cell lung cancer patients: a prospect for early diagnosis. Clin. Cancer Res. 5:2689–2692.

65. Shao ZM, Wu J, Shen ZZ, and Nguyen M. 2001. p53 mutation in plasma DNA and its prognostic value in breast cancer patients. Clin. Cancer Res. 7:2222–2227.

66. Adam BL, Qu Y, Davis JW, et al. 2002. Serum protein fingerprinting coupled with a pattern-matching algorithm distinguishes prostate cancer from benign prostate hyperplasia and healthy men. Cancer Res. 62:3609–3614.

67. Feroze-Merzoug F, Schober MS, Chen YQ. 2001. Molecular profiling in prostate cancer. Cancer Metastasis Rev. 20:165–171.

68. Petricoin EF, Ardekani AM, Hitt BA, et al. 2002. Use of proteomic patterns in serum to identify ovarian cancer. Lancet 359:572–577.

69. Duffy MJ. 1995. Can molecular markers now be used for early diagnosis of malignancy? Clin. Chem. 41:1410–1413.

6

Emerging Circulating Tumor Markers

James T. Wu

1. INTRODUCTION

Current tumor markers are limited in their clinical utilities. They are only useful for monitoring cancer patients during treatment and for detecting recurrence. Because of the lack of specificity and sensitivity, currently used tumor markers are not recommended for screening or diagnosis. Therefore, new tumor markers are being sought to improve the sensitivity for cancer detection and to improve the specificity for diagnosis. In this chapter we introduce several new tumor markers to complement currently used tumor markers. These new tumor markers may provide specificity and improved sensitivity for cancer management. Recently the importance of using tumor markers for target therapy, prognosis, and early detection has been emphasized *(1)*. Therefore, there is a need to discover new circulating tumor markers for use in these areas. Introduced in this chapter are several new tumor markers that appear to have improved clinical utilities. In addition, a new group of circulating tumor markers are also described in this chapter relating to the signal transduction pathway, cell cycle, apoptosis, angiogenesis, and adhesion. This addition is largely owing to the recent change of emphasis on tumor markers. Instead of stressing diagnosis, monitoring and early detection of recurrence, the emphasis is placed at early tumor detection, prognosis, and target therapy. Note that these new tumor markers are also detectable in blood circulation. Because their appearance in the circulation are associated with various stages of growth regulation of cells, their detection could be correlated with prognosis and to be detectable in early neoplasm, and to be identifiable as target for target therapy. As will be shown below, these new markers involve not only oncoproteins and mutated suppressor proteins but also enzymes and various factors. Although not yet fully verified, these new tumor markers described here should greatly improve the use of circulating tumor markers in cancer management.

2. CELL-SPECIFIC TUMOR MARKERS

Tumors are heterogeneous in their composition of cells. Carcinomas, although made of malignant cell mainly derived from epithelial cell, also contain other cells in the tumor. Both neuroendocrine and squamous cell have been found in carcinomas *(2,3)*, which may also proliferate and progress to malignancy. Both neuroendocrine and squamous cells can be detected with the measurement of specific tumor markers including squamous cell carcinoma-associated antigen (SCC antigen), chromogranin A (CgA), and neuron-specific enolase (NSE). Their detection is also important for the designing of proper therapeutic strategy.

From: *Cancer Diagnostics: Current and Future Trends*
Edited by: R. M. Nakamura, W. W. Grody, J. T. Wu, and R. B. Nagle © Humana Press Inc., Totowa, NJ

2.1. SCC Antigen

Elevated serum SCC antigen has been detected in tumors containing squamous cell, which include cervical cancer, lung cancer, head and neck cancer, and esophageal carcinoma. SCC antigen, a subfraction of TA-4 purified from squamous cell carcinoma tissue of the uterine cervix, is also a glycoprotein with a molecular weight of approx 48 kDa. Although elevated serum SCC can also be found in benign disease including pulmonary benign diseases, ovarian cystoma, uterine myoma, endometriosis, hepatitis, and cirrhosis, the frequency and the serum levels of SCC in these benign diseases, however, were low (4). Few of these benign diseases containing SCC exceeded 5 ng/mL. SCC appears to increase with the advance of clinical stage. SCC antigen is highest in patients with recurrent malignant diseases. Decline of serum SCC was observed in patients who respond to chemotherapy.

2.2. CgA and NSE

Both CgA and NSE are markers for neuroendocrine cells. They are useful for the diagnosis and management of patients with carcinoid-like tumors and neuroendocrine tumors such as neuroblastoma, pheochromocytoma, and small cell lung carcinoma (5).

Chromogranin A (CgA) is an acidic glycoprotein with a molecular weight of 68 kDa. CgA is present in a variety of polypeptide-secreting endocrine cells that possess secretory granules, such as in neuroendocrine cells. CgA is a more stable and thus more easily manageable marker than plasma and urinary catecholamines traditionally used for the diagnosis and management of pheochromocytoma (6).

Neuroendocrine cells, in general, have not been found in nonendocrine carcinomas. Serum CgA has not been detected in carcinomas except in those tumors whose normal counterparts contain neuroendocrine cells, such as the prostate (7). However, elevated serum CgA can frequently be detected in carcinomas at more advanced stage (6). Recently, it was found that in patients with prostate cancer undergoing hormonal serum, CgA may rise several months earlier than PSA when patients developed resistance (8). Neuron-specific enolase (NSE) is a glycolytic enzyme normally present in neurons, peripheral nerve tissues, and neuroendocrine tissues, especially in the cells of the amine precursor uptake decarboxylation (APUD) system. The dimers of αG and γG, two monomers with a molecular weight of approx 95 kDa, are expressed preferentially in neurons and neuroendocrine cells and APUD cells. NSE is a useful marker for small cell lung cancer (SCLC) (9) and elevated levels have been found in 78% of patients with SCLC but only 17% of patients with other solid malignant tumors (9). As a marker of neuroendocrine cell, NSE appears to be less sensitive in many neuroendocrine tumors than that of CgA.

3. HOMOCYSTEINE

Homocysteine (Hcy) is a sulfur-containing amino acid detected in blood circulation. Current procedures employed for the measurement of plasma homocysteine measure the total concentration of homocysteine (tHcy), which includes albumin bound, mixed disulfide linkages, and the free reduced form of homocysteine.

tHcy is a well-known risk factor for cardiovascular diseases but has been found recently as a risk factor for cancer (10,11) and can be used as a tumor marker monitoring treatment of cancer patients. It was found that the rapid proliferation rate of tumor cells would cause an elevation of circulating concentration of tHcy. Therefore, in blood circulation, the level of tHcy will reflect tumor activity. Current assays available for tHcy measurement are too expensive for use as a monitoring tool. However, new less expensive enzymatic methods will soon be available allowing the use of serum or plasma tHcy to monitor cancer patients during treatment. It should be noted that the level of serum or plasma tHcy changes with the type of drugs that affect folate status. Wu and colleagues *(11)* and Geisler et al. *(12)* have found that circulating tHcy could fluctuate in cancer patients during chemotherapy. Geisler suggested the use of circulating tHcy as a responsive indicator of leucovorin (LV) pharmacodynamics. It is important to know that measurement of tHcy has advantages over currently used monoclonal defined tumor markers such as CA 15-3, CA 125, and CA 19-9. Using cell tissue culture, we have found that the concentration of tHcy reflected cell death but not these monoclonal-defined tumor markers. The concentration of monoclonal antibody-defined tumor markers continued to rise even when cells started dying, but the level of serum tHcy declined responding to the death of tumor cells *(10)*.

4. CELL-FREE DNA

There are two types of DNA present in the circulating blood; blood lymphocyte DNA and so-called cell-free circulating DNA. Cell-free DNA can be detected in either plasma or serum. The greatest advantage of cell-free circulating DNA is its easy sampling. Sampling cell-free DNA is a non-invasive procedure, and it can be performed frequently. Unlike DNA from tissue biopsies, cell-free DNA allows use for screening and monitoring. Cell-free circulating DNA has the potential of replacing invasive and laborious tissue biopsy for detecting DNA mutations.

Cell-free DNA is elevated in cancer patients *(13)*. The clinical utility of quantifying cell-free DNA has not been established although elevated plasma cell-free DNA from cancer patients exhibited all the characteristics of the tumor DNA in the same cancer patient such as microsatellite instability, hypermethylation, and the presence of specific oncogene, tumor suppressor gene *(14)*.

Castells et al. *(15)* have concluded that analyzing *k-ras* in cell-free plasma DNA is a highly specific, low-sensitivity approach that has diagnostic and prognostic clinical implications in patients with pancreatic carcinoma. Detection of *k-ras* mutation in circulating plasma DNA has also been reported by de Kok et al. *(16)* to assess tumor burden in patients with neoplastic disease and as a tumor marker in consecutive testing after surgery or chemotherapy for detecting recurrence. The fact that small tumors of grade 1 or *in situ* carcinomas of breast could present DNA alterations in the plasma/serum at an early stage by Chen et al. *(17)* suggest that cell-free plasma or serum DNA may become a useful diagnostic tool for early and potentially curable cancer. The possibility for early diagnosis of head and neck squamous cell carcinomas was also supported by Nunes et al. *(18)*. Assaying genetic alterations in circulating cell-free plasma DNA was also believed to be a useful addition to conventional markers for the diagnosis of lung cancer, because there is no satisfactory tumor marker for cancer of lung.

Conceivably one should be able to sample cell-free DNA in an asymptomatic population to measure early mutations to detect early neoplasm. One can also measure mutations in cell-free DNA to predict prognosis and to identify target for target therapy. Detecting residual tumor should also be possible with cell-free DNA to determine the success of therapy including surgery. In addition, coupled with specific PCR, detection of tumor-specific mutations in cell-free DNA can be treated as having a new tumor marker of high specificity for tumor. It is believed that a combined measurement of the cell-free DNA with currently used tumor markers will improve the sensitivity and specificity for cancer management.

5. INFLAMMATION MARKER

Inflammation plays a major part in tumorigenesis *(19,20)*. Among many markers for inflammation, C-reactive protein (CRP) is the most sensitive and can be frequently detected in the blood circulation of various cancer patients *(21,22)*. Fluctuation of serum CRP can also be found in serial specimens from cancer patients undergoing treatment. It appears that a combination of CRP with currently used tumor markers will improve the sensitivity of tumor detection.

5.1. CRP

CRP is an acute phase globulin with a molecular weight of approx 105 kD. In tumor, CRP is synthesized only by hepatocytes upon stimulation by interleukins from activated monocytes and macrophages at the inflammation site. CRP is the most dynamic and easily measured among acute phase reactants. Appearance of elevated cytokines, and acute phase proteins such as CRP in circulation has been observed in many cancer patients *(22–24)*. In colon cancer, a preoperative serum CRP was found to be an indicator of the malignant potential of the tumor as well as a predictor of the prognosis *(24)*. Serum level of CRP also appears to have prognostic value and is useful to help make treatment decision. One study found that patients with elevated pretreatment serum CRP would benefit from cytoreductive surgery, and those in whom serum CRP decreased to within normal limits would expect longer survival when surgery is combined with postoperative immunotherapy *(21)*.

Cancers of the liver, nasopharyngeal, and gastric carcinomas, commonly prevailing in Asia countries, were found to be associated with high percentages of elevated serum CRP. The percent of elevation of serum CRP in leukemia and lymphoma was comparable to that found in carcinomas. In breast cancer, a 70% elevation was found with elevated serum CRP, a 97.5% elevation was found in liver cancer, 88.5% in nasopharygeal carcinoma, 90.3% in gastric carcinoma, 58.1% in colon carcinoma, 82.6% in lymphoma, and 73.5% in leukemia (Wu JT, et al., unpublished data). Individuals with elevated serum CRP should be treated to reduce inflammation to avoid risk for cancer.

5.2. COX-2

Cyclooxygenase-2 (COX-2) is one of two COX enzymes catalyzing the first step in the conversion of arachidonic acid to prostaglandin. A detailed description of COX-2 can be found in Chapter 14. COX-2 is a marker of inflammation and could be a new tumor marker for early detection of tumorigensis.

6. PROTEINASES AND THEIR INHIBITOR

6.1. MMP-2 and 9

Matrix metalloproteinases (MMPs) are zinc-dependent endopeptidases implicated in cancer invasion and metastasis. MMPs are capable of degrading most components of the extracellular matrix such as collagens, elastins, laminins, fibronectins, and the protein core of prodeoglycans. MMP activity is a hallmark of tumor metastasis. Because the degradation and penetration of extracellular matrices, particularly basement membranes, are critical for cancer cell metastasis, MMP-2 and MMP-9 are unique in their ability to cleave the helical domains of type IV collagen (type IV collagenases), a principle structural component of the basement membrane. Consequently, these enzymes have been implicated in tumor cell invasion and metastasis, as well as angiogenesis and other normal cellular scenarios involving basement membrane remodeling.

Elevated MMP-2 and MMP-9 have been found in many human cancers such as breast, colon, prostate, and ovarian and have been associated with increased metastatic potential. They may be secreted by tumor cell themselves or secreted by host cells within the tumor stroma *(25)*.

6.2. TIMP

Because MMPs are all produced as latent proenzymes from tumor cells, they undergo proteolytic cleavage of an amino terminal domain during activation. The net activity of MMPs is determined by the amount of proenzyme expressed, the extent to which the proenzyme is activated, and the local concentration of specific tissue inhibitors of MMPs (MMPI). Four different tissue inhibitors of metalloproteinases (TIMP) exist. They are TIMP-1, TIMP-2, TIMP-3, and TIMP-4 *(6)*. They regulate the MMPs activity in the extracellular space. It is conceivable that the imbalance between MMPs and TIMPs determines the invasive potential in cancer cells. During tumor invasion, the balance between MMPs and TIMPs is often shifted in favor of the proteases. Studies have shown an inverse correlation between TIMP levels and the invasive potential of murine and human tumor cells *(27)*. Increased levels of TIMP-1 were found in patients with advanced cancer *(28)* and correlated with the level of invasion in malignant melanomas *(29)*.

7. ASSOCIATION WITH SIGNAL TRANSDUCTION PATHWAY

The signal transduction pathway is the major biological pathway controlling cell growth *(1)*. Many of the proteins involved in these multiple pathways are oncoproteins that can be used as tumor markers, specifically related to target identification, prognosis, and early detection. Described below are several well-studied new tumor markers

7.1. TGF-β1

All activities relating to cell growth start with the interaction of cytokines or growth factors with their receptors *(1)*. Transforming growth factor-β (TGF-β1), a cytokine, is believed to play a dual role in carcinogenesis. It is a multifunctional peptide that controls the proliferation, differentiation, and other functions in many cell types. Several inhibitory as well as stimulating activities were found to be associated with TGF-β. TGF-β1 is expressed higher in low grade and stage of bladder transitional cell carcinoma than in the high grade and stage tumors suggesting that TGF-β1 expression may be specific to early stage human bladder cancer. However, serum TGF-β1 levels were significantly elevated in patients with invasive bladder cancer compared to healthy controls TGF-β *(30)*, In addition, elevated TGF-β1 has been found in about 20% of liver cancer patients. Some patients with elevated TGF-β1 did not show elevation of serum AFP *(31)*. Elevated TGF-β1 has also been detected in cervical cancer *(32)* and in ovarian carcinoma *(33)*. Plasma TGF-β levels were markedly elevated in men with prostate cancer metastatic to regional lymph nodes and bone *(34)*. Pretreatment TGF-β1 levels were a significant prognostic factor for survival and local control. The pretreatment TGF-β1 levels reflect tumor burden and are a significant prognostic factor for survival *(32)*.

7.2. TNF-α

Tumor necrosis factor-α (TNF-α), a cytokine, belongs to the family including TNF-β or lymphotoxin. TNF-α is produced mainly by monocytes and/or macrophages, whereas TNF-β is a product of lymphoid cells. TNF-α and TNF-β are grouped among the major inflammatory cytokines. They are produced at the sites of inflammation by infiltrating mononuclear cells. Serum TNF-α levels were detected in 36.5% of patients with pancreatic cancer patients with metastasis. Patients with metastatic disease had significantly higher positive serum TNF-α rate compared to those with nonmetastatic disease. Serum TNF-α levels were found to inversely correlated with body weight, body mass index, hematocrit, hemoglobin, and serum protein and albumin levels *(35)*.

7.3. C-erbB2 Oncoprotein (p185)

The importance of the interaction between growth factors and their receptors is first illustrated in c-erbB-2 oncoprotein (p185). The protein encoded by c-*erb*B-2 gene is a 185 kDa transmembrane receptor; also a glycoprotein having intracellular, transmembrane, and extracellular domains *(36)*. The c-erbB-2 protein shows structural and functional homology with the epidermal growth factor receptor (EGFR). The cytosolic tyrosine-kinase domain of these two receptors differs only at the ectodomain of the molecule.

This transmembrane receptor is presumably involved in the regulation of cell growth and cell transformation through signal transduction pathway. The oncoprotein sits in the cell membrane and transmits signals by interacting with growth factor outside the cell membrane, which activates its cytosolic tyrosine kinase, and passes the message (signal) via a specific pathway to the nucleus to initiate biosynthesis. Overexpression of p185 has been found in breast, ovarian, gastric, endometrial carcinoma, NSCL adenocarcinoma and prostate cancer. Both amplification and overexpression of c-*erb*B-2 oncoprotein was associated with poor prognosis and with short survival and recurrence *(37,38)*.

The ectodomain of the c-erbB-2 oncoprotein can be proteolytically cleaved from the intact receptor and released as soluble molecule *(38,39)*. In blood circulation, only the ectodomain of the c-erbB-2 protein exist *(38)*. There is no p185 molecule present in the serum. Because c-*erb*B-2 gene alterations have been detected in mammary tumors as early as in stage I or II and also in ductal carcinomas *in situ* suggesting that the overexpression of c-erbB-2 oncoprotein and the appearance of serum ectodomain may be an early event in tumorigenesis *(40)*. In other words, serum ectodomain could be used as an early marker to detect tumor at benign stage, especially for breast and ovarian cancers.

The first successful example of "target therapy" was the treatment of women with metastatic breast cancer with Herceptin, a humanized monoclonal antibody against the ectodomain of c-erbB2 oncoprotein. Detecting the overexpression of c-erbB-2 oncoprotein has been used to identify women with metastatic breast cancer for Herceptin treatment *(41)*. Overexpression of c-erbB2 protein could also be used to define a subgroup of breast cancer patients with estrogen receptor-positive primary tumors, who are less likely to respond to the endocrine therapy.

7.4. EGFR

Epidermal growth factor receptor (EGFR) is another important receptor that has been used as one of the risk factors in tumor tissue cytosol for breast cancer. EGFR belongs to class I subfamily, which include the products of the *erbB2/neu, erbB3,* and *erbB4* genes.

EGFR is also a transmembrane glycoprotein with tyrosine kinase activity, which transmits the mitogenic action of the EGF family of growth factors including EGF, TGFβ1, and amphiregulin.

Overexpression of the EGFR has been reported in a number of human malignancies, including cancer of the breast, brain, bladder, head, and medulloblastomas. High levels of expression of this receptor also have been associated with poor survival in some of these patients. Like c-erbB-2, the ligand-induced activation of cells also acts primarily via receptors on the cell surface. EGFR may also form a suitable target for monoclonal antibody-directed therapy *(42)*. The fact that this receptor is not found in normal tissue also makes it an attractive candidate for various anti-tumor strategies.

7.5. IGF-1 and IGF-1R (IGFBP-3)

The insulin-like growth factors (IGFs) are a ubiquitous family of growth factors, binding proteins, and receptors that are involved in normal cell growth and development. High serum concentrations of IGF1 are associated with an increased risk of breast, prostate, colorectal, and lung cancers. Because IGF1 is the major mediator of the effects of the growth hormone, it has a strong influence on cell proliferation and differentiation and is a potent inhibitor of apoptosis *(43)*. Measurement of the level of circulating IGF-1 and IGF binding protein-3 appears to be most useful for cancer management. Plasma levels of IGF-I and IGFBP-3 were found as predictors of advanced-stage prostate cancer *(44)*. This family of growth factors, especially the IGF-I receptor, is also an excellent target for new therapeutic agents in the treatment of cancer and other disorders of excessive cellular proliferation *(45)*.

Risk for prostate cancer is increased in men with elevated plasma IGF-I. This association was particularly strong in younger men in this study, suggesting that circulating IGF-I may be specifically involved in the early pathogenesis of prostate cancer *(46)*. Significantly higher IGF-I and intact IGFBP-3 levels were found in carcinoma of the prostate (CaP) vs benign prostate hyperplasia (BPH). IGF-I and IGFBP-3 (intact and total) correlated significantly and inversely with free PSA in BPH, but not in CaP. Increases in IGF-I and intact IGFBP-3 levels were positively associated with the presence of CaP in one group of patients with low to moderately elevated PSA and that their measurements in relation to PSA might help improve diagnostic discrimination between BPH and prostate cancer *(47)*.

7.6. IL-2R

Interleukin-2 (IL-2), is a lymphokine, secreted by T lymphocytes upon antigen stimulation for normal immune responsiveness. Even though it is secreted exclusively by T cells, IL-2 stimulates all lymphoid cells to proliferate and differentiate via binding to its receptor (IL-2R). IL-2R is a transmembrane receptor with extracellular, membrane, and cytosolic domains *(48)*. Three forms of the receptor are recognized with different affinity for IL-2 binding. The high affinity receptor is a hetero-trimer composed of α, β, and γ (c)-polypeptide chains. The 55 kDa α-chain, also known as the T-cell activation (Tac) antigen or CD-25, is a unique subunit of the high affinity IL-2 receptor (IL-2R α), which is readily shed from the cell surface.

A rising serum soluble IL-2R (sIL-2R) level in serial samples from patients with hairy cell leukemia indicates increased risk of relapse *(49,50)*. In all stages of melanoma the mean values of sIL-2R were significantly higher than in normal controls and correlated with the disease progression. In patients with head and neck cancer, high serum concentrations of sIL-2Rα at diagnosis were highly correlated with a shorter survival. In addition, patients who had low serum sIL-2R concentrations at diagnosis were less likely to develop distant metastasis. Serum sIL-2R αcould be considered an independent serum biomarker *(51)*.

Levels of serum s1L-2R in the patients with stage III and IV breast cancer were significantly higher than in normal controls, and patients with stage I and II breast cancer. Serum levels of IL-2R in patients with distant metastasis were also significantly higher than patients without distant metastasis *(52)*. sIL-2Rα showed the strongest correlation with the tumor burden in non-Hodgkin's lymphoma (NHL) *(53)*.

7.7. Ras Protein (ras p21 or p21^{ras})

Ras protein is a crucial regulator of cell growth in eukaryotic cells. It is activated most frequently by receptors along the signal transduction pathways with various functions. There are several *ras* genes including *k-ras, H-ras,* and *N-ras*. The *ras* genes give rise to a family of related proteins with a molecular weight of 21 kDa (hence p21) that have strong transforming potential. *Ras* gene family is one of the most commonly mutated genes in both solid tumors and hematological neoplasm, and *k-ras* gene is the most prone to mutation *(54)*.

At least a third of tumors contain mutated *ras* genes, therefore, 30% of human cancers, including the common colon, bladder, and pancreatic cancer are caused by the presence of activated ras protein. Mutant, constitutively activated forms of ras proteins, are frequently found in cancer. In leukemia and solid tumors, aberrant ras signaling can be induced directly by *ras* gene mutation or indirectly by altering genes that associate with *ras* or its signaling pathways.

Because *k-ras* gene is most prone to mutation, elevation of *k-ras* protein or *ras p21* are frequently observed in various cancers including 30 to 50% of colorectal carcinoma *(55)*, prostate carcinoma *(56)*, NSCLC (30 to 50%) *(57)*, gastric carcinoma *(58)*, endometrial carcinoma *(59)*, ovarian carcinoma *(60)*, duodenal adenocarcinomas *(61)*, and 90 to 95% in pancreatic carcinoma.

7.8. C-Myc

At the end of the signal transduction pathway the signal needs to enter the nuclei to activate the transcription factor in the nuclei. C-myc is one of the more important transcription factors located in the nucleus that is also a nuclear oncogene. There are three characterized members of the myc gene family including *c-myc, N-myc,* and *L-myc*. Their coded proteins are myc oncoproteins that act as sequence-specific transcription factors that regulate a variety of genes important in normal cellular growth and differentiation processes. Aberrant expression of all three members of the *myc* gene family has been implicated in the development of a wide variety of tumors. The best characterized member of the family is the c-myc gene, which was originally isolated by virtue of its homology to the v-myc oncogene carried by avian myelocytomatosis virus. The protein product of the three myc genes are closely related to each other *(62)*. All these myc proteins modulate cell proliferation by functioning as transcription factors.

Overexpression of any one of the myc family member is a feature of over 95% of SCLC cell lines and in SCLC tumor specimens *(63)*. There is ample evidence that the elevated myc gene expression is associated with cell proliferation and can help induce a transformed phenotype. Approximately 70% of colon carcinomas and adenomatous polyps also over express the *c-myc* gene *(64)*.

8. ASSOCIATION WITH CELL CYCLE

Regarding cell growth, the cell cycle represents the most important biological process controlling cell proliferation. Many oncogenes and suppressor genes encode proteins operating throughout the cell cycle, leading eventually to uncontrolled cell growth. For example, some cyclins behave like oncoproteins whereas certain cell cycle inhibitors behave as proteins encoded by tumor suppressor genes. Products of the tumor suppressor gene may suppress cell growth by interacting with the cyclins and negatively regulating progression through the cell cycle. Mutations in the cyclin gene have been found in a variety of cancers.

8.1. Cyclin D1

Cyclin D1 is a protooncogene that plays a critical role in G_1 progression of the cell cycle. Overexpression of the cyclin D1 locus was found in many human cancers as a result of gene amplification or translocations *(65)*. Cyclin D1 is also the most frequently overexpressed in tumor. Because there is evidence that cell cycle derangement becomes worse as tumors progress to a more malignant state, the detection or measurement of cell cycle proteins has been used to determine a patient's prognosis. Amplification of *Cyclin D1* gene has been observed in carcinomas of the breast, and head and neck, and translocated in parathyroid adenomas and centrocytic lymphomas *(65)*. More than one-third of human breast cancers may contain excessive levels of cyclin D1, which accumulate through the deregulated expression of cyclin D1 without an apparent increase in gene copy number, indicating the prognostic significance of cyclin D1 protein.

Overexpression of cyclin D1 also occurs in most invasive ductal cancers of the breast, which can distinguish invasive breast caners from nonmalignant lesions. Abnormal coexpression of cyclin D1 and p53 protein contributes to the development of endometrial carcinoma *(66)*.

8.2. Cyclin E

Cyclin E is another G_1 cyclin which can be severely expressed in many tumor cells. Altered expression of cyclin E protein (as oncogene) occurs in most of the breast tumor and increases with increase of grade and stage of the tumor. Alteration of cyclin E was also observed in other types of solid tumors as well as leukemia. It appears that cyclin Eprotein (not cyclin D protein) is the most consistent marker for determining the prognosis of early-stage node-negative ductal carcinomas. In breast cancer, the alteration in cyclin E expression becomes progressively worse with increasing stage and grade of the tumor, suggesting its potential as a new prognostic marker. Cyclin E alteration is reported as a more consistent event then c-*erb* B2 overexpression in breast cancer *(67)*. Cyclin E protein overexpression was also found associated with *p53* alteration and it was suggested that a simultaneous overexpression of both *cyclin E* and *p53* is related to poor prognosis *(66,68)*. According to Gong et al. *(69)* the expression of *cyclin E*usually peaked at the time of cell entrance to S phase. Cyclin E will accumulate up to certain critical level before the initiation of DNA replication.

8.3. Cyclin-Dependent Kinase Inhibitor

The cell cycle is regulated by cyclin-dependent kinases (CDKs). Complexes of CDKs and their partner cyclins drive the cell through the cell cycle. Each complex phosphorylates a distinct set of proteins at a particular check-point or phase of the cycle. In addition, there are inhibitors for CDKs. Normal control of cellular growth requires a balance between the activators (cyclins) and the inhibitors of the CDKs. Several inhibitors of CDK can also be used as tumor markers. The several most common inhibitors of CDKs are listed below.

8.3.1. p16

Mutation of *p16* has been reported in several malignancies. Alteration in the *p16* gene and its mutant protein have been found in several tumor cell lines and tumors, which include squamous cell carcinoma of the head and neck, esophageal squamous cell carcinoma, NSCLC, familial melanoma kindreds, primary bladder carcinoma, acute adult T-cell leukemia, T-cell acute lymphoblastic leukemia, and B-cell acute lymphoblastic leukemia *(70)*.

8.3.2. p27

Although mutation in *p27* is rare, reduced expression of *p27* correlates with poor survival in cohorts of breast and colorectal carcinoma patients have been reported *(71)*. High cyclin E and low p27 expression is associated with about 20% survival among all women tested and approx 30% survival in the node-negative subgroup.

Other cyclin dependent kinase inhibitors involving in malignancies include *p21* in NSCLC and pancreatic adenocarcinoma, and *p15* in leukemia, melanoma and metastatic lung cancer, and *p57* in sarcomas and Wilms' tumors. Additional studies are needed in the future will verify their clinical utilities as tumor markers.

9. ASSOCIATION WITH APOPTOSIS

As cell cycle controls the cell proliferation the process of apoptosis regulates the number of cells. There are several proteins involved in apoptosis including *Bcl-2, p53* protein, *sFas*, and *sFasL*.

9.1. Bcl-2 Protein

The Bcl-2 protein is an intracellular, integral membrane protein found primarily in the nuclear envelope, endoplasmic reticulum, and outer mitochondrial membrane. *Bcl-2* may contribute to tumorigenesis by blocking apoptosis and prolonging cell survival without necessarily affecting the rate of cell proliferation. Overexpression of *Bcl-2* not only may promote neoplastic transformation but may also confer resistance of tumor (such as in ovarian carcinoma) to chemotherapy by enabling cells to avoid apoptosis. *Bcl-2* expression has been demonstrated in solid tumors, including NSCLC, thyroid, prostate, colon, uterine cervix, bladder, and breast. *Bcl-2* expression is usually associated with a survival advantage for tumor *(72)*.

In certain cancers, Bcl-2 protein is strongly associated with a good prognosis, and with several favorable prognostic features such as lack of p53 protein expression (inversely related to *p53* expression) in cancer of the breast, lung, and ovarian carcinoma *(73)*.

9.2. p53 Mutant Protein

p53 is a suppressor gene. Wild-type p53 protein suppresses cell growth and plays a crucial role in maintaining genomic stability in both normal and tumor cells. The p53 tumor suppressor protein induces cell-cycle arrest, or cell death by triggering apoptosis in response to DNA-damaging agents, such as radiation and many of the chemotherapeutics used in cancer therapy. Mutation of *p53* gene (through mis-sense point mutation or allelic loss) causes functional inactivation of the gene, which appears to be the commonest genetic alteration encountered in human malignancy. More than 50% of human cancers contain p53 mutation including breast, bladder, esophageal, gastric, head and neck, hepatocellular, laryngeal, lung, ovarian, pancreatic, prostate, thyroid and chronic myelogenus leukemia, glioblastoma, B-cell lymphoma, melanoma, neuroblastoma, nephroblastomas, and sarcomas (most commonly occurring cancers). Detection of p53 mutant proteins has been shown to be associated with aggressive tumor phenotypes while normal cells, in contrast, typically have undetectable concentrations of mutant p53 protein. Consequently mutant p53 protein is the single most important predictive indicator for recurrence and death for breast cancer patients.

Several reports have indicated that p53 protein may be used as an early tumor marker. Mutant p53 protein was detected in esophageal precancerous lesions. Wang et al. *(74)* suggested that accumulation of p53 protein might be a promising early biomarker for identifying high-risk subjects for esophageal cancer. Mutant p53 protein was also found in patients with early stage laryngeal carcinoma by Narayana et al. *(75)*, and mutant p53 protein overexpression was found in patients with early gastric cancer *(76)*.

9.3. P53 Autoantibody (p53 Ab)

Certain cancer patients with elevated circulating concentration of mutated p53 protein (released from dying tumor cells) may mount a humoral immune response producing antibody against mutant protein p53 (p53 Ab). Serum antibodies against the p53 mutant protein have been found in about 20% of patients with breast, lung, and lymphoreticular cancers *(77)*. p53-Abs are found predominantly in human cancer patients with a specificity of 96%. Such antibodies are predominantly associated with *p53* gene missense mutations and p53 accumulation in the tumor, but the sensitivity of such detection is only 30%. The clinical value of these antibodies remains subject to debate, but consistent results have been observed in breast, colon, lung, oral, and gastric cancers, and in children with B-lymphomas in which they have been associated with high-grade tumors and poor survival.

9.4. sFas

Fas (Apo-1, CD95) is a cell-surface receptor, a member of the tumor necrosis factor/nerve growth factor receptor superfamily. Fas exists in two forms, transmembrane and soluble form. Cell-surface Fas is widely expressed in normal and malignant cells. The soluble form of Fas (sFas) lacks the transmembrane domain of the full-length Fas, which has five variants produced via alternative mRNA splicing. sFas inhibits Fas-mediated apoptosis by neutralizing FasL *(78)*. Binding of sFas with cell-surface Fas will prevent signal transduction by Fas.

Serum sFas levels are elevated in patients with leukemia, colon cancer, breast cancer, and bladder cancer. The suppression of apoptosis contributes to carcinogenesis, as well as to a resistance to chemotherapy and radiotherapy. sFas may be a useful tumor marker in that it may reflect cancer status. A decrease in serum sFas levels has been found to occur after surgical resection in breast cancer.

Elevated sFas can also be detected in bladder carcinoma, gastric carcinoma, hepatoma, osteosarcoma *(79)*, gynecological malignancies (ovarian, cervical, endometrial), T- and B-cell leukemia, lymphoma and non-Hodgkin's lymphoma *(80)*. They are usually associated with poor prognosis.

9.5. sFasL

It is likely that soluble forms of Fas ligand (sFasL) are derived from the membrane bound FasL after the cleavage by a metalloproteinase(s). FasL belongs to the growing tumor necrosis factor family. FasL induces apoptosis by binding to its receptor, Fas. FasL is predominantly expressed in activated T cells and natural killer cells, whereas Fas is ubiquitously expressed in various cells.

Patients with Ta bladder carcinoma with a low level of serum sFasL (less than the median value) had a longer postoperative tumor-free interval than patients with a high sFasL level (greater than the median value) in the 5-yr follow-up. Elevated serum sFasL levels may be associated with a greater risk of disease progression and recurrence in patients with bladder carcinoma *(81)*. There was an apparent inverse correlation between the level of serum sFasL and antiautologous tumor cytotoxic activity. Therefore, the level of serum sFasL correlates with both disease progression and increase in the tumor grade. An elevated serum sFasL level predicted early recurrence in patients with Ta bladder carcinoma.

The sFasL levels are also significantly increased in patients with gastric carcinoma in a manner reflective of the disease stages such as the depth of tumor invasion, lymph node metastasis, and distant metastasis. Patients with high sFasL levels had a worse prognosis than those with low levels. It was found that sFasL concentrations could be a prognostic tumor marker for the assessment of the progression of advanced gastric carcinoma.

10. ASSOCIATION WITH ANGIOGENESIS

10.1. Angiogenic Factor

Angiogenesis, the development of new blood vessels from pre-existing vasculature, is a prerequisite for tumor growth and metastasis. Several potential regulators of angiogenesis have been identified, including vascular endothelial growth factor (VEGF), acidic fibroblast growth factor (aFGF), basic fibroblast growth factor (bFGF), transforming growth factor-α (TGF-α, TGF-β, hepatocyte growth factor/scatter factor (HGF/SF), tumor necrosis factor-α (TNF-α), and angiogenin. Only those factors that have been studied in detail are presented here.

10.1.1. bFGF

Basic fibroblast growth factor is produced by a wide variety of normal and malignant cells and has been shown to be a potent inducer of angiogenesis. Elevated bFGF concentration in serum and urine has been found in many cancers in addition to breast, head and neck cancer, and myoloma *(82)*.

The serum levels of bFGF and VEGF were found to be significantly higher in patients with renal cancer compared to healthy subjects. bFGF and VEGF values were significantly higher in patients with disseminated cancer compared to those with undisseminated cancer. Elevated serum levels of VEGF, bFGF, and IL-8 were strongly correlated with a poor overall and progression-free survival, respectively *(83)*.

10.1.2. VEGF

Vascular endothelial growth factor is an endothelial cell-specific mitogen. VEGF is potent angiogenic factor specific for vascular endothelial cells and, unlike bFGF, freely diffusible. VEGF has anti-apoptotic, mitogenic, and permeability-increasing activities specific for vascular endothelium. VEGF plays a pivotal role in the development of neovascularization in both physiological and pathological processes, e.g., developmental and reproductive angiogenesis, proliferative retinopathies, and cancers. Several solid tumors produce ample amounts of VEGF, which stimulates proliferation and migration of endothelial cells, thereby inducing neovascularization by a paracrine mechanism. Measurements of circulating VEGF have diagnostic and prognostic value not only in malignancies but also in cardiovascular failures and inflammatory diseases.

Elevated VEGF can be detected in various cancers including colon *(84–88)*. VEGF can be measured to determine the risk of cancer development, screen for early tumor detection, distinguish benign from malignant disease, and distinguish between different types of malignancies. In patients with established malignancies VEGF can be used to determine prognosis, predict the response to therapy, and monitor the clinical course *(89)*. The study of multiple angiogenic factors in melanoma cell lines demonstrated the importance of measuring VEGF, bFGF, IL-8, and platelet-derived endothelial cell growth factor simultaneously. Apparently, a unique expression pattern associated with each cell line and multiple angiogenic factors are involved in the promotion of angiogenesis in the most angiogenic melanoma lines, whereas angiogenesis in the least angiogenic melanoma lines was possibly promoted solely by VEGF.

It is important to note that inhibiting a single angiogenic factor may not be effective in the prevention of angiogenesis. To achieve an efficient anti-angiogenic treatment of melanoma therefore, may require identification and blocking of common functional features of several angiogenic factors *(90)*. Combining VEGF with *p53* status resulted in better prognostic prediction. The results significantly correlated with a worse outcome for patients with estrogen receptor-positive tumors receiving adjuvant tamoxifen. Combining VEGF and *p53* determinations also provided additional prognostic information in terms of relapse-free survival and overall survival in breast cancer *(86)*.

11. ASSOCIATION WITH ADHESION

Cellular adhesion molecules are implicated in tumor progression and metastasis. They exist in both soluble and membrane bound forms. All soluble biologically active forms of adhesion molecules including E-cadherin, CD 44, L-selectin, E-selectin, VCAM-1, and ICAM-1 can be found in vivo and in vitro. Adhesion molecules also help disguise tumor cells to look and act like normal lymphocytes. This disguise allows tumor cells to avoid immune attack in the blood circulation to be able to spread throughout the body via lymphatic and blood vessel. These molecules appear to be useful tumor markers for predicting prognosis.

11.1. E-Cadherin

E-cadherin, a distant member of the immunoglobulin superfamily, is important in maintaining homophilic cell–cell adhesion in epithelial tissues. Loss of normal E-cadherin contributes to progression in breast cancer and other solid tumors by increasing proliferation, invasion, and/or metastasis *(91)*. Therefore E-cadherin behaves as a therapeutic agent capable of suppressing tumor invasion and/or metastasis.

Soluble fragments of E-cadherin molecule, on the other hand, have been reported to increase in the sera in 67% of patients with gastric cancer. Serum soluble E-cadherin is regarded as a potential valid prognostic marker for gastric cancer *(92)*.

11.2. CD 44

CD44 is a tightly regulated cell adhesion molecule present on leukocytes and implicated in their attachment to endothelium during an inflammatory immune response. CD44 is a transmembrane glycoprotein involving in the cell–cell and cell–substrate interactions. Ectodomain of CD44 can shed from the cell surface and release as a soluble molecule. High serum levels of CD44 have been demonstrated in some solid tumors such as advanced gastric and colon cancer. Serum CD44 concentration is correlated with tumor metastasis.

Elevated soluble CD 44 has been detected in a variety of cancers including ovarian carcinoma *(93)*, non-Hodgkin lymphoma and B-cell chronic lymphocytic leukemia *(94)*. Soluble CD44 can be used for monitoring therapy in patients with low grade NHL and CLL who have received interferon-α (IFN-α).

11.3. ICAM-1

Intercellular adhesion molecule-1 (ICAM-1, CA 54) belongs to the immunoglobulin gene superfamily and is the ligand for the β2-integrins, and the leucocyte function associated antigen-1. The expression of ICAM-1 on the cell surface can be induced by several cytokines such as IFN-γ, TNF-α and also by lipopolysaccharid, oxygen radicals, and hypoxia.

ICAM-1is involved in metastatic spread. It has been shown that ICAM-1, both cell surface bound form and soluble form, increased in a variety of carcinoma cell lines, including those of the stomach, colon, liver, lung, and pancreas. Elevated sICAM-1 has also been detected in breast *(95)* and gastric carcinomas, *(96)*, and in Hodgkin disease *(97)*. Elevated levels of sICAM-1 in serum have been shown to be associated with poor prognosis in Hodgkin disease and non-Hodgkin lymphomas. High serum sICAM-1 levels were significantly associated with advanced stage and poor response to therapy *(98)*.

11.4. VCAM-1

Vascular cell adhesion molecule1 (VCAM-1) is expressed on endothelial cells as a result of VEGF stimulation. In early breast cancer serum VCAM-1 correlated closely with the microvessel density in tumors. Women who developed early recurrence had higher preoperative levels of serum VCAM-1. Serum VCAM-1 levels rose in women with advanced breast cancer whose disease progressed; but remained unchanged or fell in women with advanced breast cancer whose disease remained stable or showed a partial response to hormonal therapy. Women with lymph node-positive and high-grade tumors had higher levels of serum VCAM-1 than women with lymph node-negative and low-grade tumors. Serum VCAM-1 is a surrogate marker of angiogenesis in breast cancer and its measurement may help in the assessment of anti-angiogenic drugs *(99)*.

12. MISCELLANEOUS

There are a few promising tumor markers, which do not fit into the categories listed above.

12.1. LPA

The plasma level of total lysophosphatidic acid (LPA) has been shown to be a new, potential biomarker for ovarian cancer and other gynecological cancers. Total LPA is composed of different LPA species with distinct fatty acid chains. Because lysophosphatidylinositol (LPI) co-migrates with LPA, ratio of LPA/LPI has been analyzed and compared with disease status. Results suggested that increased LPA/LPI species with unsaturated fatty acid chains might be associated with late-stage or recurrent ovarian cancer *(99)*.

12.2. Telomere and Telomerase

Telomerase activity is a potential new tumor marker. Telomeres are the specialized DNA/ protein structures located at the end of eukaryotic chromosomes consisting of small, tandemly repeated DNA sequences (TTAGGG). The telomeres shorten with each round of DNA replication, and cells stop dividing when telomeres reach a critical length. Telomerase is a ribonucleoprotein, which is also called telomerase reverse transcriptase. The telomerase enzyme acts as a reverse transcriptase that uses part of human telomerase-associated RNA (hTR) (on which the TTAGGG repeats at the ends of chromosome can be synthesized) as a template for telomeric repeat synthesis *(100)*. Most somatic cells switch off the activity of telomerase after birth. By contrast, many cancer cells reactivate telomerase. The telomerase rebuilds chromosomes' ends (telomeres) and allows tumor cells to replicate indefinitely. Telomerase has been detected in a majority of tumor cells *(101)*. The presence of telomerase activity is correlated with poor clinical outcome in cancer patients. For example, telomerase activity is strongly associated with prostate cancer but not benign prostatic hyperplasia (BPH) or the normal gland *(102)*. Similarly significant levels of telomerase activation frequently occurred in ovarian and pancreatic cancer but rarely in premalignant and benign lesions *(103,104)*.

REFERENCES

1. Wu JT. 2002. Circulating tumor markers of the new millennium. Target therapy, early detection, and prognosis. AACC Press, Washington DC.
2. Wu JT, Erickson AJ, Tsao K-C, Wu T-L, Sun C-F. 2000. Elevated serum CgA is detectable in carcinomas at advanced stage. Ann. Clin. Lab. Sci. 30:175–178.
3. Molina R, Filelia Z, Torres MD, et al. 1990. SCC antigen measured in maliganat and nonmalignant diseases. Clin. Chem. 36: 251–254.
4. Collazos J and Rodriguez J. 1993. Squamous cell carcinoma antigen in patients with cirrhosis. Clin. Chem. 39:548–553.
5. Deftos LJ and Chromogranin A. 1991. Its role in endocrine function and as an endocrine and neuroendocrine tumor marker. Endocr. Rev. 12:181–186.
6. Wu T-L, Chang CP-Y, Tsao K-C, Sun C-F, Wu JT. 1999. Development of a microplate assay for serum chromogranin A (CgA): establishment of normal reference values and the detection of elevated CgA in carcinomas. J. Clin. Lab. Anal. 13:312–319.
7. Tsao KC and Wu JT. 2001. Development of an ELISA for the detection of serum chromogranin A (CgA) in prostate and non-neuroendocrine carcinomas Clin. Chim. Acta. 313:21–29.
8. Wu JT, Wu T-L, Chang CP-Y, Tsao K-C, Sun C-F. 1999. Different patterns of serum chromogranin A in patients with prostate cancer with and without undergoing hormonal therapy. J. Clin. Lab. Anal. 13:308–311.
9. Burghuber OC, Worofka B, Schernthaner G, et al. 1990. Serum neuron-specific enolase is a useful tumor marker for small cell lung cancer. Cancer 65:1386–1390.
10. Sun C-F, Haven TR, Wu T-L, Tsao K-C, Wu JT. 2002. Serum total homocysteine increases with the rapid proliferation rate of tumor cells and decline upon cell death: a potential new tumor marker Clin. Chim. Acta. 321:55–62.
11. Wu LL and Wu JT. 2002. Hyperhomocysteinemia is a risk factor for cardiovascular disease and a marker for cancer risk: biochemical bases. Clin. Chim. Acta. 322:21–28.
12. Geisler J, Geisler SB, Lonning PE, et al. 1998. Changes in folate status as determined by reduction in total plasma homocysteine levels during leucovorin modulation of 5-fluorouracil therapy in cancer patients. Clin. Cancer Res. 4:2125–2128.
13. Wu TL, Ju-Hsin Chia JH, Zhang D, Tsao K-C, Sun C-F, Wu J.T. 2002. Cell-free DNA: normal reference range, elevation in cancer and correlation with tumor markers. Clin. Chim. Acta. 321:77–87.

14. Anker P, Mulcahy H, Chen XQ, Stroun M. 1999. Detection of circulating tumour DNA in the blood (plasma/serum) of cancer patients. Cancer Metastasis Rev. 18:65–73.
15. Castells A, Puig P, Mora J. et al. 1999. K-ras mutations in DNA extracted from the plasma of patients with pancreatic carcinoma: diagnostic utility and prognostic significance. J. Clin. Oncol. 17:578–584.
16. de Kok JB, van Solinge WW, Ruers TJ, et al. 1997. Detection of tumour DNA in serum of colorectal cancer patients. Scand. J. Clin. Lab. Invest. 57:601–604.
17. Chen X, Bonnefoi H, Diebold-Berger S, et al. 1999. Detecting tumor-related alterations in plasma or serum DNA of patients diagnosed with breast cancer. Clin. Cancer Res. 5: 2297–2303.
18. Nunes DN, Kowalski LP, Simpson AJ. 2001. Circulating tumor-derived DNA may permit the early diagnosis of head and neck squamous cell carcinomas. Int. J. Cancer 92:214–219.
19. Shacter E and Weitzman SA. 2002. Chronic inflammation and cancer. Oncology 16:217–226.
20. Fitzpatrick FA. 2001. Inflammation, carcinogenesis and cancer. Int. Immunopharmacol. 1:1651–1667.
21. Fujikawa K, Matsui Y, Oka H, Fukuzawa S. Takeuchi H. 1999. Serum C-reactive protein level and the impact of cytoreductive surgery in patients with metastatic renal cell carcinoma. J. Urol. 162:1934–1937.
22. Kodama J, Miyagi Y, Seki N, et al. 1999. Serum C-reactive protein as a prognostic factor in patients with epithelial ovarian cancer. Eur. J. Obstet. Gynecol. Reprod. Biol. 82:107–110.
23. Legouffe E., Rodriguez C, Picot MC, et al. 1998. C-reactive protein serum level is a valuable and simple prognostic marker in non Hodgkin's lymphoma. Leuk. Lymphoma 31:351–357.
24. Nozoe T, Matsumata T, Kitamura M, Sugimachi K. 1998. Significance of preoperative elevation of serum C-reactive protein as an indicator for prognosis in colorectal cancer. Am. J. Surg. 176:335–338.
25. Remacle AG, Noel A, Duggan C, et al. 1998. Assay of matrix metalloproteinases types 1,2,3 and 9 in breast cancer. Br. J. Cancer 77:926–931.
26. Greene L, Wang M, Xiao G, Liu,YE, Shi YE. 1996. Loss of expression of TIMP-4, a novel human tissue inhibitor of metalloproteinases, in human breast cancer progression. Pros. Am. Assoc. Cancer Res. 37:91–95.
27. Stetler-Stevenson WG, Brown PD, Onisto M, Levy AT, Liotta LA. 1990. Tissue inhibitor of metalloproteinases-2 (TIMP-2) mRNA expression in tumor cell lines and human tumor tissues. J. Biol. Chem. 265:13933–13938.
28. Holten-Andersen MN, Murphy G, Nielsen HJ, et al. 1999. Quantitation of TIMP-1 in plasma of healthy blood donors and patients with advanced cancer. Br. J. Cancer. 80:495–503.
29. Airola K, Karonen T, Vaalamo M, et al. 1999. Expression of collagenases-1 and -3 and their inhibitors TIMP-1 and -3 correlates with the level of invasion in malignant melanomas. Br. J. Cancer. 80:733–743.
30. Eder IE, Stenzl A, Hobisch A, et al. 1996. Transforming growth factors-b1 and b2 in serum and urine from patients with bladder carcinoma. J. Urol. 156:953–957.
31. Sacco R, Leuci D, Tortorella C, et al. 2000. Transforming growth factor beta1 and soluble Fas serum levels in hepatocellular carcinoma. Cytokine. 12:811–814.
32. Dickson J, Davidson SE, Hunter RD, West CM. 2000. Pretreatment plasma TGF beta 1 levels are prognostic for survival but not morbidity following radiation therapy of carcinoma of the cervix. Int. J. Radiat. Oncol. Biol. Phys. 48:991–995.
33. Francis-Thickpenny KM, Richardson DM, van Ee CC, et al. 2001. Analysis of the TGF beta functional pathway in epithelial ovarian carcinoma. Br. J. Cancer. 85:687–691.
34. Shariat SF, Shalev M, Menesses-Diaz A, et al. 2001. Preoperative plasma levels of transforming growth factor beta(1) (TGF-beta(1) strongly predict progression in patients undergoing radical prostatectomy. J. Clin. Oncol. 19:2856–2864.
35. Karayiannakis AJ, Syrigos KN, Polychronidis A, Pitiakoudis M, Bounovas A, Simopoulos K. 2001. Serum levels of tumor necrosis factor-alpha and nutritional status in pancreatic cancer patients. Anticancer Res. 21:1355–1358.

36. Akiyama T, Sudo C, Ogawara H, et al. 1986. The product of the human c-erbB-2 gene: a 185-kilodalton glycoprotein with tyrosine kinase activity. Science 232:1644–1646.
37. Slamon DJ, Clark GM, Wong SG, et al. 1987. Human breast cancer correlation of relapse and survival with amplification of the HER-2/cerbB-2 oncogene. Science 235:177–181.
38. Wu JT. 2002. C-*erb*B2 oncoproein and its soluble ectodomain: a new patental tumor marker for prognosis early detection and montoring patients undergoing Herceptin treatment. Clin. Chim. Acta. 322:11–19.
39. Langton BC, Crenshaw MC, Chao LA, et al. 1991. An antigen immunologically related to the external domain of gp185 is shed from nude mouse tumors overexpressing the c-erbB-2 (HER-2/neu) oncogene. Cancer Res. 51:2593–2598.
40. McCann AH, Dervan PA, O'Regan M, et al. 1991. Prognostic significance of c-erbB-2 and estrogen receptor status in human breast cancer. Cancer Res. 51:3296–3303.
41. Pegram MD, Lipton A, Hayes DF, et al. 1998. Phase II study of receptor-enhanced chemosensitivity using recombinant humanized anti-p185HER2/neu monoclonal antibody plus cisplatin in patients with HER2/neu-overexpressing metastatic breast cancer refractory to chemotherapy treatment. J. Clin. Oncol. 16:2659–2671.
42. Moyer JD, Barbacci EG, Iwata KK, et al. 1997. Induction of apoptosis and cell cycle arrest by CP-358,774, an inhibitor of epidermal growth factor receptor tyrosine kinase. Cancer Res. 57:4838–4848.
43. Furstenberger G and Senn HJ. 2002. Insulin-like growth factors and cancer. Lancet Oncol. 3:298–302.
44. Chan JM, Stampfer MJ, Ma J, et al. 2002. Insulin-like growth factor-I (IGF-I) and IGF binding protein-3 as predictors of advanced-stage prostate cancer. J. Natl. Cancer Inst. 94:1099–1106.
45. Werner H and Le Roith D. 2000. New concepts in regulation and function of the insulin-like growth factors: implications for understanding normal growth and neoplasia. Cell. Mol. Life. Sci. 57:932–942.
46. Stattin P, Bylund A, Rinaldi S, et al. 2000. Plasma insulin-like growth factor-I, insulin-like growth factor-binding proteins, and prostate cancer risk: a prospective study. J. Natl. Cancer Inst. 92:1910–1917.
47. Khosravi J, Diamandi A, Mistry J, Scorilas A. 2001. Insulin-like growth factor I (IGF-I) and IGF-binding protein-3 in benign prostatic hyperplasia and prostate cancer. J. Clin. Endocrinol. Metab. 86:694–699.
48. Waldmann TA. 1991. The interleukin-2 receptor. J. Biol. Chem. 266:2681–2684.
49. Gebauer G, Rieger M, Jager W, Lang N. 1999. Prognostic relevance of soluble interleukin-2 receptors in patients with ovarian tumors. Anticancer Res. 19:2509–2511.
50. Arun B, Curti BD, Longo DL, et al. 2000. Elevations in serum soluble interleukin-2 receptor levels predict relapse in patients with hairy cell leukemia. Cancer J. Sci. Am. 6:21–24.
51. Tartour E, Mosseri V, Jouffroy T, et al. 2001. Serum soluble interleukin-2 receptor concentrations as an independent prognostic marker in head and neck cancer. Lancet 357:1263–1264.
52. Murakami S, Hirayama R, Satomi A, et al. 1997. Serum Soluble Interleukin-2 Receptor Levels in Patients with Breast Cancer. Br. Cancer 4:25–28.
53. Perez-Encinas M, Quintas A, Bendana A, Rabunal MJ, Bello JL. 1999. Correlation and prognostic value of serum soluble ICAM-1, beta-2 microglobulin, and IL-2alphaR levels in non-Hodgkin's lymphoma. Leuk. Lymphoma 33:551–558.
54. Ram PT and Iyengar R. 2001. G protein coupled receptor signaling through the Src and Stat3 pathway: role in proliferation and transformation. Oncogene 20:1601–1606.
55. Carpenter KM, Durrant LG, Morgan K, et al. 1996. Greater frequency of K-ras val-12 mutation in colorectal cancer as detected with sensitive methods. Clin. Chem. 42:904–909.
56. Viola MV, Fromowitz F, Oravez S, et al. 1986. Expression of *ras* oncogene p21 in prostate cancer. N. Engl. J. Med. 314:133–137.
57. Fujino M, Dosaka-Akita H, Harada M, et al. 1995. Prognostic significance of p53 and ras p21 expression in nonsmall cell lung cancer. Cancer 2457–2463.

58. Czerniak, S, Herz Gorczyca GW, Koss LG. 1989. Expression of ras oncopene p21 protein in early gastric carcinoma and adjacent gastric epithelia. Cancer 64:1467–1473.
59. Duggan BD, Felix JC, Muderspach LI, Tsao J-L, Shibata K. 1994. Early mutational activation of the c-Ki-ras in encometrial carcinoma. Cancer Res. 54:1604–1607.
60. Cuatrecasas M, Villanueva A, Matias-Guiu X, Prat J. 1997. K-ras mutations in mucinous ovarian tumors. Cancer 79:1581–1586.
61. Younes N, Fulton N, Tanaka R, et al. 1997. The presence of K-12 ras mutations in deudenal adenocarcinomas and the absence of ras mutations in other small bowel adenocarcinomas and carcinoid tumors. Cancer 79:1804–1808.
62. Melhem MF, Meisler AI, Finley GG, et al. 1992. Distribution of cells expression myc proteins in human colorectal epithelium, polyps, and malignant tumors. Cancer Res. 52:5853–5864.
63. Plummer H 3rd, Catlett J, Leftwich J, et al. 1993. c-myc expression correlates with suppression of c-kit protooncogene expression in small cell lung cancer cell lines. Cancer Res. 53: 4337–4342.
64. Melhem MF, Meisler AI, Finley GG, et al. 1992. Distribution of cells expressing myc proteins in human colorectal epithelium, polyps, and malignant tumors. Cancer Res. 52:5853–5864.
65. Sherr CJ. 1996. Cancer cell cycles. Science 274:1672–1677.
66. Nikaido T, Li S-F, Shiozawa T, Fujii S. 1996. Coabnormal expression of cyclin D1 and p53 protein in human uterlin endometrial carcinomas. Cancer 78:1248–1253.
67. Keyomarsi K, O'Leary N, Molnar G, Lees E, Fingert HJ, Pardee AB. 1994. Cyclin E, a potential prognostic marker for breast cancer. Cancer Res. 54:380–385.
68. Furihata M, Ohtsuki Y, Sonobe H, et al. 1998. Prognostic significance of cyclin E and p53 protein overexpression in carcinoma of the renal pelvis and ureter. Br. J. Cancer. 77:783–788.
69. Gong J, Traganos F, Darzynkiewicz Z. 1995. Threshold expression of cyclin E but not D type cyclins characterizes normal and tumour cells entering S phase. Cell. Prolif. 28:337–346.
70. Hatta Y, Hirama T, Takeucyhi S, et al. 1995. Alterations of the p16 (MTS1) gene in testicular, ovarian and endometrial malignancies. J. Urol. 154:1959–1957.
71. Porter PL, Malone KE, Heagerty PJ, et al. 1997. Expression of cell-cycle regulators p27 and cyclin E, alone and in combination, correlate with survival in young breast cancer patients. Nat. Med. 3:222–225.
72. Herod JJO, Eliopoulos AG, Warwick J, et al. 1996. The prognostice significance of Bcl-2 and p53 expression in ovarian carcinoma. Cancer Res. 56:2178–2184.
73. Joensuu H, Pylkkanen L, Toikkanen S. 1994. Bcl-2 protein expression and long-term surviaal in breast cancer. Am. J. Pathol. 145:1191–1198.
74. Wang L-D, Hong J-Y, Qiu S-L, Gao H, Yang CS. 1991. Accumulation of p53 protein in human esophageal precancerous lesions: a possible early biomarker for carcinogenesis. Cancer Res. 53:1783–1787.
75. Narayana A, Vaughan ATM, Gunaratne A. 1998. Is p53 an independent prognostic factor in patients with laryngeal carcinoma. Cancer 82:286–291.
76. Oiwa H, Maehara Y, Ohno S, et al. 1995. Growth pattern and p53 overexpression in patients with early gastric cancer. Cancer 75:1454–1459.
77. Harris CC and Holistein M. 1993. Clinical implications of the p53 tumor-suppressor gene. N. Engl. J. Med. 329:1318–1327.
78. Cascino I, Fiucci G, Papoff G, Ruberti G. 1995. Three functional soluble forms of the human apoptosis-inducing Fas molecule are produced by alternative splicing. J. Immunol. 154: 2706–2713.
79. Mizutani Y, Yoshida O, Bonavida B. 1998. Prognostic significance of soluble Fas in the serum of patients with bladder cancer. J. Urol. 160: 571–576.
80. Hara T, Tsurumi H, Takemura M, et al. 2000. Serum-soluble fas level determines clinical symptoms and outcome of patients with aggressive non-Hodgkin's lymphoma. Am. J. Hematol. 64:257–61.

81. Mizutani Y, Hongo F, Sato N, et al. 2001. Significance of serum soluble Fas ligand in patients with bladder carcinoma. Cancer 92:287–293.

82. Sezer O, Jakob C, Eucker J, et al. 2001. Serum levels of the angiogenic cytokines basic fibroblast growth factor (bFGF), vascular endothelial growth factor (VEGF) and hepatocyte growth factor (HGF) in multiple myeloma. Eur. J. Haematol. 66:83–88.

83. Ugurel S, Rappl G, Tilgen W, Reinhold U. 2001. Increased serum concentration of angiogenic factors in malignant melanoma patients correlates with tumor progression and survival. J. Clin. Oncol. 19:577–583.

84. Davies MM, Jonas SK, Kaur S, Allen-Mersh TG. 2000. Plasma vascular endothelial but not fibroblast growth factor levels correlate with colorectal liver mestastasis vascularity and volume. Br. J. Cancer 82:1004–1008.

85. Cheng WF, Chen CAm, Lee CN, et al. 1999. Vascular endothelial growth factor in cervical carcinoma. Obstet. Gynecol. 93:761–765.

86. Linderholm BK, Lindahl T, Holmberg L, et al. 2001. The expression of vascular endothelial growth factor correlates with mutant p53 and poor prognosis in human breast cancer. Cancer Res. 61:2256–2260.

87. Feldman AL, Tamarkin L, Paciotti GF, et al. 2000. Serum endostatin levels are elevated and correlate with serum vascular endothelial growth factor levels in patients with stage IV clear cell renal cancer. Clin. Cancer Res. 6:4628–4634.

88. Boss EA, Massuger LF, Thomas CM, et al. 2001. Vascular endothelial growth factor in ovarian cyst fluid. Cancer 91:371–377.

89. Kuroi K and Toi M. 2001. Circulating angiogenesis regulators in cancer patients. Int. J. Biol. Markers 16:5–26.

90. Rofstad EK and Halsor EF. 2000. Vascular endothelial growth factor, interleukin 8, platelet-derived endothelial cell growth factor, and basic fibroblast growth factor promote angiogenesis and metastasis in human melanoma xenografts. Cancer Res. 60:4932–4938.

91. Hiraguri S, Godfrey T, Jakamura, H., et al. 1998. Mechanisms of inactivation of E-cadherin in breast cancer cell lines. Cancer Res. 58:1972–1977.

92. Chan AO, Lam SK, Chu KM, et al. 2001. Soluble E-cadherin is a valid prognostic marker in gastric carcinoma. Gut 48:808–811.

93. Stickeler E, Vogl,FD, Denkinger T, Mobus VJ, Kreienberg R, Runnebaum IB. 2000. Soluble CD44 splice variants and pelvic lymph node metastasis in ovarian cancer patients. Int. J. Mol. Med. 6:595–601.

94. Sasaki K and Niitsu N. 2000. Elevated serum levels of soluble CD44 variant 6 are correlated with shorter survival in aggressive non-Hodgkin's lymphoma. Eur. J. Haematol. 65:195–202.

95. Altomonte M, Fonsatti E, Lamaj E, et al. 1999. Differential levels of soluble intercellular adhesion molecule-1 (sICAM-1) in early breast cancer and benign breast lesions. Breast Cancer Res. Treat. 58:19–23.

96. Nakata B, Hori T, Sunami T, et al. 2000. Clinical significance of serum soluble intercellular adhesion molecule 1 in gastric cancer. Clin. Cancer Res. 6:1175–1179.

97. Lei KI and Johnson PJ. 2000. The prognostic significance of serum levels of soluble intercellular adhesion molecules-1 in patients with primary extranodal non-Hodgkin lymphomas. Cancer 89:1387–1395.

98. Byrne GJ, Ghellal A, Iddon J, et al. 2000. Serum soluble vascular cell adhesion molecule-1: role as a surrogate marker of angiogenesis. J. Natl. Cancer Inst. 92:1329–1336.

99. Shen Z, Wu M, Elson P, et al. 2001. Fatty acid composition of lysophosphatidic acid and lysophosphatidylinositol in plasma from patients with ovarian cancer and other gynecological diseases. Gynecol. Oncol. 83:25–30.

100. Buys C. 2000. Telomeres, telomerase, and cancer. N. Engl. J. Med. 342: 1282–1283.

101. Kim NW, Piatyszek MA, Prowse KR, et al. 1994. Specific association of heman telomerase activity with immortal cells and cancer. Science 266:2011–2015.

102. Sommerfeld HJ, Meeker AK, Piatyszek MA, Bova GS, Shay JW, Coffey DS. 1996. Telomerase activity: a prevalent marker of malignant human prostate tissue. Cancer Res. 56:218–222.
103. Kyo S, Takakura M, Tanaka M, et al. 1998. Qantitative differences in telomerase activity among maliganat, premalignant, and benign ovarian lesions. Clin. Cancer Res. 4:399–405.
104. Hiyama E, Kodama T, Shinbara K, et al. 1997. Telomerase activity is detected in pancreatic cancer but not in benign tumors. Cancer Res. 57:326–331.

7

Prostate Cancer Markers

From Discovery to the Clinic

Judith A. Finlay, Stephen D. Mikolajczyk, Thomas M. Pribyl, R. Bruce Wallace, and Harry G. Rittenhouse

1. INTRODUCTION

In 1936 prostatic acid phosphatase (PAP) became the key serum marker for monitoring prostate cancer (PCa) treatment *(1–3)*. Approximately 50 yr later, prostate-specific antigen (PSA) emerged as the most useful serum marker for PCa management followed a few years later by the watershed application for early detection. In spite of the many tumor marker candidates proposed and studied for over 50 yr, these two prostate proteins remained the most clinically requested PCa serum tests (Table 1). With the accumulation of human genome sequence knowledge and extraordinary methodological advances in gene arrays and proteomics, new PCa molecular tests appear to be on the horizon. Although the biological rationale for a marker's function may not be known when research is initiated, marker candidates with biological basis for their function, will likely be the most useful. Therefore, the biological function of a marker is an important factor to consider when assessing the potential of new markers. Table 2 and Fig. 1 illustrate PCa markers catagorized by biological activity. What are the clinical utilities and deficiencies for PSA today and what are the features of PAP and PSA, which contribute to the long standing utility of these markers? These properties will be important when assessing the potential of new markers for PCa.

1.1. Current Practice of PCa Diagnosis

Following Food and Drug Administration(FDA) approval of PSA for monitoring PCa relapse in 1986, PSA has surpassed PAP as a clinical test for PCa. After radical prostatectomy (RP), it was hypothesized that PSA would drop to undetectable concentrations. Patients usually exhibit serum PSA of less than 0.1 ng/mL after surgically disrupted PSA is cleared from the body. Concentrations of PSA above 0.1 ng/mL signal "biochemical relapse" followed by clinical relapse. Studies using ultrasensitive PSA detection have shown that the "biological zero" (the lowest level of PSA which can be attained after RP) is less than 0.008 ng/mL *(4)*. Among other ramifications, this result indicates that nonprostate sources of PSA do not contribute to blood PSA concentrations, including the periurethral glands, which express PSA *(4)*.

Apparently the PSA from periurethral glands leaks directly into the urinary tract confounding the use of urine as a specimen source for clinical testing *(5,6)*. The availability of ultrasensitive PSA assays require a three month postoperative period before PSA testing to

From: *Cancer Diagnostics: Current and Future Trends*
Edited by: R. M. Nakamura, W. W. Grody, J. T. Wu, and R. B. Nagle © Humana Press Inc., Totowa, NJ

Table 1
Milestones for PAP and PSA

1936	PAP discovered
1970s	Immunoassay for PAP
1972	γ-Seminoprotein (γSP) identified as forensic marker for semen
1976	p30 Identified as forensic marker for semen
1978	PSA discovered as potential PCa marker
1981	First immunoassay for PSA
1986	FDA approval of PSA to monitor PCa relapse
1990	γSP, p30, and PSA reported as identical 30K protein
1990	PSA forms (free/complex) discovered in blood
1994	FDA approval of PSA for early detection of PCa
1995	FDA approval of complex PSA (cPSA) for monitoring
1998	FDA approval of FPSA for use with total PSA to increase specificity for PCa detection
2000	Identification of molecular forms of FPSA in serum, BPSA, proPSA

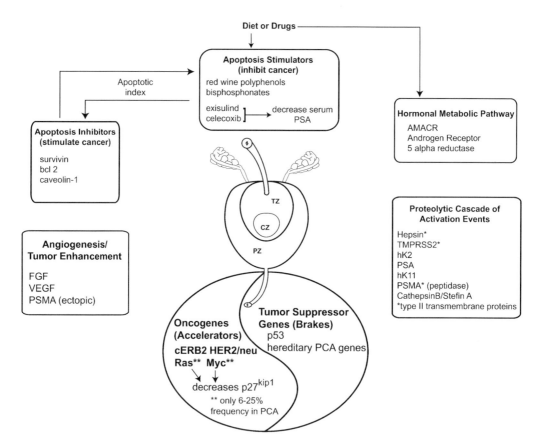

Fig. 1. Current and potential markers for PCa with a biological basis for their use. Selected current and potential future PCa markers are categorized into indicated groups on the basis of biological activity. A cancer marker, which is linked to a biological process, may have more potential for utility. For details and references *see* Table 2.

Table 2
Classification of Future and Current PCa Markers by Biological Activity

Biological function/effect	Example markers	Ref.
Apoptosis inhibitors	survivin	*(230,284)*
	bcl-2	*(284)*
	caveolin-1	*(146)*
Apoptosis stimulators (chemoprevention)	red wine polyphenols	*(285)*
	Bisphosphonates	*(286)*
	Exisulind	*(287)*
	Celecoxib	*(288)*
Factors involved in hormonal or metabolic pathways	α-methylacyl-CoA racemase (AMACR)	*(72)*
	androgen receptor	*(289,290)*
	5-α reductases	*(291)*
Angiogenesis/tumor enhancement	fibroblast growth factor (FGF)	*(269,270)*
	vascular endothelial growth factor (VEGF)	*(119,268,269)*
	prostate-specific membrane antigen (PSMA) (ectopic expression)	*(77,205,292)*
Factors involved in proteolytic cascade of activation events	Hepsin	*(91,124)*
	transmembrane protease receptor speract/scavenger family 2 (TMPRSS2)	*(293)*
	human kallikrein 2 (hK2)	*(40,197,198)*
	Prostate-specific Antigen (PSA)	*(29,40,53)*
	human kallikrein 11 (hK11)	*(294)*
	PSMA *(77,205,292)* cathepsin B/ stefin A	*(295)*
Tumor suppressor genes/proteins	p53	*(266,267,296)*
Oncogenes/ oncoproteins	c-erbB-2 (equivalent to HER-2/neu)	*(212,215,216,218)*
	ras	*(297)*
	myc	*(297)*

allow clearance of residual preoperative PSA *(7)*. With the advent of the ultrasound-guided sextant biopsy as an outpatient procedure in the late 1980s, the paradigm to use PSA for biopsy decisions began to emerge *(8–10)*. Clinical studies of PSA in the early 1990s led to the first tumor marker approved by the US FDA for early cancer detection. One of the most compelling facts leading to the use of PSA in conjunction with digital rectal exam (DRE) for early detection of PCa was the superior predictive value of PSA over DRE *(11–14)*.

The relatively high positive predictive value of approx 25% for men with PSA greater than 4.0 ng/mL has led to an unprecedented number of PCas detected in the last 10 yr. This has resulted in a significant migration to lower clinical stage at diagnosis and has significantly reduced the number of patients presenting with PSA concentrations higher than 10 ng/mL. Recent studies have indicated that the cancer mortality for PCa is decreasing slightly *(15–19)*. The combination of PSA testing with sextant biopsy has revolutionized the detection of PCa *(20–22)*. Monitoring PCa patients with PSA following treatment has become the gold standard to detect cancer relapse.

The rise in the use of PSA has essentially eclipsed the use of PAP. Is there still a clinical role for PAP? Some studies have indicated that PAP may be a more accurate indicator of micrometastatic disease than PSA and should be used for monitoring patients after radiation treatment *(23)*. A study at Walter Reed Medical center showed that PAP testing significantly added prognostic information and was an independent predictor of recurrence *(24)*. The use of neural net analysis or other algorithm approaches may benefit from the inclusion of PAP. Nevertheless PAP has been completely surpassed by PSA and is infrequently used *(25)*. PAP has the potential to regain importance in PCa as a therapy target. Recent studies have identified T-cell epitopes from PAP leading to its potential use for directing immunotherapy in advanced PCa *(26–28)*.

Although PSA has been in routine use for well over 10 yr and the analyte has completed a standardization process *(29)* differences between PSA assays from different manufacturers still exist *(30)*. Furthermore, the issues of standardization will only get more complicated as multiple markers come into use. For instance, if a certain cutpoint is recommended for %FPSA with two assays from one manufacturer, will this cutpoint still be valid if a different manufacturer's PSA assay is used in the denominator? This depends on how close the two PSA assays correlate. These types of standardization and correlation issues will become more important as more markers are used and become available from a variety of manufacturers.

1.2. Current Unmet Clinical Need

What are the unmet diagnostic needs and current dilemmas of the frequent and multiple uses of PSA? Although valuable nomograms to predict organ-confined disease using PSA have been developed, *(31)* PSA is not related to tumor volume nor does it accurately predict aggressive PCa in the "diagnostic gray zone" from 4–10 ng/mL *(32–34)*. Currently, no blood test can definitively tell how aggressively a man, who has been diagnosed with apparently localized PCa should be treated *(35)*. It is well known that most PCa patients will die with the disease and not from it *(36)*. The potential for over treatment exists along with the possibility of dying from the cancer in the absence of proper treatment *(36)*.

A blood test is needed to significantly aid in the management of localized PCa. The detection of cancer cells in blood is being examined to detect micrometastatic disease. Reverse transcriptase polymerase chain reaction (RT-PCR) of PSA for the detection of cells expressing PSA mRNA in blood of PCa patients has been demonstrated in a number of studies. However, most studies, including a large consortium study, have concluded that the method does not provide significant information for clinical staging and can not be used for therapy decisions *(37–39)*. The current failure of the test for staging may be the lack of discrimination between normal prostate cells and cancer cells. Both cells will express mRNA for PSA and be detected, leading to confusing results. In addition, the test does not discriminate between different types of prostate cancer cells, such as cells with high vs low metastatic potential. Quantitative RT-PCR may enhance this technique; knowing the number of circulating PSA containing cells may be crucial. In men with low PSA concentrations, for example, below 2 ng/mL, the test works well in screening populations to indicate which men will have a low probability of prostate cancer. However, marker(s) to increase cancer specificity in the 2–10 ng/mL range are needed *(40–42)*. Using the standard 4.0 ng/mL "cut-off," the goal of the primary value PSA is to spare biopsies for the majority of men with lower cancer risk. For every 100 men going into the clinic for PCa screening about 80–85 men will have PSA values lower than 4.0 ng/mL and are not routinely biopsied. Nevertheless, the 15–20 remaining men with PSA greater than 4 ng/mL are candidates for biopsy even though greater than 60% of these men do not have clinical prostate cancer. This results in a large number of biopsies and many millions of dollars in medical expense. Various methods to enhance PSA specificity are currently in use including factoring the size of the prostate gland (PSA density), rate of increase of PSA with time (PSA velocity), and age specific cutoffs for PSA *(35,40–43)*.

Perhaps the most practical and frequent method to increase cancer specificity is to measure uncomplexed or free PSA (FPSA) and use the free to total PSA ratio *(40,43–46)*. FPSA in serum is higher in benign prostatic hyperplasia (BPH), resulting from the higher concentrations of inactive PSA in the BPH tissues *(47)*. FPSA has been shown to reduce 20% of unnecessary biopsies *(45)*, only missing 5% of the cancers (they tend to be the less aggressive cancers).

However, the clinical diagnostic challenge of detecting PCa in men with moderately elevated PSA concentrations may be growing. PSA may have created its own clinical dilemma. For more than 10 yr, millions of men have been screened with PSA. In 2001 about 16–25 million PSA tests were done in the United States *(48,49)*. A significant portion of these men will have PSA in the 4–10 ng/mL range. Some of these men will be biopsy positive for cancer, but the majority will be biopsy negative. The biopsy-negative men will likely continue to have a PSA greater than 4 unless benign prostatic hyperplasia (BPH) therapy is undertaken and reduces the PSA. This group with elevated PSA will be screened again for PCa. Even if no cancer develops in the interim period, their PSA will likely remain high owing to the chronic benign prostate condition that led to the original elevation. As this pool of men with suspicious PSA concentrations resulting from benign disease increases, repeat biopsies become a serious challenge to the patient and the physician. Total PSA is not helpful in this situation. FPSA is useful for a minor portion of the patients but when to do a repeat biopsy has not been clearly established. No satisfactory marker is available to select the appropriate patients for biopsy in men who have PSA 4–10 ng/mL, a previous negative biopsy and a %FPSA of 10–25%. New markers could be helpful for this ever-growing patient group.

Although the combination of PSA and biopsy is a practical method to detect early PCa in men with PSA greater than 4.0 ng/mL, a significant number of men missed by this procedure are becoming more evident. The initial normal range limit of 4.0 for PSA was determined in 1986 in a small population of 472 men without a history of prostate disease *(50)*. Later studies containing larger and more clinically relevant populations to define the optimum "cutoff" value combining both sensitivity and specificity for cancer detection fluctuated between 2.8 and 4.0 *(11,13,51)*. The screening study of 6630 men aged 50–74 led to FDA approval of PSA for early detection and assessed the efficacy of the 4.0 cutoff and derived an upper limit of 3.9 in the 50–54 age group *(52)*. Consequently >4.0 ng/mL has been used most frequently for recommending biopsy.

Recently a number of studies have focused on the 2.5–4.0 ng/mL range resulting in a growing consensus that as many as 40% of PCa patients have PSA below 4.0 *(53)*. FPSA can help select some of these patients but the majority will be undetected unless biopsy of this group of men is completed *(53)*. The problem is that more men with benign prostate disease without clinical PCa are in the 2–4 ng/mL PSA range. More specific and sensitive markers are needed to justify routine biopsy of men in this lower PSA range.

Although PSA is the gold standard for detection of PCa relapse after therapy and before clinical symptoms develop, there remains uncertainty regarding the concentration of PSA that should be used to initiate further treatments *(16,54,55)*. The availability of ultrasensitive methods that detect less than 0.05 ng/mL PSA can lead to anguish for the patient whereas appropriate secondary treatment protocols are often given only after the PSA reaches concentrations higher than 0.1 ng/mL *(55)*. Markers, which provide information about the velocity of the clinical relapse, would augment the current test.

PSA is not a tumor-specific marker, which limits its usefulness for PCa detection. However, PSA does accurately reflect the integrity of the prostate and this key property may expand the clinical applications. More evidence is accumulating that 5-α-reductase inhibitor drugs like finasteride (Proscar) diminish symptoms for some BPH patients by decreasing the size of the prostate *(56,57)*. Patients with PSA values greater than 1.8 are more likely to respond to Proscar and decreases in PSA with duration of treatment may be a positive indicator of drug efficacy*(56–58)*.

Proscar treatment may also complicate PSA testing for PCa. PSA levels in serum drop approx 50% with continued Proscar treatment *(59)*. A correction method has been used that multiplies the observed PSA value by 2. Although a group of men will show a 50% mean reduction of serum PSA, there is significant variation from individual to individual *(60)*. In contrast, the free to total PSA ratio does not change significantly with Proscar treatment and may provide a superior method to detect cancer in men treated with Proscar *(61)*. The recent report from the Prostate Cancer Prevention trial with a study cohort of almost 19,000 men has demonstrated that Proscar prevents or delays prostate cancer *(62)*. This striking result has enormous ramifications and will likely lead to millions of men taking Proscar or related drugs in the near future. The current diagnostic algorithm using PSA for PCa detection will need to be reexamined and alternative diagnostic algorithms may be needed.

A growing number of drugs require specific laboratory tests to guide their use. For example, before a woman receives Herceptin therapy for breast cancer a test must be run on the breast cancer tissue to determine if it contains significant expression of the human epidermal growth factor receptor (HER2); the protein product of the HER-2/neu oncogene. The therapeutic efficacy depends upon a significantly elevated concentration of the protein. A test specifically coupled to therapy is referred to as a theranostic. The theranostic use of PSA and of new markers for therapy selection and for monitoring treatment course is likely to increase in the future. Prostate markers, which may be predictive of "prostate health"(i.e., smaller volumes and architecturally intact prostates may be valuable to monitor chemopreventive trials and individual dietary regimens). The effect of several drugs and herbal treatments on serum PSA has already been documented (Table 3). Many epidemiological studies point to a significant positive association between saturated fat intake and PCa risk *(63–69)*. Conversely, certain trace minerals and antioxidants correlate with decreased incidence of PCa, indicating some cancers may have been chemoprevented or at least chemodelayed *(63–70)*. Several of the dietary antioxidants correlating with decreased PCa incidence including lycopene have been recently reported to decrease PSA concentration *(71)*. Markers that can be used to guide positive dietary effects on overall prostate health would be valuable to resolve the complex and often confusing results from the many studies

Table 3
Drugs, Herbal Treatments, and Dietary Factors
That May Effect Serum PSA Concentration

Drug or herbal treatment	Dosage	Use	Effect on serum PSA concentration	Ref. (s)
Lycopene		chemo-prevention?	decreases approx 20%	*(71)*
PC-SPES		treat PCA	decreases 50% or greater	*(68)*
Finasteride (Propecia)	1 mg/d	decrease baldness, chemo-prevention?	decreases by approx 50%	*(298)*
Finasteride (Proscar)	5 mg/d	treat BPH	decreases by approx 50%	*(299)*
Dutasteride	0.5 mg/d	treat BPH, chemo-prevention?	decreases by approx 50%	*(291)*
Saw palmetto		treat BPH	no effect	*(67)*
cernitin, saw palmetto, B-sitosterol and vitamin E		treat BPH	no effect	*(300)*
Exisulind		treat PCA PSA progression after Radical prostatectomy	inhibited the rise of PSA	*(287)*
Docetaxel		treat hormone refractory PCA	significant decrease in PSA	*(301)*

to date. Biomarkers which signal fatty acid metabolic pathway activities may also be useful in this regard (e.g., the recently reported overexpression of the α-methylacyl-CoA racemase (AMACR) gene in prostate tumors) *(72)*.

1.3. PCa Markers for Bone Metastases

An exciting and emerging research focus on the cellular and molecular mechanisms that lead to the specific targeting of PCa cells to bone with subsequent osteoblastic lesions may reveal an entirely new set of PCa markers *(73,74)*. For several years, bone specific alkaline phosphatase and other bone matrix derived components have been investigated as more specific markers than total alkaline phosphatase for assessment of PCa metastasis *(75)*. An intriguing hypothesis that PCa cells mimic osteoblast cells and acquire "bone-like" properties in order to effectively succeed in bone metastasis, has stimulated investigations of the ectopic expression of bone proteins in PCa cells *(75,76)*. PCa cells have now been reported to secrete several bone extracellular matrix proteins including osteopontin, osteocalcin, and bone sialoprotein *(75,76)*. Future methodologies that allow the specific and practical capture of prostate cells in blood or urine may provide the targets for selective probes of bone-associated proteins to estimate metastatic potential and provide valuable clinical staging information.

1.4. Special Properties of PAP and PSA That Have Contributed to Their Prevalent Clinical Diagnostic Use

Both PAP and PSA are secretory proteins produced by the prostate. The level of PAP is more than 200-fold higher in prostate than other tissues *(41)*. PSA is highly localized to the prostate and is expressed more than 1 million-fold higher in prostate tissue and seminal plasma *(40,41)* than in blood. Two key shared properties are the secretory nature and prostate tissue localization. Secretory proteins are more likely to leak into the blood in a relatively intact form than cytosolic or membrane bound proteins. Prostate-specific membrane antigen (PSMA), which is highly enriched in prostate and up regulated in hormonally resistant PCa, is a good target for antibody-labeled imaging (ProstaScintR) and a potential target for antibody therapy *(77)*. PSMA has also been investigated as a serum marker, but studies have not revealed significant sensitivity or specificity for PCa *(78,79)* over and above that of PSA. One possible explanation is the transmembrane property of PSMA. Unless the extracellular portion of a transmembrane protein is released into blood, as is the case for Her-2/neu in breast cancer *(80)* and possibly CA125 in ovarian cancer *(81)*, these types of proteins are not consistently released into the blood in an easily measurable form. The tissue enrichment and localization of a protein appears to play a major role in the utility of some markers. The significantly greater clinical utility of PSA may result from its increased prostate specificity over PAP.

Today the role for PAP has all but disappeared. The abundance of PSA in the prostate and seminal plasma and its extreme compartmentalization away from the blood is an important property for clinical utility. Elevations of PSA usually signal a significant disturbance of the prostate. The prostate compartmentalization of PSA model can now be used to partially explain the relative increase of uncomplexed or FPSA in benign prostate disease compared with PCa *(82)*. A distinct enzymatically inactive PSA form, benign PSA (BPSA), is associated with nodular hyperplasia in the prostate transitional zone, which is characteristic of BPH. BPSA is released as one of the forms of FPSA in blood *(82,83)*.

A similar paradigm exists for troponin I which is compartmentalized to the heart muscle and appears in the blood if muscle damage occurs *(84–86)*. Unlike the troponin I model, perturbations of the prostate can occur by multiple mechanisms and diseases, including prostatitis *(87)*, chronic BPH, and even vigorous bicycle riding before blood draw *(88,89)*, as well as PCa. The multiple mechanisms leading to PSA elevations hinder its diagnostic accuracy.

1.5. The Search for New PCa Markers

The search for new markers with powerful tools like gene arrays and protein chips may identify candidate markers that are more specific to prostate tumors compared with normal prostate tissue *(90–105)*. It may be important to determine if the genomic and proteomic approaches would have identified either PAP or PSA. Both of these genes are not overexpressed in cancer, which probably rules out the gene array methodologies. In theory, the proteomics approach would identify both protein markers. However, proteomic testing of serum using two-dimensional (2D)-gel electrophoresis or mass spectrometry techniques like surface enhanced laser desorption/ionization (SELDI) will detect the abundant serum proteins before the detection of minor amounts of tumor proteins *(106)*. Tumor markers like

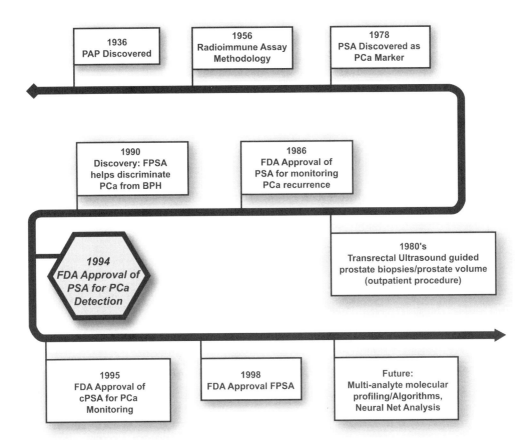

Fig. 2. Milestones in PCa testing. Some important events and dates in PCa testing are shown. As illustrated here it can take a long time for a marker to move from discovery and use in research labs to routine clinical practice. The adoption rate for markers that are completely new in methodology or concept can be expected to take longer to adopt to routine clinical practice than markers that are a variation on what is already accepted practice as is seen here for PSA and FPSA.

CA125, CEA, or PSA are usually present at picomolar concentrations, therefore the ability of a proteomic approach to detect these markers in the presence of the abundant serum proteins sets a limit on the usefulness of these approaches *(107)*. For a particular methodology the technical approach may fail to identify proteins derived from the tumor and detect instead host-response proteins (e.g., haptoglobin) that are elevated owing to the presence of the tumor *(108,109)*.

The discovery technologies available today may lead to significant improvements in PCa diagnostics. Some of the diagnostic gaps for PSA may close in the near future. Will new markers replace PSA as rapidly and completely as PSA replaced PAP? This is unlikely because of the millions of patients tested with PSA and the enormous clinical experience using this marker. The PSA database will probably continue to be used as a reference assay even if superior markers are discovered. If a methodology provides a superior result from previous methodologies, the adoption rate often takes years for a test to be incorporated into standard clinical laboratory testing (Fig. 2).

For instance, urologists began to use PSA to screen patients for PCa in clinical research studies long before the clinical trial data was obtained to gain FDA approval. The adoption rate of approx 15 yr for PSA use in PCA early detection is relatively rapid for a new marker. On the other hand, a related test like FPSA may have a faster adoption rate because the testing paradigm already exists. It is likely that new markers will be developed to complement and augment PSA to cover the significant unmet clinical needs, e.g., an accurate serum test to predict cancer aggressiveness. In addition, remember that the development and practical application of new markers is a formidable time-consuming and costly process. It should be expected that the immediate future will see improved use of PSA, as we are learning more about the relationship of serum PSA elevations and clinical parameters. Perhaps the nearest term advance will be specific assays of PSA forms in serum to get all the pieces, benign as well as malignant, of the PSA puzzle.

2. SPECIMEN SOURCES FOR PCA

Throughout the process of using markers to detect, stage, and monitor PCa, several different sources of specimens can be used. Serum and plasma are the most convenient specimens because they are easy to prepare and can be stored frozen for many years. Although storage is not important for clinical lab testing, it can be important when conducting research to determine if a test is useful. Stored clinical samples with good clinical histories are easier to use than creating a protocol where fresh samples from eligible patients are collected. PSA and FPSA are examples of markers detected primarily in serum or plasma. Serum is generally thought of as a better sample than plasma because it contains fewer proteins and is less likely to develop precipitates that will interfere in assays, especially upon freeze thaw. Nevertheless, plasma is being promoted over serum as a sample for many clinical tests because it can be prepared more quickly *(110)*. Additionally, some analytes may be more stable in plasma than serum.

Whole blood will be needed for most nucleic acid based tests. This may change how research is done on markers. Whole blood is not easily stored like serum or plasma so a test that requires whole blood must be tested in a prospective trial. This limits the ability of researchers to test a marker and later bring it into routine use in the clinic. The use of retrospective studies and archived samples makes it easier and less expensive to evaluate a marker in the research stage. In fact, our current selection of markers may be biased by this. As new tests are evaluated it will be important to take sample type into consideration and find new ways of circumventing the problems of using whole blood, cell-based assays, and labile analytes so useful clinical tests are not overlooked.

Whole blood is not routinely used for PCa testing. In the future, it may be used more frequently as new techniques, such as cell-based assays and nucleic acid testing (NAT) come into greater use. For example, MHC-tetramer detection of PCa T cell receptors and circulating cell-based PCa tests currently utilize whole blood. Epithelial cancer cells found in bone marrow, as well as cells isolated from whole blood have been used in an attempt to detect micrometastases in PCa *(111)*. Cell-based assays that detect markers on known circulating cancer cells in either blood or bone marrow could be useful in clinical decision making but so far these types of tests are not commonly used in PCa. Prostate biopsy cores and prostate tissue from prostates removed after radical prostatectomy can be examined by immunohistological or *in situ* hybridization methods. Portions of the tissue and cores may also be homogenized and the resulting proteins or nucleic acids extracted for assay by molecular methods.

Cancer specific groups of cells can be isolated by laser capture microdissection (LCM) and analyzed by a variety of molecular methods *(112,113)*. This is a powerful research application and greatly reduces the significant variability of cell types in dissected tumor tissue. The molecular testing of biopsy cores and tissue obtained after radical prostatectomy are not yet routinely used for clinical tests but research progress *(90,91,114)* indicates that significant tests for staging and therapeutic decisions are on the horizon.

Prostatic and seminal fluids can be obtained from the prostate and seminal vesicles respectively *(115)*. These fluids may be valuable sources of cancer related prostate-secreted proteins and even cancer cells. Cells, proteins, and nucleic acids from both glands are potentially valuable specimen sources for key clinical diagnostic information about the pathological state of these glands, especially with respect to the pathology and metastatic potential of PCa. Currently, no test has successfully utilized these fluids for PCa diagnostics although attempts are in progress *(116)*.

At first glance, urine appears to be the most accessible clinical specimen for urological cancers. Because it passes through the prostate on its way out of the body it might be expected to yield important diagnostic information about PCa. For example, Fluorescence *in situ* hybridization (FISH) of cells obtained from urine has recently been developed and marketed as a test for bladder cancer *(117)*. Unfortunately, several factors lead to the severe limitations for using urine as a valid specimen for PCa testing *(40)*. Analyte instability in stored urine, variability of shed cells from prostate, and the necessity to correct for volume change (creatinine index), as well as diurnal variation in analytes, contribute to the multiple challenges for urine analysis of tumor markers. Consequently, urine clinical assays for PCa are not in use. However, the shedding of PCa cells into the urinary tract does make this specimen potentially valuable if cells can be induced to be released from the prostate gland. It appears that molecular techniques on nucleic acids and/or proteins combined with cell-based assays may allow for more diagnostic utility from fluids associated with the prostate, including urine and proteomic techniques.

3. TYPES OF MARKERS

3.1. Nucleic Acids

3.1.1. Methods for Discovery

The search for nucleic acid disease-associated genes and markers fall into several approaches: linkage-association, subtractive hybridization/differential display libraries, RT-PCR, chip-based (microarray) gene expression profiling, and in vitro perturbation of gene expression. To a large extent, each of these methods has been enhanced through developments associated with the genome sequencing efforts, including single nucleotide polymorphisms (SNPs) (for linkage) and higher gene/coding sequence content for chips (microarray). In addition, the relative ease that a laboratory can now perform quantitative RT-PCR has helped both to validate gene expression data as well as provide a platform to perform the diagnostic and investigative analyses.

Some of the most detailed insights in the search for new markers have recently come from the use of DNA microarrays to analyze tumor tissue. When used in conjunction with laser capture microdissection, which can effectively isolate a relatively homogenous set of cancerous cells from the surrounding normal tissue, microarray analysis can elucidate a more discrete pattern of gene expression changes associated with PCa *(90)*.

Through these studies, a variety of genes are cataloged as either up regulated or down regulated in PCa. The total number of gene expression changes and their magnitudes are variable, and depend upon the stage and grade of the tumor, tumor tissue sample, sample heterogeneity, density of sequences on the chip, and even the assay itself. Given these differences, a twofold or greater change in expression either up or down, can be detected in anywhere from 5 to over 400 genes. Therefore, results from microarray experiments require extensive follow-up validation by more quantitative and standardized methods—usually either by RT-PCR or Northern blot.

3.1.2. Potential Nucleic Acid Markers for Use in PCa

Results from microarray analyses have detected a wide variety of prostate tumor and metastasis-associated genes. For instance, transcriptional up-regulation has been noted for *hepsin, pim-1, PSMA, c-myc, ras, fas* and *bcl-2,* whereas transcriptional down-regulation has been documented for *PTEN, CD44, Nkx3.1, p27,* GST family, *caveolin 1,* E-cadherin *(90,91,95,114,118–122).* Microarray expression validation efforts are both ongoing and time consuming, thus the following section highlights some of these genes and trends.

3.1.3. Hepsin

Hepsin has recently emerged as one of the most exciting up-regulated genes in PCa. The hepsin protein is a membrane-bound serine protease first identified by Leytus et al *(123).* The gene was cloned from a liver cDNA library *(124).* Microarray analyses have revealed that the expression of hepsin mRNA is barely detectable in normal prostate tissue, but increases between 30 and 40 fold in PCa tissue *(90,91,114).*

A similar dramatic increase is observed at the protein level, and initial immunohistochemical staining of tumor tissue sections localizes the protein to the transformed cells. Real-time quantitative PCR shows a strong overexpression in prostate cancer tissue that may be useful to assess PCa aggressiveness *(125).* The expression of hepsin by liver tissue *(123)* may pose problems for diagnostic use in plasma but the detection and localization of hepsin presents intriguing opportunities for both cancer detection and possibly therapeutics.

3.1.4. Melanoma Antigen Encoding Gene Family

The melanoma antigen encoding genes (MAGEs) are a collection of cell-surface antigens that expressed in a variety of tumors and tumor-types. Microarray and RT-PCR analyses have been performed using a set of nested primers that specifically amplify the MAGE–1, –2, –3/6, –4, and –12 genes from the MAGE-A family *(126).* Expression of these genes is absent from normal prostate and bone marrow samples. In contrast, a heterogeneous expression of MAGE genes was detected both in prostate tumor tissue and in bone marrow aspirates (containing metastatic prostate tumor cells). These data suggest that although there is no single consensus pattern of MAGE gene expression, the ability to detect MAGE gene products (and perhaps even a specific subset) in a biopsy might be highly predictive of cancer or metastasis.

3.1.5. Telomerase

Telomerase is a ribonucleoprotein complex responsible for the maintenance of the telomere length of chromosomes. The presence of active telomerase in normal adult cells and tissue is highly debated. It is present at low levels in some cells in the normal state, although in cancer and tumorigenesis, telomerase is up regulated and its activity associated with immortality of the transformed cells. Measurement of telomerase by enzyme activity utilizing the telomerase repeat amplification protocol (TRAP) assay or with RT-PCR for the RNA component of telomerase has yielded variable results, most likely resulting from the unstable nature of the RNA component of the molecule. Nevertheless, positive correlations exist between telomerase and detection of PCa *(127–129)*.

Further studies examining tumor samples by RT-PCR for mRNA of the catalytic subunit of telomerase (hTERT), have demonstrated better reliability and sensitivity, and a positive association between detection of hTERT mRNA and PCa has been noted *(130)*.

3.1.6. DD3 (PCA3)

The transcript for DD3 was first identified through differential display analysis of tumor vs normal prostate tissue. The expression of this gene is limited to the prostate and is normally expressed at low levels *(131)*. Northern blot analysis reveals that expression of this gene is dramatically increased in prostate tumor tissue compared with normal prostate tissue. DD3 with another prostate-specific gene overexpressed in PCa may represent a distinct class of prostate-specific genes that lack protein coding capacity *(132)*. Combination analysis of DD3 and hTERT expression by real time quantitative RT-PCR in tumor samples demonstrated an average of a 34-fold increase over normal tissue for DD3 and a sixfold increase for hTERT *(133)*. Although DD3 might prove to be a more sensitive marker to reveal the early stages of PCa (owing to its tissue specificity), the relationship between hTERT and tumor stage is significant *(133)*. In DD3 and hTERT, a practical PCa test will require available PCa cells captured from blood or induced by prostate massage into the urine. Saad et al. observed a high clinical specificity and moderate sensitivity for cancer detection utilizing nucleic acid sequence-based amplification (NASBA) for detection of the relative expression of the PSA and DD3 genes in shed cells in first morning voided urine following a vigorous DRE *(134)*. This study demonstrates the potential of molecular tests utilizing urine if the prostate can be manipulated to release cancer cells into the urinary tract.

3.1.7. Prostate-Specific Membrane Antigen (PSMA)

Markers to discriminate aggressive PCa from less aggressive cancers prior to therapy are an important unmet clinical need in the management of PCa. Many labs have attempted to detect circulating PCa cells in the blood of PCa patients by RT-PCR *(135–137)*. PSMA has been a mRNA target in addition to PSA and hK2. The use of these analytes to detect metastatic cancer or discriminate more aggressive PCas before radical prostatectomy has produced mediocre and conflicting results. It is not surprising that PSMA does not work well as an RT-PCR analyte since both prostatic and non-prostatic tissues express it. Nevertheless, the results with PSA and hK2 have not been more useful clinically *(137)* even though these analytes are more prostate specific. The data from studies using telomerase and/or DD3 (*see* Section 3.1.6.) are relatively compelling, and when combined with new markers entering the field (hepsin, EZH2, MAGE, for example), current attempts to develop real time quantitative RT-PCR assays may enable the formation of a clinically useful test. Nevertheless, at this time the use of RT-PCR assays to aid in detection, staging, or the aggressiveness of PCa is far from being incorporated into standard clinical practice.

3.1.8. Enhancer of Zeste Homolog 2 (EZH2)

In a recent report, Varambally et al. *(138)* described up-regulation of the EZH2 mRNA specifically associated with metastatic PCa. This mRNA product of a known regulatory gene was discovered through gene expression profiling among several genes up regulated in metastatic prostate tissue. When mRNA levels of EZH2 were decreased by transfecting cells with interfering RNA in vitro, cell proliferation was reduced. Conversely, when mRNA levels for gene were increased by transfection of the EZH2 gene into prostate cells, cell proliferation was enhanced. Thus, there is a link between the regulation of EZH2 mRNA and the tumor proliferative phenotype. Furthermore, EZH2 may represent a new marker for the progression of PCa *(138)*.

3.1.9. Hereditary Breast Cancer Genes BRCA1 and 2

Epidemiological studies show evidence of predisposition of PCa in men who have mutations in BRCA1 or 2 *(139)* but further studies indicate that BRCA genes or their protein products may only be peripherally involved in PCa *(140,141)*. There is a possibility that the link may be the result of a gene distal to BRCA1 *(142)*. Because of all the unknowns, it is unlikely that BRCA genes or their protein products will be used for PCa diagnosis and monitoring soon.

3.1.9.1. PROMOTER HYPERMETHYLATION

Microarray analyses have revealed decreased expression for CD44, E-cadherin, androgen and estrogen receptors, caveolin-1 and glutathione-*S*-transferase, among others in PCa tissue when compared with normal tissue. RT-PCR and immunohistochemical staining have confirmed these findings. Transcriptional silencing of genes is often accompanied by an increase in the methylation of the DNA in or near the 5' end of the gene (in the regulatory regions containing CpG islands). Experiments using methyl-sensitive restriction enzymes, genomic PCR amplification, and genome sequencing have demonstrated an increase in the methylation of promoter regions of these genes *(143–146)*. Although there is general agreement that methylation of these genes accompany the progression of PCa, the absolute level, heterogeneity, lack of tissue specificity, and occasionally inconsistent correlation between methylation status and expression *(147–149)*, decreases the potential of this methodology for use as a robust clinical test for PCa.

3.1.9.2. LINKAGE MAPPING AND POLYMORPHISMS

A volume of data exists in which linkage studies have been performed to determine the probable location of PCa disease genes. PCa, like most other cancers, is a complex and multifactorial disease, thus the search for the specific genes related to PCa is difficult. Evidence exists for PCa susceptibility loci on chromosome 1-CAPB in 1p36, HPC1 in 1q25-q25, PCAP in 1q42-q43; chromosome 17-HPC2/ELAC2 in 17p11; chromosome 20-HPC20 in 20q13 and X chromosome-HPCX in Xq27-q28 *(150–156)*. The use of SNPs to saturate these loci is currently used and should accelerate the identification of the specific disease-related gene(s) contained within these large chromosomal regions.

Polymorphisms and mutations have been identified in several genes believed to be involved in pathways associated with the development of PCa, including the androgen and vitamin D receptors, ribonuclease L, 5-α-reductase II, and isoforms of cytochrome P *(105,157–160)*. The weak association data highlight the fact that none of these polymorphisms represent a highly penetrant allele for PCa susceptibility. The combined result of these analyses indicates that PCa involves several distinct loci with no single major gene accounting for a major proportion of susceptibility to the disease. Thus, the search for a detection or diagnostic marker may result in the use of a combination of involved genes.

Recently, a polymorphism has been found in the *hK2* gene that correlates with prostate cancer risk *(161)*. This polymorphism is even more interesting because elevated serum concentrations of hK2 have previously been shown to correlate with increased prostate cancer risk. A combination of the gene polymorphism data along with hK2 serum concentration data was able to segregate a group of patients with a approx 14-fold higher risk of having prostate cancer in the above study.

3.1.9.3. HPC1

Hereditary forms of prostate cancer account for approx 10% of clinical prostate cancers. The most intensive effort has been focused on chromosome 1, and it has been proposed to contain at least three subchromosomal regions (HPC1, PCAP, CAPB) harboring putative PCa susceptibility gene(s). Nevertheless, one susceptibility gene, ELAC2/HPC2 at chromosome 17, has been identified. Yet, it seems to have a questionable role in PCa predisposition *(151)*.

3.1.9.4. THE RNASE L GENE (2',5'-OLIGOISOADENYLATE-SYNTHETASE DEPENDENT)

The RNase L gene codes for an enzyme that destroys RNA and may induce apoptosis in a novel way. Variants in the RNase L gene are enriched in families with mutant HPC1 that include more than two affected members and may also be associated with younger age at disease onset. This suggests a possible modifying role in cancer predisposition. The impact that the RNase L sequence variants have on PCa burden at the population level seems small *(105,153)*. Although the association of RNase L variants with mutations in the HPC1 is a provocative finding, the number of patients with the mutations is too small to be clinically useful at this time. However, if the gene(s) within HPC1 are further defined, the association of these identified genes with RNase L may be stronger, leading to a role for RNase L and an identified HPC1 gene in PCa management.

In addition to HPC1(1q24-q25), PCa susceptibility loci reported so far include PCAP (1q42-q43), HPCX (Xq27-q28), CAPB (1p36), HPC20 (20q13), HPC2/ELAC2 (17p11), and 16q23. PCa aggressiveness loci have also been reported (5q31-q33, 7q32 and 19q12). Further complicating the process is the existence of polymorphisms in several genes associated with PCa including, AR, PSA, SRD5A2, VDR, and CYP isoforms. These polymorphisms are not thought to be highly penetrant alleles in families at high risk for PCa. It is clear that PCa etiology involves several genetic loci with no major gene accounting for a large proportion of susceptibility to the disease. At this time, it is too early to predict if these or any other genes may become important tests for predicting people who will get the disease as well as those likely to have disease with a worse prognosis.

3.2. Proteins

3.2.1. Kallikrein Biochemistry

PSA is a single-chain glycoprotein with a polypeptide backbone of approx 26 kDa consisting of 237 amino acid residues. The apparent mass of PSA is approx 33 kDa, as determined both by gel filtration and by sodium dodecylsulfate-polyacrylamide gel electrophoresis (SDS-PAGE). These techniques overestimate the true mass of glycoproteins owing to the presence of the carbohydrate moiety. The true mass of PSA as determined by mass spectrometry is approx 28.4 kDa. PSA is a serine protease with chymotrypsin-like hydrolytic activity toward the carboxy-terminal side of selective tyrosine and leucine residues *(162)*. The biological function of PSA is believed to be liquefaction of the seminal clot formed by semenogelin I and II, and fibronectin in freshly ejaculated semen *(163)*, which aids in sperm motility and may have a role in fertility. These and other biochemical properties of PSA have been extensively reviewed *(40,164)*.

3.2.2. Current PSA Assays and Cancer Detection

The measurement of serum PSA is widely used for the screening and early detection of PCa *(11,164–166)*. The first clinical investigations of serum PSA established that values above 4 ng/mL were significantly correlated with an increased risk of PCa. Later it was discovered that serum contained two distinct forms of PSA: one form that was covalently attached to the serum protease inhibitor α1-antichymotrypsin (complexed PSA), and a second form that was present as the free "noncomplexed" form (FPSA) *(167,168)*. The development of immunoassays to measure these two forms of serum PSA has improved the discrimination of PCa from benign disease, such as BPH. A higher ratio of FPSA correlates with a lower risk of PCa *(45,169)*. In addition to free and total assays, an assay for complexed PSA has been developed. Because complexed PSA is the counterpart to FPSA in serum, it is not surprising that its ratio with total PSA performs comparably with FPSA. Although various advantages of this assay may be a consideration for some laboratories, the most recent and comprehensive multi-site clinical study comparing complexed PSA to FPSA and total PSA concludes that cPSA detects PCa equivalently to total PSA, and less well than ratios of free or complexed PSA (cPSA) with total PSA *(170)*.

3.2.3. Molecular Forms of PSA That Improve Prostate Disease Discrimination

The primary shortcoming of PSA as a serum marker of PCa is that PSA is also released into the serum as a result of benign prostate diseases such as BPH and prostatitis. This deficiency is compounded by the fact that benign conditions are far more prevalent than cancer. Prostates become enlarged as a result of BPH and higher volume prostates are associated with elevated serum PSA. The finding of free and complexed forms of PSA, and the finding that a higher FPSA was more positively associated with benign disease was the first signal that an understanding of the molecular forms of FPSA might add value to PSA as a diagnostic tool. Only the free form of PSA appears to be a candidate for a more detailed molecular characterization. This is a result of the single PSA form and the relative homogeneity of PSA-ACT. Only enzymatically active PSA can form a complex with protease inhibitors such as ACT, and thus it is expected that this PSA is relatively homogeneous. Peter et al. confirmed this hypothesis by analyzing PSA that was chemically released from the PSA-ACT complex and found that there were no structural differences from seminal plasma PSA *(171)*. The only hypothesis involving the PSA-ACT itself as a cancer marker, refers to the potential for intrinsic ACT complex formation in cancer tissues *(172)*. There has been little experimental evidence, however, to support this hypothesis because almost all of the PSA in tissues is found in the free form *(83,173)*. This suggests that PSA-ACT is formed almost exclusively in the blood as native PSA released from the prostate reacts with serum protease inhibitors.

However, FPSA (enzymatically inactive PSA) can result from any number of processes. These include PSA containing internal peptide bond cleavages that are known to be present in seminal plasma PSA *(40)*. In addition, PSA is expressed as the zymogen or precursor that is enzymatically inactive. The third molecular form of FPSA is a mature, intact, nonclipped form of PSA that does not form a complex with ACT *(82)*.

Therefore, the term "molecular forms of PSA" has expanded beyond reference to free and complexed PSA only. In recent years, there have been significant advances in the molecular characterization of FPSA to understand the mechanisms leading to the elevation of serum FPSA with benign disease. These efforts are directed toward a better discrimination of benign from cancerous conditions *(82)*. Implicit in FPSA forms research is the hypothesis that PSA is expressed as a homogeneous, enzymatically active protein, but that the tissue environment associated with benign or cancerous conditions plays a role in rendering the PSA inactive, possibly as a result of the action of disease-specific proteases. Understanding the disease-associated nature of FPSA may lead to better serum markers to discriminate cancer from benign disease.

3.2.4. ProPSA for Cancer Detection

The first molecular form of FPSA characterized in serum is the zymogen, or precursor form of PSA. Paradoxically, this FPSA form was found to be associated with cancer and not benign disease *(174,175)*. This contradiction can be explained by the fact that FPSA is actually a mixture of these distinct forms and has a statistical association with benign disease. It is also important to note that the correlation with benign disease is not absolute. For instance, men with greater than 25% FPSA have a 92% probability of benign disease, but still have an 8% chance of cancer *(53)*. BPH and cancer are co-existing diseases and therefore cancer can occur in men with advanced BPH. The discovery that pPSA was present in serum was the first indication that FPSA might also be comprised of cancer-associated forms of PSA and that this could potentially explain cancer patients with high % FPSA. In fact, preliminary studies have shown that pPSA is significantly elevated in PCa patients with high % FPSA *(176)*.

Although the presence of proPSA in serum was initially controversial *(177,178)*, several studies have now confirmed the presence of pPSA forms in serum *(174,175,179–181)*. Overall pPSA represents about a third of the FPSA in cancer serum, although the pPSA itself is composed of three major pPSA subforms (Fig. 3). PSA is normally secreted from prostate luminal epithelial cells as pPSA, an inactive proenzyme containing a seven amino acid pro-leader peptide (APLILSR) attached to the N-terminus of the PSA protein *(182,183)*. Studies reported that pPSA was present in several truncated pPSA forms, containing from one to five amino acids in the pro-leader peptide instead of the usual seven amino acids *(174,175,179,180)*. Three research immunoassays have been recently developed to measure the pPSA forms with both seven and five amino acid pro-leader peptides ([–5, –7]pPSA), the pPSA with the four amino acid pro-peptide ([–4]pPSA, and the two amino acid pro-peptide ([–2]pPSA) *(176)*.

A rationale for the apparent enrichment of truncated pPSA forms is that more truncated forms of pPSA are more resistant to activation than the intact pPSA *(175)*. Thus, the truncated pPSA forms are more stable as pPSA forms, and not rapidly converted to mature PSA. Studies have shown that cumulatively, the pPSA formed as a percentage of FPSA, is superior to PSA, FPSA, or complexed PSA in predicting PCa, particularly in the range between 2.5 and 4 ng/mL where the standard PSA assays are largely ineffective *(176)*. Among the pPSA forms, [–2]pPSA appears to be the most cancer associated, and also correlated with aggressive cancer. A number of studies are underway to explore the diagnostic properties of the pPSA forms.

3.2.9. Benign PSA (BPSA) in Benign Prostate Disease

The first evidence that PSA in BPH contained more enzymatically inactive species was demonstrated by Chen et al. *(47)*. In this study of BPH tissues, the PSA mixture contained a higher level of internal peptide bond cleavages. A study of BPH tissue by Mikolajczyk et al. identified a distinct degraded form of PSA termed benign PSA (BPSA) because it was present at lower levels in cancer tissue from the same prostate *(83)*. BPSA is characterized by two internal peptide bond cleavages at residues Lys145 and Lys182. Studies with specific immunoassays for BPSA have shown that BPSA represents about a third of the FPSA in serum *(82)* (Fig. 3).

Serum BPSA alone would not be expected to provide specific discrimination of PCa from BPH, because PCa and BPH frequently coexist. The ratio of BPSA (more BPH associated) and pPSA (more cancer associated) has shown some significant promise in discriminating cancer from BPH *(176)*. Thus, it is not only the % FPSA but the relative proportion of the FPSA subforms that offers the most potential to improve cancer detection.

Studies are underway to evaluate BPSA as a biomarker for clinical BPH. In preliminary studies of men undergoing drug treatment for BPH, early changes in BPSA levels may signal eventual drug response (unpublished results). Thus, BPSA may have several potential applications in the study of cancer and BPH. One striking characteristic of BPSA is that it is secreted into seminal plasma, apparently as an indicator of BPH. In normal pooled seminal plasma of healthy men, BPSA is present on average at 5–8% of the total PSA, while in older men the BPSA can represent more than 30% of the total seminal plasma PSA *(82)*. This wide range of BPSA levels in the seminal plasma may represent corresponding levels of BPSA in the prostate. Therefore, BPSA in seminal plasma may represent a direct marker of biochemical changes in the prostate and provide a means to monitor some aspects of drug therapy.

3.2.5. In PSA the Third Component of FPSA in Serum

BPSA and pPSA forms make up a substantial percentage of FPSA in serum but there is a third form designated as intact nonnative PSA (inPSA) (*see* Fig. 3). This form of FPSA has been observed in seminal plasma where a significant amount of PSA is intact, mature PSA but has been altered to prevent complex formation with exogenous ACT *(184)*. Such forms have also been observed with the PSA expressed by LNCaP cells *(185)*. The definition of inPSA in this section is defined as FPSA that is not pPSA or BPSA. Prevailing evidence suggests that inPSA represents mostly intact, nonnative (and thus inactive) PSA, though the presence of some minor percentage of PSA forms with internal cleavages such as Lysine 145 alone can not be completely ruled out. It is likely that inPSA contains PSA with missing N-terminal amino acids, which are also inactive.

An alternate approach to measuring intact forms of PSA has also been reported by Nurmikko *(186)*. This assay detects intact PSA (PSA-I), which is defined as PSA that is not clipped at Lys145. PSA-I would include both inPSA and pPSA. The FPSA forms not measured by this assay would include PSA forms clipped at Lys145 such as BPSA. Although the assay of PSA-I has both overlapping and distinct features compared to specific BPSA and pPSA assays, a common theme is emerging for studies of molecular forms of FPSA to enhance the discrimination BPH from cancer. The exact role of inPSA as a member of the triad of PSA forms in FPSA (Fig. 3) has not been established. The relationship of inPSA with pPSA and BPSA in the discrimination of cancer from BPH is complex and awaits further experimental and statistical analysis.

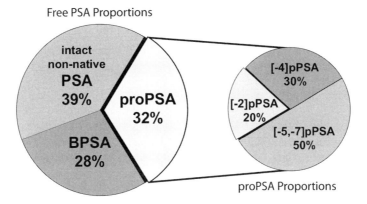

Fig. 3. FPSA is composed of three disease-associated forms of PSA. The pie chart shows typical mean proportions of these PSA forms in PCa serum containing 4–10 ng/mL total PSA. All FPSA forms are enzymatically inactive and do not complex with ACT. BPSA, "benign PSA," is associated with BPH. ProPSA (pPSA) indicates precursor forms of PSA, which are associated with PCa. pPSA is composed of native pPSA ([–7]pPSA) and truncated forms, [–5]pPSA, [–4]pPSA and [–2]pPSA. The [–2]pPSA form is most associated with cancer. The inPSA (intact, non-native PSA) in serum appears to correlate with cancer independently from pPSA. The measurement of these free forms of PSA significantly improves cancer detection over free, complexed, or total PSA, especially in the total PSA range below 4 ng/mL.

3.2.6. Human Kallikrein 2 (hK2)

Although PSA is the predominant tissue kallikrein in the prostate, a second tissue kallikrein called human kallikrein 2, hK2, has also been the subject of much investigation. PSA and hK2 share many properties, such as high amino acid sequence identity, prostate localization, androgen regulation, and gene expression but have other biochemical properties distinct from one another *(40)*. PSA and hK2 differ most in their enzymatic properties. HK2 displays the trypsin-like specificity common to most members of the tissue kallikrein family of proteases, while PSA is anomalous with chymotrypsin-like activity. HK2 is a much more active protease than PSA, with about 20,000 times more activity on its synthetic substrates than is PSA on its synthetic substrate.

HK2 appears to be more highly expressed by PCa cells than by normal prostate epithelium, as judged by immunostaining. In contrast to PSA, hK2 immunostaining increases with increasing Gleason grade, and hK2 has been proposed to be a potentially better candidate marker for cancer aggressiveness *(187)*. HK2 exhibits other potentially cancer-inducing properties such as the ability to activate single chain urokinase plasminogen activator (uPA), and to inactivate plasminogen activator inhibitor-1 (PAI-1), the major inhibitor of uPA *(188,189)*. Although the examination of PCa tissues showed that less than 1% of the PSA is complexed to inhibitors such as ACT, cancer tissues were found to contain about 10% of the hK2 as a novel complex with an intracellular serine protease inhibitor called protease inhibitor-6 *(190)*. Curiously, the major complex of hK2 in serum is with ACT even though ACT is an inhibitor of chymotrypsin-like proteases. However, preliminary data indicate the concentration of hK2-ACT in serum is at the most only 5–20% of the free hK2 *(191,192)*, almost the inverse of the typical PSA to PSA-ACT ratio. The minor protease-inhibitor complex formation of hK2 in serum may reflect a rapid inactivation of hK2 in tissue. Preliminary studies of hK2-ACT in serum have not revealed a diagnostic role for this complexed form of hK2. The tissue, hK2-PI-6 complex has not been detected at measurable levels in serum but appears to have several interesting properties in prostate tissues *(193)*.

3.2.7. Clinical Studies With hK2

Several immunoassays specific for hK2 have now been developed *(191,194–196)*. Concentrations of serum hK2 are typically less than 100 pg/mL and represent 1 to 2% of serum PSA concentration. However, the hK2 levels are not directly proportional to PSA and they do improve the discrimination of cancer in combination with total PSA and FPSA *(197,198)*. HK2 also appears to serve as a better marker for aggressiveness *(199)* and has been shown to correlate with extra-capsular extension of the cancer. It is in the area of aggressiveness, or correlation with stage, or grade of the cancer that hK2 appears to have the most distinctive diagnostic properties compared to PSA. It seems unlikely that hK2 will survive as a stand-alone diagnostic marker because it does not significantly improve cancer detection over % FPSA, the current standard for cancer detection. With PSA and other PSA forms combined with the appropriate mathematical algorithms, hK2 may find clinical utility in both the improved detection of cancer and the discrimination of more aggressive forms of cancer.

3.2.9.5. OTHER HUMAN KALLIKREINS AND CANCER

Until recently, only three members of the human kallikrein family had been identified: hK1, hK2, and hK3 (PSA). This was in contrast to the extensive kallikrein families in rats (approx 20 genes or pseudogenes) and mice (24 genes or pseudogenes) *(200)*. The next member of the human kallikrein family to be identified was prostase, hK4, though many other potential candidate kallikreins were under investigation *(201)*. All 15 kallikrein genes of the human KLK family are clustered in the gene locus 19q13.4. The most successful effort to discover and elucidate the many members of this family was mounted by the Diamandis laboratory, and these findings have been comprehensively reviewed by Yousef et al. *(202)*. Genes representing 15 members of the human kallikrein family have been identified and their protein transcripts have been at least partially characterized.

Within this family of 15 human kallikreins only hK2, hK3(PSA), and hK4 appear to be predominantly prostate localized, though hK10, hK12, hK13, and hK15 are significantly expressed in the prostate. Utilizing PCR amplification technology, almost all of these kallikreins can be found at some level of expression in several tissues throughout the body, including breast, ovary, testis, salivary gland, and pancreas. The tissue localization of these kallikreins and the diversity of function in multiple disease processes is an exciting field that is only beginning to emerge *(202)*.

PSA and hK2 have been studied fairly extensively *(40)* as the first kallikreins determined to be localized to the prostate, but hK4 has yet to receive significant attention as a serum marker. Biochemically, hK4 appears to be similar to hK2 and could potentially serve some of the putative functions ascribed to hK2, such as the activation of proPSA *(203)*. Specific and sensitive immunoassays for kallikreins hK4 to hK15 are currently being developed and it is too early to assess potential roles in PCa. However, each of these prostate localized kallikreins could offer both therapeutic as well as diagnostic value as our understanding of their role in the prostate increases. Even tissue kallikreins that are not exclusive to the prostate may turn out to have positive diagnostic value once their role in the prostate is identified.

3.2.8. Prostate-Specific Membrane Antigen

Prostate-specific membrane antigen (PSMA) is a type II membrane bound protein abundant in prostate tissue, but it is not prostate specific because it can also be found in kidney *(41)*, small intestine, and brain *(204)*. Antibodies to this protein have been used to make an FDA approved, in vivo, imaging agent (Prosta-ScintR) that is currently in use in the clinic *(205)* primarily for predicting durable complete response in postoperative patients. Nevertheless, PSMA has not attained wide spread in vitro clinical use probably because it is not sufficiently prostate specific. A novel protein-biochip immunoassay has been reported to detect significantly higher PSMA in men with PCa than men with BPH, but paradoxically the normal group of men over 50 yr of age had higher ng/mL concentrations of PSMA than the BPH men *(79)*. Interestingly this assay detects hundreds of ng/mL of PSMA in patient sera. Further studies to detect the prostate form of the protein, if it exists, are needed to evaluate its utility as a serum PCa marker.

PSMA is currently being used in a number of experimental gene and immunotherapy trials for PCa *(206,207)*. If these therapies are successful, theranostic (rather than diagnostic) tests for PSMA may become more prevalent as the therapy would be followed at the molecular level.

Interestingly PSMA has been found to be ectopically expressed on the neovasculature of renal cell *(208)*, breast and bladder *(209)* carcinoma. Neovasculature associated PSMA may be a target for the detection of angiogenesis.

3.2.9. HER-2/neu

As a result of the success of HER2/neu antibody (Herceptin) treatment for breast cancer, the association of this oncogene with PCa has been further explored *(210,211)*. Analysis of biopsies by HER-2/neu immunohistochemistry added additional prognostic information to traditional metrics during radiation therapy for PCa *(212)*. Although a clinical trial using an antibody against HER-2/neu has begun *(213)*, it is still unknown how useful this type of therapy will be for PCa nor is it yet known how to interpret HER2/neu marker data from immunohistochemistry, fluorescence, or colorimetric *in situ* hybridization (F/CISH) *(214–218)*.

3.2.10. Telomerase

Telomerase can be studied with both nucleic acid based as well as protein based tests primarily because the enzyme has a nucleic acid subunit. Most normal, noncancerous cells do not contain the ribonucleoenzyme telomerase but cancerous cells often do *(219)*. Therefore, telomerase is currently being examined for use as a cancer marker and a therapeutic target. The human telomerase enzyme requires a protein subunit: telomerase reverse transcriptase (hTRT), and an RNA subunit (hTR) for activity *(130)*. Therefore, assays to detect telomerase may be directed at the protein portion of the enzyme, the RNA portion of the enzyme, or both at once in the form of enzymatic activity assays because both properly folded RNA and protein are required for activity.

Multiple studies are underway to investigate telomerase as a therapeutic target for PCa *(219–222)*. Straub et al. attempted to use telomerase activity to aid in early planning of adjuvant therapy for PCa but found that telomerase was not more sensitive than conventional histology or PSA-RT-PCR *(223)*. Several groups are at the early stages of investigating the potential of telomerase as a marker for PCa. Ruijter and colleagues have looked at the cytological and histological changes of the enzyme with PCa *(224)* and Sakr et al. have looked at changes in telomerase between high grade prostatic intraepithelial neoplasia (HGPIN) and PCa *(225)*. Study of the HGPIN to PCa progression is important because it is well known that a finding of HGPIN upon biopsy confers increased risk of finding PCa in that patient in later prostate biopsies.

In general, many strong correlations exist between cancer and telomerase. However technical hurdles to develop robust telomerase assays have hindered rapid progress for definitive evaluations *(226)*. Conceptually, telomerase is an attractive candidate tumor marker but much work is yet to be done before the parameters for practical use are established.

3.2.11. Survivin

Survivin is a new tumor antigen identified on the basis of spontaneous cytotoxic T lymphocyte (CTL) responses in cancer patients *(227)*. Survivin has been shown to be an antiapoptosis protein and is overexpressed in most human cancers *(228)* so it has potential utility as a cancer marker. Survivin is a member of the inhibitor of apoptosis protein (IAP) family *(229)* and has homology in one baculovirus IAP repeat *(230)*. No other homologies were found between survivin and other known proteins, and survivin has little sequence homology to the other well-known anti-apoptosis protein bcl-2. Xing and colleagues have examined prostate tissue sections from patients who had under gone prostatectomy for treatment of PCa. Apoptosis could not be detected in neuroendocrine cells of the prostates but they found cells in both benign and malignant areas of the glands that overexpressed surviving *(231)*. Nevertheless, they were unable to find an association between survivin positivity and PCa progression.

3.2.12. Insulin-Like Growth Factors and Their Binding Proteins

Numerous growth factors may be involved in PCa (Table 4), but insulin-like growth factors (IGFs) and their receptors, or binding proteins (IGFBPs) have historically been studied for possible in vitro diagnostic utility and as therapeutic targets *(232)*. Measurement of serum or plasma IGFs and IGFBPs have been show to predict prostate cancer risk *(233,234)*. Recently it has been shown that IGFs and IGFBPs have limited utility as screening markers *(235)* for PCa. The cleavage of IGFBP3 by PSA has been reproduced in vitro, nevertheless the cleaved binding protein fragments that result could not be used successfully as markers *(236)*. Several labs are currently exploring the ways IGFs and their binding proteins can be used as markers for prostate cancer *(237–239)*. Recently, Latif et al. have examined the relationship between IGF-1, IGFBP-3, PSA, and C-reactive protein and have concluded that the modulations in IGF-1 and IGFBP-3 are owing to systemic inflammatory response not prostate cancer stage *(240)*. In summary, there is much research activity on the use of IGFs and IGFBPs as prostate cancer markers, but more research will need to be completed before the utility of these markers can be determined.

3.2.13. Matrix Metalloproteases and Their Tissue Inhibitors

Matrix metalloproteases (MMPs) and their tissue inhibitors (TIMPs) have been considered promising therapeutic targets for cancer for some time *(241)*. It was logical to attempt to use either of these proteins as diagnostic markers for prostate or other cancers. Indeed there is research evidence that these markers may be useful as immunohistochemical *(242)* or DNA probe tests on tumor tissue *(243)* or that TIMP-1 may find use in the future as a plasma test for PCa metastases *(244)*.

Table 4
Peptide Growth Factor Families

Name	Acronym	Relation to PCa	References
Transforming growth factor-β	TGF-β	mRNA decreased in PCa tissue	*(302)*
Fibroblast growth factors	FGFs	angiogenesis factors for PCa	*(269,270)*
Insulin-like growth factors	IGFs	may predict the risk of developing advanced- PCa Utility for screening patients with prostate limited	*(235)*
Neuropeptides: serotonin, somatostatin	not applicable	serotonin is expressed higher in benign and cancerous tissue than lymph node metastases Somatostatin receptor mRNA is up-regulated in PCa tissue when compared to BPH tissue	*(303,304)*

3.2.14. Urokinase-Type Plasminogen Activator and Plasminogen Activator Inhibitor Type-1

The association of urokinase-type plasminogen activator (uPA) with PCa metastases has been well studied and recently reviewed *(245)*. It appears that metastases are mediated by pericellular plasminogen activation. Biochemical studies have shown that prostate localized kallikrein proteases hK2 and hK4 can activate pro-uPA as well as inactivate (by complexing with it) PAI-1 *(189,203)* in vitro. The use of uPA and PAI-1 as markers is not as evolved. Plasminogen activator and its receptor were found to be more highly expressed in high grade PCa tumors *(246)* and the *uPA* gene is sometimes amplified in hormone refractory PCa *(247)*. Data from an immunoassay for both forms when combined with prostate volume indicated that increased serum concentrations were associated with overall survival *(248)*. Nevertheless, the methods need to be characterized before uPA and PAI-1 can be used successfully as markers to test for PCa metastases or prognosis.

3.2.15. Circulating Autoantibodies to PSA

Circulating antibodies to tumor antigens (autoantibodies) may be earlier and more sensitive markers for cancer detection than direct measurement of circulating cancer antigens themselves *(249)*. A small amount of tumor antigen can provoke an immune response, generating circulating antibodies that are at a higher concentration than the original antigen. However, a major obstacle to formulating immunoassays for the detection of autoantibodies to cancer antigens has been the putative low affinity and low titer of autoantibodies. For an assay to be successful there must be a clear demonstration of detection of the anti-tumor antigen specifically without nonspecific signal generated by other proteins in serum or plasma that might raise the background of the assay. For example, rheumatoid factor has a similar structure to human immunoglobin (Ig). Rheumatoid factor might substitute for antigen and give a signal in autoantibody assays without anti-tumor autoantibody being present. This type of interference would confound anti-tumor antigen immunoassays.

A few researchers have begun to generate assays for circulating antibodies to tumor antigens, but no immunoassays for these analytes has yet made it to routine clinical practice similar to established immunoassays for cancer associated antigens. However, the potential use of circulating cancer antigen antibodies is being explored and preliminary qualitative assays have been established. Experimental use of these type of assays has been explored in breast cancer and has recently been reviewed *(249)*. The autoantibodies may circulate free or bound to antigen. Although the use of circulating antibodies to breast cancer antigens is still controversial it appears to have potential in the area of screening.

Circulating antibodies to PSA have been assayed by two separate groups as a potential way of monitoring PCa immunotherapy with recombinant vaccinia virus expressing PSA. Sanda et al. made a qualitative Western blot assay for PSA antibodies by reacting patient sera with nitrocellulose that had been blotted with purified PSA. They measured the sera for response to both IgG and IgM. Interestingly, they found that most of the patients had anti-PSA antibodies before the immunotherapy had begun. Only one patient out of six had any change in anti-PSA antibody status over the course of the therapy *(250)*. Eder and colleagues have used an enzyme linked immunosorbent assay (ELISA) to measure presence of anti-PSA IgG and IgM in patients undergoing experimental therapy. Out of 33 patients, only one developed low concentrations of anti-PSA IgG *(251)*.

Although the early results for using anti-PSA antibody immunoassays do not appear overly successful, these publications do not include detail about the analytical characteristics of the assays. It is possible that the anti-PSA assays will be more successful once they are fully developed and demonstrate low nonspecific signal in the presence of common serum or plasma Ig-like molecules and can specifically and sensitively measure circulating human Ig molecules directed against PSA. If this type of assay can be constructed, as new therapies for PCa evolve, these assays may be used in different monitoring situations and find more use.

3.2.16. Polycomb Group Protein Enhancer of Zeste Homolog 2

Recently the gene encoding the EZH2 protein, a repressor of gene transcription, has been found to be up regulated in advanced prostate tumors *(138)*. Consequently, EZH2 may be a tissue marker for PCa aggressiveness. Modulation of EZH2 in PCa may cause subsequent changes in the regulation of many genes. Increased expression of EZH2 as measured by immunohistochemistry increased with tissue pathology type. It was lowest in benign prostate tissue, but expression increased in cancerous tissue and in metastatic tissue. Researchers showed that patients with clinically localized PCa that have higher expression of EZH2 also had a greater risk of recurrence of their cancer after prostatectomy.

3.2.17. Caveolin-1

The role of caveolin-1 in androgen-independent PCa, has recently been reviewed *(146)*. Caveolin-1 is a major structural protein in caveolae, which are membrane microdomains that have a role in signal transduction and membrane transport. Experiments in animals and cell lines indicate that the caveolin-1 gene is anti-apoptotic. Caveolin-1 expression progressively increases in primary cancer, metastatic cancer, and hormone resistant cancer (after androgen ablation therapy). The role of caveolin-1 in PCa is not straightforward because although the protein appears to be increased in more aggressive cancer, the promoter of the gene is more highly methylated in PCa tissue than in adjacent normal tissue *(147)*, which would be expected to decrease transcription of the gene in PCa. Caveolin-1 has been found in the serum of stage-D cancer patients *(252)*. Cumulative data indicate that the caveolin-1 gene and protein plays an important role in the progression of PCa. Caveolin-1 gene has also been found in serum, albeit in extreme disease circumstances, this protein and gene has potential to become an important PCa marker in the future.

3.2.18. Neuroendocrine Markers and PCa

Neuroendocrine cells exist in the normal prostate but not much is known about their function. It is thought that these cells are important in growth, differentiation, and homeostasis of normal prostate tissue. Some neuroendocrine differentiation is found in 30–100% of PCa and markedly neuroendocrine-like tumors are associated with poor prognosis *(253)*. Several neuroendocrine markers can currently be measured in the serum of PCa patients: neuron-specific enolase (NSE), chromogranins A and B, and pancreastatin (a breakdown product of chromogranin A). Increases in serum or tissue neuroendocrine markers generally correlate with androgen independent cancer or poor prognosis. Which neuroendocrine markers will be the most successful at predicting poor prognosis is yet to be determined.

3.3. Cellular Markers

3.3.1. T-Cell Markers

Now that the components of an effective immune response are better defined, this knowledge is used to design new therapies for PCa, involving the patient's immune system *(254)*. If the patient's dysfunctional immune system can be manipulated by therapeutic agents it may be possible to specifically redirect PCa cells with curative effect *(255)*. These new therapies for PCa will change how and what markers will be used during treatment of disease. For example, Eaton et al., in a recent clinical trial, immunized hormone refractory PCa patients with several allogenic PCa cell lines *(256)*. They monitored the therapy with PSA, intracellular cytokines, and specific humoral and cell-mediated assays. More than four different assays were needed to monitor this trial. One standard for PCa; PSA, one routinely used for immunotherapy: intracellular cytokines, and several assays derived specifically for this trial. Similarly, Heiser and colleagues treated patients with autologous dendritic cells transfected with PSA mRNA *(257)*. They analyzed the patients post therapy for production of PSA specific T cells, PSA, and circulating tumor cells. It is clear that as immunotherapy trials for PCa continue many assays will be needed to monitor them. It is too early to know if serum or plasma PSA is a useful marker for PCa immunotherapy. It is also too early to know which other assays will become most useful. What is known is that clinical trials for several types of novel PCa therapies have already begun to stimulate research into a myriad of methods and antigens to be explored for their efficacy in aiding clinical decision-making.

3.3.2. Major Histocompatability Complex Tetramers

Major histocompatability complex (MHC) tetramers are a relatively new reagent *(258)* (*see* Chapter 10) that can be used to enumerate T-cells specific for a particular peptide. Vonderheide et al. *(259)* have used MHC tetramers with a peptide found in telomerase reverse transcriptase to show increased numbers of specific T-cells after immunization of

PCa patients with autologous dendritic cells pulsed with the same telomerase peptide. As the numbers of immunotherapy trials increase, the use of MHC tetramers to follow these trials is expected to increase as well.

3.3.3. Circulating Tumor Cells

The detection and characterization of rare circulating tumor cells in blood has potential for PCa management. Moreno et al. have initiated studies to assess whether detection of circulating tumor cells will aid in PCa management *(111)*. They captured potential cancer cells with an antibody to an epithelial cell adhesion molecule and detected them with multi-parameter flow cytometry and CD45 (leukocyte marker to identify nonepithelial cells), and cytokeratin (epithelial cell marker) antibodies. They detected increased numbers of cells in men with localized PCa and in men with metastatic disease. Men with more slowly progressing disease had lower numbers of cells in their blood than men with rapidly progressing disease. They also observed that the number of circulating cancer cells fluctuated more than serum PSA during chemotherapy suggesting that measurement of circulating tumor cells may add value when monitoring for treatment response. Nevertheless, previous studies have not shown much additional information gained over conventional histology in examining either pelvic lymph nodes *(260)* or bone marrow *(261)* by cytokeratin immunohistochemistry. However, a recent study has shown that PSA RT-PCR of blood cells can help prognosticate hormone refractory prostate cancer and allow for separation of patients into groups for phase III clinical trials *(262)*. Eventually, cell-based assays may provide the greatest diagnostic utility because the cancer cell is directly measured and characterized as opposed to the "surrogate" serum markers currently used. Advances in technology to make this type of assay easier, practical, and robust will require significant resource and future studies.

3.3.4. Angiogenesis and Blood Vessel Growth

Angiogenesis or growth of new blood vessels around tumors is thought to be essential for their continued growth and eventual metastasis. Increased microvessel density was shown to be associated with PCa previously *(263)*. More recently, the protein endoglin (CD105) was found to be expressed on immature blood vessels and immunohistochemical studies indicated endoglin was prognostic for survival *(264)*. There are recent well-designed studies describing the relationship of the angiogenesis related proteins; p53, vascular endothelial growth factor (VEGF), thrombospondin 1 (TSP-1) *(265–270)*. TSP-1 is a p53-dependent inhibitor of tumor angiogenesis. VEGF mediates angiogenesis during tumor progression. These markers are associated with other markers in the angiogenesis process. Angiogenesis is critically important in tumor progression, thus any of these proteins may be important markers for PCa staging. Presently, most studies have examined the qualitative levels of microvessel density and associated markers by immunohistochemistry in PCa specimens obtained as paraffin embedded tissue after radical prostatectomy. They could be developed as prognostic indicators but they may need to be explored in other formats to become more useful to urologists making clinical decisions regarding therapy. For example, if these markers are found to be prognostic at the biopsy stage they might yield important information about outcomes before radical prostatectomy is performed. In the future, perhaps the technique of laser capture microdissection may allow these types of markers to be used in a more quantitative way, thus increasing their utility *(112,113)*. In addition to VEGF associated angiogenesis markers, the following markers have also been found to have significant associations with PCa at the immunohistochemical level: cyclooxygenase-2 *(271)*, MUC1 *(48)*, hyaluronic acid and hyaluronidase *(272)*, and endoglin (CD105) *(264)*.

Although angiogenic markers are not routinely used in the clinic at this time, a recent study reports how these markers could be used for therapeutic monitoring. Bok et al. have shown that an ELISA for urine VEGF can be predictive of survival for hormone refractory patients who were undergoing therapy with a growth factor antagonist *(269)*.

4. MULTIANALYTE TESTS

4.1. The Proteomics of PCA Markers

4.1.1. Proteomic Challenges

Proteomics is a large and growing multidisciplinary field *(273)*, and the search for PCa markers is representative of many of these applications. This section does not review the many proteomic technologies because they have been extensively reviewed *(274)*, but rather describes some approaches, findings, and future challenges as they apply to PCa.

As with genomic approaches, the search for PCa protein markers usually attempts to identify new proteins or proteins that increase or decrease in men with cancer. In the latter case, findings from genomic and proteomic technologies are not necessarily correlated. For instance, the mRNA expression of hK2 can range from 10–50% of PSA *(275)* while the actual levels of hK2 protein in prostate tissues, seminal plasma, and serum are typically only 1–2% of the PSA levels *(40)*. Thus, whereas hK2 mRNA may be expressed at significant levels, the protein may be less abundant because it is degraded rapidly. Aside from expression levels, proteins are affected by posttranslational modification, turnover rates, solubility, membrane association, and other factors such as complex formation. Gene expression alone does not always provide the relevant information for the identification of suitable protein biomarkers.

The comparison between PSA and hK2 as protein cancer markers illustrates another important challenge for proteomics; protein concentration. PSA is present at mg/mL levels in the prostate, and must be detected at ng/mL in the serum to be clinically useful. Levels of hK2 are typically present at less than 0.1 ng/mL in the serum, which is already challenging for the well-established and sensitive immunoassay technologies. Ideally, any proteomic technology should be capable of detecting and quantifying proteins in the ng/mL range while in the presence of other proteins of at least 1000-fold higher concentrations *(106)*.

4.1.2. Separation, Enrichment, and Detection of Proteins

Investigational proteomics may be split into two categories: proteins in the tissue, and proteins in the blood. At the tissue level, these technologies are not unlike some aspects of the genomic technologies. One of the more useful techniques in discriminating tissue-specific genes and proteins is laser capture microdissection (LCM) *(112)*. The ability to isolate small numbers of cells based on their common morphology greatly enhances the specificity of subsequent findings. More material is needed for protein identification because no comparable amplification techniques are available for protein enhancement such as PCR for genes. Conceptually, the study of tissues may be better suited for the discovery and identification of new cancer-related proteins. Once identified in tissue studies, antibodies can be developed, and sensitive immunoassays or other technologies developed to measure potentially low levels of the protein in the blood.

In tissues and especially in blood there is a need to enrich for the proteins of interest. Given that blood contains more than 50 mg/mL protein, and cancer related analytes would likely be present at ng/mL to pg/mL levels, a means of enriching blood samples for tumor-derived proteins is essential. For many years, 2D electrophoresis has been the standard for separating blood components, and more recently combined with mass spectrometry to identify the proteins. A wide number of studies have been undertaken utilizing 2D gels to identify new PCa markers, with mixed results *(276)*. In order to identify new proteins present at less than approx 1 ug/mL in the blood it is still necessary to apply classical protein separation technology prior to loading on 2D gels.

Another recent approach has been the use of chemically modified protein chips, a derivative of gene array chip technology. In the case of protein chips, the matrix typically contains ionic, hydrophobic, or metal binding sites. Blood or serum is incubated with the matrix and, after washing, bound proteins are analyzed by matrix-assisted laser desorption-induced mass spectrometry (MALDI-MS). A chip technology termed surface-enhanced laser desorption/ionization (SELDI) (Ciphergen Biotechnologies, Palo Alto, CA), coupled with MALDI-MS has received some prominence by automating this approach. Only a minor subset of blood proteins are theoretically bound to any given chip chemistry, although the diagnostic efficacy of one type of chip over another must be tested empirically. Many studies continue in this area *(276)*, though the translation from the finding of a new MS peak to the identification of that peak as a novel cancer-associated protein or useful tumor marker has yet to be realized. An interesting second-generation approach to the SELDI technology is the use of antibodies to bind specific components from the serum. This approach was used successfully to measure PSMA in serum where standard immunoassay techniques had been unsuccessful *(79)*.

4.1.3. Protein Profiling

Genomic approaches are typically dependent on cells and their genomic components, whether from RT-PCR of circulating cells or from the study of neoplastic tissues directly. In these cases, the cellular genesis of the signal is clear. In proteomic approaches utilizing protein profiling the signal (protein or peptide) may not derive from neoplastic cells or tissue, and the proteins in theory do not even need to be identified. Protein profiling depends on specific patterns of proteins that increase or decrease in cancer serum compared to benign serum, and depends on sophisticated algorithms to interpret these patterns. Results from such controlled studies can be impressive, with sensitivity and specificity greater than 90% *(277)*.

It remains to be seen if protein-profiling approaches can survive the rigors of diagnostic screening demands if it turns out that none of the proteins that make up the profile are tissue or tumor-specific. In blood at least, the issue of protein concentration becomes an issue even with SELDI technology. It is probable that tumors as large as a cubic centimeter could not contribute more than ng/mL serum concentrations of any diagnostic protein *(107)*. Many interfering serum proteins are at concentrations more than 1000 times higher, thus technology may necessarily be selecting for response proteins to the tumor and not from the tumor itself *(106)*. In some cases the most highly correlated serum proteins with cancer have been acute phase or inflammatory proteins such as thioredoxin and haptoglobin. Protein profiling does have one unique advantage in that it relies on a pattern of several proteins, which should minimize the effects of aberrant induction of a single component. Utilizing protein profiling, the paradigm has clearly shifted from identifying unique tumor associated proteins, to identifying protein patterns resulting from any number of biochemical processes ancillary to the tumor. Once the proteins are identified, a multiplex assay format may provide clinical labs with a practical way to offer these tests. Many challenges remain.

4.2. Methodologies for Multiple Markers

Through the explosion of new potential markers discovered through genomics and proteomics, the use of multiple markers to increase specificity will become more common. A simple example of the use of multiple markers is the ratio of FPSA to PSA or % FPSA. The use of % FPSA is already frequently used in the clinic. When the assay result for FPSA is used along with the assay result for total PSA it allows urologists to eliminate 20% of unnecessary biopsies while only missing 5% of cancers, which also tend to be low stage and grade *(45)*. Percent FPSA is used as a simple ratio of the FPSA assay result divided by the total PSA assay result. More complicated, informatics type analysis methods have been proposed but none are used commonly in the clinic.

There are several problems in PCa treatment where multiple markers and clinical parameters are known to be individually predictive of outcome but if combined these parameters might be even more predictive. Several groups have explored two methods, multivariate logistic regression (MLR) and artificial neural networks (ANN), where data can be combined. For example, O'Dowd and colleagues constructed a multivariate logistic regression algorithm including patients' age, initial biopsy diagnosis, total PSA, and free/total PSA that could predict the likelihood of cancer on the repeated biopsy with an accuracy of 70% *(278)*. Others have used ANN to improve prediction of cancer on biopsy by 20–22% over % FPSA *(279)* or to improve the prediction over standard cutoffs *(280)*. Several studies have compared ANN and MLR and neither method appears to be better than the other in general *(281,282)*. Selection between ANN, logistic regression, or other techniques will depend upon what data is being input, what the actual data distributions look like and exactly what type of clinical questions need to be answered *(283)*.

5. SUMMARY

Currently, PSA and FPSA are the only PCa markers widely used in the clinic. These assays have established a paradigm for use of markers for PCa management. Novel kallikrein or PSA forms immunoassays may be the first new markers implemented if it can be shown that they add a significant amount of additional diagnostic information over and above that provided by PSA and FPSA.

New therapies for PCa will stimulate the development of assays for clinical assessments. The successful therapies will determine which assays are used for clinical research, diagnostic, or theranostic purposes.

New markers, specimen sources, and techniques will be realized as good clinical value is shown with ability for implementation. It is a long road from noting a correlation of a biomarker to a PCa clinical parameter, to perfecting a technique, and elucidating a method robust enough for clinical or pathology labs to run the test to give urologists clear decision points.

It is our speculation that the world of PCa markers will expand from single analyte serum based immunoassays for PSA to a variety of molecular diagnostic techniques using multiple analytes of either proteins and/or nucleic acids, that utilize a variety of sample types including cells, tissues, and fluids. The data from the multiple analytes and samples will be combined with bioinformatic output to provide urologists with practical algorithmic results for spanning a variety of clinical decision points across the PCa treatment continuum from prevention through treatment of metastatic disease with experimental therapies.

ACKNOWLEDGMENTS

The authors wish to thank Susan Keenan and Sherrie Green for their expert technical and informational assistance in the preparation of this manuscript.

REFERENCES

1. Sproul EE. 1980. Acid phosphatase and prostate cancer: historical overview. Prostate 4:411–413.
2. Chu TM. 1990. Prostate cancer-associated markers. Immunology
3. Wang MC Valenzuela LA, Murphy GP, and Chu TM. 1979. Purification of a human prostate specific antigen. Invest. Urol. 17:159–163.
4. Ellis WJ, Vessella RL, Noteboom JL, Lange PH, Wolfert RL, Rittenhouse HG. 1997. Early detection of recurrent prostate cancer with an ultrasensitive chemiluminescent prostate-specific antigen assay. Urology 50(4):573–579.
5. Takayama TK, Vessella RL, Brawer MK, True LD, Noteboom J, Lange PH. 1994.Urinary prostate specific antigen levels after radical prostatectomy.J. Urol. 1:82–87.
6. Oesterling JE, Tekchandani AH, Martin SK. 1996. The periurethral glands do not significantly influence the serum prostate specific antigen concentration. J. Urol. 5:1658–1660.
7. Oh J, Colberg JW, Ornstein DK. 1999. Current followup strategies after radical prostatectomy: a survey of American Urological Association urologists. J. Urol. 2:520–523.
8. Dahnert WF, Hamper UM, Eggleston JC, Walsh PC, Sanders RC. 1986. Prostatic evaluation by transrectal sonography with histopathologic correlation: the echopenic appearance of early carcinoma. Radiology 1:97–102.
9. Shinohara K, Wheeler TM, Scardino PT. 1989. The appearance of prostate cancer on transrectal ultrasonography: correlation of imaging and pathological examinations. J. Urol. 1:76–82.
10. Hodge KK, McNeal JE, Terris MK, Stamey TA. 1989. Random systematic versus directed ultrasound guided transrectal core biopsies of the prostate. J. Urol. 1:71–74.
11. Catalona WJ, Smith DS, Ratliff TL, et al. 1991.Measurement of prostate-specific antigen in serum as a screening test for prostate cancer. N. Engl. J. Med. 324:1156–1161.
12. Prostate cancer vaccine–Northwest Biotherapeutics: CaPVax, DC1/HRPC, DCVax–Prostate. 2002. BioDrugs 3:226–227.
13. Colberg JW, Smith DS, Catalona WJ. 1993. Prevalence and pathological extent of prostate cancer in men with prostate specific antigen levels of 2.9 to 4.0 ng./mL. J. Urol. 3:507–509.
14. Catalona WJ, Richie JP, Ahmann FR, et al. 1994. Comparison of digital rectal examination and serum prostate specific antigen in the early detection of prostate cancer: results of a multicenter clinical trial of 6,630 men. J. Urol. 5:1283–1290.
15. Holmberg L, Bill-Axelson A, Helgesen F, et al. 2002. A randomized trial comparing radical prostatectomy with watchful waiting in early prostate cancer. N. Engl. J. Med. 347(11):781–789.
16. Soergel TM, Koch MO, Foster RS, et al. 2001.Accuracy of predicting long-term prostate specific antigen outcome based on early prostate specific antigen recurrence results after radical prostatectomy. J. Urol. 6:2198–2201.
17. Small EJ and Roach M III. 2002. Prostate-specific antigen in prostate cancer: a case study in the development of a tumor marker to monitor recurrence and assess response. Semin. Oncol. 3:264–273.
18. Partin AW, Pound CR, Clemens JQ, Epstein JI, Walsh PC. 1993. Serum PSA after anatomic radical prostatectomy. The Johns Hopkins experience after 10 years. Urol. Clin. North. Am. 4:713–725.

19. Walsh PC. 2002. Surgery and the reduction of mortality from prostate cancer. N. Engl. J. Med. 11:839–840.

20. Candas B, Cusan L, Gomez JL, et al. 2000. Evaluation of prostatic specific antigen and digital rectal examination as screening tests for prostate cancer. Prostate 45:19–35.

21. Grumet SC and Bruner DW. 2000. The identification and screening of men at high risk for developing prostate cancer. Urol. Nurs. 20:15–24.

22. Moul JW. 2000. Prostate specific antigen only progression of prostate cancer. J. Urol. 6:1632–1642.

23. Dattoli M, Wallner K, True L, et al. 1999. Prognostic role of serum prostatic acid phosphatase for 103Pd-based radiation for prostatic carcinoma. Int. J. Radiat. Oncol. Biol. Phys. 4:853–856.

24. Moul JW, Connelly RR, Perahia B, McLeod DG. 1998. The contemporary value of pretreatment prostatic acid phosphatase to predict pathological stage and recurrence in radical prostatectomy cases. J. Urol. 3:935–940.

25. Bunting PS. 1999. Is there still a role for prostatic acid phosphatase? CSCC Position Statement. Canadian Society of Clinical Chemists. Clin. Biochem. 8:591–594.

26. Inoue Y, Takaue Y, Takei M, et al. 2001. Induction of tumor specific cytotoxic T lymphocytes in prostate cancer using prostatic acid phosphatase derived HLA-A2402 binding peptide. J. Urol. 4:1508–1513.

27. McNeel DG, Nguyen LD, Disis ML. 2001. Identification of T helper epitopes from prostatic acid phosphatase. Cancer Res. 13:5161–5167.

28. Peshwa MV, Shi JD, Ruegg C, Laus R, van Schooten WC. 1998. Induction of prostate tumor-specific CD8+ cytotoxic T-lymphocytes in vitro using antigen-presenting cells pulsed with prostatic acid phosphatase peptide. 2:129–138.

29. Nakamura RM. 1998. Current status and future directions in standardization of prostate-specific antigen immunoassay. Urology 51:83–88.

30. Semjonow A, Brandt B, Oberpenning F, Hertle L. 1995. Different determination methods make interpretation of prostate-specific antigen more difficult. Urologe A 4:303–315.

31. Partin AW, Mangold LA, Lamm DM, Walsh PC, Epstein JI, Pearson JD. 2001. Contemporary update of prostate cancer staging nomograms (Partin Tables) for the new millennium. Urology 6:843–848.

32. Stamey TA, Johnstone IM, McNeal JE, Lu AY, Yemoto CM. 2002. Preoperative serum prostate specific antigen levels between 2 and 22 ng./mL. correlate poorly with post-radical prostatectomy cancer morphology: prostate specific antigen cure rates appear constant between 2 and 9 ng./mL. J. Urol. 1:103–111.

33. Moul JW, Connelly RR, Lubeck DP, et al. 2001. Predicting risk of prostate specific antigen recurrence after radical prostatectomy with the Center for Prostate Disease Research and Cancer of the Prostate Strategic Urologic Research Endeavor databases. J. Urol. 4:1322–1327.

34. D'Amico A, Moul JW, Kattan MW. 1999. Emerging prognostic factors for outcome prediction in clinically localized prostate cancer: prostate-specific antigen level, race, molecular markers, and neural networks, in: Comprehensive Textbook of Genitourinary Oncology,Vogelzang N, Scardino P, Shipley W, Coffey D, and Miles BJ, eds., Lippincott Williams and Wilkins: Philadelphia, pp. 680–700.

35. Stephan C, Jung K, Diamandis EP, Rittenhouse HG, Lein M, Loening SA. 2002. Prostate-specific antigen, its molecular forms, and other kallikrein markers for detection of prostate cancer. Urology 1:2–8.

36. Chodak GW, Thisted RA, Gerber GS, et al. 1994. Results of conservative management of clinically localized prostate cancer. N. Engl. J. Med. 4:242–248.

37. Ellis WJ, Vessella RL, Corey E, et al. 1998. The value of a reverse transcriptase polymerase chain reaction assay in preoperative staging and followup of patients with prostate cancer. J. Urol. 4:1134–1138.

38. Pelkey TJ, Frierson HF Jr, Bruns DE. 1996. Molecular and immunological detection of circulating tumor cells and micrometastases from solid tumors. Clin. Chem. 9:1369–1381.

39. Vessella RL, Lange PH, Blumenstein BA, et al. 1998. Multicenter RT-PCR-PSA clinical trial for pre-operative staging of prostate cancer. J. Urol. 159:292.

40. Rittenhouse HG, Finlay JA, Mikolajczyk SD, Partin AW. 1998. Human kallikrein 2 (hK2) and prostate-specific antigen (PSA): Two closely related, but distinct, kallikreins in the prostate. Crit. Rev. Clin. Lab. Sci. 35:275–368.

41. Haese A, Becker C, Diamandis EP, Lilja H. 2002. Adenocarcinoma of the prostate, in: Tumor Markers Physiology, Pathobiology, Technology and Clinical Applications, Diamandis EP, Fritsche HA, Lilja H, Chan DW, and Schartz M eds., AACC Press: Washington DC, pp. 193–237.

42. Stenman UH, Leinonen J, Zhang WM, Finne P. 1999. Prostate-specific antigen. Semin. Cancer Biol. 2:83–93.

43. Catalona WJ, Southwick PC, Slawin KM, et al. 2000. Comparison of percent free PSA, PSA density, and age-specific PSA cutoffs for prostate cancer detection and staging. Urology 56: 255–60.

44. Catalona WJ, Smith DS, Wolfert RL, et al. 1995. Evaluation of percentage of free serum prostate-specific antigen to improve specificity of prostate cancer screening. JAMA 15:1214–1220.

45. Catalona WJ, Partin AW, Slawin KM, et al. 1998. Use of the percentage of free prostate-specific antigen to enhance differentiation of prostate cancer from benign prostatic disease: a prospective multicenter clinical trial. JAMA 19:1542–1547.

46. Kroll M. 2002. Prostate Cancer Free PSA Adds Value to PSA Testing. Clin. Lab. News Apr:10–11.

47. Chen Z, Chen H, Stamey TA. 1997. Prostate specific antigen in benign prostatic hyperplasia: purification and characterization. J. Urol. 157:2166–2170.

48. Papadopoulos I, Sivridis E, Giatromanolaki A, Koukourakis MI. 2001. Tumor angiogenesis is associated with MUC1 overexpression and loss of prostate-specific antigen expression in prostate cancer. Clin. Cancer Res. 6:1533–1538.

49. The Gail Group. 2001. Endocare Expands Agreement to Distribute 15-minute PSA Test to Urologists. *Cancer Weekly* 38.

50. Myrtle JF, Klimley PG, Ivor LP, Bruni JF. 1987. Clinical utility of prostate specific antigen (PSA) in the management of prostate cancer. Adv. Cancer Diag.

51. Dalkin BL, Ahmann FR, Kopp JB. 1993. Prostate specific antigen levels in men older than 50 years without clinical evidence of prostatic carcinoma. J. Urol. 6:1837–1839.

52. Catalona WJ, Smith DS, Ornstein DK. 1997. Prostate cancer detection in men with serum PSA concentrations of 2.6 to 4.0 ng/mL and benign prostate examination. Enhancement of specificity with free PSA measurements. JAMA 18:1452–1455.

53. Catalona WJ, Partin AW, Finlay JA, et al. 1999. Percentage of Free Prostate-Specific Antigen to Identify Men with High Risk for Prostate Cancer When PSA Levels are 2.51–4 ng/mL and Digital Rectal Examination is Not Suspicious for Prostate Cancer: an Alternative Model. Urology 54:220–224.

54. Amling CL, Bergstralh EJ, Blute ML, Slezak JM, Zincke H. 2001. Defining prostate specific antigen progression after radical prostatectomy: what is the most appropriate cut point? J. Urol. 4:1146–1151.

55. Pound CR, Partin AW, Eisenberger MA, Chan DW, Pearson JD, Walsh PC. 1999. Natural history of progression after PSA elevation following radical prostatectomy. JAMA 17:1591–1597.

56. McConnell JD. 2002. Epidemiology, Etiology, Pathophysiology, and Diagnosis of Benign Prostatic Hyperplasia. Campbell's Urology. Philadelphia: W.B. Saunders Co., pp. 1429–1452.

57. Roehrborn CG, Boyle P, Gould AL, Waldstreicher J. 1999. Serum prostate-specific antigen as a predictor of prostate volume in men with benign prostatic hyperplasia. Urology 3:581–589.

58. Roehrborn CG, Oesterling JE, Olson PJ, Padley RJ. 1997. Serial prostate-specific antigen measurements in men with clinically benign prostatic hyperplasia during a 12-month placebo-controlled study with terazosin. HYCAT Investigator Group. Hytrin Community Assessment Trial. Urology 4:556–561.

59. Andriole GL, Guess HA, Epstein JI, et al. 1998. Treatment with finasteride preserves usefulness of prostate-specific antigen in the detection of prostate cancer: results of a randomized,

double-blind, placebo-controlled clinical trial. PLESS Study Group. Proscar Long-term Efficacy and Safety Study. Urol. 2:195–201.

60. Brawer MK, Lin DW, Williford WO, Jones K, Lepor H. 1999. Effect of finasteride and/or terazosin on serum PSA: results of VA Cooperative Study #359. Prostate 4:234–239.
61. Espana F, Martinez M, Royo M, et al. 2002. Changes in molecular forms of prostate-specific antigen during treatment with finasteride. BJU Int. 90:672–677.
62. Thompson IM, Goodman PJ, Tangen CM, et al. 2003. The influence of finasteride on the development of prostate cancer. N. Engl. J. Med. 3:215–224.
63. Fair WR, Fleshner NE, Heston W. 1997. Cancer of the prostate: a nutritional disease? Urology 6:840–848.
64. Thomson JO, Dzubak P, Hajduch M. 2002. Prostate cancer and the food supplement, PC-SPES. Minireview. Neoplasma 2:69–74.
65. Cohen LA. 2002. Nutrition and prostate cancer: a review. Ann. NY Acad. Sci. 963:148–155.
66. Marks LS, Hess DL, Dorey FJ, Luz MM, Cruz Santos PB, Tyler VE. 2001. Tissue effects of saw palmetto and finasteride: use of biopsy cores for *in situ* quantification of prostatic androgens. Urology 5:999–1005.
67. Marks LS and Tyler VE. 1999. Saw Palmetto Extract: Newest (and oldest) Treatment Alternative for Men with Symptomatic Benign Prostatic Hyperplasia. Urology 53:457–461.
68. Marks LS, DiPaola R, Nelson P, et al. 2002. PC-SPES: Herbak Formulation for Prostate Cancer. Urol. 60:369–377.
69. McGuire MS and Fair WR. 1997. Prostate Cancer and Diet: Investgations, Interventions, and Future Considerations. Mol. Urol. 1:3–9.
70. Willis M and Wians FJ. 2003. The role of nutrition in preventing prostate cancer: a review of the proposed mechanism of action of various dietary substances. Clin. Chim. Acta. 1–2:57–83.
71. Chen L, Stacewicz-Sapuntzakis M, Duncan C, et al. 2001. Oxidative DNA damage in prostate cancer patients consuming tomato sauce-based entrees as a whole-food intervention. J. Nat. Cancer Instit. 24:1872–1879.
72. Rubin MA, Zhou M, Dhanasekaran SM, et al. 2002. alpha-Methylacyl coenzyme A racemase as a tissue biomarker for prostate cancer. JAMA 13:1662–1670.
73. Corey E, Quinn JE, Bladou F, et al. 2002. Establishment and characterization of osseous prostate cancer models: intra-tibial injection of human prostate cancer cells. Prostate 1:20–33.
74. Lange PH and Vessella RL. 1998. Mechanisms, hypotheses and questions regarding prostate cancer micrometastases to bone. Cancer Metastasis Rev. 4:331–336.
75. Oremek GM, Kramer W, Seiffert UB, Jonas D. 1997. Diagnostic value of skeletal AP and PSA with respect to skeletal scintigram in patients with prostatic disease. Anticancer Res. 4B:3035–3036.
76. Brown JM, Corey E, Lee ZD, et. al. 2001. Osteoprotegerin and rank ligand expression in prostate cancer. Urology 4:611–616.
77. Elgamal AA, Holmes EH, Su SL, et. al. 2000. Prostate-specific membrane antigen (PSMA): current benefits and future value. Semin. Surg. Oncol. 18:10–16.
78. Sokoloff RL, Norton KC, Gasior CL, Marker KM, Grauer LS. 2000. A dual-monoclonal sandwich assay for prostate-specific membrane antigen: levels in tissues, seminal fluid and urine. Prostate 2:150–157.
79. Xiao Z, Adam BL, Cazares LH, et al. 2001. Quantitation of serum prostate-specific membrane antigen by a novel protein biochip immunoassay discriminates benign from malignant prostate disease. Cancer Res. 16:6029–6033.
80. Andersen TI, Paus E, Nesland JM, McKenzie SJ, Borresen AL. 1995. Detection of c-erbB-2 related protein in sera from breast cancer patients. Relationship to ERBB2 gene amplification and c-erbB-2 protein overexpression in tumour. Acta. Oncol. 4:499–504.
81. O'Brien TJ, Beard JB, Underwood LJ, Dennis RA, Santin AD, York L. 2001. The CA125 Gene: An Extracellular Superstructure Dominated by Repeat Sequences. Tumor Biol. 22:348–366.
82. Mikolajczyk SD, Marks LS, Partin AW, Rittenhouse HG. 2002. Free prostate-specific antigen in serum is becoming more complex. Urology 6:797–802.

83. Mikolajczyk SD, Millar LS, Wang TJ, et al. 2000. "BPSA," a specific molecular form of free prostate-specific antigen, is found predominantly in the transition zone of patients with nodular benign prostatic hyperplasia. Urology 1:41–45.

84. Apple FS. 1999. Tissue specificity of cardiac troponin I, cardiac troponin T and creatine kinase-MB. Clin. Chim. Acta. 2:151–159.

85. Collinson PO, Boa FG, and Gaze DC. 2001. Measurement of cardiac troponins. Ann. Clin. Biochem. 38:423–449.

86. Mainet GD, Sorell GL, Torres MB. 2000. The cardiac troponin I: Gold biochemical standard of myocardial damage La troponina i cardiaca: Marcador bioquimico de eleccion del dano miocardico. BIOTECNOL APL 2:77–84.

87. Bozeman CB, Carver BS, EasthamJA, Venable DD. 2002. Treatment of chronic prostatitis lowers serum prostate specific antigen. J. Urol. 4:1723–1726.

88. Oremek GM and Seiffert UB. 1996. Physical activity releases prostate-specific antigen (PSA) from the prostate gland into blood and increases serum PSA concentrations. Clin. Chem. 5:691–695.

89. Price CP, Allard J, Davies G, et al. 2001. Pre- and post-analytical factors that may influence use of serum prostate specific antigen and its isoforms in a screening programme for prostate cancer. Ann. Clin. Biochem. 38:188–216.

90. Stamey TA, Warrington JA, Caldwell MC, et al. 2001. Molecular genetic profiling of Gleason grade 4/5 prostate cancers compared to benign prostatic hyperplasia. J. Urol. 6:2171–2177.

91. Magee JA, Araki T, Patil S, et al. 2001. Expression profiling reveals hepsin overexpression in prostate cancer. Cancer Res. 15:5692–5696.

92. Jenkins RB, Qian J, Lieber MM, Bostwick DG. 1997. Detection of c-myc oncogene amplification and chromosomal anomalies in metastatic prostatic carcinoma by fluorescence *in situ* hybridization. Cancer Res. 3:524–531.

93. Hooper JD, Clements JA, Quigley JP, Antalis, T.M. 2001. Type II transmembrane serine proteases. Insights into an emerging class of cell surface proteolytic enzymes. J. Biol. Chem. 2:857–860.

94. Isaacs W and Kainu T. 2001. Oncogenes and tumor suppressor genes in prostate cancer. Epidemiol. Rev. 1:36–41.

95. Liu A., Nelson PS, van den EG, Hood L. 2002. Human prostate epithelial cell-type cDNA libraries and prostate expression patterns. Prostate 2:92–103.

96. Li PE and Nelson PS. 2001. Prostate cancer genomics. Curr. Urol. Rep. 1:70–78.

97. Platz EA, Krithivas K, Kantoff PW, Stampfer MJ, Giovannucci E. 2002. ATAAA repeat upstream of glutathione S-transferase P1 and prostate cancer risk. Urology 1:159–164.

98. Nelson KA and Witte JS. 2002. Androgen receptor CAG repeats and prostate cancer. Am. J. Epidemiol. 10:883–890.

99. Isaacs W and Coffey DS. 2002. Molecular Genetics of Prostate Cancer. In Comprehensive Textbook of Genitourinary Oncology. Vogelzang N, Scardino P, Shipley W, and Coffey D, eds. Philadelphia: Lippincott Williams and Wilkins, pp. 545–552.

100. Thompson T, Timme T, Bangma C, et al. 2002. Molecular Biology of Prostate Cancer. In Comprehensive Textbook of Genitourinary Oncology. Vogelzang N, Scardino P, Shipley W, Coffey D, eds. Philadelphia: Lippincottm Williams and Wilkins, pp. 553–564.

101. David A, Mabjeesh N, Azar I, et. al. 2002. Unusual alternative splicing within the human kallikrein genes KLK2 and KLK3 gives rise to novel prostate-specific proteins. J. Biol. Chem. 20:18,084–18,090.

102. Stapleton AM, Timme TL, Gousse AE, et. al. 1997. Primary human prostate cancer cells harboring p53 mutations are clonally expanded in metastases. Clin. Cancer Res. 8:1389–1397.

103. Aihara M, Scardino PT, Truong LD, et al. 1995. The frequency of apoptosis correlates with the prognosis of Gleason Grade 3 adenocarcinoma of the prostate. Cancer 2:522–529.

104. Furuya Y, Krajewski S, Epstein JI, Reed JC, Isaacs JT. 1996. Expression of bcl-2 and the progression of human and rodent prostatic cancers. Clin. Cancer Res. 2:389–398.

105. Carpten J, Nupponen N, Isaacs S, et al. 2002. Germline mutations in the ribonuclease L gene in families showing linkage with HPC1. Nat. Genet. 2:181–184.
106. Anderson N. andAnderson NG. 2002. The human plasma proteome: history, character, and diagnostic prospects. Mol. Cell. Proteomics 11:845–867.
107. Rittenhouse HG, Petruska JC, Hirata AA. 1984. Detection of Carcinoembryonic Antigen in Cancer Serum by Two-Dimensional Gel Electrophoresis. In: Proceedings of the Thirty-First Collequium. Bruges, GE, ed., New York: Pergamon Press, pp. 937–940.
108. Hu W, Verschraegen CF, Wu W, et al. 2002. Differential protein profile analysis of sera from normal donors and ovarian cancer patients by proteomics. Proc. Amer. Assoc. Cancer Res. Annual Meeting 43:37.
109. Rai AJ, Zhang Z, Rosenzweig J, et al. 2002. Proteomic approaches to tumor marker discovery. Arch. Pathol. Lab. Med. 12:1518–1526.
110. Chance J. 2001. Blood testing. choosing the right specimen. clinical laboratory news 7:18–20.
111. Moreno JG, O'Hara SM, Gross S, et al. 2001. Changes in circulating carcinoma cells in patients with metastatic prostate cancer correlate with disease status. Urology 3:386–392.
112. Paweletz CP, Liotta LA, Petricoin EF III. 2001. New technologies for biomarker analysis of prostate cancer progression: Laser capture microdissection and tissue proteomics. Urology 4:160–163.
113. Rubin MA. 2001. Use of laser capture microdissection, cDNA microarrays, and tissue microarrays in advancing our understanding of prostate cancer. J. Pathol. 1:80–86.
114. Dhanasekaran SM, Barrette TR, Ghosh D, et al. 2001. Delineation of prognostic biomarkers in prostate cancer. Nature 6849:822–826.
115. Lee C, Keefer M, Zhao ZW, et al. 1989. Demonstration of the role of prostate-specific antigen in semen liquefaction by two-dimensional electrophoresis. J. Androl. 6:432–438.
116. Suh CI, Shanafelt T, May DJ, et al. 2000. Comparison of telomerase activity and GSTP1 promoter methylation in ejaculate as potential screening tests for prostate cancer. Mol. Cell. Probes 4:211–217.
117. Halling KC, King W, Sokolova IA, et al. 2000. A comparison of cytology and fluorescence *in situ* hybridization for the detection of urothelial carcinoma. J. Urol. 5:1768–1775.
118. Bull JH, Ellison G, Patel A, et al. 2001. Identification of potential diagnostic markers of prostate cancer and prostatic intraepithelial neoplasia using cDNA microarray. Br. J. Cancer 11:1512–1519.
119. Chaib H, Cockrell EK, Rubin MA, Macoska JA. 2001. Profiling and verification of gene expression patterns in normal and malignant human prostate tissues by cDNA microarray analysis. Neoplasia 1:43–52.
120. Ernst T, Hergenhahn M, Kenzelmann M, et al. 2002. Decrease and gain of gene expression are equally discriminatory markers for prostate carcinoma: a gene expression analysis on total and microdissected prostate tissue. Am. J. Pathol. 6:2169–2180.
121. Luo J, Duggan DJ, Chen Y, et al. 2001. Human prostate cancer and benign prostatic hyperplasia: molecular dissection by gene expression profiling. Cancer Res. 12:4683–4688.
122. Welsh JB, Sapinoso LM, Su AI, et al. 2001. Analysis of gene expression identifies candidate markers and pharmacological targets in prostate cancer. Cancer Res. 16:5974–5978.
123. Leytus SP, Loeb KR, Hagen FS, Kurachi K, Davie EW. 1988. A novel trypsin-like serine protease (hepsin) with a putative transmembrane domain expressed by human liver and hepatoma cells. Biochemistry 3:1067–1074.
124. Tsuji A, Torres-Rosado A, Arai T, et al. 1991. Hepsin, a cell membrane-associated protease. Characterization, tissue distribution, and gene localization. J. Biol. Chem. 25:16948–16953.
125. Stephan C, Yousef GM, Scorilas A, et al. 2003. Quantitative analysis of kallikrein 15 gene expression in prostate tissue. J. Urol. 1:361–364.
126. Kufer P, Zippelius A, Lutterbuse R, et al. 2002. Heterogeneous expression of MAGE-A genes in occult disseminated tumor cells: a novel multimarker reverse transcription-polymerase chain reaction for diagnosis of micrometastatic disease. Cancer Res. 1:251–261.

127. Latil A, Vidaud D, Valeri A, et al. 2000. htert expression correlates with MYC over-expression in human prostate cancer. Int. J. Cancer 2:172–176.
128. Meid FH, Gygi CM, Leisinger HJ, Bosman FT, Benhattar, J. 2001. The use of telomerase activity for the detection of prostatic cancer cells after prostatic massage. J. Urol. 5:1802–1805.
129. Paradis V, Dargere D, Laurendeau I, et al. 1999. Expression of the RNA component of human telomerase (hTR) in prostate cancer, prostatic intraepithelial neoplasia, and normal prostate tissue. J. Pathol. 2:213–218.
130. Liu BC, LaRose I, Weinstein LJ, et al. 2001. Expression of telomerase subunits in normal and neoplastic prostate epithelial cells isolated by laser capture microdissection. Cancer 7: 1943–1948.
131. Bussemakers MJ, van Bokhoven A, Verhaegh, GW. et al. 1999. DD3: a new prostate-specific gene, highly overexpressed in prostate cancer. Cancer Res. 23:5975–5979.
132. Srikantan V, Zou Z, Petrovics G, et al. 2000. PCGEM1, a prostate-specific gene, is overexpressed in prostate cancer. Proc. Natl. Acad. Sci. USA 22:12216–12221.
133. de Kok JB, Verhaegh GW, Roelofs RW, et al. 2002. DD3(PCA3), a very sensitive and specific marker to detect prostate tumors. Cancer Res. 9:2695–2698.
134. Saad F, Aprikian AG, Dessureault J, et al. 2003. Multicenter Study of the UPM3 Test, a New Molecular Urine Assay to Detect Prostate Cancer. J. Urol. 169:121–469.
135. Su SL, Boynton AL, Holmes EH, Elgamal AA, Murphy GP. 2000. Detection of extraprostatic prostate cells utilizing reverse transcription-polymerase chain reaction. Semin. Surg. Oncol. 1:17–28.
136. Thomas J, Gupta M, Grasso Y, et al. 2002. Preoperative combined nested reverse transcriptase polymerase chain reaction for prostate-specific antigen and prostate-specific membrane antigen does not correlate with pathologic stage or biochemical failure in patients with localized prostate cancer undergoing radical prostatectomy. J. Clin. Oncol. 15:3213–3218.
137. Shariat SF, Gottenger E, Nguyen C, et al. 2002. Preoperative blood reverse transcriptase-PCR assays for prostate- specific antigen and human glandular kallikrein for prediction of prostate cancer progression after radical prostatectomy. Cancer Res. 20:5974–5979.
138. Varambally S, Dhanasekaran SM, Zhou M, et al. 2002. The polycomb group protein EZH2 is involved in progression of prostate cancer. Nature 419:624–629.
139. Rosen EM, Fan S, and Goldberg ID. 2001. BRCA1 and prostate cancer. Cancer Invest. 4:396–412.
140. Sinclair CS, Berry R, Schaid D, Thibodeau SN, Couch FJ. 2000. BRCA1 and BRCA2 have a limited role in familial prostate cancer. Cancer Res. 5:1371–1375.
141. Uchida T, Wang C, Sato T, et al. 1999. BRCA1 gene mutation and loss of heterozygosity on chromosome 17q21 in primary prostate cancer. Int. J. Cancer 1:19–23.
142. Williams BJ, Jones E, Zhu XL, et al. 1996. Evidence for a tumor suppressor gene distal to BRCA1 in prostate cancer. J. Urol. 2:720–725.
143. Goessl C, Mueller M, Heicappell R, et al. 2001. DNA-based detection of prostate cancer in urine after prostatic massage. Urology 3:335–338.
144. Kito H, Suzuki H, Ichikawa T, et al. 2001. Hypermethylation of the CD44 gene is associated with progression and metastasis of human prostate cancer. Prostate 2:110–115.
145. Lou W, Krill D, Dhir R, et al. 1999. Methylation of the CD44 metastasis suppressor gene in human prostate cancer. Cancer Res. 10:2329–2331.
146. Mouraviev V, Li L, Tahir SA, et al. 2002. The role of caveolin-1 in androgen insensitive prostate cancer. J. Urol. 168:1589–1596.
147. Cui J, Rohr LR, Swanson G, Speights VO, Maxwell T, Brothman AR. 2001. Hypermethylation of the caveolin-1 gene promoter in prostate cancer. Prostate 3:249–256.
148. Verkaik NS, van Steenbrugge GJ, van Weerden WM, Bussemakers MJ, van der Kwast TH. 2000. Silencing of CD44 expression in prostate cancer by hypermethylation of the CD44 promoter region. Lab. Invest. 8:1291–1298.
149. Vis AN, Oomen M, Schroder FH, van der Kwast TH. 2001. Feasibility of assessment of promoter methylation of the CD44 gene in serum of prostate cancer patients. Mol. Urol. 4:199–203.

150. Bock CH, Cunningham JM, McDonnell SK, et al. 2001. Analysis of the prostate cancer-susceptibility locus HPC20 in 172 families affected by prostate cancer. Am. J. Hum. Genet. 3:795–801.
151. Goode EL, Stanford JL, Peters MA, et al. 2001. Clinical characteristics of prostate cancer in an analysis of linkage to four putative susceptibility loci. Clin. Cancer Res. 9:2739–2749.
152. Nwosu V, Carpten J, Trent JM, Sheridan R. 2001. Heterogeneity of genetic alterations in prostate cancer: evidence of the complex nature of the disease. Hum. Mol. Genet. 20:2313–2318.
153. Simard J, Dumont M, Soucy P, and Labrie F. 2002. Perspective: prostate cancer susceptibility genes. Endocrinology 6:2029–2040.
154. Stephan DA, Howell GR, Teslovich TM, et al. 2002. Physical and transcript map of the hereditary prostate cancer region at xq27. Genomics 1:41–50.
155. Suarez BK, Gerhard DS, Lin J, et al. 2001. Polymorphisms in the prostate cancer susceptibility gene HPC2/ELAC2 in multiplex families and healthy controls. Cancer Res. 13:4982–4984.
156. Xu J, Zheng SL, Chang B, et al. 2001. Linkage of prostate cancer susceptibility loci to chromosome 1. Hum. Genet. 4:335–345.
157. Bousema JT, Bussemakers MJ, van Houwelingen KP, et al. 2000. Polymorphisms in the vitamin D receptor gene and the androgen receptor gene and the risk of benign prostatic hyperplasia. Eur. Urol. 2:234–238.
158. Chang BL, Zheng SL, Hawkins GA, et al. 2002. Polymorphic GGC repeats in the androgen receptor gene are associated with hereditary and sporadic prostate cancer risk. Hum. Genet. 2:122–129.
159. Hsing AW, Chen C, Chokkalingam AP, et al. 2001. Polymorphic markers in the srd5a2 gene and prostate cancer risk: a population-based case-control study. Cancer Epidemiol. Biomark. Prev. 10:1077–1082.
160. Latil AG, Azzouzi R, Cancel GS, et al. 2001. Prostate carcinoma risk and allelic variants of genes involved in androgen biosynthesis and metabolism pathways. Cancer 5:1130–1137.
161. Nam RK, Zhang WW, Trachtenberg J, et al. 2003. Single nucleotide polymorphism of the human kallikrein-2 gene highly correlates with serum human kallikrein-2 levels and in combination enhances prostate cancer detection. J. Clin. Oncol. 12:2312–2319.
162. Robert M, Gibbs BF, Jacobson E, Gagnon C. 1997. Characterization of prostate-specific antigen proteolytic activity on its major physiological substrate, the sperm motility inhibitor precursor/semenogelin I. Biochem. 36:3811–3819.
163. Lilja H. 1985. A Kallikrein-like serine protease in prostatic fluid cleaves the predominant seminal vesicle protein. J. Clin. Invest. 76:1899–1903.
164. Balk SP, Ko YJ, Bubley GJ. 2003. Biology of prostate-specific antigen. J. Clin. Oncol. 2:383–391.
165. Oesterling JE. 1991. Prostate-specific antigen: a critical assessment of the most useful tumor marker for adenocarcinoma of the prostate. J. Urol. 145:907–923.
166. Labrie F, Dupont A, Suburu R, et al. 1992. Serum prostate specific antigen as pre-screening test for prostate cancer. J. Urol. 147:846–851.
167. Lilja H, Christensson A, Dahlen U, et al. 1991. prostate-specific antigen in serum occurs predominantly in complex with alpha-1-antichymotrypsin. Clin. Chem. 9:1618–1625.
168. Stenman UH, Leinonen J, Alfthan H, Rannikko S, Tuhkanen K, Alfthan O. 1991. A complex between prostate specific antigen and a1-antichymotrypsin is the major form of prostate-specific antigen in serum of patients with prostatic cancer: assay of the complex improves clinical sensitivity for cancer. Cancer Res. 51:222–226.
169. Woodrum DL, Brawer MK, Partin AW, Catalona WJ, Southwick PC. 1998. Interpretation of free prostate specific antigen clinical research studies for the detection of prostate cancer. J. Urol. 1:5–12.
170. Okihara K, Cheli CD, Partin AW, et al. 2002. Comparative analysis of complexed prostate specific antigen, free prostate specific antigen and their ratio in detecting prostate cancer. J. Urol. 5:2017–2023.
171. Peter J, Unverzagt C, Hoesel W. 2000. Analysis of free prostate-specific antigen (PSA) after chemical release from the complex with alpha(1)-antichymotrypsin (PSA-ACT). Clin. Chem. 4:474–482.

172. Bjork T, Bjartell A, Abrahamsson PA, Hulkko S, di Sant'Agnese A, Lilja, H. 1994. Alphal-antichymotrypsin production in PSA-producing cells is common in prostate cancer but rare in benign prostatic hyperplasia. Urology 43:427–434.

173. Jung K, Brux B, Lein M, et al. 2000. Molecular forms of prostate-specific antigen in malignant and benign prostatic tissue: biochemical and diagnostic implications. Clin. Chem. 1:47–54.

174. Mikolajczyk SD, Grauer LS, Millar LS, et al. 1997. A precursor form of PSA (pPSA) is a component of the free PSA in prostate cancer serum. Urology 50:710–714.

175. Mikolajczyk SD, Marker KM, Millar LS, et al. 2001. A truncated precursor form of prostate-specific antigen is a more specific serum marker of prostate cancer. Cancer Res. 18:6958–6963.

176. Mikolajczyk SD and Rittenhouse HG. 2003. Pro PSA: a more cancer specific form of prostate specific antigen for the early detection of prostate cancer. Keio J. Med. 2:86–91.

177. Noldus J, Chen Z, Stamey T. 1997. Isolation and characterization of free form prostate specific antigen (f-PSA) in sera of men with prostate cancer. J. Urol. 158:1606–1609.

178. Hilz H, Noldus J, Hammerer P, Buck F, Luck M, Huland, H. 1999. Molecular heterogeneity of free PSA in sera of patients with benign and malignant prostate tumors. Eur. Urol. 4:286–292.

179. Mikolajczyk SD, Millar LS, Wang TJ, et al. 2000. A precursor form of prostate-specific antigen is more highly elevated in prostate cancer compared with benign transition zone prostate tissue. Cancer Res. 3:756–759.

180. Peter J, Unverzagt C, Krogh TN, Vorm O, Hoesel W. 2001. Identification of precursor forms of prostate-specific antigen in serum of prostate cancer patients by immunosorption and mass spectrometry. Cancer Res. 61:957–962.

181. Niemela P, Lovgren J, Karp M, Lilja H, Pettersson K. 2002. Sensitive and specific enzymatic assay for the determination of precursor forms of prostate-specific antigen after an activation step. Clin. Chem. 8:1257–1264.

182. Kumar A, Mikolajczyk SD, Goel AS, Millar LS, Saedi MS. 1997. Expression of pro form of Prostate-specific antigen by mammalian cells and its conversion to mature, active form by human kallikrein 2. Cancer Res. 57:3111–3114.

183. Khan AR and James MNG. 1998. Molecular mechanisms for the conversion of zymogens to active proteolytic enzymes. Prot. Sci. 7:815–836.

184. Zhang WM, Leinonen J, Kalkkinen N, Dowell B, Stenman UH. 1995. Purification and characterization of different molecular forms of prostate-specific antigen in human seminal fluid. Clin. Chem. 41:1567–1573.

185. Kumar A, Mikolajczyk S, Hill TM, Millar L, Saedi MS. 2000. Different proportions of various prostate-specific antigen (PSA) and human kallikrein 2 (hK2) forms are present in noninduced and androgen-induced LNCaP cells. Prostate 3:248–254.

186. Nurmikko P, Vaisanen V, Piironen T, Lindgren S, Lilja H, Pettersson K. 2000. Production and characterization of novel anti-prostate-specific antigen (PSA) monoclonal antibodies that do not detect internally cleaved Lys145-Lys146 inactive PSA. Clin. Chem. 10:1610–1618.

187. Darson MF, Parcelli A, Roche P, et al. 1997. Human Glandular Kallikrein 2 (hK2) expression in prostatic intraepithelial neoplasia and adenocarcinoma: a novel prostate cancer marker. Urology 6:857–862.

188. Frenette G, Tremblay RR, Lazure C, Dube JY. 1997. Prostatic kallikrein hK2, but not prostate-specific antigen (hK3), activates single-chain urokinase-type plasminogen activator. Int. J. Cancer 5:897–899.

189. Mikolajczyk SD, Millar LS, Kumar A, Saedi MS. 1999. Prostatic human kallikrein 2 inactivates and complexes with plasminogen activator. Int. J. Cancer 81:438–442.

190. Mikolajczyk SD, Millar LS, Marker KM, et al. 1999. Identification of a novel complex between human kallikrein 2 and protease inhibitor-6 in prostate cancer tissue. Cancer Res. 16:3927–3930.

191. Black MH, Magklara A, Obiezu CV, Melegos DN, Diamandis EP. 1999. Development of an ultrasensitive immunoassay for human glandular kallikrein (hK2) with no cross reactivity from prostate specific antigen (PSA). Clin. Chem. 6:790–799.

192. Becker C, Piironen T, Kiviniemi J, Lilja H, Pettersson K. 2000. Sensitive and specific immunodetection of human glandular kallikrein 2 in serum. Clin. Chem. 2:198–206.

193. Saedi MS, Zhu Z, Marker K, et al. 2001. Human kallikrein 2 (hK2), but not prostate-specific antigen (PSA), rapidly complexes with protease inhibitor 6 (PI-6) released from prostate carcinoma cells. Int. J. Cancer 4:558–563.

194. Finlay JA, Day JR, Evans CL, et al. 2001. Development of a dual monoclonal antibody immunoassay for total human kallikrein 2. Clin. Chem. 7:1218–1224.

195. Becker C, Piironen T, Pettersson K, et al. 2000. Discrimination of men with prostate cancer from those with benign disease by measurements of human glandular kallikrein 2 (HK2) in serum. J. Urol. 1:311–316.

196. Klee GG, Goodmanson MK, Jacobsen SJ, et al. 1999. A highly sensitive automated chemiluminometric assay for measuring free human glandular kallikrein (hK2). Clin. Chem. 6:800–806.

197. Partin AW, Catalona WJ, Finlay JA, et al. 1999. Use of human glandular kallikrein 2 for the detection of prostate cancer: preliminary analysis. Urology 5:839–845.

198. Kwiatkowski MK, Recker F, Piironen T, et al. 1998. In prostatism patients the ratio of human glandular kallikrein to free PSA improves the discrimination between prostate cancer and benign hyperplasia within the diagnostic "gray zone" of total PSA 4 to 10 ng/mL. Urology 3:360–365.

199. Haese A, Graefen M, Steuber T, et al. 2001. Human glandular kallikrein 2 levels in serum for discrimination of pathologically organ-confined from locally-advanced prostate cancer in total PSA-levels below 10 ng/mL. Prostate 2:101–109.

200. Clements J. 1989. The glandular kallikrein family of enzymes: tissue specific expression and hormonal regulation. Endocrine Rev. 10:393–419.

201. Clements J, Hooper J, Dong Y, Harvey T. 2001. The expanded human kallikrein (KLK) gene family: genomic organisation, tissue-specific expression and potential functions. Biol. Chem. 1:5–14.

202. Yousef GM and Diamandis EP. 2001. The new human tissue kallikrein gene family: structure, function, and association to disease. Endocr. Rev. 2:184–204.

203. Takayama TK, McMullen BA, Nelson PS, Matsumura M, Fujikawa K. 2001. Characterization of hK4 (prostase), a prostate-specific serine protease: activation of the precursor of prostate specific antigen (pro- PSA) and single-chain urokinase-type plasminogen activator and degradation of prostatic acid phosphatase. Biochemistry 50:15341–15348.

204. Tasch J, Gong M, Sadelain M, Heston WD. 2001. A unique folate hydrolase, prostate-specific membrane antigen (PSMA): a target for immunotherapy? Crit. Rev. Immunol. 21:249–261.

205. Freeman LM, Krynyckyi BR, Li Y, et al. 2002. The role of 111In Capromab Pendetide (ProstaScintR) immunoscintigraphy in the management of prostate cancer. Q. J. Nucl. Med. 2:131–137.

206. Mabjeesh NJ, Zhong H, Simons JW. 2002. Gene therapy of prostate cancer: current and future directions. Endocr. Relat. Cancer 2:115–139.

207. Gong MC, Chang SS, Watt F, et al. 2000. Overview of evolving strategies incorporating prostate-specific membrane antigen as target for therapy. Mol. Urol. 3:217–222.

208. Chang SS, Reuter VE, Heston WD, Gaudin, P.B. 2001. Metastatic renal cell carcinoma neovasculature expresses prostate-specific membrane antigen. Urol. 4:801–805.

209. Chang SS, Reuter VE, Heston WD, Bander NH, Grauer LS, Gaudin PB. 1999. Five different anti-prostate-specific membrane antigen (PSMA) antibodies confirm PSMA expression in tumor-associated neovasculature. Cancer Res. 13:3192–3198.

210. Barton J, Blackledge G, Wakeling A. 2001. Growth factors and their receptors: new targets for prostate cancer therapy. Urology 58:114–122.

211. Bergan RC, Waggle DH, Carter SK, Horak I, Slichenmyer W, Meyers M. 2001. Tyrosine kinase inhibitors and signal transduction modulators: Rationale and current status as chemopreventive agents for prostate cancer. Urology 57:77–80.

212. Fossa A, Lilleby W, Fossa SD, Gaudernack, G, Torlakovic G, Berner A. 2002. Independent prognostic significance of HER-2 oncoprotein expression in pN0 prostate cancer undergoing curative radiotherapy. Int. J. Cancer. 1:100–105.

213. James ND, Atherton J, Jones J, Howie AJ, Tchekmedyian S, Curnow RT. 2001. A phase II study of the bispecific antibody MDX-H210 (anti-HER2 x CD64) with GM-CSF in HER2+ advanced prostate cancer. Br. J. Cancer. 2:152–156.

214. Reese DM, Small EJ, Magrane G, Waldman FM, Chew K, Sudilovsky D. 2001. HER2 protein expression and gene amplification in androgen-independent prostate cancer. Am. J. Clin. Pathol. 2:234–239.

215. Shi Y, Brands FH, Chatterjee S, et al. 2001. Her-2/neu expression in prostate cancer: high level of expression associated with exposure to hormone therapy and androgen independent disease. J. Urol. 4:1514–1519.

216. Osman I, Scher HI, Drobnjak M, et al. 2001. HER-2/neu (p185neu) protein expression in the natural or treated history of prostate cancer. Clin. Cancer Res. 9:2643–2647.

217. Savinainen KJ, Saramaki OR, Linja MJ, et al. 2002. Expression and gene copy number analysis of ERBB2 oncogene in prostate cancer. Am. J. Pathol. 160(1):339–345.

218. Liu HL, Gandour-Edwards, R, Lara, PN Jr, de Vere WR, LaSalle JM. 2001. Detection of low level HER-2/neu gene amplification in prostate cancer by fluorescence *in situ* hybridization. Cancer J. 5:395–403.

219. Kim NW and Hruszkewycz AM. 2001. Telomerase activity modulation in the prevention of prostate cancer. Urology 57:148–153.

220. Elayadi AN, Demieville A, Wancewicz EV, Monia BP, Corey DR. 2001. Inhibition of telomerase by 2'-O-(2-methoxyethyl) RNA oligomers: effect of length, phosphorothioate substitution and time inside cells. Nucleic Acids Res. 8:1683–1689.

221. Schroers R, Huang XF, Hammer J, Zhang J, Chen SY. 2002. Identification of HLA DR7-restricted epitopes from human telomerase reverse transcriptase recognized by CD4+ T-helper cells. Cancer Res. 9:2600–2605.

222. Heiser A, Maurice MA, Yancey DR, et al. 2001. Induction of polyclonal prostate cancer-specific CTL using dendritic cells transfected with amplified tumor RNA. J. Immunol. 5:2953–2960.

223. Straub B, Muller M, Krause H, et al. 2002. Molecular staging of pelvic surgical margins after radical prostatectomy: Comparison of RT-PCR for prostate-specific antigen and telomerase activity. Oncol. Rep. 3:545–549.

224. Ruijter E, Montironi R, van de KC, Schalken J. 2001. Molecular changes associated with prostate cancer development. Anal. Quant. Cytol. Histol. 1:67–88.

225. Sakr WA and Partin AW. 2001. Histological markers of risk and the role of high-grade prostatic intraepithelial neoplasia. Urol. 57:115–120.

226. Lianidou E. 2002. Telomerase. In Tumor Markers Physiology, Pathobiology, Technology and Clinical Applications. Diamandis EP, Fritsche HA, Lilja H, Chan DW, and Schartz M, eds. Washington: AACC, pp. 509–511.

227. Andersen MH and Thor, S. 2002. Survivin—a universal tumor antigen. Histol. Histopathol. 2:669–675.

228. Altieri DC. 2001. The molecular basis and potential role of survivin in cancer diagnosis and therapy. Trends Mol. Med. 12:542–547.

229. LaCasse EC, Baird S, Korneluk RG, MacKenzie AE. 1998. The inhibitors of apoptosis (IAPs) and their emerging role in cancer. Oncogene 25:3247–3259.

230. Ambrosini G, Adida C, Altieri DC. 1997. A novel anti-apoptosis gene, survivin, expressed in cancer and lymphoma. Nat. Med. 8:917–921.

231. Xing N, Qian J, Bostwick D, Bergstralh E, Young CY. 2001. Neuroendocrine cells in human prostate over-express the anti-apoptosis protein survivin. Prostate 1:7–15.

232. Djavan B, Waldert M, Seitz C, Marberge, R. M. 2001. Insulin-like growth factors and prostate cancer. World J. Urol. 4:225–233.

233. Chan JM, Stampfer MJ, Giovannucci E, et al. 1998. Plasma insulin-like growth factor-I and prostate cancer risk: A prospective study. Science 279:563–565.

234. Shi R, Berkel HJ, Yu H. 2001. Insulin-like growth factor-I and prostate cancer: a meta-analysis. Br. J. Cancer. 7:991–996.

235. Chan JM, Stampfer MJ, Ma J, et al. 2002. Insulin-like growth factor-I (IGF-I) and IGF binding protein-3 as predictors of advanced-stage prostate cancer. J. Natl. Cancer Inst.14:1099–1106.

236. Koistinen H, Paju A, Koistinen R, et al. 2002. Prostate-specific antigen and other prostate-derived proteases cleave IGFBP-3, but prostate cancer is not associated with proteolytically cleaved circulating IGFBP-3. Prostate 2:112–118.

237. Ismail AH, Pollak M, Behlouli H, Tanguay S, Begin LR, Aprikian AG. 2002. Insulin-like growth factor-1 and insulin-like growth factor binding protein-3 for prostate cancer detection in patients undergoing prostate biopsy. J. Urol. 6:2426–2430.

238. Shariat SF, Lamb DJ, Kattan MW, et al. 2002. Association of preoperative plasma levels of insulin-like growth factor I and insulin-like growth factor binding proteins-2 and -3 with prostate cancer invasion, progression, and metastasis. J. Clin. Oncol. 3:833–841.

239. Lehrer S, Diamond EJ, Droller MJ, Stone NN, Stock RG. 2002. Re: Insulin-like growth factor-I (IGF-I) and IGF binding protein-3 as predictors of advanced-stage prostate cancer. J. Natl. Cancer Inst. 24:1893–1894.

240. Latif Z, McMillan DC, Wallace AM, et al. 2002. The relationship of circulating insulin-like growth factor 1, its binding protein-3, prostate-specific antigen and C-reactive protein with disease stage in prostate cancer. BJU Int. 4:396–399.

241. Coussens LM, Fingleton B, Matrisian LM. 2002. Matrix metalloproteinase inhibitors and cancer: trials and tribulations. Science 5564:2387–2392.

242. Bodey B, Bodey B Jr, Siegel SE, Kaiser HE. 2001. Immunocytochemical detection of matrix metalloproteinase expression in prostate cancer. In Vivo 15(1):65–70.

243. Wood M, Fudge K, Mohler JL, et al. 1997. *In situ* hybridization studies of metalloproteinases 2 and 9 and TIMP-1 and TIMP-2 expression in human prostate cancer. Clin Exp Metastasis 3:246–258.

244. Jung K, Nowak L, Lein M, Priem F, Schnorr D, Loening SA. 1997. Matrix metalloproteinases 1 and 3, tissue inhibitor of metalloproteinase-1 and the complex of metalloproteinase-1/tissue inhibitor in plasma of patients with prostate cancer. Int. J. Cancer 2:220–223.

245. Sheng S. 2001. The urokinase-type plasminogen activator system in prostate cancer metastasis. Cancer Metastasis Rev. 3–4:287–296.

246. Gavrilov D, Kenzior O, Evans M, Calaluce R, and Folk WR. 2001. Expression of urokinase plasminogen activator and receptor in conjunction with the ets family and AP-1 complex transcription factors in high grade prostate cancers. Eur. J. Cancer 8:1033–1040.

247. Helenius MA, Saramaki OR, Linja MJ, Tammela TL, Visakorpi T. 2001. Amplification of urokinase gene in prostate cancer. Cancer Res. 14:5340–5344.

248. Miyake H, Hara I, Yamanaka K, Gohji K, Arakawa S, Kamidono S. 1999. Elevation of serum levels of urokinase-type plasminogen activator and its receptor is associated with disease progression and prognosis in patients with prostate cancer. Prostate 2:123–129.

249. Cheung J, Graves C, Robertson J. 2002. Autoantibodies as circulating cancer markers. In Tumor Markers Physiology, Pathobiology, Technology and Clinical Applications. Diamandis EP, Fritsche HA, Lilja H, Chan DW, and Schartz M, eds. Washington: AACC, pp. 123–131.

250. Sanda MG, Smith DC, Charles LG, et al. 1999. Recombinant Vaccinia-PSA (Prostvac) can Induce a Prostate-Specific Immune Response in Androgen-Modulated Human Prostate Cancer. Urology 53:260–266.

251. Eder JP, Kantoff PW, Roper K, et al. 2000. A phase I trial of a recominant vaccinia virus expressing prostate-specific antigen in advanced prostate cancer. Clin. Cancer Res. 6:1632–1638.

252. Tahir SA, Yang G, Ebara S, et al. 2001. Secreted caveolin-1 stimulates cell survival/clonal growth and contributes to metastasis in androgen-insensitive prostate cancer. Cancer Res. 10:3882–3885.

253. Abrahamsson PA. 1999. Neuroendocrine differentiation in prostatic carcinoma. Prostate 2: 135–148.
254. Rini BI and Small EJ. 2001. Immunotherapy for prostate cancer. Curr. Oncol. Rep. 5:418–423.
255. Satthaporn S and Eremin O. 2001. Dendritic cells (II): Role and therapeutic implications in cancer. J. R. Coll.Surg. Edinb. 46(3):159–167.
256. Eaton JD, Perry MJ, Nicholson S, et al. 2002. Allogeneic whole-cell vaccine: a phase I/II study in men with hormone- refractory prostate cancer. BJU Int. 1:19–26.
257. Heiser A, Coleman D, Dannull J, et al. 2002. Autologous dendritic cells transfected with prostate-specific antigen RNA stimulate CTL responses against metastatic prostate tumors. J. Clin. Invest. 3:409–417.
258. Hampl J and Kuus-Reichel K. 2002. Measurement of Tumor-Specific T Cells with MHC Tetramer Technology. In Tumor Markers Physiology, Pathobiology, Technology and Clinical Applications. Diamandis EP, Fritsche HA, Lilja H, Chan DW, and Schartz M, eds. Washington: AACC, pp. 457–460.
259. Vonderheide RH, Domchek SM, Hahn WC, et al. 2001. Vaccination of cancer patients against telomerase: A phase I study using peptide-pulsed dendritic cells. Blood 98:508a.
260. Moul JW, Lewis DJ, Ross AA, Kahn DG, Ho CK, McLeod DG. 1994. Immunohistologic detection of prostate cancer pelvic lymph node micrometastases: correlation to preoperative serum prostate-specific antigen. Urology 1:68–73.
261. Vagunda V, Landys K, Kankkunen JP, et al. 2001. Bone marrow micrometastases in patients with stage I-II localised prostate cancer. Eur. J. Cancer 15:1847–1852.
262. Halabi S, Small EJ, Hayes DF, Vogelzang NJ, Kantoff PW. 2003. Prognostic significance of reverse transcriptase polymerase chain reaction for prostate-specific antigen in metastatic prostate cancer: a nested study within CALGB 9583. J. Clin. Oncol. 3:490–495.
263. Bigler SA, Deering RE, Brawer MK. 1993. Comparison of microscopic vascularity in benign and malignant prostate tissue. Hum. Pathol. 2:220–226.
264. Wikstrom P, Lissbrant IF, Stattin P, Egevad L, Bergh A. 2002. Endoglin (CD105) is expressed on immature blood vessels and is a marker for survival in prostate cancer. Prostate 4:268–275.
265. Mehta R, Kyshtoobayeva A, Kurosaki T, et al. 2001. Independent association of angiogenesis index with outcome in prostate cancer. Clin. Cancer Res. 1:81–88.
266. Kwak C, Jin RJ, Lee C, Park MS, Lee SE. 2002. Thrombospondin-1, vascular endothelial growth factor expression and their relationship with p53 status in prostate cancer and benign prostatic hyperplasia. BJU Int. 3:303–309.
267. Grossfeld GD, Carroll PR, Lindeman N, et al. 2002. Thrombospondin-1 expression in patients with pathologic stage T3 prostate cancer undergoing radical prostatectomy: association with p53 alterations, tumor angiogenesis, and tumor progression. Urology 1:97–102.
268. Cvetkovic D, Movsas B, Dicker AP, et al. 2001. Increased hypoxia correlates with increased expression of the angiogenesis marker vascular endothelial growth factor in human prostate cancer. Urology 4:821–825.
269. Bok RA, Halabi S, Fei DT, et al. 2001. Vascular endothelial growth factor and basic fibroblast growth factor urine levels as predictors of outcome in hormone-refractory prostate cancer patients: a cancer and leukemia group B study. Cancer Res. 61(6):2533–2536.
270. West AF, O'Donnell M, Charlton RG, Neal, DE, Leung HY. 2001. Correlation of vascular endothelial growth factor expression with fibroblast growth factor-8 expression and clinico-pathologic parameters in human prostate cancer. Br. J. Cancer 4:576–583.
271. Uotila P, Valve E, Martikainen P, Nevalainen M, Nurmi M, Harkonen P. 2001. Increased expression of cyclooxygenase-2 and nitric oxide synthase-2 in human prostate cancer. Urol. Res. 1:23–28.
272. Lokeshwar VB, Rubinowicz D, Schroeder GL, et al. 2001. Stromal and epithelial expression of tumor markers hyaluronic acid and HYAL1 hyaluronidase in prostate cancer. J. Biol. Chem. 15:11,922–11,932.

273. Kenyon GL, DeMarini DM, Fuchs E, et al. 2002. Defining the Mandate of Proteomics in the Post-Genomics Era: Workshop Report: National Academy of Sciences, Washington, D.C., USA. http://www.nap.edu/catalog/10209.html. Mol. Cell. Proteomics 10:763–780.

274. Srinivas PR, Verma M, Zhao Y, Srivastava S. 2002. Proteomics for cancer biomarker discovery. Clin. Chem. 8:1160–1169.

275. Chapdelaine P, Paradis G, Tremblay R, and Dube J. 1988. High level of expression in the prostate of a human glandular kallikrein mRNA related to prostate-specific antigen. FEBS Lett. 236:205–208.

276. Adam BL, Vlahou A, Semmes OJ, Wright GL Jr. 2001. Proteomic approaches to biomarker discovery in prostate and bladder cancers. Proteomics 10:1264–1270.

277. Adam BL, Qu Y, Davis JW, et al. 2002. Serum protein fingerprinting coupled with a pattern-matching algorithm distinguishes prostate cancer from benign prostate hyperplasia and healthy men. Cancer Res. 13:3609–3614.

278. O'dowd GJ, Miller MC, Orozco R, Veltri RW. 2000. Analysis of repeated biopsy results within 1 year after a noncancer diagnosis. Urology 4:553–559.

279. Stephan C, Cammann H, Semjonow A, et al. 2002. Multicenter evaluation of an artificial neural network to increase the prostate cancer detection rate and reduce unnecessary biopsies. Clin. Chem. 8:1279–1287.

280. Horninger W, Bartsch G, Snow, PB, Brandt JM, Partin AW. 2001. The problem of cutoff levels in a screened population: appropriateness of informing screenees about their risk of having prostate carcinoma. Cancer 8:1667–1672.

281. Borque A, Sanz G, Allepuz C, Plaza L, Gil P, Rioja LA. 2001. The use of neural networks and logistic regression analysis for predicting pathological stage in men undergoing radical prostatectomy: a population based study. J. Urol. 5:1672–1678.

282. Djavan B, Remzi M, Zlotta A, Seitz C, Snow P, Marberger M. 2002. Novel artificial neural network for early detection of prostate cancer. J. Clin. Oncol. 4:921–929.

283. Zhang Z. 2002. Combining Multiple Biomarkers in Clinical Diagnostics: A review of methods and issues, in: Tumor Markers Physiology, Pathobiology, Technology and Clinical Applications, Diamandis EP, Fritsche HA, Lilja H, Chan DW, Schartz M, eds., AACC Press: Washington, pp. 133–139.

284. McEleny K, Watson R, Fitzpatrick J. 2001. Defining a role for the inhibitors of apoptosis proteins in prostate cancer. Prostate Cancer Prostatic Dis. 4:28–32.

285. Damianaki A, Bakogeorgou E, Kampa M, et al. 2000. Potent inhibitory action of red wine polyphenols on human breast cancer cells. J. Cell. Biochem. 3:429–441.

286. Berruti A, Dogliotti L, Tucci M, Tarabuzzi R, Fontana D, Angeli A. 2001. Metabolic bone disease induced by prostate cancer: rationale for the use of bisphosphonates. J. Urol. 6: 2023–2031.

287. Goluboff ET. 2001. Exisulind, a selective apoptotic antineoplastic drug. Expert Opin. Investig. Drugs 10:1875–1882.

288. Hsu AL, Ching,TT, Wang DS, Song X, Rangnekar VM, Chen CS. 2000. The cyclooxygenase-2 inhibitor celecoxib induces apoptosis by blocking Akt activation in human prostate cancer cells independently of Bcl-2. J. Biol. Chem. 15:11397–11403.

289. Debes J and Tindall D. 2002. The role of androgens and the androgen receptor in prostate cancer. Cancer Lett. 1–2:1.

290. Small EJ, Prins G, Taplin M. 2000. The androgen receptor and the physiology and endocrinology of the prostate, in: Comprehensive Textbook of Genitourinary Oncology. Vogelzang NJ, Scardino PT, Shipley W, and Coffey DS, eds., Lippincott Williams and Wilkins: Philadelphia, pp. 565–586.

291. Roehrborn C, Boyle P, Nickel J, Hoefner K, Andriole G. 2002. Efficacy and safety of a dual inhibitor of 5-alpha-reductase types 1 and 2 (dutasteride) in men with benign prostatic hyperplasia. Urology 3:434.

292. Burger MJ, Tebay MA, and Keith PA, et al. 2002. Expression analysis of delta-catenin and prostate-specific membrane antigen: their potential as diagnostic markers for prostate cancer. Int. J. Cancer. 2:228–237.

293. Paoloni-Giacobino A, Chen H, Peitsch MC, Rossier C. 1997. Antonarakis, S.E. Cloning of the TMPRSS2 gene, which encodes a novel serine protease with transmembrane, LDLRA, and SRCR domains and maps to 21q22.3. Genomics 3:309–320.

294. Diamandis EP, Okui A, Mitsui S, et al. 2002. Human kallikrein 11: a new biomarker of prostate and ovarian carcinoma. Cancer Res. 1:295–300.

295. Sinha AA, Quast BJ, Wilson MJ, et al. 2001. Ratio of cathepsin B to stefin A identifies heterogeneity within Gleason histologic scores for human prostate cancer. Prostate 4:274–284.

296. Al Maghrabi J, Vorobyova L, Chapman W, Jewett M, Zielenska M, Squire JA. 2001. p53 Alteration and chromosomal instability in prostatic high-grade intraepithelial neoplasia and concurrent carcinoma: analysis by immunohistochemistry, interphase *in situ* hybridization, and sequencing of laser-captured microdissected specimens. Mod. Pathol. 12:1252–1262.

297. Qian J, Hirasawa K, Bostwick DG, et al. 2002. Loss of p53 and c-myc overrepresentation in stage T(2-3)N(1-3)M(0) prostate cancer are potential markers for cancer progression. Mod. Pathol. 1:35–44.

298. Finasteride Male Pattern Hair Loss Study Group. 2002. Long-term (5-year) multinational experience with finasteride 1 mg in the treatment of men with androgenetic alopecia. Eur. J. Dermatol. 1:38–49.

299. Pannek J, Marks LS, Pearson JD, et al. 1998. Influence of finasteride on free and total serum prostate specific antigen levels in men with benign prostatic hyperplasia. J. Urol. 159:449–453.

300. Preuss HG, Marcusen C, Regan, J, Klimberg IW, Welebir TA, Jones WA. 2001. Randomized trial of a combination of natural products (cernitin, saw palmetto, B-sitosterol, vitamin E) on symptoms of benign prostatic hyperplasia (BPH). Int. Urol. Nephrol. 2:217–225.

301. Ryan CW, Stadler WM, Vogelzang NJ. 2001. Docetaxel and exisulind in hormone-refractory prostate cancer. Semin. Oncol. 28:56–61.

302. Chetcuti A, Margan S, Mann S, et al. 2001. Identification of differentially expressed genes in organ-confined prostate cancer by gene expression array. Prostate. 2:132–140.

303. Bostwick DG, Qian J, Pacelli A, et al. 2002. Neuroendocrine expression in node positive prostate cancer: correlation with systemic progression and patient survival. J. Urol. 3:1204–1211.

304. Hansson J, Bjartell A, Gadaleanu V, Dizeyi N, Abrahamsson PA. 2002. Expression of somatostatin receptor subtypes 2 and 4 in human benign prostatic hyperplasia and prostatic cancer. Prostate 1:50–59.

8

Serum Tumor Marker Test Profile in Testicular Germ-Cell Tumors

Frank J. Liu, Robert M. Nakamura, C. Howard Tseng, and Kevin S. Liu

1. INTRODUCTION

1.1. Histologic Classification of Testicular Cancer

The primary testicular cancers are classified as testicular germ-cell tumors and non-germ-cell tumors of the testis. The testicular germ-cell tumors constitute approx 90 to 95% of all testicular cancers, whereas the incidence of non-germ-cell tumors of testes is usually less than 10% *(1)*. The testicular germ-cell tumors include seminoma, embryonal carcinoma, and teratoma with or without malignant transformation, choriocarcinoma, and yolk sac tumor (also known as endodermal sinus tumor, or embryonal adenocarcinoma of the prepubertal testis) *(1)*.

1.1.1. Histopathologic Classification of Testicular Germ-Cell Tumors

Histopathologic classifications of neoplasia and clinical staging evaluations of cancer have provided an important clinical basis for therapeutic decision-making *(1)*. Surgical pathology diagnoses of the surgically removed tumor tissue provide the most accurate skills of identifying and classifying a tumor and predicting and estimating its possible occurrence of local extent or metastasis into other organ systems *(1)*. There is a close relationship between serum tumor markers and histologic types of testicular germ-cell tumors; therefore, while applying the serum tumor marker tests, it is necessary to understand the interrelationship between the histologic types of testicular germ-cell tumors and the serum tumor markers *(1)*. The following four histologic classifications are listed for understanding the association of the histologic types of testicular germ-cell tumors with each serum tumor marker that is clinically useful for the management of patients with testicular germ-cell tumors.

1.1.1.1. REVISED WORLD HEALTH ORGANIZATION (WHO) CLASSIFICATION OF GERM-CELL TUMOR OF THE TESTIS

The WHO classification of testicular germ-cell tumors categorizes the tumors into three main groups:

1. Precursor lesion.
2. Tumors of one histologic type including seminoma, spermatic seminoma, embryonal carcinoma, yolk sac tumor, polyembryoma, trophoblastic tumors (choriocarcinoma: pure, mixed or placental-site implantation tumor), teratoma (mature teratoma, immature teratoma, and teratoma with malignant areas).

From: *Cancer Diagnostics: Current and Future Trends*
Edited by: R. M. Nakamura, W. W. Grody, J. T. Wu, and R. B. Nagle © Humana Press Inc., Totowa, NJ

3. Tumors of more than one histologic type *(2)*.

Relative frequency of histologic types of testicular germ-cell tumors are 35–70% for seminoma, 3–6% for embryonal carcinoma, 3% for teratoma in adults, and 38% for childhood, 1% for choriocarcinoma, and 60% for mixed tumors of more than one histologic type *(2)*. The majority of cases being the mixed tumor reflect the pluripotential nature of testicular germ-cell tumors *(1,2)*. The occurrence of different histologic types in the metastatic site compared to the primary tumor is evidence of the pluripotential nature of testicular germ-cell tumors, and in particular nonseminomatous tumors, more than half of which display different morphologies in primary vs metastatic sites, although pure choriocarcinoma invariably spreads unaltered *(1,2)*. For example, postmortem studies indicate that 30 to 45% of patients dying with seminoma in the primary tumor had nonseminomatous metastases; this is another evidence to reflect this nature *(1,2)*.

1.1.1.2. DIXON AND MOORE PATHOLOGICAL CLASSIFICATION OF TESTICULAR GERM-CELL TUMORS

Based on the clinical and pathological characters of testicular germ-cell tumors, Dixon and Moore classified testicular germ-cell tumors into five histopathological groups: group I, pure seminoma; group II, embryonal carcinoma, pure, or with seminoma; group III, teratoma, pure, or with seminoma; group IV, teratoma, with either embryonal carcinoma or choriocarcinoma or both, and with or without seminoma; and group V, choriocarcinoma, pure, or with embryonal carcinoma or seminoma or both *(3)*.

In the group of 166 patients with stage I, II, and III testicular germ-cell tumors at the University of Texas MD Anderson Cancer Center (UTMDACC), 18 (11%) patients had group I, pure seminoma; 67 (40%) had group II, embryonal carcinoma, pure, or with seminoma; 2 (1%) had group III, teratoma, pure, or with seminoma; 63 (38%) had group IV, teratoma, with either embryonal carcinoma or choriocarcinoma or both, and with or without seminoma; and 16 (10%) had group V, choriocarcinoma, pure, or with embryonal carcinoma or seminoma or both *(4,5)*.

1.1.1.3. BROAD CLASSIFICATION OF TESTICULAR GERM-CELL TUMORS

Testicular germ-cell tumors are broadly classified pathologically into two groups, as pure seminoma and nonseminomatous testicular germ-cell tumors *(1,6)*. The nonseminomatous testicular germ-cell tumors are further classified as embryonal carcinoma, teratoma, and choriocarcinoma *(1,6)*. Nonseminomatous testicular germ-cell tumors are often mixtures of more than one histologic type, sometimes including seminoma *(1,6)*. The classification is important, convenient, and significant for the management and treatment of patients, because each histological type should have different treatments and has its specific biological behavior, clinical outcome, and special association with different tumor markers *(1,6)*. Most clinical studies for tumor markers have classified the patients into these two groups and analyzed the impact of the use of tumor markers on each histologic morphology *(1,6)*.

1.1.1.4. CLASSIFICATION OF PREPUBERTAL TESTICULAR TUMORS

Seminoma and choriocarcinoma are extremely rare in children, therefore, adult classification for testicular tumors are not adequate for children *(7)*. The section on urology of the Academy of Pediatrics has developed the classification of prepubertal testis tumors *(7)*. It categorizes child testicular tumors as:

1. Germ-cell tumors that include yolk sac tumor, teratoma, teratocarcinoma, and seminoma.
2. Gonadal stromal tumors.

3. Gondablastoma.
4. Tumors of supporting tissues (fibroma, leiomyoma, and hemangioma).
5. Lymphomas and leukemia.
6. Tumor-like lesion (epidermoid cyst, hyperplasic nodule attributable to congenital adrenal hyperplasia).
7. Secondary tumors.
8. Tumors of adnexa *(7)*.

There is a difference of incidence of testicular germ-cell tumors between children and adults; only 60–75% of children's testicular tumors are germ-cell tumors, whereas 95% of all testicular tumors in adults are germ-cell tumors *(1,7)*. Another difference between adults and children is that the children have the higher incidence of benign tumors. Overall, the yolk sac carcinoma is the most common prepubertal testicular tumor *(7)*. This tumor is also known as an endodermal sinus tumor, orchidoblastoma, embryonal carcinoma, infantile adenocarcinoma of the testis, and a testicular adenocarcinoma with clear cells *(7)*.

1.2. Incidence of Testicular Cancer

The American Cancer Society (ASC) estimated that about 7600 new cases of testicular cancer were diagnosed in the year 2003 in the United States and an estimated 400 men died of testicular cancer in the year 2003 *(8)*. Testicular cancer is relatively rare when compared to the leading cancer types for the estimated new cancer cases in 2003 in the United States. Leading tyes of cancers include prostate, lung and bronchus, colon and rectum, urinary bladder, melanoma of skin, non-Hodgkin's lymphoma, leukemia, kidney, oral cavity, liver, esophagus, and pancreatic cancer as estimated by the ASC *(8)*.

1.2.1. Age-Specific Incidence

Testicular cancer is relatively rare, however, it represents the most common malignancy in men in the 15- to 35-yr-old age group and the second most common malignancy from age 35 to 40 in the United States *(1)*. Although testicular cancer may be seen at any age, it usually occurs in three distinct age groups: infants and children between 0 and 10 yr, young adults between the age of 20 and 40 yr, and older adults over the age of 60 yr *(1)*.

1.2.2. Histologic Types and Age Distribution

Different histologic types tend to occur at different age groups. Seminoma is the most common histologic type overall with a peak incidence between the age of 35 and 39 yr, however, it is rare under the age of 10 yr and above the age of 60 yr *(1,9)*. Choriocarcinoma constitutes only 1–2 % of testicular germ-cell tumors and is extremely rare in infancy but occurs more often between the ages of 20 and 30 yr *(1,2,9)*. Embryonal carcinoma and teratocarcinoma are present predominantly in the age group of 25 to 35 yr *(1,9)*. Yolk sac carcinomas are the predominant lesion of infancy and children, but are frequently found in combination with other histologic elements in adults *(1,7)*. Histologically, benign pure teratoma occurs most often in the pediatric age but frequently appears in combination with other elements in adults *(1,7,9)*.

1.3. Survival Improvement of Testicular Germ-Cell Tumor Patients

There have been improvements during the past three decades in survival of patients with testicular germ-cell tumors *(1,9)*. The survival of patients with testicular germ-cell tumors in the 1970s was only 10% with survival rates improving to 90% in the 1990s *(1,9)*. The advances in survival have resulted from combinations of accurate and sensitive imaging diagnostic techniques such as computed tomography (CT) scans and X-ray examinations; the successful integration of multimodal therapies including effective platinum-based combination chemotherapy regimens accompanied by improved and effective antimicrobial treatments with advanced general supportive therapy; improved radiation treatment, newly modified surgical procedures; and development and availability of clinically useful and relatively specific serum tumor marker tests in testicular germ-cell tumors *(1,6,9)*. A decrease in morbidity and mortality as a result of all these advances has resulted in an overall survival for patients with all stages of testicular germ-cell tumors of well over 80% and of almost 100% for patients with low stages of disease *(1,9)*. The overall 5-yr survival rates for all stages of disease for testicular germ-cell tumors are higher than that for any other cancers *(1,9)*. The modern approach to this disease with the above improved and effective multimodalities exemplifies the requirement of an effective cooperation and collaboration among the surgeon, oncologist, radiation therapist, radiologist, and clinical laboratory physician and scientist *(1,9,10)*.

1.4. Advancements of Serum Tumor Marker Tests for Testicular Germ-Cell Tumors

Research and development of serum tumor marker tests for testicular germ-cell tumors during the past four decades has resulted in better understanding of the biomolecular and clinical characteristics of current serum tumor markers; which help aid and confirm the diagnosis, facilitate case finding at the higher risk population, staging improvement, assist differential diagnosis of histologic types, prognostic prediction with outcome estimation, monitoring the response of the patients toward therapy, and early detection of recurrence *(1,9–11)*. These advancements allow careful follow-up with intervention and modification of therapy earlier in the course of disease, resulting in the survival improvement *(1,9–11)*.

1.4.1. Serum α-Fetoprotein, Serum Human Chorionic Gonadotropin, and Serum Lactate Dehydrogenase

Accumulated clinical data show that serum α-fetoprotein (AFP), serum human chorionic gonadotropin (HCG), and serum lactate dehydrogenase (LD) are well-established tumor markers integral to the successful management of patients with testicular germ-cell tumors *(11)*. Based on detailed review of published reports on germ-cell tumor markers followed by critical appraisal by a multi-specialty group of experts and finally validation of the draft guidelines by specialists in medical oncology, seven medical societies and organizations including the Association of Clinical Biochemists in Ireland (ACBI), the American Joint Committee on Cancer (AJCC), the European Association of Urology (EAU), the European Group on Tumor Markers (EGTM), the European Society of Medical Oncology (ESMO), the National Academy of Clinical Biochemistry (NACB), and the Scottish Intercollegiate Guideline Network (SIGN) have individually developed "Practice Guidelines for Tumor Marker use in Germ-cell Tumors" *(11)*. These reports, presenting guidelines for tumor marker usage in germ-cell tumors, provide useful and comprehensive summaries of relevant literatures *(11)*. Except for the ACBI and the AJCC guidelines, the other five organizations' guidelines recommend the three tumor-marker profiles of serum AFP, serum HCG, and serum LD as the gold standard for the management of testicular germ-cell tumor patients *(11)*. The ACBI guideline recommends only serum AFP and serum HCG without including serum LD for staging, prognosis, detecting recurrence, and monitoring therapy only *(11)*.

The AJCC guidelines suggest the use of serum AFP and serum HCG without serum LD and indicate the markers are useful for staging and prognosis only *(11)*.

1.4.2. Serum Lactate Dehydrogenase Isoenzyme 1

Studies have shown that the predominant and most important isoenzyme fraction of serum LD; which is associated with testicular germ-cell tumors, is the lactate dehydrogenase iso-enzyme 1 (LD-1) *(4,5,12–20)*. Total serum LD is a highly nonspecific test *(5,14)*. Serum LD-1 test is a more sensitive and specific test as a tumor marker than total serum LD for testicular germ-cell tumors *(4,5,12–20)*. Serum LD-1 is a useful adjuvant tumor marker for diagnosis, staging, monitoring the response to therapy, detection of recurrence, and prognostic estimation for patients with testicular germ-cell tumors *(4,5,12–20)*.

2. STAGING SYSTEMS OF TESTICULAR GERM-CELL TUMORS

Most testicular germ-cell cancers metastasize first along the lymphatic channels to the lymph nodes in the retroperitoneum, along the aorta and inferior vena cava *(1,6,9)*. Embryologically, the testicles develop within the abdominal cavity of the fetus and therefore derive their blood and lymph vessels from retroperitoneal, not the scrotal sources *(1,6,9)*. Blood borne metastases usually are a late event and the lungs are the most common metastatic organs *(1,6,9)*. At later stages, the tumors may metastasize to visceral organs; liver, brain, bone, or other organs *(1,6,9)*. Brain involvement is often not recognized at the early stage *(1,9)*. The stage of cancer at the time of diagnosis defines the extent of cancer involvement in a particular patient *(1,6,9)*. Clinical staging is performed preoperatively, whereas pathologic staging allows post-surgical assessment of the tumor size and location *(1,6,9,10)*. Disease staging dictates the treatment protocol *(1,6,9)*. Early stage disease, with the cancer confined to the organ of cancer origin, is effectively treated by surgery with or without adjuvant therapy including additional post-surgical treatments with cytotoxic drug administration and/or radiation therapy *(1,6,9,10)* Pre-operative chemotherapy may be given to reduce the tumor size prior to the surgery *(1,6,9)*. Regional extension of the cancer may determine the surgical treatment along with adjuvant radiation therapy or chemotherapy *(1,6,9)*. Patients with metastases to distant organs require systemic treatment with cytotoxic agents *(1,6,9,45)*. In testicular germ-cell tumors, the clinical staging is usually assessed following the orchiectomy with pathological confirmation of the histologic diagnosis. The patient is evaluated on the basis of noninvasive diagnostic procedures and techniques including physical examination, radiologic, and other diagnostic imaging techniques, such as chest X-ray, CT of abdomen, pelvis, brain or chest, laboratory studies including serum tumor marker tests *(1,9)*. Pathologic staging systems are based on surgical procedures, including retroperitoneal lymph node dissection, supraclavicular lymph node biopsy, and occasionally more invasive surgery. To determine the extent of the disease, detectable masses are dissected for cytoreductive operations for pathological examination *(1,6,9)*.

Clinical studies of serum tumor markers at different medical centers often examine the extent of the disease in patients with testicular germ-cell tumors and correlate the clinical significance of the tumor marker status with the prognostic outcome and treatment modality decision. Therefore, it is relevant to be familiar with commonly used staging systems used by different institutions that reported their studies on the tumor marker on testicular germ-cell tumor patients *(1,9,10)*.

Almost all current commonly used staging systems divide patients into three groups: stage I or A includes those with tumor confined to the testis, stage II or B includes those with tumor metastasis in the retroperitoneum, and stage III or C includes those with tumor gone beyond the retroperitoneum *(10)*.

2.1. Skinner and Water Reed Pathological Staging System

Skinner staging systems for testicular germ-cell tumors divide the disease into stage A, stage B, and stage C. Stage A includes those with tumor confined to testis *(10)*. Stage B includes those with metastasis in retroperitoneum lymph nodes only; further divided into: stage B1 with less than six positive nodes and nodes less than 2 cm; stage B2 with more than six positive nodes or any node greater than 2 cm and stage B3 with bulk disease, greater than five cm *(10)*. Stage C has disease beyond retroperitoneum *(10)*. Walter Reed staging systems are similar to the Skinner staging systems *(10)*. They use stage I for stage A, stage II for stage B, stage IIA for stage B1, stage IIB for stage B2, stage IIC for stage B3 and stage III for stage C in the Skinner staging systems *(10)*.

2.2. University of Texas MD Anderson
Cancer Center Clinical Staging System

Clinical staging at the University of Texas MD Anderson Cancer Center (UTMDACC) is done according to the following criteria based on the method of Samuels and associates: stage I patients had disease confined to the testes; stage IIA patients had microscopic evidence of metastasis in retroperitoneal lymph nodes; and stage IIB patients had gross evidence of metastasis in retroperitoneal lymph nodes; and stage IIC patients had extracapsular involvement of retroperitoneal lymph nodes *(21,22)*. Stage IIIA patients had metastatic disease confined to supraclavicular nodes; stage IIIB-1 patients had gynecomastia with or without elevation of serum AFP and serum HCG, but had no gross tumor detectable; stage IIIB-2 patients had minimal pulmonary disease, with total size of metastatic lung masses less than 40 cm^3; stage IIIB-3 patients had advanced pulmonary disease with any mediastinal or hilar mass, and neoplastic pleural effusion or intrapulmonary masses greater than 40 cm^3; stage IIIB-4 patients had advanced abdominal mass and ureteral displacement with obstructive uropathy *(21,22)*. Stage IIIB-5 patients had visceral disease (excluding the lungs) with metastasis to visceral organs such as the liver, gastrointestinal tract, brain, and inferior vena cava *(21,22)*. One difference from the other staging system is that the advanced abdominal disease is classified as a very advanced disease as stage IIIB-4 *(21,22)*.

2.3. International Germ-Cell Consensus Classification

The International Germ-Cell Collaboratory Group (IGCCC) developed a new staging classification of independent prognostic variables to predict survival for patients with metastatic testicular germ-cell tumors following analysis of a large population of over 5000 patients designated as the International Germ-cell Consensus Classification (IGCCC) *(23)*. The prognostic variables in the IGCCC staging system included the number of metastatic sites as well as concentrations of three serum tumor markers including serum LD, serum AFP, and serum HCG *(23)*. This staging system has three new features compared with previous classification systems: first, patients with seminoma have a better prognosis than patients with nonseminomatous germ-cell tumor; second, that patients with distant extrapulmonary metastases have a poor prognosis; and third, it includes three serum tumor markers of serum

LD, serum AFP, and serum HCG. The IGCCC separated patients into three categories based on the prognostic variables including the pretreatment concentrations of three serum tumor markers that contribute to the classification of metastatic germ-cell tumors as having good prognosis disease, intermediate prognosis disease, or poor prognosis disease *(23)*. The staging system has been supported by many studies. The IGCCC recommends oncologists use serum LD, serum AFP, and serum HCG as the "gold standard" in the staging of patients together with sites of metastases for patients with metastatic testicular germ-cell tumors *(23)*. Treatment strategy may be based on three categories of patients with metastatic testicular germ-cell tumors. Patients with a good prognosis receive the standard regimen with less toxicity and fewer side effects, whereas patients with poor prognoses receive more intensive chemotherapy to obtain a chance of cure even with the risk of higher toxicity *(24)*.

2.4. The International Union Against Cancer TNM Staging System

The fifth edition of the International Union against Cancer (UICC) TNM Staging System includes the prognostic value of the pretreatment marker concentrations of serum LD, serum AFP, and serum HCG established by the International Germ-cell Collaboratory Group. Additionally the conditions of T (primary tumor), N (lymph node metastasis), and M (distant metastasis) in the staging of patients with metastatic testicular germ-cell tumors *(25)* are included. It appears that the IGCCC was the bone frame of the fifth edition of the TNM staging classification *(23,25)*. Using these criteria, the patients are grouped into three stages. Pretreatment marker concentrations contribute to the classification of patients with metastatic germ-cell tumors as having low-, intermediate-, or high-risk subgroups similar as in the IGCCC *(25)*.

3. BIOMOLECULAR AND CLINICAL CHARACTERISTICS OF TUMOR MARKERS

Understanding the biomolecular and clinical characteristics of each clinical useful serum tumor marker is essential for appropriate use of the tumor marker tests to gain the best benefits for patients and reach the maximum effective treatment outcome. The biomolecular and clinical characteristics of the four clinically useful tumor markers including serum AFP, serum HCG, serum LD and, serum LD-1 isoenzyme are shown below. Although there are other tumor markers that have been reported to be elevated in some patients with testicular germ-cell tumors, these tumor markers did not provide significant clinical decision making information and are not recommended for clinical use for the management of patients.

3.1. Biomolecular and Clinical Characteristics of AFP

AFP is an oncofetal protein. AFP was the first tumor associated antigen to be used as a tumor marker in the clinical management of human malignancies. AFP is a glycoprotein with molecular weight of 61,000 to 70,000 Da, similar to albumin chemically and physically with a single polypeptide chain with interior regions homologous with human albumin. It has an isoelectric point of 4.8 and migrates as a homogeneous α-globulin on electrophoresis in an alkaline media. Chemically, it consists of 95% protein and 5% carbohydrate. AFP is synthesized in the liver, yolk sac, and gastrointestinal tract of the fetus and is a normal component of serum protein in human fetus older than 6 wk. The peak fetal serum AFP concentrations may reach 3–4 mg/dL by wk 12 to 15 of gestation. The predominant fetal serum protein serves many functions in fetus, as albumin does in the postnatal period. At birth, serum AFP declines to 30 µg/mL. At 1 yr of age, serum AFP decreases to normal adult value. The normal serum AFP range in adult is 2–10 ng/mL. Each laboratory should study, evaluate, and establish its own reference value independently, depending on the individual assay kit. The biological circulating metabolic half-life of serum AFP is 5 d. Using the sensitive and specific RIA or EIA assays, elevated serum AFP may be observed in a wide variety of both malignant and benign disorders. Serum AFP elevations have been reported in the following malignant disorders: hepatoma, testicular, and ovarian germ-cell tumors, malignant mixed Mullerian tumor of the ovary, gastric cancer, pancreatic carcinoma, male breast cancer, renal cell carcinoma, colonic carcinoma, and bronchogenic carcinoma. Increased serum AFP concentrations have been reported in benign conditions with viral hepatitis, chronic active hepatitis, postnecrotic and primary biliary cirrhosis, tyrosinemia, ataxia telangiectasia, and normal and abnormal pregnancy *(26–44)*.

3.2. Biomolecular and Clinical Characteristics of HCG

Measurement of elevated HCG in serum or urine has been used to diagnose pregnancy. HCG is a glycoprotein with molecular weight of 45,000 Da with branched carbohydrate side chains that terminate with sialic acid. HCG is normally composed of two dissimilar subunits, α and β polypeptide subunits. The α subunit of HCG has a molecular weight of 15,000–20,000 Da and is identical to and indistinguishable from that of pituitary hormones, including luteinizing hormone (LH), thyroid stimulation hormone (TSH), and follicular stimulation hormone (FSH). α-Subunit serves only as a carrier for the β-subunit chain. The β-subunit of HCG, which has molecular weight of 25,000–30,000 Da is a biologically active component. The β-subunit or C-terminal part of the β-subunit of HCG is structurally and antigenically distinct from that of the three pituitary hormones and therefore is specific immunogenically. During pregnancy, HCG is synthesized and secreted by the syncytiotrophoblastic cells of normal placenta. HCG is also secreted by various malignant neoplasms. HCG is normally absent or present in minimal amounts in the sera of nonpregnant women. The circulating half-life of serum HCG is between 24 and 36 h. The availability of sensitive and specific immunoassays for serum HCG using antibody against the β-subunit of HCG that do not crossreact with pituitary hormones including LH, TSH, and FSH has improved the diagnosis and management of normal and abnormal pregnancy, trophoblastic disease, and various malignant diseases. Malignant diseases with increased serum HCG are testicular and ovarian germ-cell tumors, breast cancer, melanoma, gastrointestinal tract cancer, hepatoma, pancreatic carcinoma, sarcoma, lung cancer, renal cancer, multiple myeloma, and other hematopoietic malignancies *(39,40,45–60)*.

3.3. Biomolecular and Clinical Characteristics of LD

LD is a ubiquitous cellular enzyme with molecular weight of 134,000 Da. It is present in the cytoplasm of all the cells and tissues in human body. It is a zinc containing enzyme that is part of the glycolytic pathway *(61)*. It is particularly abundant in smooth, cardiac, and skeletal muscles; liver, kidney, and brain *(14,61)*. Serum LD test is a highly nonspecific test; an abnormal elevation in serum can be caused by damage to any organs or by proliferation of any tissues *(61)*. Therefore, elevations of total serum LD do not provide clinically specific diagnostic information without the correlation of additional clinical and/or laboratory test findings *(61)*. Elevations of total serum LD may be seen in myocardial injury, pneumocytis carinii pneumonia, toxic or ischemic liver injury, megaloblastic anemia, hemolytic anemia, sepsis, or other causes of shock causing multiple organs damages and cardiopulmonary arrest, skeletal muscle injury, renal cortical infarct, and advanced malignant diseases including lymphoma, leukemia, multiple myeloma, renal cell carcinoma, ovarian dysgerminoma and testicular germ-cell tumors *(5,14,61)*. Total serum LD concentrations have been used as one of the three tumor marker profiles for testicular germ-cell tumors and reported to be a clinically useful tumor marker in diagnosis; monitoring the patient's clinical course, in staging, and for prognostic prediction for patients *(11,23,25)*. However, because of its low specificity, serum LD test results must be correlated with other clinical and laboratory findings for diagnosis and management of the patient *(4,5,61)*.

3.4. Biomolecular and Clinical Characteristics of LD-1

LD appears in serum and is present in tissues as five distinct isoenzymes that are tetramers of two active subunits, H designated for heart and M designated for muscle. These five isoenzymes are represented by LD-1 (HHHH), LD-2 (HHHM), LD-3 (HHMM), LD-4 (HMMM), and LD-5 (MMMM) *(14, 61)*. They can be separated by electrophoretic technique on the basis of their mobility *(14,61)*. LD-1 is the fastest anodally migrating isoenzyme and LD-5 is the slowest *(14)*. Relative percentage of these five isoenzymes in the serum and various tissues is different and is useful in differential diagnosis of elevated total serum LD *(14,61)*. The half-lives of LD isoenzymes are different for each LD isoenzymes *(61)* The half-life for LD-1 is approx 4–4 1/2 d, whereas that of LD-5 is from 4 to 6 h *(61)*. The LD isoenzymes are present in many human tissues with various percent of distributions *(14,61)*. Heart, kidney, brain, and erythrocytes have abundant LD-1, whereas liver, skeletal muscle and skin show the highest activity of LD-5 *(14,61)*.

Elevation of serum LD-1 is observed in patients following myocardial infarction, renal infarction, hemolytic anemia, and megaloblastic anemia *(14,61)*. An increase in serum LD-5 is observed in diseases associated with hepatic cell or skeletal muscle damage *(14,61)*. Three different types of LD isoenzyme patterns have been observed in a variety of malignancies. An elevated LD-5 to LD-1 ratio has been noted in malignant prostatic tumor, prostatic fluids, and in the serum of patients with prostatic carcinoma *(14,61)*. A general increase in LD-2, LD-3, and LD-4 isoenzymes has been observed in the serum of patients with leukemia, malignant lymphoma, metastatic carcinoma, neuroblastoma, and oral cancer *(14,61)*. Serum LD-1 isoenzymes have been found elevated in the serum of patients with osteosarcoma and germ-cell tumors of the testis and the ovaries *(14,61)*. If further identification of the source of the abnormal increase of total serum LD is indicated, electrophoretic separation of the five isoenzymes and the isoenzyme patterns may provide more specific clinical information, if alternative clinical and laboratory means cannot help differentiate the cause of abnormality *(14,61)*.

4. ASSOCIATION OF TUMOR MARKERS AND HISTOLOGIC TYPES OF TESTICULAR GERM-CELL TUMORS

4.1. Demonstration of Tumor Markers in Testicular Germ-Cell Tumor Tissues of Specific Histological Type

Various tumor markers have been shown to be present in the tumor cells or the cytosol of tumor tissues of specific histologic types of testicular germ-cell tumors using immunohistochemical staining *(12,62–68)*.

4.1.1. AFP in Testicular Germ-Cell Tumor Tissues of Various Histologic Types

Utilizing indirect immunoperoxidase technique, AFP was shown positive in the tumor tissue of 13 of 15 cases of yolk sac tumors, in 3 of 11 cases of teratoma, and in 3 of 14 cases of embryonal carcinoma *(62)*. Another study using an immunoperoxidase technique shows that AFP positivity was not found in the tumor tissue of 30 patients with seminoma; however, AFP was positive in 12 cases with endodermal sinus tumor elements, and additionally, in solid cell clusters in embryonal carcinoma areas, arising as a component of a mixed germ-cell tumor *(63)*. The same study also shows AFP-positivity in 54% of 37 cases with nonseminomatous tumors *(63)*. Simultaneous measurements of AFP concentrations in the peripheral serum and tumor cytosol of 40 patients with nonseminomatous testicular cancer show that serum AFP levels were normal in 13 of these 40 patients but AFP levels were elevated in 7 (54%) of 13 tumor cytosols from these 13 patients with normal serum AFP levels, indicating that tumor cytosols are more likely to have elevated levels of AFP than are sera in patients with testicular tumors *(64)*.

4.1.2. HCG in Testicular Germ-Cell Tumor Tissues of Various Histologic Types

The use of immunoperoxidase technique to localize HCG to specific histologic types of testicular germ-cell cancers, HCG was positive for syncytiotrophoblasts in 14 of 15 cases of nonseminomatous testicular germ-cell tumors, and for syncytiotrophoblasts in two of two cases of choriocarcinoma *(62)*. Another study using an immunoperoxidase technique shows HCG-positivity in 51% of 37 nonseminomatous tumors *(63)*. The same study shows that the HCG was localized in syncytiotrophoblastic-like giant cells, occurring in chorio-carcinomatous elements and as single cells in embryonal carcinomas, teratocarcinomas, and yolk sac tumors *(63)*. In the tumor tissues of 30 patients with seminomas, only one case of HCG positive giant cells was observed *(63)*. The status of immunohistochemical expression of HCG was examined in 45 seminoma tumor tissues and immunohistochemical expression of HCG was observed in syncytiotrophoblastic giant cells in 11 tumors and a few mono-nuclear seminoma cells in 36 tumors *(65)*. HCG positivity is also seen in mononuclear embryonal carcinoma cells *(66)*. Simultaneous measurements of HCG in the peripheral serum and tumor cytosol of 40 patients with nonseminomatous testicular cancers show that serum HCG levels were normal in 16 of 40 patients but HCG levels were elevated in 13 of 16 (81%) tumor cytosols from these patients with normal serum HCG levels. These findings indicate that tumor cytosols are more likely to have elevated levels of HCG than are sera in patients with testicular germ-cell tumors *(64)*.

4.1.3. LD-1 in Testicular Germ-Cell Tumor Tissues of Various Histologic Types

Elevated LD-1 isoenzyme pattern was demonstrated in both the tumor tissue and the serum of patients with seminoma and dysgerminoma as reported by Zondag in 1964 *(12)*. Using antiserum to LD-1, Murakami and Said determined immunohistochemical pattern of local-ization of LD-1 in the tumor tissues in several histopathologic types of testicular germ-cell tumors. LD 1 was found to be positive in the tumor tissues of all 29 seminomas and terato-carcinomas and four of seven embryonal carcinomas *(67)*. These results suggest that elevated serum LD 1 found in patients with testicular germ-cell tumors is synthesized and secreted into the circulation directly from the tumor cells as evidence of the association of serum LD-1 levels with the testicular germ-cell tumor. In addition, the levels of serum LD-1 may be related to the tumor burden *(67)*.

In addition, a study of LD isoenzyme patterns in both the tumor tissues and the serum of children with yolk sac tumors showed an elevated LD-1 in both the tumor tissues and the serum of the patients. On the basis of these findings, it is easy to assume that increased LD-1 in the serum of patients with yolk sac tumors is derived from tumor tissues, suggesting that serum LD-1 is useful as a tumor marker for yolk sac tumors, although it is not specific, and associated with other histologic types of testicular germ-cell tumors *(68)*.

4.2. Abnormal Serum Tumor-Marker Concentrations in Patients With Different Histologic Types

4.2.1. Association of Serum AFP and Histopathology of Testicular Germ-Cell Tumor

Highly elevated serum AFP concentrations are present in patients with tumors containing endodermal sinus (yolk sac) tumor elements irrespective of the location of the neoplasm or presence or absence of metastatic disease *(69,70)*. There is good correlation between the presence and quantity of endodermal sinus (yolk sac) tumor elements within the primary tumor or its metastases and elevated levels of serum AFP *(69,70)*. All patients with tumors composed of pure seminoma or dysgerminoma, and teratoma have normal serum AFP levels *(69)*. Slight elevations of serum AFP up to 60 ng/mg are observed in a few patients with testicular tumors composed of pure embryonal carcinoma, whereas patients with tumors composed of or containing endodermal sinus (yolk sac) tumor elements have serum AFP levels measured up to 100s or 1000s of ng/mL. Serum AFP would be elevated only in patients with active disease *(69)*. Serum AFP in all patients with gonadal tumors of non germ-cell origin is normal *(69)*. Serum AFP is a useful tumor marker for nonseminomatous testicular germ-cell tumors. Serum AFP was elevated in 67% of patients with advanced nonseminomatous germ-cell testicular tumors *(71)*.

4.2.2. Association of Serum HCG and Histopathology of Testicular Germ-Cell Tumor

Elevated serum HCG is correlated and relatively specific to choriocarcinoma *(39,40, 70–72)*. In one report on patients with advanced nonseminomatous testicular germ-cell tumors, patients with choriocarcinoma always have elevated HCG *(72)*. However, serum HCG elevations are also observed in seminoma, and all other histologic subtypes of nonseminomatous testicular germ-cell tumors *(39,40,65,66)*. The frequency of elevated serum HCG measured by immunoassays has been estimated to be 15% for seminoma, 50% for embryonal carcinoma, 42% for teratocarcinoma, and 100% for choriocarcinoma *(39,40)*.

4.2.3. Association of Serum LD-1 and Histopathology of Testicular Germ-Cell Tumor

Elevated serum LD-1 has been shown in patients with seminomas *(12,13)*. Serial determinations of serum LD-1 in eight children with yolk sac tumors show seven had elevated serum LD-1 and one without serum LD-1 abnormality had early stage of disease *(68)*. Abnormal levels of serum LD-1 activity have been observed in 34 of 42 patients (81%) with stage III testicular germ-cell malignancy *(14)*. Serum LD-1 elevation occurred in 4 of 6 patients (67%) with group I-pure seminoma, 17 of 21 patients (81%) with group II-embryonal carcinoma, pure, or with seminoma, 8 of 10 patients (80%) with group IV-teratoma with either embryonal carcinoma or choriocarcinoma or both, and all (100%) of the five patients with group V-choriocarcinoma, pure or with embryonal carcinoma or seminoma, or both *(14)*. In another group of 166 patients with stage I, stage II, and stage III testicular germ-cell tumors, abnormal serum LD-1 was observed in 11 of 18 patients (61%) with group I-pure seminoma; 39 of

67 patients (58%) with group II-embryonal carcinoma, pure, or with seminoma; 1 of 2 patients (50%) with group III-teratoma, pure, or with seminoma; 29 of 63 patients (46%) with group IV-teratoma, with either embryonal carcinoma or choriocarcinoma or both, and with or without seminoma; and 8 of 16 patients (50%) with group V-choriocarcinoma, pure, or with embryonal carcinoma or seminoma or both *(4,5)*.

4.3. Summary: Association of Tumor Markers and Histological Types

Based on the findings of the association of tumor markers both in tumor tissues and in the serum with the histologic types of testicular germ-cell tumors, the relationship between the tumor markers and the histologic types of testicular germ-cell tumors is summarized below.

Pure seminoma is associated with serum-HCG, serum-LD, and serum-LD 1 and must not have elevated serum AFP. If a patient, diagnosed by a surgical pathologist to have a pure seminoma, has elevated serum AFP; he must have nonseminomatous germ-cell components either in the primary tumor undetected and/or in undetected metastatic sites. Further studies with step sectioning of the tumor tissue or other means would usually find the nonseminomatous germ-cell tumor components; therefore, treatment has to be modified and treated the same as for the nonseminomatous germ-cell tumors. The embryonal carcinoma or mixed germ-cell tumor containing the embryonal components may have elevation of serum AFP, serum HCG, serum LD, and serum LD-1, yolk sac tumor is associated with increased serum AFP, serum LD, and serum LD-1, whereas choriocarcinoma is associated with serum HCG, serum LD, and serum LD-1. Mature teratoma does not have good tumor markers.

5. CLINICAL ROLE AND SIGNIFICANCE OF TUMOR MARKERS

The serum tumor-marker test profile of serum AFP, serum HCG, serum LD, and serum LD-1 play a significant role in diagnosis, staging, estimation of prognosis, monitoring the clinical course, and detection of recurrence of the patients with testicular germ-cell tumors *(4,5,11–20)*. Clinical role and significance of serum tumor markers for testicular germ-cell tumors are discussed below.

5.1. Diagnostic Purposes

Ideally, serum tumor marker tests for testicular germ-cell tumors should have the diagnostic ability to detect and diagnose all patients with testicular germ-cell cancers in all age groups of men and have the ability of providing a negative test result in all men without testicular germ-cell tumors, but may have other benign or malignant disorders and conditions. Unfortunately, like other currently available serum tumor marker tests, none of the four serum tumor marker tests for testicular germ-cell tumors possesses these characteristics of making a diagnosis easily. Therefore, the clinical usage of these serum tumor-marker tests, though very valuable in the management of testicular germ-cell cancer patients, is of limited value and may have greater value in other certain applications.

5.1.1. Screening for General Asymptomatic Population: Not Recommended

Because of insufficient clinical diagnostic sensitivity and clinical diagnostic specificity, all four currently available serum tumor marker tests may produce a significant degree of false-positive and false-negative test rates, which leads to the inability of these serum tumor marker tests to be used independently for cancer screening in the asymptomatic general population or as the sole criterion for making or ruling out a diagnosis of testicular germ-cell tumors *(11,73)*. Therefore, they are not recommended as screening tools to independently detect and diagnose testicular germ-cell cancers for the general asymptomatic population of men. None of the seven published "Practice Guidelines for Tumor Marker Use in Germ-Cell Tumors" recommends that the three tumor-marker tests including serum AFP, serum HCG, and serum LD be used as screening tools for general asymptomatic populations *(11)*. The same principle can be applied to serum LD-1 tumor marker test, because of its similar limited clinical diagnostic sensitivity and specificity *(4,5,14,15)*. However, an increasing understanding of cancer biology based on advances in basic sciences and technology has led to proper uses of these serum tumor-marker tests in correlation with clinical findings, other laboratory findings, and diagnostic imaging findings. This in turn, has provided a positive impact in the areas of cancer diagnosis and management, including case findings on symptomatic or high-risk individuals, diagnosis in patients with cancer, staging of diseases, correction of histopathological types and selecting the therapeutic modality, monitoring the clinical course of patients, and estimation of prognosis and outcome *(11,73)*.

5.1.2. Case Findings on Symptomatic Patients or High-Risk Individuals

Cancer screening using only serum tumor-marker tests should not be performed on the asymptomatic general population but can be done for symptomatic and high-risk individuals in conjunction with other diagnostic means *(11,73)*. For example, serum total PSA is now considered the best screening tumor-marker test for prostate cancer for high-risk age populations and symptomatic individuals *(11,73)*. It is accepted as an important component in the diagnostic algorithm used in early detection of prostate cancer in combination with the digital rectal examination *(73)*. The serum PSA screening program detects cancer at the earlier stages *(73)*. There is increasing evidence of its success in efficacy of radical prostatectomy and to reduce prostate cancer mortality rates *(73)*. Serum AFP is also used as a screening tool for primary hepatoma in China, because of high incidence of hepatoma in that country *(73)*. Ovarian cancer is often discovered and diagnosed at the advanced stage, therefore the use of serum CA 125 as a screening tool to detect ovarian cancer is being studied for early detection of ovarian cancer for the high-risk population *(73)*. Serum tumor-marker tests for testicular germ-cell tumors may be used in combination with physical examination (palpitation of the scrotum) and ultrasound examination for detection of the scrotal mass for case findings in the high-risk population, particularly in patients with symptoms and signs suggestive of testicular germ-cell tumors *(11)*. Five of the seven published "Practice Guidelines for Tumor Marker Use in Germ-Cell Tumors" including those by the EAU, EGTM, ESMO, NACB and SIGN, recommend the use of serum AFP, serum HCG, and serum LD for detection purposes *(11)*. Serum LD-1, which reports similar diagnostic specificity for testicular germ-cell tumors as serum AFP and serum HCG, can be used for this purpose *(4,5,12–20)*.

5.1.3. Diagnosis in Patients With Cancer

The serum tumor-marker tests for testicular germ-cell tumors cannot be used as the sole criterion to make a diagnosis of testicular germ-cell cancer resulting from the lack of acceptable clinical diagnostic specificity. Serum AFP, serum HCG, serum LD, and serum LD-1 are not specific for testicular germ-cell cancers, and they may be elevated in benign and malignant conditions other than testicular germ-cell tumors (*see* Section 3.). However, in patients with suspicion of testicular germ-cell tumors, the serum tumor-marker tests, particularly serum AFP, and serum HCG are specific and only rarely do patients with elevations of these tumor markers not have testicular germ-cell tumors *(6,45)*. A young male patient with a hard mass in one of his testicles with an elevation of either or both serum AFP and serum HCG is highly suggestive of testicular germ-cell cancer and most likely has a testicular germ-cell tumor. Rarely, this young man will be ruled out for that disease *(6,45)*. Serum LD-1 elevations also have the similar ability to provide this degree of relative diagnostic specificity *(4,5,12–20)*.

Although serum tumor-marker tests for testicular germ-cell tumors cannot be used independently to make a diagnosis of testicular germ-cell tumor, they can serve as a confirmatory aid in the diagnosis of symptomatic patients *(11)*. As an adjuvant in cancer diagnosis, these serum tumor-marker tests offer an opportunity to provide an early diagnosis *(11)*. In early diagnosis, when the cancer is still localized to the testis, patients can receive curative treatment earlier and easier. Normal serum tumor-marker test results must not be used to rule out a diagnosis of testicular germ-cell cancer, because a portion of patients with cancer do not have elevation of serum tumor markers *(6,45)*. Surgical exploration and histopathological examination and diagnosis remain the most insured method of diagnosis *(6)*. Five of the seven published "Practice Guidelines for Tumor Marker Use in Germ-Cell Tumors" including those by the EAU, EGTM, ESMO, NACB and SIGN, recommend the use of serum AFP, serum HCG, and serum LD for the purpose of diagnosis in testicular germ-cell tumors *(11)*. To improve the clinical diagnostic sensitivity and diagnostic specificity, use of multiple serum tumor-marker tests is observed and recommended for all cancer markers *(73)*.

5.1.3.1. TUMOR-MARKER PROFILE OF SERUM AFP AND SERUM HCG

The tumor-marker test profile of serum AFP and serum HCG has been shown to be the best tumor-marker system in human oncology, even though serum AFP and serum HCG are also elevated in the circulation of patients with other malignant and benign disorders *(6,45)*. Simultaneous assay of both serum AFP and serum HCG for patients with nonseminomatous germ-cell tumors has shown to increase clinical diagnostic sensitivity *(40)*. Serum AFP was abnormal in only 58% of patients with nonseminomatous germ-cell tumors and serum HCG was positive in 77% of the same group of patients. If both serum AFP and serum HCG were used together, 91% of these patients showed either serum AFP or serum HCG or both elevations *(40)*. Combined use of both serum AFP and serum HCG increases the clinical diagnostic sensitivity and when both markers are positive for a patient, the diagnostic specificity is also increased because rare disorders in men cause increase of both serum AFP and serum HCG concurrently *(6,45)*.

5.1.3.2. TUMOR-MARKER PROFILE OF SERUM AFP, SERUM HCG, AND SERUM LD

A study of 62 patients with advanced nonseminomatous testicular germ-cell tumors by measurements of serum HCG, serum AFP, serum LD, and serum carcinoembryonic antigen (CEA) shows that serum CEA was determined not a useful tumor marker for testicular germ-cell tumors *(71)*. Serum HCG was elevated in 64% of the patients, serum AFP elevation was observed in 67%, and serum LD was increased in 62% *(71)*. Either serum HCG or serum AFP was elevated in 86% of the patients *(71)*. We examined and recalculated the data included in the study and found that 41 patients had simultaneous assays of all the three tumor markers of serum HCG, serum AFP, and serum LD. Of these 41 patients, 16 (39%) had all the three markers, serum HCG, serum AFP, and serum LD elevations, 5 (12%) had both serum HCG and serum AFP increases, 2 (5%) had both serum HCG and serum LD abnormalities, 4 (10%) had both serum AFP and serum LD elevations, 3 (7%) had elevation of serum HCG only, 5 (12%) had an increase of serum AFP only, and 3 (7%) had a serum LD abnormality only *(71)*. Addition of serum LD to the serum tumor-marker test profile of serum HCG and serum AFP has increased the clinical diagnostic sensitivity of 7% *(71)*. Combined use of all three marker tests shows that at least one of these three tumor markers was elevated in 91% of patients *(71)*. There is still 9% of patients with diseases that have normal serum tumor-marker levels *(71)*. Another prospective study of 80 patients with testicular germ-cell cancers by simultaneous and serial determinations of serum LD, serum AFP, and serum HCG shows serum LD elevation in 78% of the stage III patients, serum AFP abnormality in 78.6%, and serum HCG elevation in 76.2% *(74)* Serum HCG and serum AFP concentrations were always elevated in the presence of elevated serum LD levels except in one patient when serum LD was the only elevated tumor marker, in which case changes of serum LD values correlated with clinical disease *(74)*. These two reports indicate that addition of total serum LD test as a tumor-marker test to the profile of serum AFP and serum HCG improves clinical diagnostic sensitivity *(71,74)*.

5.1.3.3. Tumor-Marker Profile of Serum AFP, Serum HCG, and Serum LD-1

Simultaneous measurements of serum AFP and serum HCG and serum LD-1 were done in 166 patients with stage I, stage II, and stage III testicular germ-cell tumors to evaluate the clinical usefulness of serum LD-1 levels as an additional tumor-marker test *(4,5)*. Serum AFP level was elevated in 90 of 166 patients (54%), serum HCG level was increased in 101 of 166 patients (61%), and serum LD-1 level was abnormal in 88 of 166 patients (53%) *(4,5)*. Of these 166 patients, 35 (21%) had elevations of all three tumor markers, 30 (18%) had elevations of both serum AFP and serum HCG levels, 13 (8%) had elevations of both serum AFP and serum LD-1 values, 25 (15%) had an increase of both serum HCG and serum LD-1 concentrations, 12 (7%) had elevations of serum AFP only, 11 (7%) had elevation of serum HCG only, and 15 (9%) had elevation of serum LD-1 only *(4,5)*. At least one of these three tumor markers was elevated in 141 (85%) of the 166 patients *(4,5)*. Adding serum LD-1 to the tumor-marker test profile of serum AFP and serum HCG increased the clinical diagnostic sensitivity from 76 to 85% *(4,5)*. Fifteen of these 166 patients (9%) who did not have either serum AFP or serum HCG abnormality benefited from having serum LD-1 as a tumor marker for management and treatment *(4,5)*. Serum LD-1 is a useful tumor-marker test for testicular germ-cell cancers *(4,5,12–20)*. The addition of serum LD-1 to the test profile of serum AFP and serum HCG not only has increased the diagnostic sensitivity but has increased the clinical diagnostic specificity when multiple tumor markers are elevated in one patient *(4,5,12–20)*. Serum LD-1 is a useful tumor marker for testicular germ-cell tumors *(4,5,12–20)*. In another group of 18 patients with pure seminomatous testicular germ-cell tumors, 10 patients (55%) had elevations of serum HCG and 11 patients (61%) had elevation of serum LD-1 *(5)*. When these two serum tumor-marker tests were used together, 9 (50%) had elevations of both serum HCG and serum LD-1, 1 patient (5%) had only serum HCG elevation, and 2 (10%) had only serum LD-1 abnormality *(5)*. At least one of these two serum tumor-marker tests would be elevated in 13 of the 18 patients (65%) *(5)*. Therefore, the combined use of serum LD-1 and serum HCG as the tumor-marker test profile has increased the clinical diagnostic sensitivity for seminoma *(5)*.

5.1.3.4. Tumor-Marker Profile of Serum AFP, Serum HCG, Serum LD, and Serum LD-1

Fifty-eight patients, with histologically confirmed testicular germ-cell tumors, were evaluated with simultaneous assays of all the four tumor markers including serum AFP, serum HCG, serum LD, and serum LD-1 *(15)*. Postsurgically, 21 of these 58 patients had no evidence of diseases, whereas 37 had evidence of disease. Of these patients, 19 had stage II and 18 had stage III diseases *(15)*. Serum HCG, serum LD, and serum LD-1 (except serum AFP) were all within the normal limits in the 21 patients who had no evidence of diseases *(15)*. However, 2 of the 21 disease-free patients had elevated serum AFP immediately after the surgery *(15)*. The elevated serum AFP values in these two patients declined to normal level in the follow-up *(15)*. In this study, the serum LD-1 abnormality was defined in three criteria; serum LD-1 absolute value expressed in absolute enzyme activity as U/L, greater than the upper limit of reference values; serum LD-1/total serum LD ratio greater than 0.25; and the third abnormality defined as serum LD-1/serum LD-2 ration greater than 0.8 *(15)*. Of the 37 patients with stage II and stage III testicular germ-cell tumors, 21 (57%) had elevations of serum LD, 14 (38%) had elevations of serum AFP, 25 (67%) had elevations of serum HCG, and 22 (60%) had serum LD-1 abnormality *(15)*. Twenty of the 22 patients with serum LD-1 abnormality had elevated serum LD-1 absolute value *(15)*. The elevation of serum LD-1 absolute values overlapped significantly with the elevated serum LD *(15)*. Twenty of 21 patients with elevated serum LD had elevated serum LD-1 absolute values *(15)*. Of the 20 patients with elevated serum LD-1, absolute values also included most patients with elevated serum LD-1/serum LD ratios and elevated serum LD-1/serum LD-2 ratios *(15)*. Of the 37 patients with stage II and stage III testicular germ-cell tumors, 9 had seminoma and 28 had nonseminomatous germ-cell tumors *(15)*. Serum HCG level was elevated in 6 of 9 patients (67%) with seminoma and serum LD-1 value was elevated in 7 of 9 patients (78%) with seminomas *(15)*. Further analysis shows that 5 of 9 (56%) patients with seminoma had elevations of both the serum HCG level and the serum LD-1 value, 1 of 9 patients (11%) had elevation of serum HCG only, and 2 of 9 patients (22%) had serum LD-1 elevation only *(15)*. When the two serum tumor-marker tests were used simultaneously, the clinical diagnostic sensitivity increased to 8 of 9 (88%) patients from 67% for serum HCG and 78% for serum LD-1 *(15)*. In the group of 28 patients with nonseminomatous germ-cell tumor, 19 patients (68%) had serum HCG elevations, 14 (50%) had serum AFP elevations and 13 (46%) had serum LD-1 elevations *(15)*. Of these 28 patients, 7 (25%) had elevations of all the serum AFP, serum HCG, and serum LD-1, 3 (11%) had elevations both serum AFP and serum HCG, 2 (7%) had elevations of both serum AFP and serum LD-1, 2 (7%) had elevations of both serum HCG and serum LD-1, 2 (7%) had elevations of serum AFP only, 7 (25%) had elevations of serum HCG only, and 2 (7%) had elevations of serum LD-1 only *(15)*. When all serum tumor-marker tests were assayed simultaneously, the clinical diagnostic sensitivity increased to 25 of 28 patients (89%) from the range of 46 to 68% when a simple serum tumor-marker test was used *(15)*.

5.1.4. Summary of the Role of Tumor-Marker Test for Diagnostic Purposes

In summary, the currently available serum tumor-marker tests for testicular germ-cell tumors should include serum AFP, serum HCG, serum LD, and serum LD-1. The serum tumor-marker tests should not be used in screening the general asymptomatic population for the purpose of making or ruling out a diagnosis of testicular germ-cell tumors. The serum tumor-marker tests may be applied for case findings on symptomatic patients and high-risk individuals. When they are utilized for diagnosis, they should not be used as the only criterion or utilized independently to make a diagnosis because of potential false positive test results or rule out a diagnosis because the test results are negative because of high false-negative results. They should be used as a confirmatory aid in diagnosis in patients with disease. Finally, when used for diagnostic purposes, simultaneous assays of multiple tumor-marker tests are the current recommended practice to enhance both clinical diagnostic sensitivity and specificity.

5.2. Tumor Markers and Stage of Diseases

Serum tumor-marker tests for testicular germ-cell tumors play a useful clinical role of improving staging accuracy, although the clinical role of serum tumor markers in staging is limited *(1,6,11,19,39,45–47)*. Despite the limitations, serum tumor-marker tests are helpful in staging and should be adopted as one of several modalities used for evaluation of the patient's extent of disease more accurately *(1,6,11,19,39,45–47)*.

5.2.1. Correlation of Frequency of Serum Tumor-Marker Abnormality With Stages of Diseases

A significant relationship is suggested between stage of disease and frequency of serum tumor-marker elevations in patients with testicular germ-cell tumors *(5,6,14,39,70,74)*. The frequency of serum AFP elevations in patients with nonseminomatous testicular germ-cell tumors correlates with the advance of disease stages *(39)*. Only 2 of 11 of patients (18%) with stage I disease had elevated serum AFP, while 11 of 19 (58%) stage II patients and 42 of 48 (87%) stage III patients with nonseminomatous testicular germ-cell tumors had abnormal serum AFP *(39)*. Frequency of elevations of serum AFP and/or serum HCG tests increases as the stage of disease increases *(70)*.

Serum LD and serum LD-1 were elevated more frequently with increasing tumor burden and increasing clinical staging *(4,5,14,74)*. The clinical values of serum tumor-marker tests for staging of patients with testicular germ-cell tumors are limited; because approx 60% of patients with microscopically positive lymph nodes in the retroperitoneum had normal preoperative serum tumor-marker levels and 45% of patients with grossly positive lymph nodes in the retroperitoneum also had normal preoperative serum tumor marker values. Additionally, 10% of patients with bulky retroperitoneal node diseases or distant metastatic disease had normal preoperative serum tumor-marker levels *(45)*. When the three serum tumor-marker tests including serum AFP, serum HCG, and serum LD-1 were assayed simultaneously, 50% of stage I testicular germ-cell tumor patients, 30% of stage II testicular germ-cell tumor patients, and 10% of stage III testicular germ-cell patients had normal serum tumor-marker test results of all the three tumor markers *(4)*. Therefore, normal serum tumor-marker test results do not indicate the absence of diseases *(4,6,14, 45)*.

5.2.2. Correcting Clinical Staging Error and Implementing the Proper Therapy

Despite the fact that the clinical role of serum tumor markers tests is of limited value in staging patients with testicular germ-cell tumors, they are of some value in patient staging *(1,11,19,39,40,46,47)*. The significant impact of serum tumor-marker tests in the staging of patients with nonseminomatous testicular germ-cell tumors has been the reduction of clinical staging errors, especially in the cases of understaging of the patients with non-seminomatous testicular germ-cell tumors *(1,11,19,39,40,46,47)*.

Serial measurements of both serum AFP and serum HCG postoperatively following orchiectomy have corrected and reduced the staging errors ranging from 28 to 59%, to 9 to 50% in clinical stage I patients with nonseminomatous testicular germ-cell tumors *(39,40,46,47)*. Persistent increases of serum AFP and/or serum HCG above the normal metabolic decay curve after orchiectomy in clinical stage I patients always indicate that the patients have actually stage II disease or stage III disease *(39,40,46,47)*. The clinical implication of correcting the clinical stage I error is important in selecting patients to receive adjuvant chemotherapy or other proper treatment modalities pertaining to the patient's true disease stage *(1,9)*. Similarly, persistently elevated serum AFP and/or serum HCG following a successful retroperitoneal lymph node dissection for patients with clinical stage II diseases indicate that patients have stage III disease *(47)*. These patients identified to have erroneous understaging can then receive proper and more intensive therapeutic regimens *(47)*. All seven published "Practice Guidelines for Tumor Marker Use in Germ-Cell Tumors" established by the ACBI, AJCC, EAU, EGTM, ESMO, NACB, and the SIGN recommend that both serum AFP and serum HCG are helpful in the staging of nonseminomatous germ-cell tumors *(11)*. However, only five of the seven guidelines including those published by the EAU, EGTM, ESMO, NACB, and the SIGN also recommend that the total serum LD test is a useful serum tumor marker for staging *(11)*.

Serial measurements of serum LD-1 tumor-marker test following orchiectomy in patients with clinical stage I nonseminomatous germ-cell tumors have also been reported to detect 2 of 10 patients originally classified as clinical stage I nonseminomatous germ-cell tumor of having pathological stage II diseases by evidence of persistent elevation of serum LD-1 postoperatively *(19)*.

Normal serum tumor-marker values or normal serum tumor-marker concentrations that fall at the normal decay rate during the postoperative period do not assure absence of residual diseases or disseminated disease *(47)*. A negative serum tumor-marker test result must not be used to rule out the presence of residual disease or the diagnosis of testicular germ-cell tumor *(6,45)*.

5.3. Correction of Histopathological Diagnosis Error and Selecting the Right Therapeutic Modality

Serum AFP and serum HCG tumor markers are closely related to the histopathological classification of testicular germ-cell tumors *(1,62,63,65,69–71,75,76)*. The broad classification of testicular germ-cell tumors into two groups as pure seminoma and nonseminomatous testicular germ-cell tumors has impacted choice of treatment modalities and other clinical management strategies for patients with testicular germ-cell tumors *(1,6)*. Treatment modalities for pure seminoma and nonseminomatous testicular germ-cell tumor are different based on their biological nature *(1,6,9,45)*. Usually, seminoma is sensitive to radiation therapy, therefore patients with stage I seminoma undergo conventional therapy for pure seminoma with orchiectomy and subsequent radiation therapy. The treatment of choice of for patients with nonseminomatous tumors receive chemotherapy after orchiectomy *(1,6,9,45)*. Studies have confirmed that pure seminoma does not produce AFP and only occasionally produces HCG. The majority of choriocarcinoma patients show elevated serum HCG. The adult type of embryonal carcinoma synthesizes AFP only or both AFP and HCG, pure endodermal sinus tumor produces only the AFP and mature teratoma does not produce any markers *(1,2,62,63,65,66,70–72)*.

Surgical diagnosis of testicular germ-cell tumors often shows a tumor containing two or more histopathological types within the primary tumor mass or one histopathological type in the primary tumor while another histopathological component may be found in the metastatic site, reflecting the pluripotential origin of the testicular germ-cell tumor *(1,2)*. The nonseminomatous germ-cell cancers may contain a seminomatous component in addition to an embryonic component *(1)*. If a patient with a histopathological diagnosis of a pure seminoma shows an elevated serum AFP, this patient must have nonseminomatous germ-cell cancer component undetected during surgical pathological examination *(1,6,10,11,75,76)*. Because a surgical pathological diagnosis is based on one or two small parts of tumor tissue sampled from the entire tumor mass, the nonseminomatous tissue component may not be included in tissue taken from the tumor for morphological diagnosis at the initial examination *(1,6)*. More sectioning of the primary tumor submitted for morphological examination often reveals the presence of nonseminomatous germ-cell neoplasm *(1)*. In many cases, the initial diagnosis of pure seminoma from institutions with little experience in diagnosing testicular germ-cell tumors, made a misdiagnosis of embryonal carcinoma as a pure seminoma *(6)*. Elevated serum AFP level helps correct the missing histological diagnosis of nonsemi-nomatous germ-cell tumors *(1,6,10,11,75,76)*. This corrected diagnosis helps to select the proper therapy resulting in the better outcome. Seminoma is a radiation sensitive cancer, although the nonseminomatous testicular germ-cell carcinoma is more susceptible to che-motherapy *(1,6)*. However, only four of the seven "Practice Guidelines for Tumor Marker Use in Germ-Cell Tumors" including those published by the EAU, EGTM, ESMO, and NACB recommend that elevated serum AFP be used for the differential diagnosis of histo-pathology for nonseminomatous testicular germ-cell tumors *(11)*.

5.4. Monitoring the Clinical Course of Patients

The most important role of serum tumor-marker tests is observing the changes of disease activities and serving as a guide to further therapeutic strategy for patients with nonseminomatous testicular germ-cell tumors *(4–6,11,14,45,69)*. Serial serum tumor-marker test profiles before, during, and after treatment in patients with testicular germ-cell cancers have been useful for determining the efficacy of surgery, the response of patients to postoperative radiotherapy and/or chemotherapy, for predicting prognosis, and for early detection of disease recurrence *(4–6,11,14,20,45,52,69,77)*.

5.4.1. Assessing the Response of Patients to Therapy

The greatest values and impact of serum AFP and serum HCG in the management and treatment of patients with nonseminomatous testicular germ-cell tumors is monitoring the clinical course of patients after surgery, after a completion of chemotherapy and/or radio-therapy, and during the therapy *(6,11,45,52,69,77)*. After successful and complete surgical removal of a tumor from stage I patients with preoperatively increased serum AFP and/or serum HCG, the serum AFP and/or serum HCG levels decline to normal according to the theoretical decay half-life of the tumor markers *(52,77)*. However, negative serum AFP and/or serum HCG results after chemotherapy do not necessarily mean that the patient is disease free, because serum AFP and/or serum HCG values often return to normal before the tumor cells are completely eradicated *(45,52)*. Therefore, normal serum AFP and serum HCG values after therapy must not be a signal to stop planned chemotherapy *(45,47,52)*. During chemotherapy, sustained and elevated serum AFP and/or serum HCG values indicate persis-tent disease and continuous escalation of serum AFP and/or serum HCG concentrations accompany progression of the disease, suggesting that the current chemotherapy is ineffec-tive and alternative treatments should be considered *(45,47,52,69)*.

Studies of total serum LD as a tumor-marker test for stage B and stage C testicular germ-cell tumor patients show that serum LD has similar clinical characteristics in monitoring and evaluation of the clinical course of patients as serum AFP and serum HCG *(11,71,74,78)*. Serial determinations of total serum LD reflect that decreasing disease activity is accompanied by the decline of the initially increased total serum LD; and when the patients are resistant to therapy or have progression in disease activity, the stationary or progressive disease activity is associated with sustained or progressively increasing levels of total serum LD *(78)*. As reported by Lieskovsky and Skinner, all patients with persistent elevations of total serum LD after treatment have either died or experienced progression of diseases *(78)*. Serum LD tests provide a similar clinical role as serum AFP and/or serum HCG does in monitoring the clinical course of patients with testicular germ-cell tumors *(78)*. In addition, a portion of patients with diseases have normal total serum LD values emphasizing false negative results cannot be used to rule out the presence of a residual diseases *(74,78)*. Six of the seven published "Practice Guidelines for Tumor Marker Use in Germ-Cell Tumors" including those developed by the ACBI, EAU, EGTM, ESMO, NACB, and SIGN recommend that two tumor markers of serum AFP and serum HCG be used in the monitoring of the clinical course of diseases for testicular germ-cell tumors *(11)*. Five of these six guidelines established by the EAU, EGTM, ESMO, NACB, and SIGN also suggest that serum LD test is a useful serum tumor marker for monitoring the disease course of the testicular germ-cell tumor patients *(11)*.

Studies of serum LD-1 tumor-marker test for testicular germ-cell tumors have shown that the serum LD-1 test is a useful tumor marker for monitoring the clinical course of patients *(4,5,14)*. Serial measurements of serum LD-1 in patients with testicular germ-cell tumors have clinical value in monitoring the patients' disease activity in relation to their response to therapy *(4,5,14)*. Again, there are patients who have active disease and normal concentrations of serum LD-1 indicating that there are also false negative results of serum LD-1 in patients with active diseases *(4,5,14)*.

5.4.2. Detection of Recurrent Disease or Metastatic Diseases

Serum AFP and serum HCG test profiles are indispensable in testicular germ-cell cancer patients for detecting disease recurrence and metastasis *(45,47,52,69,79)*. Serial measurements of serum AFP and serum HCG in testicular germ-cell cancer patients on surveillance predict disease recurrence several months earlier than do radiographic or other diagnostic methods *(9,45,52)*. A retrospective study proposed that more frequent monitoring to ensure detection of all recurrences at a minimal disease state is necessary *(80)*. Serial and simultaneous determinations of serum AFP, serum HCG, and serum LD for follow-up purposes show that the earliest indicator of recurrence was the elevated serum tumor-marker levels for patients with nonseminomatous testicular germ-cell tumors in those cases that serum tumor-marker test results detect the recurrence of the disease; whereas the earliest indicator of disease recurrence for patients with pure seminomas is the radiologic change *(81)*. Early detection of recurrence should not rely only on serum tumor-marker levels because not all the patients with disease or recurrence had elevated tumor markers *(81)*. Six of the seven current "Practice Guidelines for Tumor Marker Use in Germ-Cell Tumors" including those established by the ACBI, EAU, EGTM, ESMO, NACB, and SIGN, have recommended that serum AFP and serum HCG be used in detecting the recurrence of diseases, whereas five of these six guidelines also include total serum LD test in addition to serum AFP and serum HCG as a useful tumor marker for detection of recurrence *(11)*. Serum LD-1 tests were elevated in 11 of 21 patients with testicular germ-cell tumors at the time of relapse of the disease *(20)*. Seven of these 11 patients had elevations of serum LD-1 with a median time of 2 mo ranging from 1.4 mo to 4.5 mo preceding other means of detection or evidence of relapse of the disease *(20)*. Serum LD-1 tests as a serum tumor-marker test for testicular germ-cell tumors can help detect the relapse of the cancer earlier in some cases complementary to serum AFP and serum HCG, and diagnostic imaging techniques *(20)*.

5.4.3. Transient Rise in Tumor Marker

Some patients with advanced testicular germ-cell cancers with bulky tumor masses, have an acute transient increase of serum AFP and/or serum HCG during the initial induction phase of chemotherapy, even though radiographic and other evidence shows that the tumor is responding to the therapy and reducing in size *(82–85)*. This discordance between the serum AFP and/or serum HCG values and disease status by imaging results from tumor cytolysis followed by release of AFP and/or HCG into the circulation *(47)*. This phenomenon is called "paradoxical elevation" of serum tumor markers or marker surge. A paradoxical elevation of serum tumor marker requires definite radiologic or other diagnostic imaging evidence of reduction in tumor masses followed by the decline of serum tumor marker concentration; even if the serum tumor marker level may or may not rebound at a later date. This condition should not be considered as an adverse prognostic factor indicating a progression of disease because of the sudden escalation of the serum tumor-marker levels. Frequent monitoring of the serum tumor-marker level is required to observe the patient's disease activity in either cure or recurrence.

5.5. Estimation of Prognosis and Predicting the Outcome

Pretreatment serum tumor marker concentrations and patterns of serum tumor marker level changes during and after treatments in patients with testicular germ-cell tumors are of value in estimating the prognosis and predicting the outcome *(11,14,16,17,23,25, 49,50,70,74,77,84,86–105)*.

5.5.1. Pretreatment Serum Tumor-Marker Levels

Initial concentrations of the four serum tumor markers of serum AFP, serum HCG, serum LD, and serum LD-1 before the treatment have prognostic values for patients with testicular germ-cell tumor, particularly in patients with advanced stages of diseases.

5.5.1.1. PRETREATMENT SERUM AFP, SERUM HCG, AND SERUM LD VALUES AS PROGNOSTIC PREDICTOR

Pretreatment serum AFP and serum HCG values are independent prognostic variables for patients with advanced nonseminomatous testicular germ-cell tumors *(11,23,25,70,86–96)*. Serum AFP greater than 500 ng/mL and/or serum HCG greater than 10,000 mL U/mL are considered to have unfavorable prognosis *(86)*. The genitourinary consensus conference of the 1990 European Organization for Research on Treatment of Cancer (EORTC) reported that seven of the eight larger studies summarized that the pretreatment serum HCG value was a significant prognostic factor and four of the eight studies considered that serum AFP greater than 500 ng/mL predicted a poor prognosis *(87)*. It is best to use serum tumor marker values together with a clinical staging system *(88,89)*. For example, a favorable minimum lung presentation may be unfavorable with high serum tumor marker values and an unfavorable advanced abdominal presentation may actually be favorable if both serum AFP and serum HCG values are low *(88,89)*. Using different cutoff values of serum AFP and/or serum HCG, many investigators report that pretreatment concentrations of these two serum tumor maker levels can provide the prognostic values as well *(70,90–95)*. The pretreatment serum LD levels have been reported useful prognostic predictor for metastatic testicular germ-cell tumors *(74,96)*. In a study of 43 patients with testicular germ-cell tumors with normal total serum LD levels prior to therapy; mean survival time was 15.5 mo; while another group of 26 patients who had pretreatment elevated total serum LD levels had a shorter mean survival time of 9.2 mo *(74)*. Serial determinations of total serum LD in 44 patients with non seminomatous germ-cell tumors of the testis show that a poor prognosis was associated with abnormal elevations of total serum LD, whereas 92% of patients with normal total serum LD level had a survival time longer than 5 yr, no patient with elevated total serum LD had a survival time longer than 4 yr suggesting that the initial total serum LD concentrations are of prognostic value.This difference was especially significant in patients with advanced stages of disease *(96)*. Serial measurements of total serum LD are of value as prognostic indicator and when elevated, might be utilized as a guide for response to therapy *(96)*.

The prognostic significance of the pretherapy serum AFP, serum HCG, and serum LD levels for patients with metastatic testicular germ-cell tumors discussed above has been confirmed by studies of the International Germ-cell cancer Collaborative Group (IGCCCG) that developed the International germ-cell consensus classification system (IGCCC) *(23)*. Pretreatment marker concentrations are included as one of variables for classification of metastatic germ-cell tumors into three categories; good, intermediate, or poor prognosis *(11,23,25)*. The UICC TNM staging system stratifies the three serum tumor marker values into four categories designed as S0, S1, S2, and S3 *(25)*. The S0 category has all three serum marker levels within normal limits; S1:Serum LD is <1.5 × ULR (upper limits of reference values) and serum HCG is <5000 mIU/mL and serum AFP is <1000 ng/mL; S2:serum LD is 1.5–10 × ULR or serum HCG is 5000–50,000 mIU/mL or serum AFP is 1000–10,000 ng/mL; and S3: serum LD is >10 × ULR or serum HCG is >50,000 mIU/mL or serum AFP is >10,000 ng/mL *(25)*. The international classification included only two cutoff points to predict the outcome of patients with metastatic testicular germ-cell tumors *(25)*. Low levels of the serum tumor markers, the S0 and S1 categories, for patients with metastatic testicular germ-cell tumors indicate a standard risk for death of tumor *(25)*. High levels of the serum tumor markers, the S2 and S3 categories, indicate two levels of increased risk *(25)*. The IGCCC incorporates the S0 into the S1 with cutoff points of the three serum tumor markers being separated as S1, S2, and S3 categories. S1 is designated as a good prognosis marker level, S2 as an intermediate prognosis marker level, and S3 as a poor prognosis marker level *(23)*. All the seven "Practice Guidelines for Tumor Marker Use in Germ-Cell Tumors" developed by the ACBI, AJCC, EAU, EGTM, ESMO, NACB, and SIGN recommend that serum AFP and serum HCG are useful markers for prognosis *(11)*. Only five of the seven guidelines suggest that serum LD can be used in prognosis evaluation *(11)*.

5.5.1.2. Pretreatment Serum LD-1 Values as Prognostic Predictor

Pretreatment serum LD-1 concentrations can also provide some prognostic values and are useful in predicting the clinical outcome of patients *(14,16,17)*.

In a study of 42 patients with advanced testicular germ-cell cancers, abnormal levels of serum LD-1 were observed in 34 patients (81%) with stage III germ-cell malignancy of the testis *(14)*. All (100%) of the 8 patients with pretreatment normal serum LD-1 levels responded to the therapy and achieved complete remission and remained free of disease with serum LD-1 values remained normal *(14)*. Only 16 patients (47%) with pretreatment elevated serum LD-1 achieved complete remission and remained free of diseases with return of the abnormal serum LD-1 levels to normal. A total of 18 (53%) patients either did not respond to therapy or achieved partial remission and complete remission during the disease course followed by recurrent diseases with sustained, progressive or recurrent elevations of serum LD-1 *(14)*. Interestingly, 14 patients with metastatic diseases to the liver had elevated serum LD-1 instead of serum LD-5 elevations. Logically, metastatic disease to the liver should result in the increase of the LD-5 isoenzyme secondary to damage of the liver parenchyma *(14)*. This observation suggests that testicular germ-cell tumors synthesize predominantly the LD-1 isoenzyme and release into the circulation *(14)*.

Eighty-one patients with metastatic testicular germ-cell tumors were monitored with all four serum tumor markers including serum LD-1, serum LD, serum HCG, and serum AFP according to the criteria set by the IGCCCG for serum LD, serum AFP, and serum HCG *(16)*. Forty-two of 81 patients (52%) had an increased serum LD-1 and 41 of these 42 patients also had an elevated total serum LD level *(16)*. However, an additional 8 patients had an increased total serum LD with a normal serum LD-1 level *(16)*. A total of 39 patients with normal serum LD-1 concentrations had the best survival *(16)*. This favorable survival was not related to whether total serum LD was normal (31 patients) or total serum LD was elevated (8 patients) *(16)*. Serum LD-1 provided better prognostic information for the metastatic testicular germ-cell tumor patients than total serum-LD levels *(16)*. These results indicate that pretherapy serum LD-1 is better than total serum LD to predict the survival of patients with metastatic testicular germ-cell tumors. Accordingly, if the increase of total serum LD is not a result of the increase of serum LD-1, the prognostic implication of elevated total serum LD may not be grave because elevation of total serum LD is not caused by the elevation of serum LD-1 *(16)*. The results of this study suggest that serum LD-1 offers a greater difference in survival between the subgroups of patients with the best and the worst survival than the IGCCCG classification *(16)*. Overall, serum LD, serum HCG, and the prognostic classification of the IGCCCG study also showed predictive value for the survival, although serum AFP did not provide prediction for survival *(16)*.

The IGCCC staging system, which includes the prognostic variables of serum LD, serum AFP, and serum HCG, indicates that these three serum tumor markers could predict the death of patients with metastatic testicular germ-cell tumors from tumors *(23)*. In a study of 44 patients with metastatic germ-cell tumors, serum LD-1 levels using univariate analysis were shown to be a better predictor than criteria established by the international classification for the other three serum tumor markers *(17)*. In this evaluation, serum LD-1 levels greater than the upper limit of reference value are considered to be abnormally elevated *(17)*. A total of 100% of patients with a normal serum LD-1 had the survival rate of 5 yr; 81% of patients with a normal total serum LD had the survival rate of 5 yr; 75% of patients with a normal serum AFP had the survival duration of 5 yr, and 77% of patients with a normal serum HCG had the survival duration of 5 yr *(17)*. An elevated serum LD-1 had a predictive value of 46% for death from tumors in 5-yr; an elevated total serum LD had the predictive value of 46% for death from tumor in 5-yr; an elevated serum AFP had the predictive value of 25% for death from tumors in 5 yr; and an elevated serum HCG had the predictive value of 40% for death from tumor in 5-yr *(17)*. Of the patients who died of tumor, 100% had an elevated serum LD-1; 46% had an elevated total serum LD; 9% had an elevated serum AFP; and 18% had an elevated serum HCG *(17)*. Of the patients who did not die of tumors, 61% had a normal serum LD-1; 81% had a normal total serum LD, 94% had a normal serum AFP; and 94% had a normal serum HCG. These data indicate that an increased value of serum LD-1 classified more patients to a subgroup having an impaired survival than of serum LD, serum AFP, and serum HCG (17).

The prognostic value of pretreatment serum LD-1 was evaluated in 110 patients with testicular seminoma clinical stage I diseases followed with surveillance after orchiectomy (106). The patients with elevated serum LD-1 and those with normal serum LD-1 had a similar relapse or free survival (106). Elevated serum LD-1 did not predict a relapse during follow-up with surveillance in clinical stage I seminoma patients (106). The pretreatment serum LD-1 values do not provide a prognostic value for patients with seminoma in the early stage of disease (106).

5.5.2. Serum Tumor-Marker Decline Rate (Marker Half-Lives)

The clearance rates of a biological substance in the circulation are usually expressed as metabolic half-lives (31,48). The rate at which the serum tumor-marker values decrease after surgical removal of the tumor, during or after chemotherapy or radiation therapy, is designated as the actual half-life (AHL), marker decline, or marker half-life (MHL) (77,84,95,97–105). The metabolic clearance rates of serum AFP and/or serum HCG have been reported to be a significant prognostic factor for nonseminomatous testicular germ-cell tumor patients (77,84,95,97–105). The MHL of serum AFP and serum HCG is a useful prognostic factor in postoperative follow-up studies for patients with clinical stage I testicular germ-cell tumor patients (77,97,98). Following orchiectomy in patients with clinical stage I testicular germ-cell tumors, an increased or prolonged MHL of serum AFP and/or serum HCG usually indicates a residual active tumor after surgical resection (77,97,98). The MHL of AFP may be more sensitive than serial monitoring of AFP in detecting preclinical recurrence after surgical resection of AFP-secreting tumors (77,97,98). A normal MHL may suggest that surgical removal of the tumor is complete, but not all patients with normal MHL are completely free of a residual active tumor, because patients may still have the germ-cell tumor component of other histological subtypes (77). Therefore, abnormally prolonged MHL of serum tumor markers postoperatively is a significant prognostic variable indicating the presence of a residual cancer that requires further treatments (77,97,98).

Many studies have indicated that the MHL of serum AFP and serum HCG during the initial phase of chemotherapy is a prognostic indicator reflecting tumor burden and predicting the clinical outcome and dividing the patients between good prognosis and bad prognosis, which in turn can help make therapeutic decisions (77,84,95,97,99–105). These studies usually use 3 or 3.5 d as cutoffs for MHL of serum HCG and 7 d for serum AFP as the upper limit of the reference values for the MHL (77,84,95,97,99–105). When MHL of serum HCG is equal to or less than 3 or 3.5 d, it is considered normal AHL, normal MHL, or satisfactory marker decline (77,84,95,97,99–105). If the MHL of serum HCG is longer than 3 or 3.5 d, the MHL is prolonged, abnormal, increased AHL, prolonged, abnormal, increased MHL, or an unsatisfactory marker decline (77,84,95,97,99–105). The same parameters are applied to estimation of MHL of serum AFP using the cutoff of 7 d (77,84,95, 97,99–105). Prolonged, increased, or abnormal MHL, or a prolonged, abnormal; or increased AHL or unsatisfactory marker decline during the initial phase of chemotherapy, reflects ineffective chemotherapy indicating the presence of residual disease. It is recommended that patients require alternative and more intensive therapy if an acute transient rise of the serum tumor marker resulting from tumor cytolysis can be ruled out (77,84,95,97,99–105). A normal MHL usually indicates that the therapy is effective; disease activity is reducing; patients are responding to treatments, and have a better prognosis with greater chance of achieving complete remission and cure *(77,84,95,97,99–105)*. Studies using the similar principle but a modified criteria of serum HCG in patients with disseminated testicular germ-cell tumors and elevated serum HCG value during the first cycle of chemotherapy show that the ratio of d 22 serum HCG value to d 1 serum HCG value below 1:200 was highly predictive of a complete response, a ratio above this level suggested an incomplete response *(49,50)*. Although a significantly prolonged MHL likely suggests failure to therapy and the presence of chemotherapy resistant cells, many patients with a normal MHL fail to respond to the treatment *(47)*.

The prognostic value of the MHL of serum AFP and serum HCG has been debated and controversial. Several reports indicated that only the MHL of serum AFP is a useful prognostic predictor, but the MHL of serum HCG did not discriminate between patients remaining well or those who relapsed after chemotherapy nor did the prolonged MHL of serum HCG half-life adversely affect event-free survival and overall survival *(107,108)*. A few reports argued that the MHL patterns of serum AFP or serum HCG did not predict the outcome of chemotherapy with certainty; evaluation of the MHL of serum AFP and serum HCG during the initial chemotherapy did not predict patients at higher risk of progression and also was a poor guide to long-term prognosis; and MHL patterns were inaccurate parameters for the prediction of treatment failure *(94,109–111)*. In response to arguments regarding discrepant results on the prognostic significance of the MHL of serum AFP and serum HCG during the early phase of chemotherapy in testicular germ-cell tumor patients, one of the groups that initially published favorable results on this subject *(100–102)* re-evaluated the prognostic values of the MHL of serum AFP and serum HCG together with IGCCC staging system developed by the IGCCCG and studied both the patients with normal MHL and with prolonged MHL regarding their prognostic significance *(105)*. They evaluated 189 germ-cell cancer patients with elevated levels of serum AFP and serum HCG treated with platinum-based chemotherapy *(105)*. Based on the IGCCC criteria, the patients were classified into three groups: as good prognosis disease, intermediate prognosis disease, or poor prognosis disease groups and patients were separated into two groups as having normal MHL; and prolonged MHL *(105)*. The IGCCC staging classification and the MHL status of the patients were correlated with response, event-free survival, and overall survival *(105)*. Patients with normal MHL had statistically significant better complete response (CR) rates and better event-free and better overall survival ($p < 0.0001$) *(105)*. Ninety two percent of patients with normal MHL and 62% of patients with a prolonged MHL achieved CR; 91% of patients with normal MHL and 69% of patients with a prolonged MHL had 2-yr event-free survival; and 95% of patients with normal MHL and 72% of patients with a prolonged MHL had 2-yr overall survival *(105)*. MHL was still a significant variable for all three end-points when adjusted for the IGCCC staging groups ($p < 0.01$) with outcome differences most pronounced in the poor-prognosis disease group *(105)*. The authors concluded that the MHL of serum AFP and serum HCG during chemotherapy has prognostic value independent of the IGCCC prognosis staging and may play a significant role in the management of poor-prognosis disease patients *(105)*.

6. RECOMMENDED PROCEDURES FOR MEASUREMENTS OF SERUM TUMOR-MARKER TESTS AND INTERPRETATION OF TUMOR-MARKER TEST RESULTS

The following test-ordering procedures and interpretation guidelines of the serum tumor-marker test results are recommended based on the knowledge of biomolecular and clinical characteristics, interrelationship between the histologic subtypes of testicular germ-cell tumors, and the clinical role and significance of the serum tumor markers for the testicular germ-cell cancers. These recommendations may be applied when using the serum tumor-marker tests in daily practice.

6.1. Uses of Multiple Markers to Improve the Diagnostic Sensitivity and the Diagnostic Specificity Both at the Time of Diagnosis and During Monitoring

It is generally recommended that multiple marker tests be determined for improving both the clinical diagnostic sensitivity and specificity *(73)*. To improve the clinical diagnostic sensitivity and specificity, it is recommended that all four serum tumor-marker tests include serum AFP, serum HCG, serum LD, and serum LD-1 be tested at time of diagnosis and during monitoring for testicular germ-cell tumors. None of these tumor-maker tests have perfect clinical diagnostic sensitivity or specificity, and heterogeneous expressions of tumor markers by cancer cells of the same histologic type will maximize the clinical diagnostic sensitivity and specificity.

It is generally thought that only initially elevated tumor markers prior to surgery be selected for monitoring recurrence *(73)*. However, both serum AFP and serum HCG should be tested regularly at various intervals dependant upon the histology, stage, and postorchid-ectomy treatment chosen regardless of the serum tumor-marker level as markers may be normal at presentation *(6,11,81)*. The reason for this is as follows: one serum tumor marker may be initially elevated and the other tumor marker normal, later during the course of disease the elevated serum tumor marker may return to normal and the other initially normal serum tumor marker may rise *(6,81)*. This type of discordant expression of the serum tumor marker not only provides useful information regarding the tumor activity but also may reflect the different histologic subtypes or tumor cell populations in relation to the tumor-marker production *(1,6,11,81)*. Therefore, both serum AFP and serum HCG tumor-marker tests should be included in the follow-up studies for detection of recurrence and monitoring the response to the therapy, even if the initial serum tumor-marker level is normal *(6,81)*. A study with simultaneous and serial measurements of serum AFP, serum HCG, and serum LD in 794 patients with germ-cell tumors shows that 123 of 754 patients developed a first recurrence with recorded serum tumor-marker test results *(81)*. Of these123 patients with first recurrence, 79 (64%) had elevated serum tumor markers at the time of diagnosis and 76 (62%) had elevated tumor markers at the time of first recurrence *(81)*. An elevated serum tumor-marker level was present at first recurrence in 58 of 79 patients (73%) with initially positive serum tumor markers at the time of diagnosis and also in 18 of 44 patients (41%) with initially negative serum tumor markers at the time of diagnosis *(81)*. In 84 of 123 patients (68%), the same marker pattern with positive or negative results was present at the time of diagnosis and at first recurrence, 78% in seminoma and 64% in nonseminomatous germ-cell tumors *(81)*. Thirty patients developed a second recurrence, 27 of these patients (90%) had the same marker pattern as at first recurrence *(81)*. These data indicate that serum tumor-marker evaluation in follow-up monitoring of patients should include all the serum tumor markers regardless of serum tumor-marker levels at time of diagnosis *(81)*. Therefore, all the serum tumor markers for testicular germ-cell tumors should be included for both diagnosis and monitoring *(6,11,81)*.

6.2. Serial Determinations of Serum Tumor Markers Are Mandatory to Monitor the Response of Patients to Therapy and Detection of Recurrence

The development of effective and curative chemotherapy combined with improved surgical techniques and radiation therapy may predict the potential of tumor recurrence shortly after therapy renders not only the pretreatment serum tumor-marker measurements necessary but also posttreatment determinations of serum tumor markers mandatory for monitoring the disease course, estimation of effectiveness of therapy, detection of tumor recurrence, and prognostic prediction with serial determinations of several serum tumor-marker tests *(1,9–11)*.

Follow-up monitoring schedules are decided based on different stages of disease, type of treatments involved, monitoring purposes, and the histology, and postorchidectomy treatment chosen *(11)*. There are variations among the follow-up schedules at different institutions even in the same category of the monitoring *(11)*. Several protocols and testing frequency schedules have been developed and used by different medical centers over the years *(2,6,9–11,45)*. However, there is no single one thought to be optimal.

6.2.1. Tumor-Marker Tests Should Be Ordered Before and After Surgery

Both serum AFP and serum HCG should be tested before and after orchiectomy and retroperitoneal lymph node dissection *(6)*. However, even if all marker levels are normal, the diagnosis of malignancy should not be ruled out *(6,47)*. When one or both of the serum AFP and serum HCG are elevated before surgery, the elevated serum tumor markers can be measured daily for 1–2 wk following orchiectomy or retroperitoneal lymph node dissection to calculate the metabolic decline rate of the serum tumor marker *(6)*. After the initial daily measurements of the serum tumor markers, both serum tumor markers should be determined regularly at an interval of one month for at least 2 yr until the patient has been free of disease *(6)*. Usually, testicular germ-cell tumors relapse within first 2 yr after orchiectomy *(6)*. Should the serum tumor marker's MHL be prolonged, incomplete removal of the tumor is indicated suggesting that the patient has higher stage of disease and requires further investigation and treatment with chemotherapy or other treatment modality *(6)*. The cutoff normal MHL of serum HCG is 3 d and normal MHL for serum AFP is 7 d *(11)*. The return of serum tumor-marker levels to normal according to the rate of the normal MHL does not necessarily mean that the patient is completely free of tumor *(47)*. The patient should still be monitored with serum tumor-marker measurements and radiographic examination, chest X-ray, and CT scan of abdomen and pelvis and/or sonogram regularly *(6,11,45,47)*. The serum LD and serum LD-1 determinations are also recommended to improve the diagnostic sensitivity and regularly tested weekly for the first 2 mo and monthly thereafter for the first year and bimonthly for the second year until the patient is tumor-free *(4,5,14,20)*.

6.2.2. Serial Determinations of Serum Tumor Markers for Patients With Advanced Disease and Receiving Chemotherapy in Monitoring

It has been discussed previously that the first 6 wk can predict the potential for relapse when the MHL is prolonged *(77,84,95,97,99–105)*. For calculating the MHL, weekly measurements of elevated serum HCG and/or serum AFP are recommended during chemotherapy *(11,77,84,95,97,99–105)*. Generally, after the completion of chemotherapy, serum tumor markers including serum AFP, serum HCG , serum LD, and serum LD-1 levels can be determined monthly for the first year and every 2 mo for the second year after the patient appears to be free of disease *(11,45)*. If further monitoring is indicated, serum tumor markers may be tested every 2 or 3 mo during the third year, and then every 6 mo up to 5 yr *(11)*. There is no optimal follow-up protocol agreed upon by all the guidelines *(11)*.

6.2.3. Role of Serum Tumor Markers on Surveillance Protocols for Stage I Testicular Germ-Cell Tumor

Approximately 30% of clinical stage I patients with nonseminomatous germ-cell tumors would develop progression of diseases without retroperitoneal lymph node dissection, because the stage of disease of these patients is originally understaged and disease is not confined to the testis only *(9,10)*. Before the availability of the effective and curative chemotherapy for advanced testicular germ cell, almost all clinical stage I testicular germ-cell tumor patients underwent retroperitoneal lymph node dissection routinely for fear of progression of diseases *(9,10)*. Obviously, 70% of clinical stage I patients, who have their cancer truly confined to the testis and have pathologically negative lymph nodes, receive no benefit from routine retroperitoneal lymph node dissection *(9,10)*. Instead, these patients with true stage I diseases suffered from the side effects of anejaculation and infertility caused by the full bilateral retroperitoneal lymph node dissection *(9,10)*.

After effective chemotherapy had become available, several investigators doubted the clinical efficiency of the role of routine retroperitoneal lymph node dissection for nonseminomatous germ-cell tumor patients with early stage of disease *(9,10)*. To keep these 70% of patients from getting the unnecessary operation, careful observation procedures were designed and studied by several large medical centers reserving effective and curative chemotherapy and retroperitoneal lymph node dissection for the 30% of patients who later developed clinical manifestation of disease progression *(9,10)*. The results of many studies were reported from the mid-1980s to the mid-1990s *(10)*. The study concluded that 25 to 35% of patients developed metastasis on surveillance protocols. Overall survival of the patients on surveillance is 98%, similar to primary retroperitoneal lymph node dissection; 50 to 75% of cancer relapses appears in the retroperitoneum with the rest occurring in the lung or other organs suggesting the necessity of the inclusion of CT scan of abdomen and pelvis in follow-up observation protocols. Many patients with late recurrence at 6 yr and 9 yr respectively have been observed indicating that long term follow-up is required *(9,10)*. Several surveillance protocols have been developed with variations; despite the fact the optimal follow-up observation protocol has not been determined *(2,9–11)*. Three different surveillance protocols are listed below for reference.

The surveillance protocol for testicular germ-cell tumor stage I patients developed by Steele and Richie, suggests that patients have physical examination, serum tumor markers, CT scan of abdomen and pelvis, and chest X-rays every 4 mo for the first 3 yr and have physical examination, CT scan abdomen and pelvis, and chest X-ray every 6 mo for the next 4 yr. In this protocol, serum tumor markers are not included during the last 4 yr of observation *(2)*.

The protocol used by Richie et al. recommends that patients have physical examination, chest X-ray, and serum tumor-marker tests every month for the first year, every 2 mo for the second year and every 3 to 6 mo per year after the second year. CT scan of abdomen and pelvis for evaluation of the retroperitoneum should be done every 2 to 3 mo for the first 2 yr and at least every 6 mo after the second year *(9)*. Observation duration of 5 yr or even 10 yr is recommended following orchiectomy *(9)*.

Skinner and Skinner design and recommend their surveillance protocol as follows: patients have serum tumor markers of serum AFP and serum HCG together with chest X-ray and physical examination every month for the first year and CT scan of abdomen and pelvis every 3 mo. For the second year, patients have chest X-ray, serum tumor markers, physical examination every 2 mo, and CT scan of abdomen and pelvis every 4 mo. From years 3 to 5, patients should have chest X-ray, serum tumor markers, physical examination every 3 mo and CT scan of abdomen and pelvis every 6 mo. Patients should have chest X-ray, serum tumor markers, physical examination every 6 mo, CT of abdomen and pelvis every year for yr 6 and thereafter *(10)*.

Serum tumor markers play an important role on the surveillance studies *(2,9–11)*. However, the serum tumor markers mentioned in the surveillance protocols often include serum AFP and serum HCG only; it is recommended that the serum tumor-marker test profile should add serum LD and serum LD-1 in order to increase the clinical diagnostic sensitivity of detecting the progression of diseases.

6.3. Be Aware of Limitations of Tumor-Marker Tests

The serum tumor-marker tests for testicular germ-cell tumors have limitations in both clinical diagnostic sensitivity and specificity and in the analytical accuracy, precision, sensitivity, and specificity. Awareness of the limitations in both areas should raise caution in interpreting the test results, which might give erroneous information regarding diagnosis, prognosis, assessment of therapeutic effectiveness, and lead to ineffective treatment of the patients with unnecessary toxic agents or tissue damage resulting from unjustified surgical removal of normal organ or nonneoplastic tissue.

6.3.1. Limitations of the Diagnostic Sensitivity and the Diagnostic Specificity

Serum tumor-marker tests for testicular germ-cell tumors have a high false-negative test results in patients with early stage of diseases and approx 10% of patients with advanced diseases have false-negative test results *(6,45)*. All four serum tumor markers are also elevated in benign and malignant disorders other than testicular germ-cell tumors that are considered to be false-positive results for testicular germ-cell tumors. Although serum tumor markers, when applied in the population of patients with high incidence of testicular germ-cell tumors, had no false-positive results in one study *(39)*, the possibility of encountering false-positive results in patients with testicular germ-cell cancer is not impossible *(39,112,113)*.

6.3.1.1. FALSE-NEGATIVE RESULTS IN PATIENTS WITH DISEASES WHO DO NOT HAVE ABNORMAL SERUM TUMOR-MARKER TEST RESULTS

Although the use of serum tumor marker has reduced the understaging of patients with clinical stage I diseases from 47 to 37%, 37% of patients with stage II or higher do not have elevations of serum tumor markers *(39)*. This false-negative test result makes the marker test unable to correctly diagnose testicular germ-cell tumors *(39)*. Another study of patients with testicular germ-cell tumors shows a falsely negative incidence of 38% in patients found to have retroperitoneal metastases at lymphadenectomy *(114)*. Serum tumor-marker levels during chemotherapy are often normal even in the presence of residual tumor *(114)*. Resulting from false-negative test results, the serum tumor-marker tests have a limited role in the early detection of residual disease in patients treated systematically with prophylactic chemotherapy *(114)*. To cope with this problem of false-negative marker results, efforts should focus on using other diagnostic tool such as CT scan of abdomen and pelvis to detect the residual mass and followed by a retroperitoneal lymph node dissection to confirm the presence of viable caner cells in the retroperitoneum *(114)*. The findings indicate that a meticulous retroperitoneal lymphadenectomy is the most important and effective mean in deciding the use of adjuvant chemotherapy *(114)*.

6.3.1.2. FALSE-POSITIVE TEST RESULTS DUE TO OTHER DISORDERS

It may not be difficult to recognize other disorders with elevation of these serum tumor markers in patients without testicular germ-cell cancers. However, it may be confusing when patients with testicular germ-cell cancers are complicated with another disorder that causes the serum tumor-marker elevation. This type of serum tumor-marker elevations, if not interpreted carefully, may be misused as a sign to indicate the progression of the germ-cell cancer activity resulting in implementing unnecessary and harmful therapy to the patients *(112,113)*. Nine patients with testicular germ-cell cancers that had serum AFP elevation without progression or recurrence of the testicular germ-cell cancers were reported *(112)*. The elevated serum AFP was caused by liver damage secondary to medication by chemotherapy, anesthetics, or antiepiletics *(112)*. These patients do not have any clinical or surgical evidence of testicular germ-cell cancer activity *(112)*. Another 11 patients with disseminated testicular cancer had elevation of serum AFP during induction chemotherapy of the VAB-6 regimen *(113)*. However, these patients had elevations of the markers of liver damage including serum AST, ALT, and serum LD *(113)*. The elevations of the liver markers and serum AFP were induced by liver damage caused by the VAB-6 regimen, immediately after the end of induction chemotherapy *(113)*. Similar to the acute transient elevation of serum tumor markers resulting form cytolysis secondary to the effective chemotherapy *(82–85)*, the elevation of serum AFP in patients with germ-cell tumors produced by liver dysfunction should not be interpreted as progression of cancer activity *(112,113)*. These elevations must be interpreted with caution to avoid unnecessary treatments. Whenever the elevation of serum AFP is suspected as a result of liver damage, it is recommended to review the serum tumor markers of serum HCG and serum LD-1 concentration. Serum HCG and serum LD-1 are not associated with the liver damage, therefore they may somewhat be useful for differential diagnosis.

6.3.1.3. NEVER USE THE SERUM TUMOR-MARKER TEST RESULTS AS THE ONLY CRITERIA TO MAKE OR RULE OUT A DIAGNOSIS

Serum AFP, serum HCG, serum LD, and serum LD-1 tests can be negative in a substantial number of patients with testicular germ-cell tumors; for patients with seminoma, the incidence of positive serum tumor-marker elevation is much lower than that of nonseminomatous testicular germ-cell tumors *(5,6,14,39,40,45)*. In seminoma, only serum HCG, serum LD, and/or serum LD-1 may be elevated, and only 10% to 50% of patients with seminoma will have elevations of serum tumor markers *(5,6,14,15,39,40,45,65)*. This high degree of false-negative rates of serum tumor marker tests leads to the inability of serum tumor-marker tests to be used to rule out a diagnosis of testicular germ-cell tumor *(5,6,14,15,39,40,45,65)*. The four serum tumor-marker tests including serum AFP, serum HCG, serum LD, and serum LD-1 for testicular germ-cell tumors are associated with a variety of other malignant diseases and benign disorders or conditions. Therefore, the serum tumor-marker positive results can be a false-positive for germ-cell tumors. Because of the possibility of false positivity of the tests, the serum tumor-marker tests must not be used as the sole criterion for making a diagnosis of testicular germ tumor. The bottom line is to never rely on the result of a single test to make any clinical decision regarding diagnosis and treatment modality. This issue can never be over-emphasized.

6.3.2. Consideration of Analytical Limitations

If the tumor-marker results do not match the clinical conditions of the patients, review potentially inaccurate analytical variables that may be causing the discordant test results. Always investigate the sources of errors during the test procedures including the pre-analytical phase, analytical, and post-analytical errors.

6.3.2.1. PAY ATTENTION TO THE ANALYTICAL PERFORMANCE CHARACTERISTICS OF THE ASSAY KIT

The keys to providing efficient and effective monitoring, evaluating patient response to therapy, early detection of the cancer recurrence and metastasis, and detection of a minimal residual disease by the serum tumor-marker test rely on analytically and clinically valid sensitivity (or detection limit), reliable assay precision and accuracy of each of serum tumor markers. Detection limit (DL) is the lowest or smallest detectable tumor-marker concentration or minimum amount of a tumor marker that can be distinguished from the zero concentration or value *(115)*. A clinically and analytically valid DL should be able to separate patients with detectable and undetectable concentrations of the tumor markers *(115)*. Test results may be falsely detectable or falsely undetectable owing to a poorly established DL that is inaccurate and/or imprecise. Both conditions may lead to an incorrect diagnosis and mismanagement of patients with testicular germ-cell cancers. A persistent and truly elevated marker level above the low upper limits of normal reference value indicates that there is still residual cancer, which would alert further necessary treatment, whereas a falsely detectable level will cause unnecessary procedures and therapy, causing a damaging outcome of the patient. Similarly, a falsely undetectable elevated tumor marker concentration will miss detection of a recurrent disease or a residual cancer delaying the necessary therapy and may result in progression of the disease into advanced and/or terminally refractory stage. The importance of establishing an analytically and clinically valid DL or evaluating and confirming the DL of the commercial tumor-marker test kits cannot be overemphasized *(115)*. It is important to know the reliable assay precision and accuracy of the serum tumor-marker tests to correctly interpret that the scope of changes between serial-measurement results truly reflects changes of the patient's disease activity instead of analytical variations due to assay imprecision *(115)*.

6.3.2.2. WHEN ORDERING SERIAL TESTING, BE CERTAIN EACH TEST IS DONE BY USING THE SAME ASSAY KIT

Serum AFP and serum HCF are usually measured by immunoassays. Each different commercial immunoassay kit or methodology may generate different results on the same serum sample, even though all the kits are designed for the same tumor marker *(73)*. Ordering from the same laboratory consistently guarantees a more consistent performance *(73)*. In some instances, the same laboratory may switch from one assay kit to another assay kit for some reason. Should this happen, the practitioners should always inquire if the test result is inconsistent with the previous test result on the same patient. It is important to ensure that any marker concentration change observed during the monitoring process is truly owing to the change of tumor burden or other disease activity and not to the result of test methodological variability *(73)*.

6.3.2.3. HETEROPHILIC ANTIBODY-INDUCED FALSELY ELEVATED RESULTS

Falsely elevated serum HCG resulting from human anti-mouse IgG or heterophilic antibodies has been reported in a number of women treated with unnecessary chemotherapy and/or surgery with a suspected diagnosis of trophoblastic disease or postgestational choriocarcinoma *(116)*. These women suffered from adverse side effects from unnecessary chemotherapy and/or surgery *(116)*. The falsely elevated test results may occur in any immunoassay using animal anti-human IgG antibody in the assay systems, when the assay systems are designed to block heterophilic antibodies insufficiently to produce an analytical accuracy *(116)*. A case report of a young man with elevated serum HCG and a testicular mass by palpation, was suspected to have testicular cancer *(117)*. After the surgical removal of one of a testicle, his abnormal serum HCG did not decline *(117)*. This patient had a heterophilic antibody that had caused a falsely elevated serum HCG result and the testicular mass was found to be a benign cyst rather than malignancy *(117)*. The patient's serum was reassayed on another immunoassay instrument and bovine serum added to the patient's sample with reassay by the original method *(117)*. Addition of bovine serum to the patient's serum had a dramatic effect showing that his serum HCG was normal *(117)*. The heterophilic antibody-induced false test result by immunoassays was documented in the literature more than two decades ago, it has been still causing problems by producing false laboratory results in some immunoassay systems as described above *(118)*. This fact indicates that the pathological diagnosis of the tissue still remains the best, and only certain, method of diagnosis *(1,6,45)*. It is always important to keep in mind that possible assay errors could occur, particularly when patient's clinical status does not match the tumor-marker test result.

6.3.2.4. BE AWARE THAT LOW TEST RESULTS INCONSISTENT WITH PATIENT'S CONDITION MAY BE CAUSED BY A HOOK EFFECT

When the test result of a sandwich immunoassay for serum AFP and/or serum HCG is too low to be consistent with the patient's clinical advanced disease status, suspect errors that may be caused by a hook effect *(73)*. The sample should be retested and measurement of the tumor marker be repeated with a 10-fold diluted serum sample *(73)*. It is not uncommon with a sandwich immunoassay, that when the concentration of the serum sample exceeds the assay dynamic range *(73)*.

7. DISCUSSION

Serum tumor-marker tests for testicular germ-cell tumor are the best tumor-marker system in modern medical oncology *(6,45)*. The serum tumor-marker tests have provided excellent clinical values in diagnosis; significantly reduce staging errors, prognostic prediction, better defined the histopathological typing, monitored the response of the treatment and detection of the recurrent disease, and avoided unnecessary procedures and treatment and implemented appropriate therapy in patients *(1,4–6,11–20,23,25,39,40,45–47,74–77,84, 86–105)*. Additionally, the development of effective and curative chemotherapy, more sensitive imaging techniques, improved surgical procedures, advances in microbiology, antibiotics therapy, and technically improved general supportive therapy and management have contributed to the improvement of survival for patients with testicular germ-cell tumors *(1,9–11,23,25)*.

The clinical value of serum tumor markers of serum AFP, serum HCG, and serum LD has been well established and documented *(11)*. These three serum tumor markers are now included in the IGCCC staging system, the fifth edition of the UICC TNM staging system, and the staging system of the American Joint Committee on Cancer (AJCC) as prognostic variables, and also listed in the five of seven published "Practice Guidelines for Tumor Marker Use in Germ-Cell Tumors" for several different clinical functions *(11,23,25)*. Serum LD-1 test as a tumor marker for testicular germ-cell cancer is a useful adjuvant tumor-marker test for testicular germ-cell tumors *(4,5,12–20)*. Addition of serum LD-1 to the marker test profile of serum AFP, serum HCG, and serum LD, not only has increased the clinical diagnostic sensitivity and specificity, but also demonstrated its clinical value in prognostic estimation, staging, monitoring the response of the patient toward the therapy, and early detection of recurrent diseases *(4,5,12–20)*. Serum LD-1 has also shown that it is more specific than serum LD in diagnosis and prognostic prediction *(16,17)*. Some patients with elevated values of serum LD combined with a normal value of serum LD-1 had survival similar to that overall for patients with a normal serum LD-1, and did not show inferior survival caused by elevated serum LD *(16)*. The prognostic value of serum LD-1 surpassed that of serum LD, serum HCG, or serum AFP *(4,5,12–20,119)*.

Univariate analyses of patients with metastatic testicular germ-cell tumor show both the IGCCC and serum LD 1 highly and significantly predicted survival *(16)*. In this evaluation, serum LD-1 was categorized into three prognostic subgroups: patients with serum LD-1 <1.0 × upper limit of reference value (ULR) had a good prognosis, those with serum LD-1 1.0–10 × ULR had an intermediate prognosis and those with serum LD-1 >10 × ULR had a poor prognosis. Using these criteria, serum LD-1 predicted the survival as well as IGCCC staging *(16)*. A recent study, based on 81 patients with metastatic testicular germ-cell tumors from two different medical centers using multivariate analysis, examined whether the IGCCC, serum LD-1, main histology (seminoma vs nonseminomatous testicular germ-cell tumors), serum LD, serum AFP, serum HCG, treatment center, and other prognostic factors, and combinations of these variables predict the survival for patients with metastatic testicular germ-cell tumors *(119)*. The results showed that the addition of serum LD-1 in three stratified levels, to the IGCCC staging system improved the efficiency of the IGCCC in the survival prediction. Addition of the IGCCC to a model consisting of only serum LD-1 in three stratified levels also enhanced the ability to predict the survival more accurately *(119)*. Adding the other prognostic variables such as the third TNM classification, treatment center, and serum HCG to the IGCCC, the prognostic value of the system was not improved *(119)*. The study concluded the combination of the IGCCC and serum LD-1 in three categories to form a new model of staging system is a significant improvement for the prognostic staging classification *(119)*. This new prognostic model provides a better survival prediction than either the IGCCC or serum LD-1 alone *(119)*. One of the limitations of this study is that it analyzed a small number of patients *(119)*. Further studies with larger number of patients are necessary because serum LD-1 appears to be a useful tumor marker for testicular germ-cell tumors *(119)*.

Testicular germ-cell cancer is one of the few currently curable malignancies; it will continue to be the most curable solid cancer in men *(1,9,10)*. The serum tumor-marker test profile of serum AFP, serum HCG, serum LD, and serum LD-1 has contributed greatly to the management and treatment of patients with testicular germ-cell cancer *(4,5,11–20,119)*. The serum tumor-marker test profile will continue to provide clinically important and useful information offering the benefit of maintaining the excellent cure rate of this disease *(1,4,5, 9–20,119)*.

Molecular diagnostic testing for testicular germ-cell tumors is still in the early stage of development *(1,120–124)*. Molecular diagnostics appears to be promising, although clinical application has not been established. Using reverse transcription-polymerase chain reaction (RT-PCR), the expression of melanoma antigen (MAGE) has been shown in testicular cancer *(120)*. MAGE 1–3 genes were found in both seminomas and nonseminomatous germ-cell tumors with various incidences ranging from 30 to 91.7% with more frequent presence in seminomas suggesting MAGE genes might be useful tumor markers for molecular staging of testicular germ-cell tumors particularly for seminoma *(120)*. Wilms' tumor associated gene *WT1* was also demonstrated in some testicular cancers *(120)*. This gene was frequently expressed in patients of advanced stage of diseases, but less frequently in the low stage patients suggesting that WT1 gene may be a tumor marker for high stage testicular germ-cell tumors *(120)*. Investigation of proto-oncogenes in testicular germ-cell tumors shows N-*myc* expression in 94% of seminomas and 83% of embryonal carcinomas *(1)*. Immature teratoma has a high level of *c-erb*B-1 expression *(1)*. c-Ki-*ras* or N-*ras* was seen in all histologic subgroups of testicular germ-cell tumors and also normal testis which suggests a switch of proto-oncogene expression during differentiation *(1)*. Expression of c-kit proto-oncogenes has been reported in seminoma but not in nonseminomatous testicular germ-cell tumors *(1)*. Studies of *p53* in testicular germ-cell tumors have shown controversial results by immunostaining suggesting a positive role of *p53* in detecting the aggressiveness of the tumor but negative results using denaturant gel electrophoresis and single-strand conformation polymorphism *(1)*. Chromosomal abnormalities have been described in testicular germ-cell tumors, usually chromosome 1 and chromosome 12 abnormalities *(121–123)*. The rearrangements in both the short and long arms of chromosome 1 have been reported *(121)*. The testicular germ-cell tumors have characteristic chromosomal abnormalities with a high copy number of the short arms of chromosome 12, 12p, with or without an isochromosome 12p *(122,123)*. Correspondingly, the gene locus for the H subunits of LD is localized to the short arms of the chromosome 12, 12p *(124)*, whereas the gene locus for the M subunits of LD is localized to the short arms of chromosome 11, 11p *(124)*. Becuase LD-1 isoenzyme is a homogeneous tetramer of the H subunits of LD consisting of all four H subunits *(14,61)*, the positive relationship between the elevated serum LD-1 and the high copy number the short arms of chromosome 12p in testicular germ-cell tumor reflects the molecular biology of this tumor *(124)*. The high copy number of chromosome 12p in testicular germ-cell tumors is the cause of the predominant elevation of serum LD-1 in patients with testicular germ-cell tumors *(124)*.

Using multiple serum tumor marker tests for patients with testicular germ-cell tumors, there are still approx 30–50% of stage I patients with testicular germ-cell tumors and 10% of advanced stage patients have no elevation of anyone of these serum tumor markers *(4,5,11,14,15,39,40,45,71,114)*. The search for new sensitive and specific serum tumor markers for improving clinical diagnostic sensitivity and specificity is an important responsibility of the medical scientists and researchers.

REFERENCES

1. Richie JP. 1998. Neoplasms of the Testis. In: Campbell's Urology, 7th ed., vol. 3, Walsh PC, Retik AB, Vaughan DE, Wein AJ, eds. Philadelphia: W.B. Sanders, pp. 2411–2452.
2. Steele G and Richie JP. 2001. Testicular Tumors. In: Comprehensive Urology, 1st ed., Weiss RM, George N Jr, O'Reilly PH, eds. London: Mosby, pp. 425–449.

3. Dixon FJ and Moore RA. 1953. Testicular tumors: a clinicopathological study. Cancer 6: 427–454.
4. Liu FJ, Fritsche HA, Trujillo JM, et al. 1983. Serum AFP, β-hCG, and LD-1 in patients with germ-cell tumors of the testis. Am. J. Clin. Pathol. 80–120.
5. Liu FJ, Fritsche HA, Trujillo JM, et al. 1985. Lactate dehydrogenase (LDH) isoenzyme 1 in germ-cell tumors. Cancer Bull. 34:67–70.
6. Lange PA. 1981. The clinical value of α-fetoprotein (AFP) and human chorionic gonadotropin in the management of testicular cancer. In: Alpha-Fetoprotein: Laboratory Procedures and Clinical Applications, Kirkpatrick AM and Nakamura RM, eds. Masson Publishing USA, New York, NY, pp. M, 107–113.
7. Snyder HM, D'Angio GJ, Evans A, et al. 1998. Pediatric oncology, in: Campbell's Urology, 7th ed, vol. 3, Walsh PC, Retik AB, Vaughan DE, Wein AJ, eds., WB Sanders: Philadelphia, pp. 2210–2256.
8. Jemal A, Murray T, Samuels A, et al. 2003. Cancer statistics CA. J. Clin. Cancer 53:5–26.
9. Richie JP. 1997. Nonseminomatous germ-cell tumors: management and prognosis, in: Urologic Oncology, Oesterling JE and Richie JP, eds. WB Sanders: Philadelphia, pp. 481–495.
10. Skinner EC and Skinner DG. 1998. Surgery of testicular neoplasms, in: Campbell's Urology, 7th ed., vol. 3, Walsh PC, Retik AB, Vaughan DE, Wein AJ, eds., WB Sanders: Philadelphia, pp. 3410–3432.
11. Sturgeon C. 2002. Practice guidelines for tumor marker use in the clinic. Clin. Chem. 48: 1151–1159.
12. Zondag HA. 1964. Enzyme activity in dysgerminoma and seminoma - a study of malignant diseases. Rhode Island Med. J. XLVII 273–281.
13. Zondag HA and Klein F. 1968. Clinical application of lactate dehydrogenase isoenzymes: alterations in malignancy. Ann. NY Acad. Sci. 151:578–586.
14. Liu F, Fritsche HA, Trujillo JM, et al. 1982. Serum lactate dehydrogenase isoenzyme 1 in patients with advanced testicular cancer. Am. J. Clin. Pathol. 78:178–183.
15. von Eyben FE, Liu FJ, Amato RJ et al. 2000. Lactate dehydrogenase isoenzyme 1 is the most important LD isoenzyme in patients with testicular germ-cell Tumor. Acta. Oncol. 39:509–517.
16. von Eyben FE, Madsen EL, Liu F, et al. 2000. Serum lactate dehydrogenase isoenzyme 1 as a prognostic predictor for metastatic testicular germ-cell tumours. Br. J. Cancer 83:1256–1258.
17. von Eyben FE, Blaabjerg O, Hyltoft-Petersen P, et al. 2001. Serum lactate dehydrogenase isoenzyme 1 and prediction of death in patients with metastatic testicular germ-cell tumors. Clin. Chem. Lab. Med. 39:38–44.
18. Lippert M, Papadopoulos N, Javadpour N. 1981. Role of lactate dehydrogenase isoenzymes in testicular cancer. Urology 18:50–55.
19. von Eyben FE, Blaabjerg O, Petersen PH, et al. 1988. Serum lactate dehydrogenase isoenzyme 1 as a marker of testicular germ-cell tumor. J. Urol. 140:986–990.
20. Edler von Eyben F, Lindegaard Madsen E, Blaabjerg O, et al. 1995. Serum lactate dehydrogenase isoenzyme 1. An early indicator of relapse in patients with testicular germ-cell tumors. Acta. Oncol. 34:925–929.
21. Samuels ML, Johnson DE, Brown B et al. 1979. Velban plus continuous infusion bleomycin (VB-3) in stage III advanced testicular cancer: 99 patients with a note on high dose velban and sequential *cis*-paltinum, in: Cancer of the Genitourinary Tract, Johnson DE and Samuels ML, eds., Raven Press: New York, pp. 159–172.
22. Samuels ML, Holoye PY, Johnson DE. 1975. Bleomycin combination chemotherapy in the management of testicular neoplasia. Cancer 36:318–326.
23. Mead GM and Stenning S. 1997. (for the International Germ-cell cancer Collaboratory Group). International germ-cell consensus classification. A prognostic factor-based staging system for metastatic germ-cell cancers. J. Clin. Oncol. 15:594–603.
24. Bajorin DF, Mazumdar M, Meyers M, et al. 1998. Metastatic germ-cell tumors: modeling for response to chemotherapy. J. Clin. Oncol. 16:707–715.

25. Sobin LH and Wittekind C. 1997. TNM classification of malignant tumours, in: International Union Against Cancer. 5th ed., Wiley-Liss: New York, pp. 1–227.

26. Abelev GI, Perova DS, Khramkova NI, et al. 1963. Production of embryonal alpha-globulin by transplantable mouse hepatomas. Transplantation 1:174–180.

27. Bacchus H. 1977. Serum glycoproteins and malignant neoplastic disorder. CRC Crit. Rev. Clin. Lab. Sci. 8:333–362.

28. Brummund W, Arvan DA, Mennuti MT, et al. 1980. Alpha-fetoprotein in the routine clinical laboratory: Evaluation of a simple radioimmunoassay and review of current concepts in its clinical application. Clin. Chim. Acta. 105:25–39.

29. Abelev GI. 1971. Alpha-fetoprotein in oncogenesis and its association with malignant tumors. Adv. Cancer Res. 14:295–358.

30. Gitlin D and Boseman M. 1967. Sites of serum alpha-fetoprotein synthesis in the human and in the rat. J. Clin. Invest. 46:1010–1016.

31. Gitlin D and Boseman M. 1966. Serum alpha-fetoprotein, albumin and gamma-G-globulin in the human conceptus. J. Clin. Invest. 45:1826–1838.

32. Waldman TA and McIntire KR. 1974. The use of a radioimmunoassay for alpha-fetoprotein in the diagnosis of malignancy. Cancer 34:1510–1515.

33. Talerman A, Haije WG, Baggerman L. 1977. Alpha-1-antitrypsin (AAT) and alpha-fetoprotein in sera of patients with germ-cell neoplasms: Value as tumor markers in patients with endodermal sinus tumor (yolk sac tumor). Int. J. Cancer 19:741–746.

34. Bloomer JR, Waldman TA, McIntire KR, et al. 1973. Serum alpha-fetoprotein levels in patients with non-neoplastic liver disease. Gastroenterology 65:530.

35. Wepsie HT. 1981. Alpha-fetoprotein: its quantitation and relationship to neoplastic disease, in: Alpha-Fetoprotein: Laboratory Procedures and Clinical Applications, Kirkpatrick AM and Nakamura RM, eds., Masson Publishing USA: New York, pp. 115–129.

36. Kelstein ML, Chan DL, Bruzek DJ, et al. 1988. Monitoring hepatocellular carcinoma by using a monoclonal immunoenzymetric assay for alpha-fetoprotein. Clin. Chem. 34:76–81.

37. Seppala M and Ruoslahti E. 1973. Alpha-fetoprotein: physiology and pathology during pregnancy and application to antenatal diagnosis. J. Perinat. Med. 1:104–113.

38. Ruoslahti E and Seppala M. 1971. Studies of carcino-fetal proteins III. Development of radioimmunoassay for alpha fetoprotein in serum of healthy human adults. Int. J. Cancer 8:374–384.

39. Bosl GJ, Lange PH, Fraley EE. 1981. Human chorionic gonadotropin and alphafetoprotein in the staging of nonseminomatous testicular cancer. Cancer 47:328–332.

40. Scardino PT, Cox PD, Waldman TA, et al. 1977. The value of serum tumor markers in the staging and prognosis of germ-cell tumors of the testis. J. Urol. 118:994–999.

41. Poulakis V, Witzsch U, de Vries R, et al. Alpha-fetoprotein-producing renal cell carcinoma. Urol. Int. 2001. 67:181–183.

42. Morimoto H, Tanigawa N, Inoue H, et al. Alpha-fetoprotein-producing renal cell carcinoma. Cancer 1988. 61:84–88.

43. Matsunou H, Konishi F, Jalal RE, et al. 1994. Alpha-fetoprotein-producing gastric carcinoma with enteroblastic differentiation. Cancer 73:534–540.

44. Sarui H, Nakayama T, Takeda N, et al. 2001. Alpha-fetoprotein-producing male breast cancer accompanied with hepatocellular carcinoma: assessment by lectin-affinity profile. Am. J. Med. Sci. 322:369–372.

45. Lange PH. 1985. Tumor markers in germ-cell malignancy. Cancer Bull. 37:65–66.

46. Javadpour N. 1980. Improved staging for testicular cancer using biologic tumor markers: a prospective study. J. Urol. 124:58–59.

47. Barlett NL, Freiha FS, Torti FM. 1991. Serum markers in germ-cellneoplasms. Hematol. Oncol. Clin North Am. 5:1245–1260.

48. Rizkallah T, Gurpide E, Vande Weil RL. 1969. Metabolism of HCG in man. J. Clin. Endocrinol. Metab. 29:92–100.

49. Picozzi VJ, Freiha FS, Hannigan JF, et al. 1984. Prognostic significance of a decline in serum human chorionic gonadotropin levels after initial chemotherapy for advanced germ-cell carcinoma. Ann. Intern. Med. 100:183–186.

50. Amato R, Ogden S, Dexeus F, et al. 1990. Beta-HCG slope as a predictor of favorable response to chemotherapy for patients with metastatic NSGCTT. Proc. Ann. Meet. Am. Soc. Clin. Oncol. 9:A565.

51. Falkson G, Bohmer RH, Adam M, et al. 1986. Hepatitis-B as a prognostic discriminant in patients with primary liver cancer. Cancer 57:812–815.

52. Lange PH, Waldman TA, McIntire KR. 1980 Tumor markers in testicular tumors: current status and future prospects, in: Testicular Tumors: Management and treatment, Einhorm LE, ed., Masson Publishing USA: New York, pp. 69–81.

53. Morgan FJ, Briken S, Canfield RE. 1973. Human chorionic gonadotropin: a proposal for the amino acid sequence. Mol. Cell. Biochem. 2:27–99.

54. Carlsen RB, Bahl DP, Swaminathan N. 1973. Human Chorionic gonadotropin: linear amino acid sequence of the B-subunit. J. Biol. Chem. 248:6810–6827.

55. Vaitukaitis JL, Braunstein GD, Ross GT. 1972. A radioimmunoassay which specifically measures human chorionic gonadotropin in the presence of human luteining hormone. Am. J. Obstet. Gynecol. 113:751–758.

56. Schlaerth J, Morrow P, Kletyky O, et al. 1981. Prognostic characteristics of serum human chorionic gonadotropin titer regression following molar pregnancy. Obstet. Gynecol. 58:478–482.

57. Skinner DG, Scardino PT, Daniels JR. 1981. Testicular cancer. Ann. Rev. Med. 32:543–557.

58. Bohn H and Dati F. 1983. Placental-related proteins, in: Proteins in Body Fluids, Amino Acids, and Tumor Markers: Diagnostic and Clinical Aspects Ritzman SE and Killingsworth LM, eds., Alan, R. Liss: New York, pp. 333–374.

59. Braunstein GD, Vaitukaitis JL, Carbone PP, et al. 1973. Ectopic product of human chorionic gonadotropin by neoplasms. Ann. Int. Med. 78:39–45.

60. Rosen SW, Weintraub BD, Vaitukaitis JL, et al. 1975. Placental proteins and their subunits as tumor markers. Ann. Intern. Med. 82:71–83.

61. Dufour DF, Lott JA, Henry JB. 2001. Clinical enzymology, in: Clinical Diagnosis and Management by Laboratory Methods, 20th ed., Henry JB, ed., WB Saunders: Philadelphia, pp.281–303.

62. Fowler JE Jr, Sesterhenn I, Stutzman RE, et al. 1983. Localization of alpha-fetoprotein and human chorionic gonadotropin to specific histologic types of nonseminomatous testicular cancer. Urology 22:649–654.

63. Wittekind C, Wichmann T, von Kleist S. 1983. Immunohistological localization of AFP and HCG in uniformly classified testis tumors. Anticancer Res. 3:327–330.

64. Javadpour N, Woltering E, Soares T. 1980. Simultaneous measurement of tumor cytosol and peripheral serum levels of human chorionic gonadotropin and alpha-fetoprotein in testicular cancer. Invest. Urol. 18:11–12.

65. Hori K, Uematsu K, Yasoshima H, et al. 1997. Testicular seminoma with human chorionic gonadotropin production. Pathol. Int. 47:592–599.

66. Suurmeijer AJ, De Bruijn HW, Oosterhuis JW, et al. 1982. Nonseminomatous germ-cell tumors of the testis. Immunohistochemical localization and serum levels of human chorionic gonadotropin (HCG) and pregnancy-specific beta-1 glycoprotein (SP-1); value of SP-1 as a tumor marker. Oncodev. Biol. Med. 3:409–422.

67. Murakami SS and Said JW. 1984. Immunohistochemical localization of lactate dehydrogenase isoenzyme 1 in germ-cell tumors of the testis. Am. J. Clin. Pathol. 81:293–296.

68. Kinumaki H, Takeuchi H, Nakamura K, et al. 1985. Serum lactate dehydrogenase isoenzyme-1 in children with yolk sac tumor. Cancer 56:178–181.

69. Talerman A, Haije WG, Baggerman L. 1980. Serum alphafetoprotein (AFP) in patients with germ-cell tumors of the gonads and extragonadal sites: correlation between endodermal sinus (yolk sac) tumor and raised serum AFP. Cancer 46:380–385.

70. Norgaard-Pedersen B, Schultz HP, Arends J, et al. 1984. Tumour markers in testicular germ-celltumours. Five-year experience from the DATECA Study 1976–1980. Acta. Radiol. Oncol. 23:287–294.
71. Bosl GJ, Lange PH, Nochomovitz LE, et al. 1981. Tumor markers in advanced nonseminomatous testicular cancer. Cancer 47:572–576.
72. Bosl GJ, Geller N, Cirrincione C, et al. 1983. Interrelationships of histopathology and other clinical variables in patients with germ-cell tumors of the testis. Cancer 51:2121–2125.
73. Wu JT. 2001. Diagnosis and management of cancer using serologic tumor markers. In: Clinical diagnosis and management by laboratory methods, 20th ed., Henry JB, ed. Philadelphia: W.B. Saunders, pp. 1028–1042.
74. Lippert MC and Javadpour N. 1981. Lactic dehydrogenase in the monitoring and prognosis of testicular cancer. Cancer 48:2274–2278.
75. Javadpour N. 1980. Significance of elevated serum alphafetoprotein (AFP) in seminoma. Cancer 45:2166–2168.
76. Lange PH, Nochomovitz LE, Rosai J, et al. 1980. Serum alpha-fetoprotein and human chorionic gonadotropin in patients with seminoma. J. Urol. 124:472–478.
77. Lange PH, Vogelzang NJ, Goldman A, et al. 1982. Marker half-life analysis as a prognostic tool in testicular cancer. J. Urol. 128:708–711.
78. Lieskovsky G and Skinner DG. 1980. Significance of serum lactic dehydrogenase in stages B and C nonseminomatous testis tumors. J. Urol. 123:516–517.
79. William MP, Husband JE, Heron CW. 1987. Stage 1 nonseminomatous germ-cell tumors of the testis: Radiologic follow up after orchiectomy. Radiology 164:671–674.
80. Seckl MJ, Rustin GJS, Bagshawe KD. 1990. Frequency of serum tumor marker monitoring in patients with nonseminomatous testicular cancer. Br. J. Cancer. 61:916–918.
81. Trigo JM, Tabernero JM, Paz-Ares L, et al. 2000. Tumor markers at the time of recurrence in patients with germ-cell tumors. Cancer 88:162–168.
82. Wolf DJ and Williams JJ. 1982. Transient rise in tumor marker after initial adjuvant chemotherapy for testicular cancer. Urology 20:50–52.
83. Grips H, Vahrson H, Korte K. 1980. AFP CEA HCG and its beta subunit in metastatic choriocarcinoma. Oncology 37:157–162.
84. Vogelzang NJ, Lang PH, Goldman A, et al. 1982. Acute changes of alpha-fetoprotein and human chorionic gonadotropin during induction chemotherapy of germ-cell tumors. Cancer Res. 42:4855–4861.
85. Horwich A and Peckman MJ. 1986. Transient tumor marker elevation following chemotherapy for germ-cell tumors of the testis. Cancer Treat. Rep. 70:1329–1331.
86. Medical research council working party. 1985. Testicular tumors. prognostic factors in advanced nonseminomatous germ-cells testicular tumors: results of a multicenter study. Lancet 1:8–11.
87. Stoter G, Bosl GJ, Droz JP, et al. 1990. Prognostic factors in metastatic germ-cell tumors. Prog. Clin. Biol. Res. 357:313–319.
88. Samuels ML. 1991. Evolution of curative chemotherapy for testicular cancer. Cancer Bull. 43:439–455.
89. Vugrin D, Friedman A, Whitmore WF Jr. 1984. Correlation of serum tumor markers in advanced germ-cell tumors with responses to chemotherapy and surgery. Cancer 53:1440–1445.
90. Newlands ES, Begent RH, Rustin GJ, et al. 1983. Further advances in the management of malignant teratomas of the testis and other sites. Lancet 1:948–951.
91. Horwich A, Easton D, Husband J, et al. 1987. Prognosis following chemotherapy for metastatic malignant teratoma. Br. J. Urol. 59:578–583.
92. Aass N, Fossa SD, Ous S, et al. 1990. Prognosis in patients with metastatic nonseminomatous testicular cancer. Radiother. Oncol. 17:285–292.
93. Aass N, Klepp O, Cavallin-Stahl E, et al. 1991. Prognostic factors in unselected patients with nonseminomatous metastatic testicular cancer: a multicenter experience. J. Clin. Oncol. 9: 818–826.

94. de Wit R, Sylvester R, Tsitsa C, et al. 1997. Tumour marker concentration at the start of chemotherapy is a stronger predictor of treatment failure than marker half-life: a study in patients with disseminated nonseminomatous testicular cancer. Br. J. Cancer 75:432–435.

95. Koshida K, Kadono Y, Konaka H, et al. 1998. Chemotherapy of metastatic testicular germ-cell tumors: relationship of histologic response to size reduction and changes in tumor markers. Int. J. Urol. 5:74–79.

96. Canal P, Villeneuve G, Bugat R, et al. 1998. Plasma lactate dehydrogenase and its isoenzymes in nonseminomatous germ-cell tumors of the testis. Pathol. Biol. (Paris) 32:245–250.

97. Bassetto MA, Franceschi T, Lenotti M, et al. 1994. AFP and HCG in germ-cell tumors. Int. J. Biol. Markers. 9:29–32.

98. Han SJ, Yoo S, Choi SH, et al. 1997. Actual half-life of alpha-fetoprotein as a prognostic tool in pediatric malignant tumors. Pediatr. Surg. Int. 12:599–602.

99. Raghavan D, Peckham MJ, Heyderman E, et al. 1982. Prognostic factors in clinical stage I nonseminomatous germ-cell tumours of the testis. Br. J. Cancer 45:167–173.

100. Toner GC, Geller NL, Tan C, et al. 1990. Serum tumor marker half-life during chemotherapy allows early prediction of complete response and survival in nonseminomatous germ-cell tumors. Cancer Res. 50:5904–5910.

101. Bosl GJ and Head MD. 1994. Serum tumor marker half-life during chemotherapy in patients with germ-cell tumors. Int. J. Biol. Markers. 9:25–28.

102. Murphy BA, Motzer RJ, Mazumdar M, et al. 1994. Serum tumor marker decline is an early predictor of treatment outcome in germ-cell Tumor patients treated with cisplatin and ifosfamide salvage chemotherapy. Cancer 73:2520–2526.

103. Gerl A, Lamerz R, Clemm C, et al. 1996. Does serum tumor marker half-life complement pretreatment risk stratification in metastatic nonseminomatous germ-cell tumors? Clin. Cancer. Res. 2:1565–1570.

104. Gerl A, Lamerz R, Mann K, et al. 1997. Is serum tumor marker half-life a guide to prognosis in metastatic nonseminomatous germ-cell tumors? Anticancer Res. 17:3047–3049.

105. Mazumdar M, Bajorin DF, Bacik J, et al. 2001. Predicting outcome to chemotherapy in patients with germ-cell tumors: the value of the rate of decline of human chorionic gonadotropin and alpha-fetoprotein during therapy. Clin. Oncol. 19:2534–2541.

106. von Eyben FE, Madsen EL, Blaabjerg O, et al. 2002. Serum lactate dehydrogenase isoenzyme 1 in patients with seminoma stage I followed with surveillance. Acta. Oncol. 41:77–83.

107. Horwich A and Peckham MJ. 1984. Serum tumour marker regression rate following chemotherapy for malignant teratoma. Eur. J. Cancer Clin. Oncol. 20:1463–470.

108. Inanc SE, Meral R, Darendeliler E, et al. 1999. Prognostic significance of marker half-life during chemotherapy in nonseminomatous germ-cell testicular tumors. Acta. Oncol. 38:505–509.

109. Willemse PH, Sleijfer DT, Schraffordt Koops H, et al. 1981. The value of AFP and HCG half-lives in predicting the efficacy of combination chemotherapy in patients with nonseminomatous germ-cell tumors of the testis. Oncodev. Biol. Med. 2:129–134.

110. Gerl A, Clemm C, Lamerz R, et al. 1993. Prognostic implications of tumour marker analysis in nonseminomatous germ-celltumours with poor prognosis metastatic disease. Eur. J. Cancer 7:961–965.

111. Stevens MJ, Norman AR, Dearnaley DP, et al. 1995. Prognostic significance of early serum tumor marker half-life in metastatic testicular teratoma. J. Clin. Oncol. 13:87–92.

112. Germa JR, Llanos M, Tabernero JM, et al. 1993. False elevations of alpha-fetoprotein associated with liver dysfunction in germ-cell tumors. Cancer 7:2491–2494.

113. Hida S, Kawakita M, Oishi K, et al. 1986. False-positive elevation of alpha-fetoprotein during induction chemotherapy in patients with testicular cancer. Hinyokika Kiyo 32:1859–1866.

114. Skinner DG and Scardino PT. 1980. Relevance of biochemical tumor markers and lymphadenectomy in management of nonseminomatous testis tumors: current perspective. J. Urol. 123:378–382.

115. Elkins R and Edward P. 1998. On the meaning of sensitivity: a rejoinder. Clin. Chem. 44:1773–1778.

116. Cole LA, Rinne KM, Shahabi S, et al. 1999. False-Positive HCG Assay Results Leading to Unnecessary Surgery and Chemotherapy and Needless Occurrences of Diabetes and Coma. Clin. Chem. 45:313–314.

117. Johnson GF, Feld RD, Bernard JM, et al. 2000. Two cases of immunoassay interference with clinical consequences. Clin. Chem. 46:A37–A38.

118. Vladutiu AO, Sulewski JM, Pudlak KA, Stull CG. 1982. Heterophilic antibodies interfering with radioimmunoassay. A false-positive pregnancy test. JAMA 248:2489–2490.

119. von Eyben FE, Madsen EL, Fritsche H, et al. 2003. R. A new prognostic model for testicular germ-cell tumours. APMIS 111:100–105.

120. Nonomura N, Imazu T, Harada Y, et al. 1999. Molecular staging of testicular cancer using polymerase chain reaction of the testicular cancer-specific genes. Hinyokika Kiyo 45:593–597.

121. Chagantirsk R, Rodriquez E, Bosl GJ. 1993. Cytogenetics of male germ-cell tumors. Urol. Clin. North Am. 20:55–56.

122. de Jong B, Oosterhuis JW, Castedo SMMJ, et al. 1990. Pathogenesis of adult testicular germ-cell tumors. A cytogenetic model. Cytogenet. Cell. Gene. 48:143–167.

123. Suijkerbuijk RF, Looijenga L, de Jong, B, et al. 1992. Verification of isochromosome 12p and identification of other chromosome 12 aberrations in gonadal and extragonadal germ-cell tumors by bicolor double fluorescence in situ hybridization. Cancer Genet. Cytogenet. 63:8–16.

124. von Eyben FE, de Graaff W, Marrink J, et al. 1992. Serum lactate dehydrogenase isoenzyme 1 activity in patients with testicular germ-cell tumors correlates with the total number of copies of the short arms of chromosome 12 in the tumors. Mol. Gen. Genet. 235:140–146.

9

Autoantibodies, Autoimmunity, and Cancers

Markers for Identification of Early Stages of Tumors

Robert M. Nakamura and Eng M. Tan

1. INTRODUCTION

There is a significant association between neoplastic cancers and autoimmune diseases. Many autoimmune phenomena have been observed in cancers. Conversely, cancers have been diagnosed with increased frequency in autoimmune diseases *(1–4)*.

Several studies have shown a relationship between rheumatic diseases, autoimmune phenomena, and cancers *(1–6)*. Patients with malignant diseases may develop autoimmune phenomena and rheumatic diseases resulting from generations of autoantibodies to various autoantigens, oncoproteins, tumor suppressor genes, proliferation associated antigens, onconeural antigens, cancer/testes antigens, mRNA-binding proteins, and rheumatic disease-associated antigens *(1–4)*.

1.1. Autoantibodies as Predictors of Disease

Autoantibodies are markers of disease activity and under certain circumstances should be able to help define the nature of the disease and provide markers to classify the disease, i.e. type I diabetes may be autoimmune or not autoimmune based on the existence of the specific disease-associated antibodies *(7)*. Additionally, they should have the ability to predict the presence of the specific disease. The goal is to prevent the manifestations of the disease in high-risk patients.

Autoimmune diseases, which affect 5% of the population, may be prevented by avoiding environmental factors that trigger the disease or by use of therapy that modulates the destructive pathogenesis. Screening populations for susceptibility to autoimmune disease may be feasible at this time. Similarly, the testing for autoantibodies may be used to screen populations for persons who may be at increased risk of manifesting clinically significant cancers.

1.2. Autoantibodies and Cancers

In a study of liver diseases that develop into hepatocellular carcinoma, Imai et al. *(8)* found that one-third of patients with chronic hepatitis and/or liver cirrhosis demonstrated increasing titers and changing specificities of anti-nuclear antibodies (ANA) at or before transition to development of hepatocellular carcinoma. It should be emphasized that sudden changes in titers and alterations of antibody specificities of the ANA are seen infrequently in classical systemic rheumatic diseases.

From: *Cancer Diagnostics: Current and Future Trends*
Edited by: R. M. Nakamura, W. W. Grody, J. T. Wu, and R. B. Nagle © Humana Press Inc., Totowa, NJ

There have been reports that antibodies to certain oncoproteins and tumor suppressor gene antigens, such as *p53*, are detected before the diagnosis of the cancer or in the early stages of the malignant disease *(9)*. Tan et al. *(3,10–12)* have observed that antibodies against aberrantly expressed tumor antigens (such as p62, CENP-F, and p53, for example) appear before tumors are detected by conventional diagnostic tests. In this chapter, the use of specific autoantibody assays for serological screening and use as a diagnostic tool for the early detection of cancers is described.

2. AUTOIMMUNITY AND TUMOR IMMUNITY

2.1. Autoimmunity

The body is normally endowed with immune mechanisms that distinguish "self" from "non-self." There are several pathways and alterations of control mechanisms underlying self-recognition that result in an autoimmune response *(13,14)*. The autoimmune response with similar antibodies can also be found in patients with various cancers. In addition, antibodies with specificities unique to the cancerous process have been observed; such antibodies may be involved in the immune surveillance that recognizes the neoepitopes on tumors as foreign *(15–17)*.

Autoimmunity can be pathologic and induce immunological injury of the host with diseases, such as systemic lupus erythematosus. However, currently, it is known that autoimmune responses are not rare, and self-antigens may elicit a "natural autoimmunity" of the host without an accompanying autoimmune disease. Some of these benign autoimmune responses may serve a regulatory function within the immune network of the host *(13,14)*.

The association of cancers and autoimmunity has been described with increased frequency during the last two decades *(1–6,18)*. Also, autoantibodies have been observed in sera of patients with epithelial and hematologic malignancies *(19)*. Through the use of immunofluorescent assays, elevated titers of ANA have been seen in 27% of cancer patients *(19)*.

The incidence of autoantibodies to normal tissue constituents was studied in 250 cancer patients *(20)*. Utilizing indirect immunofluorescent microscopy methods, Tannenberg et al. *(20)* observed the presence of autoantibody in 15% of 250 patients with malignant disease as compared with 24% of patients with general non-neoplastic disease and 8% in normal blood donors. In patients with lymphoma or leukemia, the incidence of anti-smooth muscle antibodies was 15% compared with 4% in the control population. There was no increase of anti-smooth muscle antibodies in patients with other malignant tumors.

In contrast to the above observations, Swiss et al. *(21)* studied 164 patients with various malignant diseases, the authors did not observe an increased incidence of ANA in malignant conditions. The patients' sera were analyzed for ssDNA, dsDNA, poly(I), poly (G), cardiolipin, histones, RNP, Sm, SS-A/Ro, and SS-B/La by the enzyme-linked immunosorbent assay (ELISA) technique. We acknowledge that a limited number of autoantibody specificities were examined and these antibodies are largely seen within the rheumatic disease group of patients. It is widely known that cancer patients have different autoantibodies from rheumatic disease patients.

2.2. Identifications of Specific Immune Responses in Cancers

During the past decade new techniques have been developed to identify various oncoproteins and glycoproteins. A methodology called the serological identification of antigens by recombinant expression cloning (SEREX), which is a modification of immuno-screening cDNA expression libraries *(13)*, was used to identify more than 400 autoantigens *(15,16)*. The antibodies to a given antigen were usually confined to patients with the same tumor type. Sahin et al. *(15,16)* have observed that human tumors elicit multiple specific immune responses in the autologous host and help provide diagnostic and therapeutic approaches to human cancer. The challenge has been to find ways to harness the autoimmune response to eliminate tumor cells by the use of immunostimulants or by vaccination with tumor-specific antigens.

3. RHEUMATIC SYNDROMES ASSOCIATED WITH CANCERS

An extensive search for occult or hidden malignancy in most rheumatic syndromes is not recommended unless accompanied by specific "clues" or findings suggestive of malignancy *(5,6)*.

There is a definite association of cancers or malignances with certain rheumatic syndromes, such as rheumatoid arthritis or Sjögren's syndrome with monoclonal gammopathy and Lambert-Eaton myasthenic syndrome (paraneoplastic rheumatic disorder). Certain long-standing rheumatic syndromes may behave like "premalignant conditions." The cancer may emerge because of immune dysregulation.

The relative risk of cancer is increased in long standing rheumatoid arthritis, Sjögren's syndrome, dermatomyositis, systemic sclerosis, systemic lupus erythematosus, and temporal arteritis *(5,6)*. However, the risk of cancer is not increased in polymyositis and polymyalgia rheumatica *(5)*. Rheumatoid arthritis with monoclonal gammopathy carries a high risk for development of cancer *(6)*. Sjögren's syndrome associated with monoclonal antibody isotype 17–109 is present in all patients undergoing development of malignancy *(22)*.

Cancer-associated rheumatic disorders may be classified as, paraneoplastic syndrome induced by mediators from a distant tumor, host-altered immune surveillance system resulting in both the rheumatic and neoplastic diseases, and rheumatic disorder which arises as an adverse reaction to anti-cancer therapy *(5,6)*. Cancer-associated rheumatic syndromes occur at a distance from the primary tumor or metastasis and are induced by the malignancy through hormones, protein mediators, antibodies, and cytotoxic lymphocytes *(5,6)*.

These cancer-associated rheumatic disorders may precede, appear concomitantly with, or follow the clinical diagnosis of cancer. It should be noted that patients who are already diagnosed with a malignant disease might develop a systemic rheumatic autoimmune disease after chemotherapy treatment *(4)*. Treatment of malignancies with immunomodulating agents may induce autoimmunity and autoimmune disease. Interferon treatment of myeloproliferative disorders, such as chronic myelogenous leukemia, can often develop rheumatic symptoms and trigger the development of autoimmunity. The rheumatic syndromes after chemotherapy have been observed in patients with breast cancer, ovarian cancer, and non-Hodgkin's lymphoma.

4. PARANEOPLASTIC SYNDROMES

Paraneoplastic syndromes are organ/tissue disorders associated with cancer. The autoimmune response in paraneoplastic syndromes is triggered by specific antigens and often affects the nervous system. These paraneoplastic neurological degenerative (PND) syndromes are associated with lung, breast, and ovarian cancers *(23–28)*.

The PND syndromes with symptoms related to disorders of the nervous system show antoantibodies that react with nuclear and cytoplasmic components in neuronal cells. The associated malignant tumor may have aberrant expression of neuronal type tissues. The neurological disorders include sensory neuropathy, opsoclonus myoclonus ataxia, cerebellar degeneration, and brain stem encephalitis.

Anti-Hu/anti-neuronal nuclear antibody-1 (ANNA-1) antibodies have been detected in 90% of patients with small cell lung cancer (SCLC). The Hu antibody has been associated with encephalomyelitis, sensory neuropathy, and cerebellar degeneration. The Hu antigens are 35–40 kDa proteins and expressed in neurons. The Hu antigens constitute a family of RNA binding proteins with an RNA recognition motif of 80 amino acids *(24,25)*.

Anti-Yo/anti-Purkinje cell antibody (PCA) is an autoantibody that reacts with an onconeural antigen in the cytoplasm of Purkinje cells in the malignant cells of breast and gynecological cancers. The Yo antibody is associated with the development of cerebellar degeneration with clinical symptoms of ataxia and dysphagia *(23–25,29)*. There are three types of Yo antigen and their corresponding genes are clones.

Antibody to Ri/ANNA-2 protein antibody to Ri has been observed in sera of patients with breast, SCLC, gynecological, and other cancers *(23–28)*. The antibody to Ri binds neuron-specific RNA nuclear proteins with molecular weight of 55–80 kDa. Clinical features observed in patients with anti-Ri are cerebellar degeneration and myoclonus. The genes encoding two Ri proteins have been cloned, sequenced, and called neuronal onconeural ventral nervous system antigen *Nova-1* and *Nova -2* by Darnell and colleagues *(25,30)*.

Amphiphysin is a vesicle-associated protein on the synaptic terminal that binds the vesicle core protein adaptor AP2 and dynamin *(25)*. Antibodies to amphiphysin may prevent the release of neurotransmitters at the synaptic junction. The antibody may occur in patients with breast, lung, and other neoplasms *(25,31)*. The clinical disorders associated with anti-amphiphysin are stiff man syndrome with diffuse muscle rigidity and less frequently, encephalomyelitis.

Lambert-Eaton syndrome is a neuromuscular syndrome initiated by immune response against neuron-like components of the tumor cells. There is high frequency of calcium-channel antibodies found in patients with Lambert-Eaton syndrome. These antibodies react with voltage gated calcium channels (VGCC) *(23–28,32–34)*. The VGCC antibodies are found in small cell lung cancer (SCLC) and cause a paraneoplastic disorder. The VGCC of the P/Q type is present at the presynaptic cholinergic-synapse and in Purkinje cells of the cerebellum *(32,33)*. Clinical symptoms may improve if the patient's IgG is removed and replaced by plasma exchange treatment *(34)*. The autoantibodies to Tr antigen have been observed in sera of patients with Hodgkin's disease associated paraneoplastic cerebellar degeneration (PCD). The Tr antibody reacts with the cytoplasm and proximal dendrites of the Purkinje cells of the human cerebellum in a pattern similar to the Yo antibodies *(35)*.

Cancer-associated retinopathy (CAR) is rare and is associated with SCLC, melanoma, or gynecologic tumors. The symptoms include impaired visual changes, night blindness, photosensitivity, and the symptoms often precede the diagnosis of cancer *(24,25)*. Serum antibodies that react with retinal photoreceptor layer or ganglion cells have been observed. Antibodies to recoverin, a photoreceptor protein, have been characterized in some cases of CAR *(36)*. Also, patients with CAR develop autoantibodies to α enolase. A small percentage of healthy subjects without evident tumor or visual symptoms may have serum antibodies against α enolase *(37)*.

5. AUTOANTIBODIES TO ONCOPROTEINS

Oncoproteins are encoded by oncogenes and/or tumor suppressor genes and participate in the regulation of cell growth and differentiation. Mutations of the oncogenes or abnormal overexpression of the oncoproteins are involved in the genesis and initiation of malignant tumors *(3,4,38)*.

5.1. Autoantibodies to L-myc, c-myc, and c-myb Proteins

The *L-myc* gene is a human oncogene with structural homology to *c-myc* and *c-myb (39)*. The L-myc protein is overexpressed in 10–40% of tumors with neuroendocrine characteristics. The *L-myc* gene is important in normal development of the brain, kidney, and lungs, and in combination with *c-myc* and *c-myb* plays a role in differentiation and proliferation *(39,40)*.

Because *L-myc* oncogene product is a nuclear protein, antibodies to *L-myc* could be considered as anti-nuclear antibodies. Antibodies to *L-myc* were observed in 10% (7/70) of lung cancer patients. Of the lung tumors, there were five non-small cell lung carcinomas, two adenocarcinomas, two squamous cell carcinomas, and one large cell carcinoma *(39)*. *C-myc* oncogene product is another nuclear protein involved in cell proliferation. Ben-Mahrez et al. *(40)* have shown the presence of antibodies to *c-myc* in patients with cancers of various types, including colorectal, breast, and ovarian cancers. *C-myc* antibodies were found in patients with African Burkitt's lymphoma in Ghana and also in normal Ghanians. Thus, *c-myc* antibodies may reflect an autoimmune phenomenon prevalent in the endemic region of Ghana *(41)*.

The *c-myb* gene is a normal cellular gene homologous to the avian myeloblastosis virus oncogene. The human *c-myb* gene product is a 80 kD nuclear protein associated with the chromatin and nuclear matrix *(42)*. *C-myb* antibodies were found in many types of cancers. However, the *c-myb* antibodies were also observed in normal controls (healthy volunteers). The percentage of positive sera varied depending upon the cancer type, and breast cancer patients showed a frequency of 43% seropositivity for anti *c-myb* antibodies; however, the control patients had an incidence of 24% positivity *(42)*.

The antibodies to *L-myc* was detected only in sera of cancer patients *(39)*. The antibodies to *c-myc* and *c-myb* are not specific for cancer and have been found in healthy patients and patients with systemic lupus erythematosus *(40–44)*.

5.2. Autoantibody to HER-2/neu Protein

HER-2/neu is a proto-oncogene that encodes a transmembrane tyrosine kinase human epidermal growth factor receptor protein *(45)*. Overexpression of HER-2/neu protein is seen in 20–33% of breast cancers *(46,45)* and at a lower frequency in other solid tumors, such as ovarian cancers. The HER-2/neu protein consists of three domains, an extracellular receptor binding site, a lipophilic transmembrane segment, and an intracellular segment with tyrosine kinase activity. The HER-2/neu receptor has an important role in cellular growth. Disis et al. *(46)* studied the antibody response to HER-2/neu in 107 newly diagnosed breast cancer patients. The sera was analyzed for the presence of HER-2/neu specific antibodies with a capture enzyme-linked immunosorbent assay (ELISA) and verified by a Western blot assay. Serum HER-2/neu antibodies correlated with the presence of breast cancer. The HER-2/neu antibodies at titers of 1/100 or greater were detected in 12 of 107 (11%) breast cancer patients vs none of 200 (0%) normal controls. Titers of greater than 1/5000 were detected in 5/107 (5%). A total of 20% (9/44) patients with HER-2/neu positive breast cancers demonstrated serum antibodies to HER-2/neu. A total of 5% of patients with HER-2/neu negative breast tumors had the antibodies present in their sera *(46)*.Ward et al. *(45)* studied 57 patients with colorectal cancers in various stages for the presence of serum HER-2/neu antibody titer of 1/100 or greater as compared to zero titer in the control population. The HER-2/neu antibody response detected in the serum of patients with colorectal cancer was primarily IgG and IgA.

The data suggest that detection of antibody to HER-2/neu in cancer patients may be useful, since the antibody was seen in the early stages of breast cancer patients.

5.3. Autoantibodies ras Proteins

The *ras* oncogenes are cancer-related genes that can be activated by specific point mutation and found in many different types of cancer *(47)*. Three *ras* genes have been identified as H-*ras*-1, *k*-*ras*-2, and N-*ras*. The *ras* genes encode a highly conserved group of 21,000 M.W. proteins *(47)*.

Mutated ras proteins have been associated with malignant transformation of many human cancers. The ras mutations have been seen in 45% of colon adenocarcinomas.

In a study of 160 colon cancer patients, Takahashi et al. *(47)* detected IgA antibodies in 32% of the patients reactive with mutated p21 ras-D12 protein and only in one of 40 so-called normal patients. Thus, the data suggest that the presence of antibody to the ras protein is highly correlated with the presence of colon cancer. The major antibody response to the p21 ras protein was an IgA response to epitopes located in the non-mutated carboxy terminus segment rather than to the mutated segments of the mutated rasprotein.

5.4. Autoantibodies to Abl and Bcr Proteins

Formation of an aberrant Abl-Bcr protein is the hallmark marker of Philadelphia chromosome (ph)-positive leukemia. Abl and Bcr are intracellular molecules that are biologically important in many cell functions *(48)*. Talpaz et al. *(48)* studied cases of Philadelphia chromosome-positive leukemia, Philadelphia chromosome-negative leukemia, and normal patients. A positive antibody response was observed in the above three groups, including healthy individuals and Philadelphia chromosome-negative cases of leukemia. Thus, it appears that serum assays for antibodies to Abl and Bcr proteins do not have a significant correlation to the leukemia group with a positive Philadelphia chromosome.

6. AUTOANTIBODIES TO TUMOR SUPPRESSOR PROTEINS

6.1. p53 Antibodies in Cancer Patients

The tumor suppressor gene *p53* is a phosphoprotein in the nucleus of normal cells. The *p53* has certain properties that can activate genes involved in cell-cycle regulation and can arrest cell-cycle progression and allow damaged DNA to be repaired *(9)*.

In various types of cancers, an incidence of 50% mutations in the *p53* gene have been observed *(9)*. Approximately 30 to 40% of cancer patients with p53 mutations will develop p53 antibodies. The specificity of serum assay for p53 antibodies in cancer is 96% *(9,49,50)*. The *p53* mutations are the most frequent genetic event in human cancers. The most common mutations of p53 in human cancers are missense point mutations within the coding sequences of the gene *(9,50,51)*. These mutant p53 proteins are usually inactive and have increased stability and accumulate in the nucleus of neoplastic cells. The half-life of the mutant p53 protein is several hours as compared with a 20 min half-life for the wild type of p53 protein.

The p53 mutations have been found in cancers of the colon, stomach, breast, lung, brain, and esophagus *(52)*. There is a positive correlation between the frequency of p53 mutations in certain types of cancer *(9)*. However, there are three types of cancers, hepatoma, testicular carcinoma, and melanoma that are devoid of p53 mutations and are also negative for antibodies to the p53 protein *(53–55)*.

Esophageal and oral cancers have a high rate of p53 mutations and a high frequency of antibodies. The one exception is gliomatous tumor of brain that has a low incidence of p53 antibodies despite a high frequency of p53 mutations *(9,56)*. Rainnov et al. *(56)* found p53 mutations in 24 to 60 glioblastomas and none of the patients demonstrated p53 serum antibodies. The blood–brain barrier may inhibit the induction of the humoral immune response to p53.

The specificity analysis of the p53 antibodies has revealed that antibody reacts with amino and carboxy terminal regions away from the central regions of p53 containing the mutations *(9,50,57)*. As seen in many autoimmune diseases, the p53 antibodies are equally reactive with the wild type and mutated forms of p53 proteins. The mutated forms of p53 have a longer half-life than the wild type and demonstrate an increased expression.

The mutated forms of p53 with overexpression and aberrant localization in the nucleus and cytoplasm help trigger the autoimmune response. The antibody response to p53 is mainly of IgG1 and IgG2 subclasses and some patients show an IgM antibody response *(9)*. No IgG3 or IgG4 isotypes of p53 antibody was detected in the patients.

The detection of serum p53 antibodies can be useful for early detection of cancer in high-risk patients. Anti-p53 antibodies were found in sera of workers exposed to vinyl chloride, who developed angiosarcoma of the liver and in the sera of heavy smokers who developed lung cancer *(57)*. In these individuals exposed to vinyl chloride, serum anti-p53 antibodies were detected before the diagnosis of the malignant disease. Anti-p53 antibodies in serum have been detected several months before clinical diagnosis of cancers in heavy smokers and in patients with chronic obstructive pulmonary diseases *(58,59)*. Cawley et al. *(60)* have studied patients with Barrett's esophagus and esophageal carcinoma and found that the presence of serum p53 antibodies may pre-date the clinical diagnosis of cancer. Thus, the data suggest that anti-p53 antibodies are found in sera of patients with cancer. The antibodies to p53 are generated in association with *p53* gene missense mutation. It has a specificity of 96% and is useful as a marker for the early detection of carcinoma in patients who are at high risk for developing malignancy.

6.2. Antibody to Retinoblastoma Suppressor Protein

The retinoblastoma (*RB*) gene product Rb is a cell-cycle regulator protein. The overexpression of Rb leads to hypermethylation of the cellular DNA and modulates DkA replication in the cell cycle *(61)*. The inactivating mutation of the RB gene is seen in a variety of tumors *(61,62)*.

Matsumoto et al. *(62)* published the first report describing the presence of RB antibodies in several patients with small cell carcinoma and non-small cell carcinoma of the lung. The presence of antibody reactive with an RB fusion protein was not detected in 30 normal patients. The usefulness and significance of antibodies to RB suppressor protein needs to be studied further.

7. AUTOANTIBODIES TO PROLIFERATION-ASSOCIATED ANTIGENS

Cancer patients may develop antibodies reactive with antigens that are involved in cell-cycle regulation. Antibodies to nuclear and cytoplasmic antigens associated with splicing processes and ribosome biosynthesis have been reported *(3,4)*.

Covini et al. *(63)* reported that antibodies to the nuclear protein cyclin B1 (protein expressed in the S and G2 phases of the cell cycle) have been found in 15% (15/100) of patients with hepatocellular carcinoma (HCC). In the same study, no antibodies were detected to cyclin D1 and E and only one patient had antibodies to cyclin A. Anti-cyclin B1 was also detected in the sera of patients with chronic active hepatitis and cirrhosis.

A novel nuclear protein called SG2NA (S/G2 nuclear antigen) was found to be expressed in S and G2 phase cells *(64,65)*. The SG2NA antigen was characterized from sera obtained from a patient with lung cancer. The SG2NA is involved in regulating nuclear function associated with cell cycles. CENP-F, also known as P330, is a cell cycle-associated nuclear antigen that is expressed in low amounts in G0/G1 cells and accumulates in the nuclear matrix during the S phase with a maximal expression in G2/M cells *(66,67)*. CENP-F is associated with the centromeres and the nuclear matrix.

Anti-CENP-F antibodies were found to be associated with cancer *(67,68)*. The most common tumors were breast and lung cancers. Autoimmunity to CENP-F is not associated with systemic rheumatic diseases. The antibodies to CENP-F were present in rare cases of chronic liver disease, and chronic rejection of renal allografts and Crohn's disease *(69)*. Thus, it appears that autoimmunity to CENP-F may be related to events of altered or abnormal cells proliferation.

Antibodies to antigens associated with splicing processes and ribosomal biosynthesis have been found in cancer patients *(3,70,71)*. When the eukaryotic cells divide, the nucleoli disperse before mitosis and reform in the daughter cells at the sites of ribosomal RNA gene clusters called nucleolus organizer regions (NOR) *(70)*.

Tightly bound to NOR during mitosis is the hUBF (human upstream binding factor), a critical factor in the regulation of RNA transcription. Imai and co-workers *(71–73)* have found that sera from patients with hepatocellular carcinoma have antibodies that bind NOR-90/hUBF, the U3-RNP associated fibrillarin, DNA topoisomerase II, and other proteins that are involved in the ribosomal biosynthesis.

8. AUTOIMMUNE RESPONSES TO mRNA-BINDING PROTEINS p62 AND KOC IN DIFFERENT TYPES OF CANCER

8.1. p62 and KOC Antigens

In hepatocellular carcinoma (HCC), autoantibodies to intracellular antigens are detected in 30 to 40% of patients *(10–12)*. Further studies *(8,11)* have shown that when patients with chronic hepatitis or liver cirrhosis develop HCC, patients develop new autoantibodies with different immuno-specificities.

In 1999, Zhang et al. *(10)* described a putative cancer antigen called p62. p62 is a 62-kD protein containing two types of RNA-binding motifs, the consensus sequence RNA-binding domain (CS-RBD) and four hn RNP K homology (KH) domains.

The *koc* gene was identified by Mueller-Pillasch et al. *(74)* and the protein they called hKOC was observed to be overexpressed in pancreatic cancer. Additional experiments have shown that *koc* gene and overexpression of the messenger RNA were present in a variety of other cancers besides cancer of the pancreas.

Nielsen et al. *(75)* reported three IGF-II mRNA-binding proteins, which they called IMP-1, IMP-2, and IMP-3. They demonstrated that IMP-1, 2 and 3 were able to bind IGF-11 mRNA and alter the translatability of IGF-II mRNA.

Several proteins of this family bind to and alter the expression of insulin-like growth factor II (KGF-II) messenger RNA. IGF-II has been implicated as a secondary oncogene and its overexpression has been demonstrated in cytoplasm of cells of many different types of cancer. Studies by Tan and colleagues *(10–12)* have shown that p62 (a splice variant of IMP2) is overexpressed in the cancer nodules of hepatocellular carcinoma (HCC). In addition, p62 mRNA was found in fetal livers and not detected in normal adult livers *(76)* and immunohistochemical assay on liver sections confirmed protein expression in fetus but not in adult tissue. Thus, p62 is developmentally regulated, expressed in fetal, but not in adult liver and aberrantly expressed in HCC. The p62 protein is cytoplasmic in location and autoantibodies were found in 21% of a cohort of HCC patients. The reported evidence shows that IGF-II may play an important role in carcinogenesis.

8.2. Autoantibody Responses to p62 and KOC

Zhang et al. *(12)* have demonstrated that with use of recombinant polypeptide antigens, autoantibodies to both p62 and KOC antigens can be detected. They studied sera from 777 patients with ten different types of cancers. Autoantibodies to p62 were found in 11.6% and to KOC in 12.2% and cumulatively to both antigens in 20.5% with significant differences from control populations consisting of normal subjects and patients with autoimmune diseases without cancer.

The types of cancers and number of patients studied in each group are: breast *(98)*, colorectal *(65)*, esophageal *(119)*, gastric *(135)*, hepatocellular *(75)*, lung *(84)*, lymphoma *(72)*, pharyngeal *(56)*, ovarian *(33)*, and uterine *(40)*.

The control groups studied for the presence of p62 band KOC autoantibodies include 82 normal patients and 139 patients with autoimmune diseases. The *p* values for the group of normal patients as compared to the cancer patients was less than 0.05. The autoimmune disease group included patients with systemic lupus erythematosus (SLE) *(62)*, rheumatoid arthritis *(57)*, and Sjögren's syndrome *(20)*. The *p* value was less than 0.01 in the comparison of the autoimmune group with the patients with cancer.

The above data demonstrates that tests for autoantibodies to p62 and KOC will be helpful tumor markers to identify patients with a wide variety of cancers.

9. ANTI-CANCER/TESTIS ANTIGEN ANTIBODIES

Cancer/testes antigens refer to a large group of antigens that are expressed in various tumors *(77–79)*. Both specific cellular and humoral immune recognition of human tumor antigens have been reported. Seven cancer/testes antigens have been identified and belong to the following gene families: *MAGE, GAGE, BAGE, SSX, ESO, SCP,* and *CTT (77–79)*.

Antibodies to MAGE and tyrosinase antigens first recognized by cytotoxic T lymphocytes (CTL) have been detected in melanoma patients *(78)*. A low frequency of 5% of anti-MAGE-1 and SSX2 was found in the sera of patients with melanoma, ovarian, or lung cancer *(79)*. NY-ESO-1, a cancer-testes (CT) antigen has been identified by autologous antibody

Table 1
The Percentage of Positive Hsp27 Serum Antibodies
in Various Cancers

Ovarian cancer	50%	17/34
Endometrial cancer	38.2%	13/34
Cervical and uterine cancers	30%	3/10
Vaginal and vulvar cancers	60%	3/5

(77). In a study of 234 cancer patients, Stockert et al. *(79)* reported that the frequency of NY-ESO-1 antibody was 9.4% in melanoma patients and 12.5% in ovarian cancer patients, lung cancer (42%), and breast cancer (71%).

10. AUTOANTIBODIES TO HSP-27 (HEAT SHOCK PROTEIN) AND CATHEPSIN D IN CANCERS

Korneeva et al. *(80)* found that autoantibodies to Hsp 27 were found to be associated with cancers of the female genital tract. Antibodies to the Hsp 27 were detected in only 1 in 29 (3.4%) healthy control subjects and 1 in 23 (4.3%) women with benign lesions. In contrast, 39 of 96 (40.6%) women with gynecologic cancers had positive antibody for Hsp27 ($p = 0.004$ vs benign) (Table 1).

Besides the finding of the presence of antibodies to the Hsp27, there was no relationship between antibodies to the other shock proteins Hsp-60, Hsp-70, and Hsp90 and gynecological cancers.

Bosscher et al. *(81)* determined the presence of circulating pro and mature forms of cathepsin D and antibodies reactive to the cathepsin D enzyme by a Western immunoblot and quantitated by an enzyme immunoassay. Specific immunoreactivity with the 34 kDa and 52 kDa Cathepsin D forms were analyzed by Western blot on 40 patients with endometrial cancer and 15 normal patients. The circulating pro form of cathepsin D was detected in 31 of 40 endometrial cancer patients tested and none of the healthy controls. Serum IgG autoantibodies reactive with cathepsin D were demonstrated in 29 of 31 patients who also had circulating procathepsin D. The normal control patients did not have evidence of anti-cathepsin D antibodies.

11. SUMMARY

Malignant diseases are commonly associated with induction of autoimmunity, which results in the generation of numerous autoantibodies against a wide variety of autoantigens.

Specific autoimmune features and rheumatic manifestations are associated with a significant number of patients with cancer. The association between autoimmunity and cancer may result from a number of factors that include genetic, environmental, hormonal, and immunologic factors. Many of the autoantibodies are highly specific for various cancers and include autoantibodies to p53, p62, KOC, L-*myc*, and *ras* oncogenes. Studies of antibodies to p53, p62, and KOC have shown that the specific autoantibodies have been detected in the sera of patients several months before the clinical diagnosis of malignancy.

The studies on humoral immune responses to tumor-associated autoantigens have shown that antibodies can be useful reagents to identify aberrant cellular mechanisms involved in tumor formation. The autoantibodies to p53 have a specificity of 96% with a prevalence of

30 to 40% of cancer patients with *p53* gene mutations. The general incidence of *p53* gene mutations in cancer patients is 50%. The incidence of autoantibodies to p62 and KOC antigens were studied in 777 patients with 10 different types of cancer. Autoantibodies to p62 were found in 11.6% and to KOC in 12.2% and cumulatively in 20.5% of the cancer patients studied.

A recent study of 546 cancer sera used a multiple array of six antigens, which included p62, KOC, and p53 antigen *(3)*. They observed that 45% of the sera were positive for antibody to any one of the six antigens, as compared with 12% when a single antigen was utilized.

In the future, one can hope that a panel array of several antigens to detect various specific autoantibodies may be useful for the early detection of cancer in patients who are in a high-risk population.

The autoantibodies have been useful to provide insight into mechanisms and pathways associated with cell transformation, regulation of growth factors, and tumorigenesis.

REFERENCES

1. Tomer Y, Sherer Y, Shoenfeld Y. 1998. Autoantibodies, autoimmunity and cancer. Oncology. Rep. 5:753–761.
2. Livingston PO, Ragupathi E, Muselli C. 2000. Autoimmune and anti-tumor consequences of antibodies against antigens shared by normal and malignant tissue. J. Clin. Immunol. 20:85–93.
3. Tan EM. 2001. Autoantibodies as reporters identifying aberrant cellular mechanisms in tumorigenesis. J. Clin. Invest. 10:1411–1415.
4. Abu-Shakra M, Buskila D, Ehrenfeld M, Conrad K, Shoenfeld Y. 2001. Cancer and autoimmunity: Autoimmune and rheumatic features in patients with malignancy. Ann. Rheumatic Dis. 60:433–440.
5. Nachitz JE, Rosner I, Rozenbaum M, Zuckerman E, Yeshurun D. 1999. Rheumatic syndromes: clues to occult neoplasia. Sem. Art. Rheum. 29:43–55.
6. Nachitz JE. 2001. Rheumatic Syndromes: Clues to Occult Neoplasia. Curr. Opin. Rheumatol. 13:62–66.
7. Leslie D, Lipsky P, Notkins AL. 2001. Autoantibodies as Predictors of Disease. J. Clin. Invest. 108:1417–1422.
8. Imai H, Nakano Y, Kiyosawa K, Tan EM. 1993. Increasing titers and changing specificities of antinuclear antibodies in patients with chronic liver disease who develop hepatocellular carcinoma. Cancer 71:26–35.
9. Soussi T. 2000. p53 antibodies in the sera of patients with various types of cancer: A review. Cancer Res. 60:1777–1788.
10. Zhang JY, Chain EKL, Peng XX, Tan EM. 1999. A novel cytoplasmic protein with RNA-binding motifs is an autoantigen in human hepatocellular carcinoma. J. Exp. Med. 189:1101–1110.
11. Zhang JY, Zhu W, Imai H, Kiyosawa K, Chan EKL, Tan EM. 2001. De-novo humoral immune responses to cancer-associated autoantigens during transition from chronic liver disease to hepatocellular carcinoma. Clin. Exp. Immunol. 125:1–9.
12. Zhang JY, Chan EKL, Peng XX, et al. 2001. Autoimmune Responses to mRNA Binding Proteins p62 and Koc in Diverse Malignancies. Clin. Immunol. 100:149–156.
13. Nakamura MC and Nakamura RM. 1992. Contemporary concepts of autoimmunity and autoimmune diseases. J. Clin. Lab. Anal. 6:275–289.
14. Hang LM and Nakamura RM. 1997. Current Concepts and Advances in Clinical Laboratory Testing for Autoimmune Diseases. Crit. Rev Clin Lab Sci. 34:275–311.
15. Sahin U, Tureci O, Schmitt H, et al. 1995. Human neoplasms elicit multiple specific immune responses in the autologous host. Proc. Natl Acad. Sci. USA 92:11810–11813.

16. Sahin U, Tureci I, Pfreundschuh M. 1997. Serological identification of human tumor antigens. Curr. Opin. Immunol. 9:709–716.
17. Ditzel HJ. 2000. Human antibodies in cancer and autoimmune disease. Immunol. Res. 21: 185–193.
18. Sela O and Shoenfeld Y. 1988. Cancer in Autoimmune disease. Semin. Arthritis Rheum. 18: 77–87.
19. Fairley CH. 1972. Autoantibodies in malignant disease. Brit. J. Hematol. 23:31.
20. Tannenberg AEG, Mueller HK, Cauchi MN, Anirn RC. 1973. Incidence of autoantibodies in Cancer patients. Clin. Exp. Immunol. 15:153–156.
21. Swissa M, Amital-Teplizki H, Haim N, Cohen Y, Shoenfeld Y. 1990. Autoantibodies in neoplasia—an unresolved enigma. Cancer 65:2554–2558.
22. Shokri F, Mageed RA, Maziak BR. 1993. Lymphoproliferation in primary Sjögren's syndrome; evidence of selective expansion of a B-cell subset characterized by the expression of cross-reactive idiotopes. Arthritis Rheum. 36:1128–1136.
23. Darnell RB. 1996. Onconeural antigens and the paraneoplastic neurologic disorders: At the intersection of cancer, immunity, and the brain. Proc. Natl. Acad. Sci. USA 93:4529–4536.
24. Dalmau JO, Posner JB. 1997. Paraneoplastic syndromes affecting the nervous system. Semin. Oncol. 24:318–28.
25. Posner JB and Dalmau, J. 1997. Paraneoplastic Syndromes. Curr. Opin. Immunol. 9:723–729.
26. Inuzuka T. 2000. Autoantibodies in paraneoplastic neurological syndrome. Am J. Med. Sci. 319:217–226.
27. Lennon VA. 1994a,b. Views and reviews: Paraneoplastic autoantibodies: The case for a descriptive generic nomenclature. Neurology 44:2236–2240.
28. Nakamura RM and Hang L. 2002. Autoimmune paraneoplastic syndromes of the central nervous system, in Clinical and Laboratory Evaluation of Human Autoimmune Diseases. (Nakamura RM, Keren DA, Bylund DJ. eds., American Society of Clinical Pathologists Press, Chicago, IL, pp. 308–317.
29. Lennon VA. 1989. Anti-Purkinje cell cytoplasmic and neuronal autoantibodies aid in diagnosis of paraneoplastic autoimmune neurological disorders. J. Neurol. Neurosurg. Psych. 42: 1438–1439.
30. Buckanovich R, Posner JB, Darnell R. 1993. Nova, the paraneoplastic Ki antigen, is homologous to an RNA-binding protein and is specifically expressed in the developing motor system. Neuron 11:657–672.
31. Dropcho EJ. 1996. Antiamphiphysin antibodies with small cell lung carcinoma and paraneoplastic encephalomyelitis. Ann. Neurol. 39:659–667.
32. Lennon VA. 1996. Calcium channel and related paraneoplastic disease autoantibodies, in Autoantibodies. Peter JB and Shoenfeld Y, eds., pp. 139–147.
33. Voltz R, Carpentier AF, Rosenfeld MR, et al. 1999. P/Q-type voltage-gated calcium channel antibodies in paraneoplastic disorders of the central nervous system. Muscle Nerve. 22:119–122.
34. Posner J and Dalmau JO. 1997. Paraneoplastic syndromes affecting the central nervous system. Ann. Rev. Med. 48:157–166.
35. Graus F, Dalmau J, Valldeoriola F, et al. 1997. Immunological characterization of a neuronal antibody (anti-Tr) associated with paraneoplastic cerebellar degeneration and Hodgkin's disease. J. Neuroimmunol. 74:55–61.
36. Adamus G. 2000. Antirecoverin antibodies and autoimmune retinopathy. Arch. Ophthalmol. 11:1577–1578.
37. Adamus G, Amundson D, Seigel GM, et al. 1998. Anti-enolase-alpha autoantibodies in cancer-associated retinopathy:epitope mapping and cytotoxicity on retinal cells. J. Autoimmun. 11: 671–677.
38. Cheever MA, Disis ML, Bernhard H, et al. 1995. Immunity to oncogenic proteins. Immunol. Rev. 145:33–59.

39. Yamamoto A, Shimizu E, Ogura T, et al. 1996. Detection of auto-antibodies against *L-myc* oncogene products in sera from lung cancer patients. Int. J. Cancer. 69:283–289.

40. Ben-Mahrez K, Thierry D, Sorokine I, Danna-Muller A, Kohiyama M. 1988. Detection of circulating antibodies against *c-myc* protein in cancer patient sera. Brit. J. Cancer 57:529–534.

41. LaFond RE, Eaton RB, Watt RA, Villee CA, Actor JK, Schur PH. 1992. Autoantibodies to *c-myc* protein: elevated levels in patients with African Burkitt's lymphoma and normal Ghanians. Autoimmunity 13:215–224.

42. Sorokine I, Ben-Mahrez K, Bracone A, et al. 1991. Presence of circulating Anti-*c-myb* oncogene product antibodies in human sera. Int. J. Cancer 47:665–669.

43. Yamamoto A, Shimizu E, Takeuchi E, et al. 1999. Infrequent presence of anti-*c-Myc* antibodies and absence of *c-myc* oncoprotein in sera from lung cancer patients. Oncology 56:129–133.

44. Yamauchi T, Naoe T, Kurosawa Y, Shiku H, Yamada K. 1990. Autoantibodies to *c-myc* nuclear protein products in autoimmune disease. Immunology 69:117–120.

45. Ward RL, Hawkins NJ, Coomber D, Disis ML. 1999. Antibody immunity to the HER-2/*neu* oncogenic protein in patients with colorectal cancer. Hum. Immunol. 60:510–515.

46. Disis ML, Pupa SM, Gralow JR, Dittadi R, Menard S, Cheever MA. 1997. High-titer HER-2/*neu* protein-specific antibody can be detected in patients with early-stage breast cancer. Clin Oncol. 15:3363–3367.

47. Takahashi M, Chen W, Byrd D, et al. 1995. Antibody to ras proteins in patients with colon cancer. Clin. Cancer Res. 1:1071–1077.

48. Talpaz M, Qiu X, Cheng K, et al. 2000. Autoantibodies to Abl and Bcr proteins. Leukemia 14:1661–1666.

49. Angelopoulou K, Diamandis EP, Sutherland DJ, Kellen JA, Bunting PS. 1994. Prevalence of serum antibodies against the p53 tumor suppressor gene protein in various cancers. Int. J. Cancer 58:480–487.

50. Lubin R, Schlichtholz B, Bengoufa D, et al. 1993. Analysis of p53 antibodies in patients with various cancers define B-cell epitopes of human p53: distribution on primary structure and exposure on protein surface. Cancer Res. 53:5872–5876.

51. von Brevern MC, Hollstein MC, Cawley HM, et al. 1996. Circulating anti-p53 antibodies in esophageal cancer patients are found predominantly in individuals with p53 core domain mutations in their tumors. Cancer Res. 56:4917–4921.

52. Greenblatt MS, Bennett WP, Hollstein M, Harris CC. 1994. Mutations in the p53 tumor suppressor gene: clues to cancer etiology and molecular pathogenesis. Cancer Res. 54:4855–4878.

53. Fleischhacker M, Strohmeyer T, Imai Y, Slamon DJ, Koeffler HP. 1994. Mutations of the p53 gene are not detectable in human testicular tumors. Mod. Pathol. 7:435–439.

54. Peng HQ, Hogg D, Malkin D, et al. 1993. Mutations of the p53 gene do not occur in testis cancer. Cancer Res. 53:3574–3578.

55. Lubbe J, Reichel M, Burg G, Kleihues P. 1994. Absence of p53 gene mutations in cutaneous melanoma. J. Invest. Dermatol. 102:819–821.

56. Rainov NG, Dobberstein KU, Fittkau M, et al. 1995. Absence of p53 antibodies in sera from glioma patients. Clin. Cancer Res. 1:775–781.

57. Trivers GE, Cawley HL, DeBenedetti VM, et al. 1995. Anti-p53 antibodies in sera of workers occupationally exposed to vinyl chloride. J. Natl Cancer Inst. 87:1400–1407.

58. Trivers GE, DeBenedetti VM, Cawley HL, et al. 1996. Anti-p53 antibodies in sera from patients with chronic obstructive pulmonary disease can predate a diagnosis of cancer. Clin. Cancer Res. 2:1767–1775.

59. Lubin R, Zalcman G, Bouchet L, et al. 1995. Serum p53 antibodies as early markers of lung cancer. Nat. Med. 1:701–702.

60. Cawley HM, Meltzer SJ, DeBenedetti V, et al. 1998. Anti-p53 antibodies in patients with Barrett's esophagus or esophageal carcinoma can predate cancer diagnosis. Gastroenterology 115:19–27.

61. Pradhan S and Kim GD. 2002. The retinoblastoma gene product interacts with maintenance human DNA (cytosine-5) methyltransferase and modulates its activity. EMBO J. 21:779–788.

62. Matsumoto S, Teramoto H, Nakamoto M, Igishi T, Kawasaki H, Shimizu E. 2001. Presence of antibodies against retinoblastoma tumor suppressor protein in patients with lung cancer. Int. J. Oncol. 19:1035–1039.

63. Covini G, Chan EKL, Nishioka M, Morshed SA, Reed SI, Tan EM. 1997. Immune response to cyclin B1 in hepatocellular carcinoma. Hepatology 25:75–80.

64. Landberg G, Tan EM. 1994. Characterization of a DNA-binding nuclear autoantigen mainly associated with S phase and G2 cells. Exp. Cell. Res. 212:255–261.

65. Muro Y, Chan EK, Landberg G, Tan EM. 1995. A cell-cycle nuclear autoantigen containing WD-40 motifs expressed mainly in S and G2 phase cells. Biochem. Biophys. Res. Commun. 207:1029–1037.

66. Casiano CA, Landberg G, Ochs RL, Tan EM. 1993. Autoantibodies to a novel cell cycle-regulated protein that accumulates in the nuclear matrix during S phase and is localized in the kinetochores and spindle midzone during mitoses. J. Cell Sci. 106(Pt 4):1045–1056.

67. Landberg G, Erlanson M, Roos G, Tan EM, Casiano CA. 1996. Nuclear autoantigen p330d/CENP-F: a marker for cell proliferation in human malignancies. Cytometry 25:90–98.

68. Rattner JB, Rees J, Whitehead CM, et al. 1997. High frequency of neoplasia in patients with autoantibodies to centromere protein CENP-F. Clin. Invest. Med. 20:308–319.

69. Casiano CA, Humbel RL, Peebles C, Covini G, Tan EM. 1995. Autoimmunity to the cell cycle-dependent centromere protein p330d/CENP-F in disorders associated with cell proliferation. J. Autoimmun. 8:575–586.

70. Chan EK, Imai H, Hamel JC, Tan EM. 1991. Human autoantibody to RNA polymerase I transcription factor hUBF. Molecular identity of nucleolus organizer region autoantigen NOR-90 and ribosomal RNA transcription upstream binding factor. J. Exp. Med. 174:1239–1244.

71. Imai H, Chan EK, Kiyosawa K, Fu XD, Tan EM. 1993. Novel nuclear autoantigen with splicing factor motifs identified with antibody from hepatocellular carcinoma. J. Clin. Invest. 92:2419–2426.

72. Imai H, Fritzler MJ, Neri R, Bombardieri S, Tan EM, Chan EK. 1994. Immunocytochemical characterization of human NOR-90 (upstream binding factor) and associated antigens reactive with autoimmune sera. Two MR forms of NOR-90/hUBF autoantigens. Mol. Biol. Rep. 19:115–124.

73. Imai H, Furuta K, Landberg G, Kiyosawa K, Liu LF, Tan EM. 1995. Autoantibody to DNA topoisomerase II in primary liver cancer. Clin. Cancer Res. 1:417–424.

74. Muller-Pillasch F, Lacher U, Wallrapp C, et al. 1997. Cloning of a gene highly overexpressed in cancer coding for a novel KH-domain containing protein. Oncogene 14:2729–2733.

75. Nielsen J, Christiansen J, Lykke-Andersen J, Johnsen AH, Wewer UM, Nielsen FC. 1999. A family of insulin-like growth factor II mRNA-binding proteins represses translation in late development. Mol. Cell. Biol. 19:1262–1270.

76. Maolong L, Nakamura RM, Dent EK, et al. 2001. Aberrant Expression of Fetal RNA-Binding Protein p62 in Liver Cancer and Liver Cirrhosis. Am. J. Path. 159:945–953.

77. Chen YT, Scanlan MJ, Sahin U, et al. 1997. A testicular antigen aberrantly expressed in human cancers detected by autologous antibody screening. Proc. Nat. Acad. Sci. USA 94:1914–1918.

78. Jager E, Chen YT, Drijfhout, JW, et al. 1998. Simultaneous humoral and cellular immune response against cancer-testis antigen NY-ESO-1: definition of human histocompatibility leukocyte antigen (HLA)-A2-binding peptide epitopes. J. Exp. Med. 187:265–270.

79. Stockert E, Jager E, Chen YT, et al. 1998. A survey of the humoral immune response of cancer patients to a panel of human tumor antigens. J. Exp. Med. 187:1349–1354.

80. Korneeva I, Bongiovanni AM, Girotra M, Caputo TA, Witkin SS. 2000. Serum antibodies to the 27-kd heat shock protein in women with gynecologic cancers. Am. J. Obstet. Gynecol. 183:18.

81. Bosscher JR, Gercel-Taylor C, Watkins CS, Taylor DD. 2001. Epitope recognition by anti-cathepsin D autoantibodies in endometrial cancer patients. Gynecol. Oncol. 81:138–143.

III

CELLULAR TUMOR MAKERS

10

MHC Tetramers

A Tool for Direct Ex Vivo Detection and Enumeration of Tumor-Specific Cytotoxic T Lymphocytes

Jennie C. C. Chang, Ferdynand Kos, Charles T. Nugent, and Kristine Kuus-Reichel

1. INTRODUCTION

Recent advances in our understanding of the immune mechanisms at work in cancer vaccine therapy and our ability to precisely measure patient immune responses in association with cancer therapy have expanded the potential of cancer vaccines and immunotherapy to a new level. The emerging fields of genomics, proteomics, immunomics, and bioinformatics have provided new tools and allowed the accelerated discovery of cancer associated antigens and specific peptides already proved useful in the development of effective cancer immunotherapies. It is critical that we measure the effectiveness of potential immunotherapies to quickly determine if a new therapy has clinical potential and if individual patients are responding to specific therapies. In this chapter, we review the role of the measurement of antigen-specific T cells, using major histocompatibility complex (MHC) tetramer technology, in management of cancer vaccine therapy and cancer immunotherapy.

2. TUMOR ANTIGENS

Therapeutic cancer vaccines have been an area of intense research in recent years, as reflected by the number of clinical trials using tumor-associated antigens (TAAs). Although tumor cells or tumor lysates are the basis of vaccines in some cases, in the majority of cases, predetermined TAAs are used. TAAs are defined as antigens or antigenic determinants that are either specifically expressed or overexpressed by tumor cells. As candidates for therapeutic vaccines, TAAs not only need to be recognized by the immune system, but also to be immunogenic (i.e., to elicit an immune response). In this section, methods used to identify TAAs by cellular, serologic, and molecular approaches are described.

2.1. T-Cell-Defined Tumor Antigens

Many TAAs including *MAGE*-1 *(1)*, *MAGE*-3 *(2)*, tyrosinase *(3)* gp100 *(4,5)*, *MART*-1 *(6)* and *HER*-2/neu *(7)* were derived using immunology-based assays, where CD8[+] tumor infiltrating lymphocyte (TIL) cell lines/clones were used to define TAA. In these studies, TILs associated with clinical responsiveness and demonstrated tumor cell killing were used to identify target cells transfected with cDNA derived from tumor cells, or for reactivity with peptides eluted from MHC class I on tumor cells. Most of the molecular identification

From: *Cancer Diagnostics: Current and Future Trends*
Edited by: R. M. Nakamura, W. W. Grody, J. T. Wu, and R. B. Nagle © Humana Press Inc., Totowa, NJ

and characterization of tumor antigens has been done in association with melanoma, owing to the difficulty of establishing tumor-specific T-cell lines or clones from other types of cancer. Isolation of sufficient quantities of tumor-specific peptides from human lymphocyte antigen (HLA) class I alleles for sequencing is also technically demanding, owing to the large number of peptides represented on the cell surface that are bound to MHC molecules (up to 2000 by HLA class I alone) *(5)*.

Effort has been placed on defining the role of MHC I-restricted CD8[+] T cells in cell-mediated immunity against tumors. Evidence also suggests that CD4[+] T cells may play a role in tumor immunity. CD4[+] T cells are known to provide "help" for CD8[+] T cells, not only through cytokine production, but also by activation of antigen-presenting cells that effectively stimulate CD8[+] T cells *(8)*. Moreover, melanoma and breast cancer cell lines have been shown to express MHC class II molecules upon induction by cytokines such as interferon-γ (IFN-γ) and tumor necrosis factor-α (TNF-α) *(9)*. In humans, CD4[+] T cells reacting with tumor cells are an important subset of a TIL population *(10,11)*. There are data that demonstrate the presence of MHC class II epitopes in proteins, such as tyrosinase, gp100, MAGE-1, MAGE-3, MART-1, and NY-ESO-1 *(12–14)*, all originally defined as antigens recognized by CD8[+] T cells.

2.2. Classification of T-Cell-Defined Tumor Antigens

Recently, Renkvist et al. *(15)* compiled a comprehensive list of T-cell-defined human tumor antigens and their epitopes. The list is posted at the internet website (www.istitutotumori.mi.it). This list consists of both CD8[+] and CD4[+] T-cell-defined cancer antigens divided into the following classes:

1. Tissue-specific antigens, such as the melanocyte-specific antigens and the prostate-specific antigens. Many of the melanocyte-lineage antigens are involved in the biosynthesis of melanin. Similarly, prostate antigens in this category are also specifically expressed in prostate tissue.
2. Antigens such as MAGE proteins that are expressed only in tumors but are not tissue-specific (i.e., they are expressed by histologically different human tumors). These antigens are now called cancer/testis antigens since they are also expressed in testis or embryonic/fetal tissues *(16)*. Expression of MAGE proteins in tumors appears to result from transcriptional activation of the *MAGE* genes by nonspecific demethylation of the cell's genomic DNA *(17)*.
3. Oncogenes, such as *HER-2/neu* and telomerase reverse transcriptase (*hTRT*), are expressed in many normal tissues and in many types of tumors, with higher expression levels in the latter.
4. Tumor-specific mutated or fusion gene products. Many antigens in this category are expressed only in the individual tumor where they were defined, thus precluding them from extensive clinical development. A recently discovered TAA that falls into this last category was from a lung carcinoma patient with long survival *(18)*. Using HLA class I tetramers, high frequencies (0.1 to 0.4%) of peripheral blood CD8[+] T cells recognized the unique TAA (a mutated sequence in malic enzyme) in this patient over a span of 10 yr. Interestingly, the frequency of the TAA specific CD8[+] cells doubled within 2 wk after intradermal inoculation of lethally irradiated autologous tumor cells, which demonstrated the immunogenicity of this specific peptide.

2.3. Tumor Antigens Defined by Serology

In addition to T cells, serum antibodies in cancer patients have been used to identify cancer antigens. One strategy was to make cDNA libraries from poly(A)[+] RNA isolated from fresh tumor biopsies. The cDNA libraries were cloned into phage particles and used to screen for antibodies in patient serum. This strategy identified sp100, Ran GTPase activating protein in breast cancer patients *(19)* and TEGT from patients with brain tumors *(20)*. TEGT was overexpressed in 8 of 12 astrocytomas compared to normal human brain tissues. TEGT is a conserved gene developmentally regulated in the testis *(21)* and thus belongs to the cancer/testis antigen group described above.

As research on TAAs accumulated, tumor antigens initially defined by T-cell responses such as MAGE-1 and tyrosinase were also detected by the serological approach *(22)*. In fact, for several TAAs, including *p53, MAGE, HER-2/neu*, and *NY-ESO-1*, both T-cell mediated and antibody responses were detected in the same cancer patients *(23,24)*, suggesting an integrated immune response against tumor may exist that involves both CD4+ T cells, CD8+ T cells, and B cells. Passive immunotherapy such as administration of the humanized anti-HER2/neu antibody (Herceptin; Genentech, Inc.) has proven effective in clinical trials in patients with metastatic breast cancer. Vaccines that include HER-2/neu peptides are currently being tested in the clinic. These vaccines are based on peptides derived from HER-2/neu that were recognized by TILS derived from breast, ovarian, and pancreatic cancer patients.

2.4. Molecular Approaches to Tumor Antigen Discovery

Most TAAs identified by T-cell based assays were obtained from melanomas, resulting from the technical challenges of obtaining functionally relevant T-cell lines/clones in other cancers. Therefore, to identify TAAs in less well-characterized cancers, molecular techniques including cDNA library substraction, Serial analysis of gene expression (SAGE), and *in silico* transcriptomics have also been used to search for genes that are preferentially expressed in neoplastic cells. Using a method that coupled cDNA library subtraction with cDNA microarray, Wang et al. *(25)* reported the discovery of a new gene product (L552S) in lung adenocarcinoma. L552S is overexpressed in lung adenocarcinoma tumors with half of lung adenocarcinoma tumors expressing more than tenfold the levels compared to normal tissues. To identify TAAs for diagnosis or immunotherapy purposes, genes derived by molecular approaches need to be tested by immunological assays to determine their antigenicity. In the study by Wang et al., antibodies to L552S were detected in patients' pleural effusions, thus demonstrating the immunogenicity of L552S. However, in order to consider this antigen as a vaccine component to stimulate T-cell-mediated immunity, the presence of T-cell-specific epitopes needs to be established.

Another effort to identify TAAs with molecular approaches was recently reported by Argani et al. *(26)*. In this study, a group of SAGE libraries composed of four pancreatic cancer cell lines and two primary pancreatic adenocarcinomas were compared to a group composed of short-term cultures of normal tissues, including pancreatic duct epithelial cells, colon epithelium, and microvascular endothelial cells. SAGE is a recently described technique *(27,28)* in which cellular mRNA transcripts are converted to cDNA and then cleaved by restriction enzymes into small (14 bp) fragments, also known as tags. These tags are concatenated and sequenced as one long fragment of DNA to give digital information that correlates with the expression level of a particular gene. Each 14 bp tag uniquely identifies a specific gene transcript because it corresponds to a defined sequence near the transcript's 3'terminus. SAGE, creating a large database that is available on line (www.ncbi.nlm.nih.gov/SAGE), has now analyzed a large number of normal and neoplastic tissues. Through comparative data analysis, Argani et al. identified a new and previously unsuspected marker for pancreatic carcinoma, prostate stem cell antigen (PSCA). PCSA is a cell-surface protein that has shown promise as a target for immunotherapy of advanced cancers of the prostate *(29)*, thus raising the possibility that PCSA is a rational immune target in pancreatic cancers that overexpress PSCA.

2.5. Epitope Discovery

Through the abundance of gene products that are either specific to or overexpressed in cancer cells, a major challenge is to determine the antigenic epitopes that provide good vaccine candidates. Peptide libraries have been a major tool for this purpose. As bioinformatics began to become a discipline in biological sciences, several new tools are available to move from sequence to epitope discovery and vaccine design. Two of these programs, EpiMer and EpiMatrix, are computer-driven pattern-matching algorithms that identify T-cell epitopes. Conservatrix, BlastiMer, and Patent-Blast permit the analysis to find homology with previously patented epitopes *(30)*. Recently, a non-cell-based and/or algorithm-based technology was made available. The Epitope Discovery System (iTopra Beckman Coulter) utilizes a novel technology that provides biopharmaceutical vaccine researchers with the tools to better understand the mechanism of action for the selected protein. Characterization of peptide MHC binding is performed in vitro using a process capable of high throughput to identify promising epitope candidates and evaluate them for binding affinity and rate of dissociation. This new system has the ability to shorten the route to clinical development by allowing a systematic ranking of these candidate epitopes for subsequent functional studies. Tools that facilitate epitope discovery enable researchers to move quickly to vaccine design. However, the decisive test to determine the disease relevance of a TAA still resides in functional assays, patient testing, and clinical responses.

3. METHODS TO MONITOR T-CELL RESPONSES IN CANCER PATIENTS

A primary concern among investigators monitoring T-cell responses in cancer patients is to accurately define the magnitude and functional potential of cancer antigen-specific T cells. Several methods are currently available and in use as tools to monitor T-cell responses in cancer patients and healthy controls. This section will give a brief description of each method, outline what information each method can reveal, and consequently the information which it cannot. The remainder of this section will summarize how some of these methods have been used in tandem to monitor cancer antigen-specific T cells in cancer patients.

3.1. Limiting Dilution Analysis

Historically, the most common method used to assess antigen specificity, effector function, and frequency of cancer antigen-specific cells is limiting dilution analysis (LDA), where titrated numbers of PBL are incubated with the antigen of interest *(31)*. Over time, the T-cell precursors able to respond to antigen will proliferate and expand to numbers sufficient for detection. Theoretically, this method gives every antigen-specific T-cell precursor an equal chance of proliferation and expansion, in contrast to general or "bulk" expansion of T cells, which occasionally result in cultures that are monoclonal or of limited diversity, and obscure the true composition of the original population.

The two methods commonly used for measuring the antigen-specific response in LDA are:

1. Measurement of T-cell expansion in response to incubation with antigen, and
2. Measurement of T-cell lysis of target cells expressing the antigen of interest.

In the first approach, after culture of the T cells with antigen, radiolabeled nucleotides are added into the cultures for a short time prior to harvesting the assay. The amount of radioactive isotope incorporated into the cells represents the amount of DNA synthesized within the culture, and therefore the amount of proliferation that cells have undergone in response to antigenic stimulation. The second approach is to determine the lytic potential of T cells. In this approach, after culture of T cells and antigen, the T cells are coincubated with target cells previously labeled with ^{51}Chromium (^{51}Cr). Targets may be autologous tumor cells that naturally express the antigen of interest, or MHC-matched cell lines that express the antigen following peptide pulsing, recombinant DNA transfection, or viral infection. Targets lysed by cytotoxic T lymphocyte (CTL) release ^{51}Cr into the supernatant, and the amount of ^{51}Cr in the supernatant correlates with the magnitude of lytic activity *(32)*. Alternatively, fluorometric and colorimetric readout systems can be used instead of radiolabeling for detection of lytic activity *(33–35)*. Lytic analyses can be carried out with "bulk" T-cell cultures if information concerning the frequency of antigen-specific T cells is not required.

The strength of LDA is its reliance on statistical analysis and Poisson distribution. Through a series of calculations, the investigator may determine the original frequency of the antigen-specific T-cell precursors that are able to respond to cancer antigen(s). A weakness of this approach is that T-cell frequency may be altered following in vitro expansion, as some antigen-specific T cells are incapable of expansion or unable to expand to levels sufficient for detection. In addition, this procedure is technically challenging, requires prolonged culture in vitro, and results are highly operator-dependent.

3.2. Enzyme-Linked Immunospot Assay

In addition to lytic activity and proliferation, CD8$^+$ T cells secrete cytokines in response to antigen stimulation *(36)*. Secretion of cytokines is a primary function of CD8$^+$ T cells, and in some cases, may be the primary effector function necessary for a successful immune response to some pathogens. Enzyme-linked immunospot (ELISPOT) was developed from the principle of enzyme-linked immunosorbent assay (ELISA)-based analysis, where supernatant from cultured cells of interest is incubated with plate-bound antibody that binds the cytokine of interest, followed by incubation with an additional cytokine-specific Ab that will allow detection of the specific cytokine *(37,38)*. In ELISPOT, purified T cells are directly incubated in Ab-coated wells together with antigen for a pre-determined amount of time, usually 6–48 h. T cells able to recognize the antigen will release cytokines bound by the antibody coating the well. After the predetermined incubation time, cells are washed away, and a secondary enzyme-labeled antibody plus chromogenic substrate are added to each well. Production of cytokine is determined by visually enumerating the colored spots left behind by cells able to secrete lymphokine in response to antigenic stimulation. The limits of detection using this approach have been reported to be lower than ELISA performed on culture supernatants, and allows for single-cell resolution of effector function. This procedure requires that an investigator consider which cytokine(s) to test. ELISPOT does not give absolute enumeration of T cells able to respond to antigen—only those able to secrete the cytokine of interest will be detected.

3.3. Intracellular Cytokine Analysis

Another method to detect lymphokine production is the intracellular cytokine cytometry (ICC) assay. Both ICC and ELISPOT detect whether a certain cytokine may be produced by cells following a determined period of in vitro stimulation. In contrast to ELISPOT, ICC uses flow cytometry to detect cytokine production intracellularly, and therefore measures the cell's potential to make the cytokine of interest *(39)*. During the latter part of the stimulation period, secretion of extracellular proteins is chemically blocked, thus proteins normally secreted, such as cytokines, accumulate inside the cell. Following stimulation, cells are collected, fixed, and permeabilized prior to intracellular staining. In addition to measuring cytokine production, ICC analysis has the capability to measure cell surface expression of activation and effector proteins that further characterize the T cells. As with ELISPOT, ICC will not detect antigen-specific T cells unable to produce the cytokine of interest.

3.4. Major Histocompatability Complex Tetramer-Based Detection of Antigen-Specific T Cells

The assays described thus far have an absolute requirement for in vitro stimulation to carry out functional assessment. ELISPOT and ICC require a minimum of 6 h of stimulation before cells are harvested and processed, and LDA requires significantly more time, as cells must physically expand in numbers prior to assessment of function. In recent years, flow cytometric analysis of tetramer-stained cells has been used in experiments to enumerate T cells. Tetramer-based detection of T cells capitalizes on the observation that multimeric MHC/peptide (the primary ligand for T-cell antigen receptor) coupled with a fluorescent dye, allow detection and enumeration of antigen-specific T cells ex vivo, and in contrast to the other methods described above, do not require in vitro stimulation and manipulation *(40)*.

MHC tetramers are complexes of four MHC molecules, associated with a specific antigenic peptide and a fluorochrome. MHC tetramer specificity is conveyed in two ways: First, the four MHC molecules comprising the tetrameric complex are specific for the subject's human leukocyte antigen (HLA), and second, the peptide bound to the MHC molecules is antigen-specific. Therefore, tetramers directly enumerate the number of $CD8^+$ T cells able to interact with the antigen of interest in the patient's peripheral blood. By design, MHC tetramers enumerate all peptide-specific $CD8^+$ T cells, regardless of functionality. MHC tetramers enable accurate quantitative analysis of antigen-specific responses, even of extremely rare events that may comprise 0.01% of peripheral blood mononuclear cells (PBMCs) *(41)*. The primary strength of tetramer-based analyses is that direct enumeration of antigenic peptide/MHC allele-specific T cells can be performed directly from patient blood samples. In addition, tetramer-positive cells can be sorted by flow cytometry, expanded in vitro, and used to gather additional information on phenotype and functionality. Increasingly, tetramer-based analysis is coupled with other assays to simultaneously assess frequency and function.

In contrast to tetramer-positive T cells that respond to pathogens, cancer-reactive T cells may be of lower avidity. This phenomenon is a result of immunological tolerance mechanisms invoked against "self" epitopes, some of which are presented by tumor cells in association with their MHC complexes. Therefore, some cancer-reactive, tetramer-positive T cells may be of lower fluorescent intensity when analyzed by flow cytometry.

3.5. Comparison of Methods Used to Evaluate Cancer-Specific T-Cells

Lytic and proliferation assays, performed as stand-alone or coupled with LDA, had been the methods of choice for evaluating the functional capacity of cancer-specific T cells from patient samples. However, newer assays, such as ELISPOT, ICC, and tetramer, have some distinct advantages over the older assays. The advent of tetramer technology provides investigators the ability to easily and rapidly enumerate T cells specific for a known antigen and MHC allele combination. In addition, costaining samples with antibodies specific for various activation and adhesion markers yields additional information about the antigen-specific T-cell population. As mentioned above, tetramer staining does not yield information about the functional capacity of T cells. On the contrary, ELISPOT, and ICC assays both measure the functional capacity of T cells, but require significantly more time and technical expertise to perform *(42)*. Separately, each of these methods has definite strengths and weaknesses. Therefore, in an increasing number of cancer immune monitoring studies, investigators are using cytokine and tetramer assays in tandem.

Several published studies have dealt with direct comparison of various cytokine-based assays as well as a comparison of cytokine-based with tetramer-based analysis. In some studies, the frequency estimates given by tetramer staining exceeded those afforded by ELISPOT *(43,44)*. These results could have arisen from two possibilities:

1. Some MHC/peptide combinations used to produce tetramers tend to give higher backgrounds. In some alleles, this can be overcome by mutation of the CD8 binding region of the MHC molecule *(45)*.
2. ELISPOT analysis readily detects functional memory or effector T cells, or "primed" cells, but not naïve cells, or cells requiring additional stimulation not afforded by the ELISPOT protocol. Tetramers are able to detect primed cells, as well as additional cells that may be considered nonfunctional, naïve, or anergic.

To date, the most well-characterized cancer antigens and concordant immune responses include melanocyte/melanoma differentiation antigens MelanA/Mart-1, tyrosinase and gp100; cancer-testis antigens NY-ESO-1, CAMEL and MAGE-A10; and PR1, an antigen associated with CML *(46–50)*. Tetramer-positive lymphocytes have been detected in patient blood samples for most of these antigens. For the most part, ELISPOT and tetramer-binding studies have been in general alignment when assessing antigen-specific T-cell frequencies, but results are dependent on the type of cancer and cancer antigen being monitored *(51,52)*.

A major challenge in the field of immune monitoring of cancer patients is the ability to detect antigen-specific T cells where only few exist. Tcells specific for some cancer-specific antigens (MAGE-3) may be at a frequency that is detectable only if several rounds of in vitro stimulation are first performed, as shown by Coulie et al. *(53)*. In their study, multiple immunizations with MAGE antigen (MAGE-3.A1 peptide) raised an oligoclonal response that required in vitro expansion. Emerging technologies such as quantitative reverse transcription polymerse chain reaction analysis (qRT-PCR) are capable of specifically detecting T cells (by virtue of TCR expression) from small sample volumes, and will be a useful tool for cancer immune monitoring in the future *(42,54)*. However, not all cancer-specific responses have been difficult to detect, for example, T cells specific for Melan-A/MART-1 can be detected in the peripheral blood of non-vaccinated and even normal individuals *(55)*.

Although many methods are available to enumerate and discern the functional capability of cancer antigen-specific T cells, functional, antigen-specific T cells specific for various cancer antigens can be found in detectable (and sometimes high) frequencies in the peripheral blood, tumors, and tumor-involved nodes of cancer patients. However, the presence of tumor antigen-specific T cells may not correlate with a successful immune response to the tumor in question. Some reasons for this include the presence of antigen-specific but nonfunctional T cells or the presence of T cells that are not reactive to the appropriate tumor antigen.

4. USE OF MAJOR HISTOCOMPATABILITY COMPLEX TETRAMERS IN CANCER PATIENT MANAGEMENT

Recent developments in the molecular identification of tumor-associated antigens recognized by the immune system have renewed enthusiasm in the application of immunotherapies to treat cancer. A number of different vaccine strategies for cancer immunotherapy have been tested, including both nonspecific and tumor antigen-specific approaches *(56–60)*. T-cell-based tumor-specific vaccines with purposes ranging from the induction of protective immunity to the activation of T-cell-mediated responses currently represent the most viable approach. It is generally agreed that MHC class I-restricted CD8[+] T cells constitute the primary effector component of the adaptive immunity against pathogens and tumors.

The development of MHC tetramer technology has offered an easy and direct approach for ex vivo analysis of tumor antigen-specific CD8[+] T-cell responses in cancer patients. We are at the beginning stages of using tetramers to analyze T cells in patients, but this powerful technology may become, in the future, as useful as specific monoclonal antibodies in the studies of immunity. What are the potential utilities of MHC tetramers in cancer patient management? In this section we attempt to briefly review representative data in this field as well as to speculate and predict future applications.

4.1. Use of Tetramers in the Monitoring of Tumor Antigen-Specific T Cells in Nonvaccinated Cancer Patients

Cutaneous melanoma, one of the most immunogenic tumors, has served as the major model in the studies of tumor immunotherapy. A number of antigens expressed on melanoma cells have been identified *(61)*. Most of them, including Melan-A/MART-1, tyrosinase and gp100 are normal differentiation antigens, also present on normal melanocytes. Other antigens, such as MAGE, seem to be primarily expressed on tumor cells. Specific amino acid peptide sequences from melanoma-associated antigens bind to MHC Class I molecules, especially HLA-A2, and form epitopes recognizable by specific TCRs on CD8[+] CTLs. In some clinical trials, the inclusion of these peptides in vaccines can induce specific CTL responses in cancer patients.

In monitoring the immune responses of cancer patients, tetramers have been a useful tool to enumerate antigen-specific CD8[+] T cells ex vivo in samples of PBMCs, metastatic lymph nodes, and tumor infiltrating lymphocytes from HLA-A2 melanoma patients *(62–65)*. Staining of tumor-infiltrating lymphocytes and cells from metastatic lymph nodes with Melan-A/ MART-1 tetramers showed relatively high levels of specific CD8[+] T cells in most patients *(63,64)*. In contrast, tetramer-positive T cells were not detectable in normal lymph nodes. These observations indicate that Melan-A/MART-1-specific CD8[+] T cells accumulate in tumor inflammatory infiltrates as well as in metastatic lymph nodes, where tumor-associated antigens are present. Future development of techniques to stain tissue sections with tetramers may facilitate the analysis of distribution and interactions between antigen-specific CTLs and tumor cells *in situ.*

Tetramers have been used in studies of tolerance induction by tumors. Lee et al. have shown that MART-1- or tyrosinase-specific T cells are selectively rendered anergic in vivo and unable to control melanoma growth *(62)*. These T cells were functionally unresponsive in vitro (i.e., they were unable to lyse melanoma target cells or to secrete cytokines in response to mitogens).

MHC class I tetramers along with peptides they carry are specific ligands for their cognate TCRs. Tetramer binding to T cells ex vivo can be detected with high sensitivity using flow cytometric analysis. Its lower detection limit reaches 0.01% in peripheral blood lymphocytes in whole blood assays. Nonspecific binding is low and can be eliminated by applying exclusion staining using monoclonal antibodies to non-T-cell lineage markers, followed by appropriate gating strategies in flow cytometric analysis. Antigen-specific T cells can be precisely enumerated without the need of using more complicated and labor-intensive assays such as LDA, ELISPOT, intracellular cytokine (IFN-γ, TNF-α, MIP-1) staining, or ^{51}Cr-release cytotoxicity assay *(55,66)*. Tetramer staining can be combined with some functional assays, such as, IFN-γ production or cytotoxicity assays. In general, these combined assays are more difficult to perform and often generate less consistent results. For example, to detect IFN-γ production either by secretion or by intracellular assays, T cells need to be activated. Activation of T cells leads to significant downregulation of surface TCRs, thus compromises the detection of IFN-γ-producing T cells by tetramers unless the assay is accurately timed.

4.2. Use of Tetramers in the Monitoring of Tumor Antigen-Specific T Cells in Vaccinated Cancer Patients

It is generally accepted that cancer immunotherapy may be limited in its effects as an adjuvant treatment to the conventional therapies and in the management of minimal residual disease following surgical resection of the primary tumor load *(67)*. Nevertheless, adjuvant therapies improve survival and further understanding of antitumor immune responses provide additional advantages to cancer treatment protocols.

It has been shown in some clinical studies that vaccination of cancer patients with peptides derived from tumor antigens leads to the stimulation of CD8$^+$ T cells and, in some cases induces clinical responses. For example, Valmori et al. *(68)* showed that immunization of melanoma patients with Melan-A peptide selected high-avidity T-cell clones exhibiting increased tumor reactivity. The number of circulating Melan-A tetramer-positive CD8$^+$ T cells increased after vaccination and remained at the stable level of 1.1%–2.3% of total circulating CD8$^+$ T cells. Coulie et al. *(53)* observed a monoclonal 100-fold expansion of MAGE-3-specific CD8$^+$ T cells in a melanoma patient vaccinated with a MAGE-3 peptide presented by HLA-A1. This patient also exhibited a partial rejection of a large metastasis after vaccination. In a study by Fong et al. *(69)*, advanced colon and lung cancer patients were treated with Flt3 ligand injections to expand their dendritic cells in vivo, after which the dendritic cells were isolated from the blood, loaded with peptide derived from carcinoembryonic antigen (CEA), and injected back into the patients. Clinical response in 2 of 12 patients was found to correlate with the expansion of tetramer-positive CD8$^+$ T cells shown to recognize tumor cells expressing endogenous CEA. Molldrem et al. *(50)*, in studies of T cells specific for PR1 peptide derived from proteinase of chronic myelogenous leukemia cells, found a strong correlation between the presence of PR1-specific T cells and clinical responses in patients after the IFN-γ and bone marrow transplant therapy. PR1-specific T cells were identified with PR1-HLA-A*0201 tetramers in this study. In addition, investigators observed that PR1-specific T cells were not detected in chemotherapy-treated or untreated patients.

In addition to their use in monitoring T-cell responses in patients, MHC tetramers offer an excellent tool for the isolation of tumor-specific CD8$^+$ T cells from heterologous populations of cells such as PBMCs, tumor-infiltrating lymphocytes, or cultured cells *(70)*. The isolated tumor-specific T cells can then be activated and expanded ex vivo for transfer to cancer patients by adoptive immunotherapy. Undoubtedly, tetramers would also be of value in tracking adoptively transferred T cells to define any correlations between their number, activity, or distribution with disease progression.

Further use of tetramers may be monitoring of CD8+ T-cell repertoire during conventional cancer therapies. Conventional cancer therapies often exert immunosuppressive effects that may not be desirable in terms of the overall therapeutic efficacy; therefore, information on status of antigen-specific T cells may provide new insights on how to balance anticancer effects of chemotherapeutics with their suppressive effects on anticancer immunity.

5. SUMMARY

Recent scientific advances allowed investigators to identify TAAs associated with individual cancers at an accelerated rate. The association of TAAs identified through cellular, serologic, or molecular approaches with specific cancer cells has been confirmed. Cancer vaccines that contain these TAAs can specifically boost the immune response of patients to the relevant tumor antigens. In spite of these advances, the identification of the breadth of tumor-associated peptides in different cancers remains a challenge. In addition, the question of whether or not the measurement of immune responses to tumor peptides will correlate with clinical outcome remains unknown. Clinical trials are now underway to answer these questions.

MHC tetramer analysis, which enumerates antigen-specific T cells, provides researchers with data that reflect the status of an individual's immune response to specific tumor antigens, whether naturally induced or stimulated through administration of cancer vaccines. These data will allow investigators to monitor the specific immune response in patients in response to immune therapies and provide early evidence of the effectiveness of therapies. A recent review, published by the Society for Biologic Therapy, recommends the use of MHC tetramer analysis combined with a measurement of immune function such as Elispot or intracellular cytokine for measurement of the immune status of patients undergoing cancer vaccine therapy *(42)*.

REFERENCES

1. van der Bruggen P, Traversari C, Chomez P, et al. 1991. A gene encoding an antigen recognized by cytolytic T lymphocytes on a human melanoma. Science 254(5038):1643–1647.
2. Gaugler B, Van den Eynde B, van der Bruggen P, et al. 1994. Human gene MAGE-3 codes for an antigen recognized on a melanoma by autologous cytolytic T lymphocytes. J. Exp. Med. 179(3):921–930.
3. Wolfel T, Van Pel A, Brichard V, et al. 1994. Two tyrosinase nonapeptides recognized on HLA-A2 melanomas by autologous cytolytic T lymphocytes. Eur. J. Immunol. 24(3):759–764.
4. Cox AL, Skipper J, Chen Y, et al. 1994. Identification of a peptide recognized by five melanoma-specific human cytotoxic T cell lines. Science 264(5159):716–719.
5. Henderson RA, Cox AL, Sakaguchi K, et al. 1993. Direct identification of an endogenous peptide recognized by multiple HLA-A2.1-specific cytotoxic T cells. Proc. Natl. Acad. Sci. USA 90(21):10275–10279.
6. Kawakami Y, Eliyahu S, Sakaguchi K, et al. 1994. Identification of the immunodominant peptides of the MART-1 human melanoma antigen recognized by the majority of HLA-A2-restricted tumor infiltrating lymphocytes. J. Exp. Med. 180(1):347–352.

7. Peoples GE, Goedegebuure PS, Smith R, Linehan DC, Yoshino I, Eberlein TJ. 1995. Breast and ovarian cancer-specific cytotoxic T lymphocytes recognize the same HER2/neu-derived peptide. Proc. Natl. Acad. Sci. USA 92(2):432–436.

8. Ridge JP, Di Rosa F, Matzinger P. 1998. A conditioned dendritic cell can be a temporal bridge between a CD4⁺ T-helper and a T-killer cell. Nature 393(6684):474–478.

9. Sotiriadou R, Perez SA, Gritzapis AD, et al. 2001. Peptide HER2(776-788) represents a naturally processed broad MHC class II-restricted T cell epitope. Br. J. Can. 85(10):1527–1534.

10. Walker BD and Korber BT. 2001. Immune control of HIV: the obstacles of HLA and viral diversity. Nat. Immunol. 2(6):473–475.

11. Dadmarz R, Sgagias MK, Rosenberg SA, Schwartzentruber DJ. 1995. CD4⁺ T lymphocytes infiltrating human breast cancer recognise autologous tumor in an MHC-class-II restricted fashion. Cancer Immunol. 40.

12. Topalian SL, Gonzales MI, Parkhurst M, et al. 1996. Melanoma-specific CD4+ T cells recognize nonmutated HLA-DR-restricted tyrosinase epitopes. J. Exp. Med. 183(5):1965–1971.

13. Zeng G. 2001. MHC class II-restricted tumor antigens recognized by CD4+ T cells: new strategies for cancer vaccine design. J. Immunother. 24(3)195–204.

14. Jager E, Jager D, Karbach J, et al. 2000. Identification of NY-ESO-1 epitopes presented by human histocompatibility antigen (HLA)-DRB4*0101-0103 and recognized by CD4(+) T lymphocytes of patients with NY-ESO-1-expressing melanoma. J. Exp. Med. 191(4):625–630.

15. Renkvist N, Castelli C, Robbins PF, Parmiani G. 2001. A listing of human tumor antigens recognized by T cells. Cancer Immunol. Immunother. 50(1):3–15.

16. Jungbluth AA, Busam KJ, Kolb D, et al. 2000. Expression of MAGE-antigens in normal tissues and cancer. Int. J. Cancer 85:460–465.

17. De Smet D, De Backer O, Faraoni I, Lurquin C, Brasseur F, Boon T. 1996. The activation of human gene MAGE-1 in tumor cells is correlated with genome-wide demethylation. Proc. Natl. Acad. Sci. USA 93(14):7149–7153.

18. Karanikas V, Colau D, Baurain JF, et al. 2001. High frequency of cytolytic T lymphocytes directed against a tumor-specific mutated antigen detectable with HLA tetramers in the blood of a lung carcinoma patient with long survival. Cancer Res. 61(9):3718–3724.

19. Hansen MH, Ostenstad B, Sioud M. 2001. Identification of immunogenic antigens using a phage-displayed cDNA library from an invasive ductal breast carcinoma tumour. Int. J. Oncol. 19(6):1303–1309.

20. Sahin U, Tureci O, Schmitt H, et al. 1995. Human neoplasms elicit multiple specific immune responses in the autologous host. Proc. Natl. Acad. Sci. USA 95(25):11810–11813.

21. Walter L, Dirks B, Rothermel E, et al. 1994. A novel, conserved gene of the rat that is developmentally regulated in the testis. Mamm. Genome 5(4):216–221.

22. Sahin U, Tureci O, Pfreundschuh M. 1997. Serological identification of human tumor antigens. Curr. Opin. Immunol. 9(5):709–716.

23. Jager E, Chen YT, Drijfhout JW, et al. 1998. Simultaneous humoral and cellular immune response against cancer-testis antigen NY-ESO-1: definition of human histocompatibility leukocyte antigen (HLA)-A2-binding peptide epitopes. J. Exp. Med. 187(2):265–270.

24. Disis ML, Calenoff E, McLaughlin G, et al. 1994. Existent T-cell and antibody immunity to HER-2/neu protein in patients with breast cancer. Cancer Res. 54(1):16–20.

25. Wang T, Fan L, Watanabe Y, et al. 2001. L552S, an alternatively spliced isoform of XAGE-1, is overexpressed in lung adenocarcinoma. Oncogene 20(53):7699–7709.

26. Argani P, Rosty C, Reiter RE, et al. 2001. Discovery of new markers of cancer through serial analysis of gene expression: prostate stem cell antigen is overexpressed in pancreatic adenocarcinoma. Cancer Res. 61(11):4320–4324.

27. Velculescu VE, Zhang L, Vogelstein B, Kinzler KW. 1995. Serial analysis of gene expression. Science 270(5235):484–487.

28. Zhang L, Zhou W, Velculescu VE, et al. 1997. Gene expression profiles in normal and cancer cells. Science 276(5316):1268–1272.

29. Saffran DC, Raitano AB, Hubert RS, Witte ON, Reiter RE, Jakobovits A. 2001. Anti-PSCA mAbs inhibit tumor growth and metastasis formation and prolong the survival of mice bearing human prostate cancer xenografts. Proc. Natl. Acad. Sci. USA 98(5):2658–2663.

30. De Groot A, Bosma A, Chinai N, et al. 2001. From genome to vaccine: in silico predictions, ex vivo verification. Vaccine 19(31):4385–4395.

31. Lefkovits I and Waldmann H. 1979. Limiting Dilution Analysis of Cells in the Immune System: Cambridge University Press:. Cambridge, UK and New York, NY.

32. Brunner KT, Mauel J, Cerottini JC, Chapuis B. 1968. Quantitative assay of the lytic action of immune lymphoid cells on 51-Cr-labelled allogeneic target cells in vitro. inhibition by isoantibody and by drugs. Immunology 14(2):181–196.

33. Korzeniewski C, and Callewaert DM. 1983. An enzyme-release assay for natural cytotoxicity. J. Immunol. Methods 64(3):313–320.

34. Sepp A, Binns RM, Lechler RI. 1996. Improved protocol for colorimetric detection of complement-mediated cytotoxicity based on the measurement of cytoplasmic lactate dehydrogenase activity. J. Immunol. Methods 196(2):175–180.

35. Larsson R. and Nygren P. 1989. A rapid fluorometric method for semiautomated determination of cytotoxicity and cellular proliferation of human tumor cell lines in microculture. Anticancer Res. 9(4):1111–1119.

36. Slifka MK and Whitton JL. 2000. Antigen-specific regulation of T cell-mediated cytokine production. Immunity 12(5):451–457.

37. Czerkinsky CC, Nilsson LA, Nygren H, Ouchterlony O, Tarkowski A. 1983. A solid-phase enzyme-linked immunospot (ELISPOT) assay for enumeration of specific antibody-secreting cells. J. Immunol. Methods 65(1–2):109–121.

38. Sedgwick JD and Holt PG. 1983. A solid-phase immunoenzymatic technique for the enumeration of specific antibody-secreting cells. J. Immunol. Methods 57(1–3):301–309.

39. Prussin C and Metcalfe DD. 1995. Detection of intracytoplasmic cytokine using flow cytometry and directly conjugated anti-cytokine antibodies. J. Immunol. Methods 188(1):117–128.

40. Altman JD, Moss PA, Goulder PJ, et al. 1996. Phenotypic analysis of antigen-specific T lymphocytes. Science 274(5284):94–96.

41. Klenerman P, Cerundolo V, Dunbar PR. T 2002. racking T cells with tetramers: new tales from new tools. Nat. Rev. Immunol. 2(4):263–272.

42. Keilholz U, Weber J, Finke JH, et al. 2002. Immunologic monitoring of cancer vaccine therapy: results of a workshop sponsored by the society for biological therapy. J. Immunother. 25(2):97–138.

43. Clay TM, Hobeika AC, Mosca PJ, Lyerly HK, Morse MA. 2001. Assays for monitoring cellular immune responses to active immunotherapy of cancer. Clin. Cancer Res. 7(5):1127–1135.

44. Gajewski TF. 2000. Monitoring specific T-cell responses to melanoma vaccines: ELISPOT, tetramers, and beyond. Clin. Diagn. Lab. Immunol. 7(2):141–144.

45. Bodinier M, Peyrat MA, Tournay C, et al. 2000. Efficient detection and immunomagnetic sorting of specific T cells using multimers of MHC class I and peptide with reduced CD8 binding. Nat. Med. 6(6):707–710.

46. Jager E, Nagata Y, Gnjatic S, et al. 2000. Monitoring CD8 T cell responses to NY-ESO-1: correlation of humoral and cellular immune responses. Proc. Natl. Acad. Sci. USA 97(9):4760–4765.

47. Valmori D, Dutoit V, Lienard D, et al. 2002. Naturally occurring human lymphocyte antigen-A2 restricted CD8SUP+ T-cell response to the cancer testis antigen NY-ESO-1 in melanoma patients. Cancer Res. 60(16):4499–4506.

48. Valmori D, Dutoit V, Rubio-Godoy V, et al. 2001. Frequent cytolytic T-cell responses to peptide MAGE-A10(254-262) in melanoma. Cancer Res. 61(2):509–512.

49. Aarnoudse CA, Van den Doel PB, Heemskerk B, Schrier PI. 1999. Interleukin-2-induced, melanoma-specific T cells recognize CAMEL, an unexpected translation product of LAGE-1. Int. J. Cancer. 82(3):442–448.

50. Molldrem JJ, Lee PP, Wang C, et al. 2000. Evidence that specific T lymphocytes may participate in the elimination of chronic myelogenous leukemia. Nat. Med. 6(9):1018–1023.

51. Yamshchikov G, Thompson L, Ross WG, et al. 2001. Analysis of a natural immune response against tumor antigens in a melanoma survivor: lessons applicable to clinical trial evaluations. Clin. Cancer Res. 7(3):909s–916s.

52. Rubio-Godoy V, Dutoit V, Rimoldi D, et al. 2001. Discrepancy between ELISPOT IFN-gamma secretion and binding of A2/peptide multimers to TCR reveals interclonal dissociation of CTL effector function from TCR-peptide/MHC complexes half-life. Proc. Nat. Acad. Sci. USA 98(18):10,302–10,307.

53. Coulie PG, Karanikas V, Culau D, et al. 2001. A monoclonal cytolytic T-lymphocyte response observed in a melanoma patient vaccinated with a tumor-specific antigenic peptide encoded by gene MAGE-3. Proc. Natl. Acad. Sci. USA 98(18):10290–10295.

54. Pilch H, Hohn H, Neukirch C, et al. 2002. Antigen-driven T-cell selection in patients with cervical cancer as evidenced by T-cell receptor analysis and recognition of autologous tumor. Clin. Diagn. Lab. Immunol. 9(2):267–278.

55. Pittet MJ, Valmori D, Dunbar PR, et al. 1999. High frequencies of naive Melan-A/MART-1-specific CD8(+) T cells in a large proportion of human histocompatibility leukocyte antigen (HLA)-A2 individuals. J Exp. Med. 190(5):705–715.

56. Toes RE, Schoenberger SP, van der Voort EIH, et al. 1997. Activation or frustration of anti-tumor responses by T-cell-based immune modulation. Semin. Immunol. 9(5):323–327.

57. Monzavi-Karbassi B and Kieber-Emmons T. 2001. Current concepts in cancer vaccine strategies. Biotechniques 30(1):170–172, 174, 176.

58. Kim CJ, Dessureault S, Gabrilovich D, Reintgen DS, Slingluff CL. Immunotherapy for melanoma. Cancer Control 9(1):22–30.

59. Borrello IM and Sotomayor EM. Cancer vaccines for hematologic malignances. Cancer Control 9(2):138–151.

60. Riddell SR, Murata M, Bryant S, Warren EH. 2002. T-cell therapy of leukemia. Cancer Control 9:152–166.

61. Boon T and Old LJ. 1997. Cancer tumor antigens. Curr. Opin. Immunol. 9:681–683.

62. Lee PP, Yee C, Savage PA, et al. 1999. Characterization of circulating T cells specific for tumor-associated antigens in melanoma patients. Nat. Med. 5(6):677–685.

63. Anichini A, Molla A, Mortarini R, et al. 1999. An expanded peripheral T cell population to a cytotoxic T lymphocyte (CTL)-defined, melanocyte-specific antigen in metastatic melanoma patients impacts on generation of peptide-specific CTLs but does not overcome tumor escape from immune surveillance in metastatic lesions. J. Exp. Med. 190(5):651–667.

64. Romero P, Dunbar PR, Valmori D, et al. 1998. Ex vivo staining of metastatic lymph nodes by class I major histocompatibility complex tetramers reveals high numbers of antigen-experienced tumor-specific cytolytic T lymphocytes. J. Exp. Med. 188(9):1641–1650.

65. Valmori D, Pittet MJ, Vonarbourg C, et al. 1999. Analysis of the cytolytic T lymphocyte response of melanoma patients to the naturally HLA-A*0201-associated tyrosinase peptide 368–376. Cancer Res. 59(16):4050–4055.

66. Tan LC, Gudgeon N, Annels NE, et al. 1999. A re-evaluation of the frequency of CD8+ T cells specific for EBV in healthy virus carriers. J. Immunol. 162(3):1827–1835.

67. Tomiyama H, Yamada N, Komatsu H, Hirayama K, Takiguchi M. 2000. A single CTL clone can recognize a naturally processed HIV-1 epitope presented by two different HLA class I molecules. Eur. J. Immunol. 30(9):2521–2530.

68. Valmori D, Dutoit V, Schnuriger V, et al. 2002. Vaccination with a Melan-A peptide selects an oligoclonal T cell population with increased functional avidity and tumor reactivity. J. Immunol. 168(8):4231–4240.

69. Fong L, Hou Y, Rivas A, et al. 2001. Altered peptide ligand vaccination with Flt3 ligand expanded dendritic cells for tumor immunotherapy. Proc. Nat. Acad. Sci. USA 98(15):8809–8814.

70. Yee C, Savage PA, Lee PP, Davis MM, Greenberg PD. 1999. Isolation of high avidity melanoma-reactive CTL from heterogeneous populations using peptide-*MHC* *tetramers*. J. Immunol. 162(4):2227–2234.

New Applications of Flow Cytometry in Cancer Diagnosis and Therapy

Sophie Song and Faramarz Naeim

1. INTRODUCTION

1.1. Overview of Clinical Flow Cytometry

Over the past two decades, clinical flow cytometry has evolved from a highly specialized research tool to an integral component of clinical practice *(1–4)*. This progress has been driven by several critical factors including the emergence of new classifications *(5–14)* of hematopoietic and lymphoid malignancies, the development of diagnostic consensus *(15–21)*, and advancement of several technological components *(22–25)*. These technical advancements include new instrumentation and software, availability of high quality fluorochromes and monoclonal antibodies, improved gating strategies, routine use of multiparameter approaches, and increased emphasis on clinicopathologic correlations.

Flow cytometry is a well-recognized powerful method of immunophenotyping in clinical diagnosis and management of hematopoietic and lymphoid malignancies. Just as immunohistochemistry revolutionized modern diagnostic pathology, many physicians predict that flow cytometry represents "the future of pathology." This statement reflects the powerful and versatile clinical role of flow cytometry in the context of clinicopathologic correlations. Nevertheless, this new era of flow cytometry does impose an unavoidable challenge upon pathologists in their routine practice.

This chapter will review the current applications of flow cytometry in cancer diagnosis and therapy, with a special focus on discussion of future trends in this field through introducing innovative and advanced technological approaches.

1.2. Practical Highlights of Basic Principles

Several outstanding reference books are available for a comprehensive understanding of the fundamental principles and technical details in clinical flow cytometry *(26–29)*. To provide a basis of understanding for clinicians and pathologists who are not used to instrumentations and software of flow cytometers for their clinical data interpretation, a few practical highlights are discussed in this section.

1.2.1. Concepts of Flow Cytometry, Cell Population, and Gating

As the term implies, flow cytometry measures cell (or particle) properties obtained when a stream of single cell (or particle) suspension passes through a set of optical detectors. Flow

From: *Cancer Diagnostics: Current and Future Trends*
Edited by: R. M. Nakamura, W. W. Grody, J. T. Wu, and R. B. Nagle © Humana Press Inc., Totowa, NJ

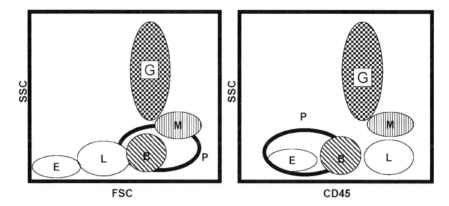

Fig. 1. Schematics of pattern recognition of hematopoietic cell clusters by flow cytometry using a combination of gating strategies. The diagram on the left shows cell population distribution using forward scatter (FSC) vs side scatter (SSC) gating. The diagram on the right represents cell population distribution using CD45 SSC gating. G,granulocytes; M, monocytes; P, plasma cells; L, lymphocytes; B,blasts; E,erythroid precursors.

cytometer recognizes particles that include cells, intracellular ultrastructures and macromolecules, isolated nuclei, debris, cell aggregates, or microsphere beads, to name a few.

To make any data analysis meaningful, specific instructions are given to the cytometer for delineating monodisperse cell populations, which under most circumstances are the target of analysis. A cell population of interest simply indicates a group of cells sharing identical characteristics creating a tendency of specific monodisperse clustering using multiparameter analysis. The use of multiparameter analysis is critical because this approach enables a multidimensional correlation between parameters, which results in significantly increased sensitivity and specificity for detecting target populations. This explains why major clinical flow cytometry laboratories quickly adopted the use of four-color and six-parameter (combination of two light scatter and four fluorescence colors) immunophenotyping in their routine diagnostic practice when cytometers with this type of analytic capacity became commercially available.

Gating is setting a population of cells in an electronic window. Gating strategies have been dramatically improved over the past several years, and some methods have been accepted as the standard by experts *(1,2,4,22,23,28)*. For example, the preferred gating strategy of human peripheral blood and bone marrow is to use CD45 vs side scatter *(22,23)* (Fig. 1). Both the sensitivity and specificity of immunophenotyping can be significantly improved when a combination of two or more gating strategies is used to complement each other. Proper gating is such a critical step in data analysis and interpretation that pathologists often offer advice to even the best-trained flow cytometry technologists.

1.2.2. Fluorochromes, Fluorescence, and Compensation

The availability of various fluorochromes and high-quality fluorochrome-conjugated monoclonal antibodies (MAbs) has enabled multiparameter immunophenotyping. Each fluorochrome has a discrete spectral pattern of light excitation and emission, therefore the use of multicolor assays results in emission spectral overlap of fluorochromes. This overlap is a spillover phenomenon of fluorescence from one fluorochrome to its neighbor fluorochrome.

Compensation is the subtraction of this fluorescence spillover. Although compensation is easily understood conceptually, it remains one of the most challenging technical aspects in data acquisition when multicolor immunophenotyping is applied. The use of new tandem fluorochromes and the most recent emergence of software compensation *(30)* have contributed to the simplification of the procedure. Several recent publications have addressed this technical challenge by providing guidance for the standardization of this complex process *(26,31–34)*.

1.3. Critical Role of Quality Assurance and Quality Control

Flow cytometry is a unique modern technology because its ultimate clinical utility relies on a highly sophisticated process involving a combination of both objective discrimination and artistic manipulation. Because of its increasing popularity and widespread use in routine clinical practice, the critical value of quality assurance and quality control of flow cytometry cannot be overemphasized. Although enormous efforts have been made to establish standards in this area by experts from Europe, the United States, and Canada *(15–18,26,35–40)*, the intra- and interlaboratory reproducibility is yet to be established *(41–43)* in two major areas: (1) the methods used for assessment of antigen expression and (2) the criteria employed for interpretation and reporting of results *(1,4)*. It is important for pathologists to identify this issue of quality assurance and quality control with a sense of urgency and professional obligation.

2. MODERN UTILITY OF FLOW CYTOMETRY IN DIAGNOSIS, CLASSIFICATION, PROGNOSTIC STRATIFICATION, AND MONITORING OF PREMALIGNANT AND MALIGNANT DISORDERS

2.1. Advantage and Limitations of Flow Cytometry in Modern Cancer Diagnosis

Immunophenotyping by flow cytometry is well recognized as an important diagnostic tool in hematopoietic and lymphoid malignancies in the context of clinicopathologic correlations, including clinical, morphologic, cytogenetic, molecular genetic, and immunohistochemical. Immunophenotyping by multiparametric flow cytometry is the only technique that permits simultaneous quantitative measurements of multiple characters in individual cells, thereby providing rapid, objective, and sensitive multivariable analysis of single-cell based cell populations (from single digit number to millions of cells).

Flow cytometry provides relatively fast service. It is able to acquire and analyze tens of thousands of cells in less than a few minutes. The time between receiving specimens and reporting results by pathologists is not more than a few hours, much faster than the conventional cytogenetic and molecular pathology services. In addition, the ability of acquiring and analyzing a large number of cells, makes it possible to detect rare events, such as minimal residual disease, where abnormal cells can be one in 10^5 cells (or 10^{-5}) or less.

The major limitation of flow cytometry is its dependence on other clinicopathologic findings, especially clinical history, morphologic examination, immunohistochemical study, cytogenetic, and molecular genetic analysis. Immunophenotyping by flow cytometry alone may not be efficient for achieving a proper pathologic diagnosis. A practical example of this argument is that flow cytometric immunophenotyping does not distinguish a lesion in the mediastinum, where normal thymic tissue, and lymphoblastic lymphoma/leukemia are all among potential differential diagnoses yet may share an identical immunophenotype.

As a result of recent technological advances in the field, some cytometrists are optimistic in clinical flow cytometry being used in a complete high-throughput and automated format. In fact, some commercial and large academic flow cytometry laboratories have already started practicing high-throughput flow cytometry by ordering a universal large panel of antibodies on high volume specimens without special emphasis on clinical and morphological correlations. Often in this type of high-throughput practice, the decision for proper gating, which is in fact a medical judgment, is left in the hands of flow cytometry technologists. It is important for pathologists to be aware of this issue and to identify the importance of their roles in data analysis and interpretation, in order to provide high quality flow cytometry service, which ultimately leads to high quality patient care.

Flow cytometry can provide clinically meaningful and accurate information, only if considered in the context of clinicopathologic correlations. Therefore, despite the rapid technological advances in the field, it is difficult to argue that the practice of clinical flow cytometry will adapt a completely automated high-throughput format independent of clinicopathologic correlations in the future.

2.2. Acute Leukemias

The new World Health Organization (WHO) classification *(44,45)* provides a guideline for the immunophenotyping of acute leukemias by flow cytometry. It is best achieved through the following sequential events:

1. Review of clinical history, morphologic evaluation, and panel selection.
2. Enumeration, lineage identification, maturation, and phenotypic aberration assessment of leukemic population.
3. Phenotypic characterization of pathologic subpopulations.
4. Additional clinicopathologic correlations, including immunohistochemistry, cytochemistry, cytogenetics, and molecular genetics.

Immunophenotypic features of leukemic/lymphomatous cells are considered as reflections of normal cells undergoing maturation arrest. However, accumulating new evidence has demonstrated aberrant immunophenotype of the pathologic cells displaying expression of cross-lineage and/or asynchronous antigens, ectopic phenotypes, as well as abnormal differentiation pathways among others *(1,46–50)*. The clinical relevance of aberrant expression and specific phenotype relies on its connection to prognostically relevant genotypic markers, because they appear to be important for identifying entities with distinct prognoses and clinical behavior *(51)*. Recent studies have focused on addressing associations between specific immunophenotypes of leukemic cells and prognostically relevant genotypic markers. The majority of the recent findings are summarized thoroughly in a review by Hrusak and Porwit-MacDonald *(52)*.

2.2.1. Acute Lymphoblastic Leukemia/Lymphoma

2.2.1.1. Precursor B-Lymphoblastic Leukemia/Lymphoma (B-ALL) Lineage

B-lineage ALLs are characterized by expression of cytoplasmic CD22 and CD79a as well as membrane CD19. In addition, it is important to assess the maturation stage of leukemic cells using CD34, TdT, CD10, CD20, cytoplasmic heavy chain (IgM), and surface light chains (κ or λ). The detection of intracellular TdT is highly specific for ALL if a B-lineage process is confirmed. If TdT is negative, attention should be directed toward Burkitt leukemia/lymphoma and other types of lymphomas, such as rare leukemic presentation of mantle

Table 1
B-Lineage ALL Immunophenotypic Groups

Type	Characteristic immunophenotypic features
Early precursor	HLA-DR, TdT, CD34, cytoplasmic CD22, CD79a and often CD19
Precursor B	HLA-DR, TdT, CD10, ±CD34, cytoplasmic CD22, CD79a and often CD20
Pre-B	HLA-DR, cytoplasmic Ig heavy chain μ, ±TdT, CD10, CD19, CD20, CD22, and CD79a
B (Burkitt type)	HLA-DR, CD19, CD20, CD22, CD79a, surface Ig, and ±CD10

Table 2
T-Lineage ALL Immunophenotypic Groups

Type	Characteristic immunophenotypic features
Early precursor	CD7, TdT, and CD34
Immature thymocyte	CD7, TdT, cytoplasmic CD3, CD2, CD5, and CD38
Intermediate thymocyte	CD7, TdT, CD38, CD1a, CD2, CD3, CD5, CD4, and CD8
Mature thymocyte	CD7, CD38, CD2, CD3, CD5, CD4 or CD8 and ±TdT

cell lymphoma *(53)*. CD34 is expressed in about 50% of the B-lineage ALL cases. The B-lineage ALLs are divided into four immunophenotypic groups (*see* Table 1).

Less than half of the precursor B-ALL patients demonstrate aberrant expression of myeloid markers such as CD13 and CD33 *(54–57)*. Although recent large clinical trial studies have not proven the clinical utility of the aberrant expression of myeloid antigens *(54,58,59)*, the expression may predict an MLL gene rearrangement *(54,60)*.

In B-lineage ALL, the genotypic marker t(12;21) (TEL/AML1) is found to be generally associated with a very good prognosis in pediatric patients *(61–65,71)*. The characteristic immunophenotype in this group is low or absent CD9, CD20, and CD45, but high CD10 *(61,65)*. The pediatric patients with t(12;21) also show more frequent expression of CD13 and/or CD33 *(53)*. In the contrary, a poor prognosis is linked to t(9;22) (BCR/ABL) and t(4;11) (MLL/AF4) genotypic markers, with specific immunophenotypes being CD34$^+$/CD38$^+$ in t(9;22) *(66)* vs NG2$^+$/CD15$^+$/CD10- in 11q23 translocations, respectively *(62,67–70)*.

2.2.1.2. Precursor T-Lymphoblastic Leukemia/Lymphoma (T-Lineage ALL)

The T-lineage ALLs are divided into four immunophenotypes (*see* Table 2) *(72)*.

The expression of CD3 (cytoplasmic or membrane) is the most helpful marker for lineage specificity. In almost 100% of the patients, CD7 is expressed on leukemic cells. The expression of CD7 is by no means specific, it is also found in about 20% AML patients *(73)*. Myeloid antigens, such as CD13 and CD33 are frequently identified in T-lineage ALL, although their clinical significance is unclear *(54–58)*.

In T-lineage ALL, it is more challenging to understand the connection between a given phenotype and prognostically relevant genotypic markers, because no cytogenetic or molecular genetic abnormality can be identified in most adult and pediatric cases *(74,75)*. Most recent trials have suggested that T-lineage ALL of intermediate differentiation (defined as expression of CD1a or combined with double positivity for CD4 and CD8) seems to be associated with a more favorable prognosis *(76–78)*. Previous indications regarding the association of CD2 and CD10 expression with a more favorable outcome have not been proven in recent trials *(76)*. A recent study described a new specific translocation t(5;14) (q35;q32), found in about 22% of pediatric T-ALL patients *(79)*. According to the study, this translocation is associated with the Hox11L2 gene expression, which is reportedly in connection with the intermediate T-ALL phenotype *(52)*.

2.2.2. Acute Myeloid Leukemia

2.2.2.1. DIAGNOSIS AND CLASSIFICATION

According to the new WHO classification, acute myeloid leukemia (AML) has four major clinical and biological categories *(44,45)*:

1. AML with recurrent genetic abnormalities.
2. AML with multilineage dysplasia.
3. AML with myelodysplastic syndromes (MDS), therapy related.
4. AML, not otherwise categorized.

This new system of classification emphasizes the critical value of clinicopathologic correlation using all available morphologic, genetic, and clinical data, in recognizing unique disease entities that are clinically and biologically meaningful. Based on the WHO criteria, the blast threshold for diagnosis of AML has also been set at ≥20%.

In addition to myeloperoxidase (MPO) as the lineage specific marker in AML *(44)*, several other myeloid antigens including CD13, CD33, CD117 are expressed in approx 65–90% or more of AML cases *(80–83)*. Practical challenges arise in enumeration and immunophenotypic characterization of leukemic cells in AML cases, owing to the widely recognized differentiation heterogeneity of these leukemic cells *(2,3,15,84)*.

To achieve accurate enumeration and phenotypic assessment of the leukemic cells, special attention should be devoted to the selection of proper gating strategies in the context of clinicopathological correlations. The standard gating method of CD45 vs side scatter is adequate in majority of the AML cases *(4)*, but a combination of several gating methods, such as forward vs side light scatter, as well as light scatter vs CD13, or CD33, or CD34, needs to be conducted to improve the sensitivity and specificity of leukemic cell detection. For example, blast cells in general express low intensity CD45, but in some cases of ALL, as well as acute monocytic and myelomonocytic leukemias, they may show high intensity CD45 expression (Fig. 2). Therefore, proper gating should allow detection of target populations including myeloblasts and their equivalents, and are exemplified by abnormal promyelocytes in acute promyelocytic leukemia (APL), as well as monoblasts and promonocytes in acute myelomonocytic leukemia.

A fundamental strategy in data analysis and interpretation is the recognition of antigen expression patterns, including lineage specific markers, maturation molecules, aberrant antigens, as well as antigen expression intensities. This strategy is more valuable when the genotypic-immunophenotypic association becomes the focus of investigation as implicated in the new WHO classification system of AML *(45)* and published in the updated review *(52)* as mentioned earlier.

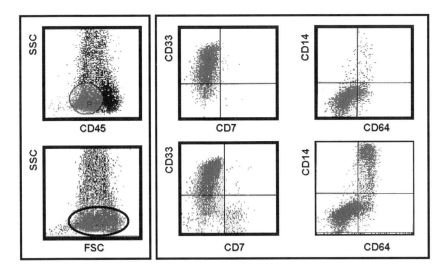

Fig. 2. Bone marrow flow cytometric analysis on a patient with acute myelomonocytic leukemia. When the gated population only represents CD45 dim cells (upper row) no CD14 positive cluster is detected. But, when the gate is expanded to also include CD45 strongly positive cells (lower row), there is clearly a population of CD14 positive cells, indicating the presence of a monocytic component. In certain leukemias, such as acute monocytic and myelomonocytic types as well as occasional cases of acute lymphoblastic leukemias, blasts and immature forms partially or totally show strong expression of CD45.

2.2.2.2. GENOTYPIC-IMMUNOPHENOTYPIC ASSOCIATIONS

Recently, efforts have been made on addressing the association between immunophenotypes and prognostically significant genotypic markers. Although conflicting results still exist, abnormal phenotypes have been detected in all AML cases carrying specific translocations discussed below *(52,85)* (Table 3).

2.2.2.2.1. AML With t(8;21) (AML1/ETO)

This translocation involves the *AML1* gene on chromosome 21q22 and *ETO* gene on chromosome 8q22 *(86)*. It is found in approx 7% of AMLs *(52)* including both adult and childhood cases, with a relatively higher incidence in younger patients. AML with this genotype is generally associated with a higher sensitivity to therapy and a better outcome *(4)*. The leukemic cells demonstrate characteristic immunophenotype expressing high-intensity MPO, CD13, and usually low-intensity CD33. Expression of CD15, CD34, CD65, CD117, and HLA-DR is identified in high proportion of the cases. In addition, lymphoid lineage markers CD19 and/or CD56 are frequently expressed. The expression of CD56 has been associated with a worse prognosis in some studies *(87)*.

2.2.2.2.2. AML With t(15;17) (PML/RARa) and Variants

Acute promyelocytic leukemia (APL) constitutes about 5–15% of all AML cases *(52)*, revealing distinct morphologic, genetic, and immunophenotypic findings (Fig. 3). The t(15;17) translocation is characteristically present in APL, involving the PML gene on chromosome 15 and the retinoic acid receptor alpha (RARα) gene on chromosome 17. About 10% of cases of APL present as microgranular variants with altered underlying genotypes

Table 3
Phenotypic and Genotypic Correlations in Acute Leukemia

Type	Immunophenotype	Chromosomes	Genes	Comments
ALL				
	Early precursor B, CD10-, plus CD15+ and/or CD65+	t(4;11)(q21;q23)	AF4/AML	50% of ALLs in infants 6–7% of all ALLs
	Precursor B phenotype CD13+ and/or CD33+	t(12;23)(p13;q22)	TEL/AML1	Undetected by routine karyotype 25% of childhood ALLs
	Precursor B phenotype plus CD9+ B phenotype, CD10± surface Ig+, and TdT	t(9;22)(q34;q11); t(8;14)(q24;q32); t(2;8)(p11;q24); t(8;22)(q24;q11)	BCR/ABL; MYC/IGH; IGK/MYC; MYC/IGL	25% of adult and 5% of childhood ALLs Burkitt leukemia/lymphoma African type EBV-associated
		t(1;19)(q23;p13)	E2A/PBX1	About 5% of ALLs
	Early precursor B, CD10- cytoplasmic IgM-, and surface Ig-	t(17;19)(q21;p13)	E2A/HLF	Rare
	Precursor B phenotype T-lineage, CD1a+, CD2+, CD5+, CD7+, CD8+	t(5;14)(q35;q32)	RanBP17/CTIP2	Approximately 20% of T-ALLs in children and adolescents
AML				
	CD34+, CD13+, CD15+, CD33+, MPO+ CD19low±, and CD56±	t(8;21)(q22;q22)	AML1/ETO	AML-M2 of FAB classification About 7% of AMLs
	CD13+, CD33+, MPO+, HLA-DR-, CD34low or CD34- CD15±, rare CD2+ and rare CD56±	t(15;17)(q22;q21)	PML/RARα	Acute promyelocytic leukemia AML-M3 of FAB classification 5–15% of AMLs
	CD13+, CD33+ CD14+ CD15+, CD11b+, CD34+, CD117+, CD4+, CD2+, and TdT+	t(16;16)(p13;q22)	CBFβ/MYH11	Acute myelomonocytic leukemia AML-M4eo of FAB classification 6–10% of AMLs
	CD41+, CD42+, CD61+, CD13±, CD33±, CD34±	t(1;22)(p13;q13)	OTT/MAL	Acute megakaryoblastic leukemia AML-M7 of FAB classification About and HLA-DR± 20% of all infant AMLs
	CD13+, CD18+, CD33+, CD34+, CD117+, HLA-DR+, plus B cell-associated markers	t(9;22)	BCR/ABL	AML-M1/M2 of FAB classification About 1% of AML

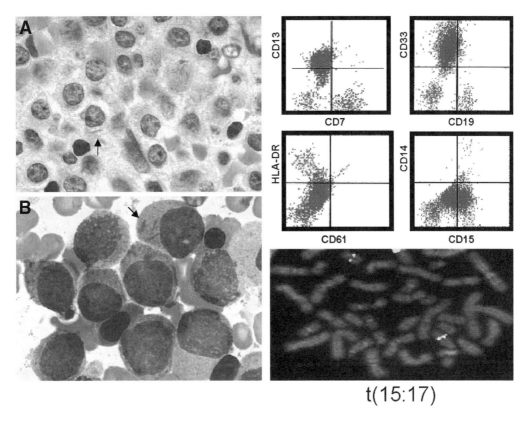

t(15:17)

Fig. 3. Multiparameter studies in a patient with acute promyelocytic leukemia (APL). The bone marrow clot section (**A**) and smear (**B**) demonstrate numerous promyelocytes, some of which contain multiple Auer rods (arrows). The diagrams of flow cytometric results show that the gated promyelocytes express CD13 and CD33, but are negative for HLA-DR and CD14. The FISH analysis demonstrates t(15;17) characteristic for APL. Color figure available for viewing at **www.humanapress.com**.

involving the RARα gene *(88,89)*. APL demonstrates highly specific scatter and immunophenotypic features, with expression of CD13, CD33, MPO, variable CD15, but absence of HLA-DR and CD34 *(90–93)*. Variable expression of CD34 is occasionally observed in microgranular variant APL *(88,94,95)*, although CD2 is often expressed in this variant *(94)*. Several studies including recent results have suggested a link between CD56 expression in APL and a worse prognosis *(96)*. The overall sensitivity and specificity of immunophenotyping in the diagnosis of t(15;17) is over 90% *(93)*. The clinical significance of the diagnosis of APL with t(15;17) is reflected by its sensitivity to treatment using all trans retinoic acid.

2.2.2.2.3. AML With inv(16) or t(16;16) (CBFβ/MYH11)

The myelomonocytic subtype of AML is often associated with inversion or translocation of chromosome 16 involving the *CBFβ/MYH11* gene, found in approx 6–10% of all AML *(52)*. This chromosome abnormality has been associated with a more favorable clinical outcome. The immunophenotype is complex yet characteristic, revealing constant maturation asynchrony and presence of both immature and differentiating blast subsets. The majority of the cases express CD4 (low-intensity), CD11b, CD13, CD14, CD15, CD33, CD34, CD64, CD65, CD117, and HLA-DR *(97–99)*. Expression of CD2 is found in about 40% of the cases *(99,100)*, CD7 is less frequently expressed *(101)*.

2.2.2.2.4. AML With 11q23 (MLL)

Genetic alterations of chromosome band 11q23 are predominantly identified in myelomonocytic and/or monocytic subtypes of AML, with involvement of the *MLL* gene. The leukemic cells display characteristic immunophenotypic features, expressing myelomonocytic-associated markers including CD4 (low-intensity), CD11b, CD13, CD14, CD15, CD33, CD64, as well as CD56 *(102–104)*.

2.2.2.2.5 AML With Aberrations of Chromosomes 5 and 7

The aberrations of chromosome 5 and 7, such as -5/del(5q), -7/del(7q), are mostly associated with AML secondary to myelodysplastic syndrome and/or AML of the elderly *(52, 137–140)*. High incidence of CD34 expression has been suggested in AML with aberrations of chromosomes 5 and 7 *(141–143)*. Expression of CD14 is observed more often in cases with aberration of chromosome 5 than in cases with aberrations of chromosome 7 *(52)*. T-cell related antigens such as CD2 or CD7 are more commonly expressed in AML cases with aberrations of chromosome 5 *(97)*. Expressions of TdT and CD7 are suggestive of multiple drug resistant phenotypes in adult AML cases with aberrations of chromosomes 5 and 7 *(144)*.

2.2.3. The Quandary of Biphenotypic Leukemia

The continuous advancement of immunophenotypic techniques along with the expansion of cells markers for the evaluation of the blast cells in acute leukemias have led to a growing incidence of leukemias that share features of more than one specific cell type. These leukemias are frequently referred to as "biphenotypic" leukemias. Biphenotypic leukemias are primarily characterized by differentiation-associated antigens, and because most of these antigens are neither tumor-specific nor lineage-restricted, there is a significant overlap in their expression in myeloid and lymphoid leukemias. A scoring system originally proposed by Catovsky and associates in 1991 *(135,136)*, has been adopted by WHO as criteria *(44)* for the inclusion of biphenotypic leukemias (Table 4). According to this scoring system, a given lineage is defined if the total score for that lineage-associated marker is greater than 2. The most definitive lineage-associated markers are cytoplasmic CD22 and cytoplamic IgM and cytoplasmic CD79a for B lymphoblasts, cytoplasmic CD3 for T lymphoblasts and myeloperoxidase for myeloblasts. In general, the majority of acute leukemias that show aberrant antigenic expressions fall into either ALL or AML subtypes without being considered biphenotypic: These leukemias are divided into two major immunophenotypic groups: AMLs expressing lymphoid-associated markers, and ALLs expressing myeloid-associated markers.

2.2.4. Minimal Residual Disease

2.2.4.1. PROGNOSTIC SIGNIFICANCE

It is well established that early response to therapy is one of the most important prognostic factors in acute leukemia. A small percentage of leukemic cells (approx 1–5% of the total marrow nucleated cells) can be detected by morphological examination alone, which provides useful information in stratification of patients achieving complete clinical remission (CR). However, many of these patients once diagnosed as CR eventually relapse, owing to the persistence of a very low percentage of leukemic cells (minimal residual disease, MRD) that are not detected by the conventional morphological examination *(105–107)*.

Table 4
The Proposed Scoring System for Lineage Association*

Score	B-cell	T-cell	Myeloid
2	cytCD22	CD3 (m/cyt)	MPO
	cytCD79a	ant-TCR	
	cyIgM		
1	CD10	CD2	CD13
	CD19	CD5	CD33
	CD20	CD8	CD65
		CD10	CD117
0.5	TdT	TdT	CD14
	CD24	CD7	CD15
		CD1a	CD64

*Adapted from ref. *44*.
Note: According to the proposed scoring system, criteria for acute biphenotypic leukemia are > 2 points from two separate lineages.

The applicability and utilization of variable sensitive and specific techniques in the past decade, has allowed many investigations focusing on the clinical relevance of MRD. Investigation of MRD is a valuable tool for predicting impending relapses before clinical and hematologic presentations, defining risk groups, and establishing patient-specific treatment modalities in acute leukemia patients *(46–49,105–115)*. It is even suggested in a recent study that MRD level is the most powerful independent prognostic factor in acute leukemia, followed by cytogenetics and number of cycles to achieve CR *(114)*.

2.2.4.2. DETECTION METHODS

Among these various technological approaches, both the PCR based molecular technique and immunophenotyping by multiparameter flow cytometry are the most commonly used methods. These two methods have shown improved sensitivity for the identification of leukemic cells when compared with *in situ* hybridization (FISH) analysis, which demonstrates high specificity but low sensitivity (at best 1/1000 cells or 10^{-3}) in identifying leukemic cells *(116)*. Using PCR based molecular technology, about 25–30% of ALL and AML cases can be monitored through detection of the gene fusion products, and about 90% of ALL can be followed up by B- or T-cell gene rearrangement studies *(2,46,47,109–112,117)*. As comparison, the multiparametric immunophenotyping approach for MRD detection can be applied in about 90% ALLs and 80% AMLs *(4,106,114,115)*. The sensitivity of this method can reach one leukemic cell among 10^5 normal cells (10^{-5}) *(106)*. Additional large studies, especially in AML cases, are being conducted. However, the present available data support multiparametric immunophenotyping as a valuable tool in the evaluation of MRD levels in acute leukemia patients.

2.2.4.3. STRATEGIC APPROACH BY FLOW CYTOMETRY

The strategic approach in the detection of MRD by multiparametric immunophenotyping is identification of aberrant phenotypes through pattern recognition, which differentiates the leukemic population from the normal hematopoietic precursors in bone marrow. As mentioned in Subheading 2.2., the concept of aberrant phenotype is now expanded to include expression of cross-lineage antigen, asynchronous antigen, ectopic antigen, altered differentiation pathways, as well as abnormal antigen intensity and light-scatter pattern.

Despite its clinical utility, MRD detection by flow cytometric immunophenotyping has two major pitfalls that would influence its sensitivity, specificity, and applicability *(67,68,118–121)*. First, the absence of well-established antibodies against leukemia-specific antigens, such as BCR/ABL and PML/RARa fusion proteins. Second, the presence of phenotypic changes occurring at relapse. Although it is not uncommon for leukemic cells to display phenotypic changes at relapse (approx 20–70% according to various studies) *(106,118–123)*, changes influencing aberrant phenotypes are less frequent (approx 16%) *(106,122)*, and at least one of the aberrances detected at the original diagnosis remained stable at relapse *(106,122)*. The practical approach in dealing with these pitfalls is a careful examination of leukemic populations and subpopulations by selecting a combination of multiple aberrant phenotypic parameters.

2.3. Myelodysplastic Syndrome

Myelodysplastic syndrome (MDS) represents a group of heterogeneous clonal abnormalities of bone marrow hematopoietic precursors. According to the new WHO classification *(124)*, MDS is divided into six subgroups: refractory anemia (RA), refractory anemia with ringed sideroblasts (RARS), refractory anemia with multilineage dysplasia (RAMD), refractory anemia with excess blasts (RAEB), unclassifiable MDS, and MDS associated with isolated del (5q) chromosome abnormality. Several factors including the percentage of blasts, cytogenetic abnormalities and cytopenia were found to be prognostically important, as suggested by the International Prognosis Scoring System *(125)*.

The diagnosis of MDS is primarily based on clinical history, morphologic findings, and cytogenetic studies. Although several studies of MDS using flow cytometric immunophenotyping have been published, their clinicopathologic significance including outcome prediction of MDS is yet to be well defined *(126–131)*. However, recent technological advances including multiparametric and pattern-recognition-based approaches in flow cytometric immmunophenotyping, have enabled phenotypic qualitative and quantitative evaluation in hematopoietic precursors and their subpopulations in MDS *(132–134)*. A recent large multicenter prospective study *(134)*, has demonstrated significant correlation between the expression of aberrant phenotypes in MDS and diagnosis, prognostic scores, as well as cytogenetic risk factors. For example, the results of this study show that the presence of a myeloid subpopulation with CD36 expression on $CD45^{low}$ or $CD45^{high}$/side scatter^{high} cells is indicative of a poor prognosis, whereas CD71 expression is associated with a good prognosis *(134)*.

Utilizing emerging new evidence, the clinical role of multiparametric immunophenotyping by flow cytometry in MDS, is being expanded from excluding other causes of cytopenia and providing blast numeration to a useful tool for diagnostic and prognostic characterization of MDS.

2.4. Lymphoproliferative Malignancies and Plasma Cell Disorders

In the past 10 yr, flow cytometric immunophenotyping has gradually gained its popularity and recognition in the diagnosis and monitoring of lymphoproliferative malignancies as well as plasma cell disorders *(2,145–152)*, a field that has historically relied on immunohistochemical analysis as the key or even sole ancillary studies. Flow cytometry is now considered a useful tool for distinguishing benign from malignant lymphoid proliferation, establishing B- or T-cell lineage and assisting the differential diagnosis of lymphoproliferative disorders *(150,151)*.

The new WHO classification *(44)* has provided an updated guideline for the diagnosis of lymphoproliferative and plasma cell malignancies. The flow cytometric immunophenotyping of lymphoid malignancies, is best achieved using multiparametric analysis that once again stresses clinicopathologic correlations including clinical history, morphologic (tissue sections, touch imprints, smears), cytogenetic, molecular genetic, and immunohistochemical findings. An updated understanding of phenotypic and genotypic correlations in non-Hodgkin's lymphoma is summarized in Table 5 *(152a)*. The correlation with immunohistochemical studies is of special interest because flow cytometry and immunohistochemistry can be relatively complimentary in lymphoid tissue immunophenotyping.

2.4.1. B-Cell Neoplasm

2.4.1.1. B-Chronic Lymphocytic Leukemia/Small Lymphocytic Lymphoma (CLL/SLL)

B-chronic lymphocytic leukemia/small lymphocytic lymphoma (CLL/SLL) is the most common adult leukemia in North America and Europe, and its nodal presentation is a common type of non-Hodgkin's lymphoma *(6,153,154)*. CLL/SLL usually has a distinct immunophenotype expressing CD5, CD19, CD21, CD23, CD43, and CD20^{low}, often lacking CD10, FMC7, and CD103 *(6,149,155,156)*. The expression of sIg is usually low, which is of IgM or IgD isotype when detectable *(6)*. When atypical phenotypes are present, such as CD5$^+$/CD23$^-$ or CD5$^-$/CD23$^+$, other types of B-cell lymphoma need to be excluded.

Although the independent prognostic utility of specific antigen phenotype is controversial *(154,157–160)*, significant correlations do exist between genotypic markers of more aggressive clinical course (e.g., involving chromosomes 17 and 12) and atypical morphology as well as phenotype (CD20^{high}, sIg^{high}, CD22$^+$, and/or CD23$^-$) *(158,161–162c)*. In addition, several recent studies have suggested an association between CD38 expression (in > 30% of CLL/SLL) and a germline mutation of the Ig gene variable segment, indicating a poor prognosis *(163,164)*. It has also been suggested that expression of Zap70 in CLL/SLL cases is associated with a worse prognosis *(164a,164b)*.

2.4.1.2. Mantle Cell Lymphoma

Mantle cell lymphoma is a clinically aggressive entity, and is characterized by t(11;14) involving the BCL1 (cyclin D1) and IgH genes *(165)*. The distinct immunophenotype is usually illustrated by CD45^{high}, sIg+ (IgD+ > IgM+/IgD+, λ+ > κ+), CD5$^+$, CD43$^+$, but CD11c$^-$, CD23$^-$, CD34$^-$, TdT$^-$ *(159, 165–168)*. In addition, pan B markers are usually strongly expressed, including CD19, CD20, CD22, and CD79α *(166,169)*. Most of the mantle cell lymphomas lack CD10, although some reports have suggested otherwise *(167,170,171)*. The availability and applicability of antibodies against BCL-1 antigen have marked a turning point for the diagnosis of mantle cell lymphoma. Expression of BCL-1 protein has been detected using immunohistochemical studies *(172–174)*, although it has also been demonstrated in recent studies using flow cytometric analysis *(175)*. The identification of the BCL-1 protein is critical in differentiating blastoid variant mantle cell lymphoma from prolymphocytic leukemia and B-lineage lymphoblastic lymphoma, as well as distinguishing atypical mantle cell lymphoma (CD5$^-$/CD23$^+$) from atypical CLL/SLL (CD5$^-$ or CD23$^-$).

2.4.1.3. FOLLICULAR LYMPHOMA

Follicular lymphoma is a common type of non-Hodgkins' lymphoma in North America and Europe. Most of the follicular lymphomas have an indolent course and patients usually present with advanced stage of disease. Occasionally, it can present a leukemic phase especially in the later phases of the disease. The immunophenotype of follicular lymphoma includes strong expression of major pan B antigens and sIg, with coexpression of CD10 at variable intensities in 70–96% of the cases *(29)*. The expression of CD23[low to moderate] is seen in a minority of follicular lymphoma cases. Virtually all follicular lymphoma cases lack CD5, BCL-1, CD11c, and CD103 *(29)*. BCL-6 is often helpful in identifying the follicular center origin of the neoplastic cells. BCL-2 is strongly expressed in subgroups of follicular lymphomas, although it is not specific because it is also expressed in other B-cell lymphomas and leukemias as well as normal T-cells *(176)*.

2.4.1.4. MARGINAL ZONE LYMPHOMA

Marginal zone lymphoma (MZL) includes marginal zone lymphoma of mucosa-associated lymphoid tissue (MALT) type, nodal marginal zone lymphoma with/without monocytoid B-cells, and splenic marginal zone lymphoma. The immunophenotypic features of MZL are rather unique, because they lack CD5, CD10, CD23, and CD43 in more than 90% of cases *(2,170,172,176–178)*, in addition to absence of BCL-1. It is important to note that very rare cases of MZL have been reported positive for CD5 or CD103 *(178)*.

2.4.1.5. HAIRY CELL LEUKEMIA

Although it is rarely encountered in general practice *(179)*, hairy cell leukemia (HCL) is important as proper treatment has enabled a durable remission in a large proportion of patients *(153,179,180)*. The immunophenotypic characters include increased forward scatter resulted from an increase in cell size and strong expression of major B-cell antigens including CD19, CD20, CD22, and sIg. The unique immunophenotypic features include strong expression of CD11c, CD103, and FMC7, where the concomitant strong expression of CD11c and CD103 is highly specific for HCL in the setting of a monoclonal B-cell proliferation *(155,181–183)*. Expression of CD25 is found in approx 70–80% of the cases and is of low to moderate intensity *(182)* (Fig. 4).

2.4.1.6. BURKITT LYMPHOMA

It is an aggressive form of lymphoma with good response to modern chemotherapy. Immunophenotyping is important in assessment of differentiation. The typical immunophenotypic features of Burkitt lymphoma are reflected by uniform and strong expression of CD19, CD20, CD45, and immunoglobulin light chains, with CD10[low] expression found in majority of the cases *(29)* (Fig. 5). Rare cases have been reported as CD5[+] *(184)*. In the event of one or more "blast"-associated immature antigens, such as CD34 and/or TdT, plus CD10[high] and sIg-, the diagnosis of precursor B-cell lymphoblastic lymphoma/leukemia should be confirmed in the absence of the characteristic MYC translocations (Table 5).

2.4.1.7. PLASMA CELL MYELOMA

Immunophenotyping of plasma cell myeloma by multiparametric flow cytometry is an attractive approach for diagnostic and prognostic evaluation of the disease. It allows discrimination between myelomatous plasma cells and normal plasma cells *(185–189)* based upon the distinct phenotypic aberrations that occur in more than 90% of the myelomatous plasma cells *(190)*. The normal plasma cells are defined as CD38[high], CD138[high], CD56-,

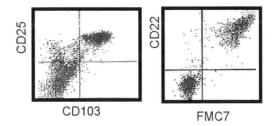

Fig. 4. Bone marrow flow cytometric studies on a patient with hairy cell leukemia. The leukemia cells characteristically coexpress CD25 and CD103. They are also strongly positive for CD22 and FMC7.

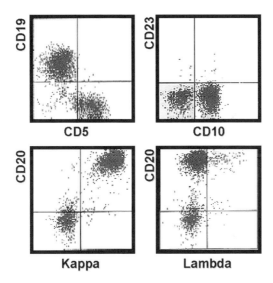

Fig. 5. Flow cytometric analysis on a lymph node biopsy sample from a patient with Burkitt lymphoma. The gated lymphoid cells express CD10 and CD19, and are Kappa light chain restricted. The neoplastic cells in Burkitt lymphoma are negative for TdT (not shown).

CD45[low], CD20−, CD28−, CD33−, and CD117− *(190–192)*. The most frequent aberrant phenotypic features consist of CD19−, strong expression of CD56, and decreased intensity of CD38. In addition, aberrant expression of CD10, CD20, CD22, CD28, CD117, and CD33 or other myelomonocytic markers are identified in neoplastic plasma cells. Although the prognostic utility of myeloma immunophenotyping is yet to be defined, recent investigations have indicated that about 35% abnormal plasma cells are present in monoclonal gammopathy, whereas nearly all plasma cells are abnormal in plasma cell myeloma *(191)*. Furthermore, it was suggested in a recent study that the presence of at least 30% normal plasma cells post therapy correlates with a significantly longer progression-free survival *(190)*.

2.4.2. T-Cell Neoplasm

2.4.2.1. T-Cell Large Granular Lymphocytic (T-LGL) Leukemia

T-LGL is one of the two most common forms of mature T-cell leukemias in North America *(153,179)*. Morphologically, LGL is characteristic, and is phenotypically divided into T-

Table 5
Phenotypic and Genotypic Correlations in Non-Hodgkin Lymphomas

Type	Immunophenotype	Chromosomes	Genes	Frequency(%)
B-cell lymphoma				
Follicular	CD19$^+$, CD20$^+$, CD22$^+$, CD10$^+$, BCL2$^+$, BCL6$^+$, CD5$^-$, CD10$^-$, CD43$^-$	t(14;18)(q32;q31)	IgH/BCL2	90
Burkitt	B phenotype, CD10$^\pm$, sIg$^+$, TdT$^-$, BCL2$^-$	t(8;14)(q24;q32) t(2;8)(p11;q24) t(8;22)(q24;q11)	MYC/IGH IGK/MYC MYC/IGL	75 16 9
Mantle cell	CD19$^+$, CD20$^+$, CD5$^+$, FMC7$^+$, CD43$^+$, BCL1$^+$ CD10$^-$, CD23$^-$, BCL-6$^-$	t(11;14)(q13;q32)	CCND1/IgH	70
Lymphoplasmacytic	CD19$^+$, CD20$^+$, CD22$^+$, CD79a$^+$, CD5$^-$, CD10$^-$, CD23$^-$, CD43$^\pm$	t(9;14)(p13;q32)	PAX5/IGH	50
Diffuse large cell	CD19$^+$, CD20$^+$, CD22$^+$, CD79a$^+$, CD5$^\pm$, CD10$^\pm$	3q27	BCL6	40
Marginal zone	CD19$^+$, CD20$^+$, CD79a$^+$, CD43$^\pm$, CD11c$^\pm$, CD5$^-$ CD10$^-$, CD23$^-$	t(11;18)(q21;q21)	AP12/MLT	40
Small lymphocytic	CD19$^+$, CD23$^+$, CD5$^+$ CD20^{low}, CD22^{low} CD79a^{low}, CD10$^-$, FMC7$^-$	del(13q14)		50
T-cell lymphoma				
Anaplastic Large cell	CD30$^+$, ALK$^+$, EMA$^+$ CD2$^+$, CD4$^+$, CD43$^+$, TIA-1$^+$, granzyme B$^+$	t(2;5)(p23;q35)	NPM/ALK	35

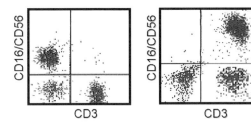

Fig. 6. The large granular lymphocytes are of two major types: natural killer (NK) cell and cytotoxic T cell. Both types express CD16 and or CD56, but NK cells are CD3-negative (*left*) and T cells are CD3-positive (*right*).

and NK-subtypes (Fig. 6) demonstrating strong correlations with clinical presentation, therapy, and prognosis *(149)*. The T-LGL is usually a very low-grade leukemia, although its NK counterpart has a much more aggressive clinical course.

Immunophenotyping of T-LGL reveals mature T-cell lymphoproliferation, with expression of pan T markers including CD2, CD3, CD5, and CD7, as well as CD8+/CD4– profile and TCR gene rearrangement. Occasional loss of a pan T antigen can be present. Usually, one or more NK-associated antigens, such as CD16, CD56, CD57, are present with the expression of CD57 being most commonly reported *(29)*. It has been suggested that CD56+ T-LGL is associated with a more aggressive clinical course, although it is not definitive *(194–196)*. The NK-LGL shares the CD2, CD7, CD8 antigen profile with the T-LGL, but does not express T-specific antigens such as CD3, CD5, and TCR. However, the NK-LGL cannot be differentiated from benign NK lymphoproliferation by immunophenotypic features.

2.4.2.2. Sézary Syndrome / Mycosis Fungoides

Mycosis fungoides (MF) is a malignant cutaneous T-cell lymphoma, and Sézary syndrome (SS) is defined when MF neoplastic cells are present in peripheral blood. MF/SS and T-LGL together represent the most prevalent forms of mature T-cell leukemia in North America *(153,179)*. Morphologically, MF/SS neoplastic cells demonstrate distinct features. These cells display abnormal T-cell phenotype, with expression of CD4+/CD8– profile in most cases, and CD4+/CD8+ or CD4–/CD8+ in less than 10% of the cases *(29)*. In addition, partial or total loss of CD7 is usually present *(156,197–199)*, which by itself, is not a definitive indication of MF/SS nor a clonal/neoplastic T-cell population, because it can also be observed in reactive T lymphocytosis *(200)*.

2.4.3. CD4⁺ CD56⁺ Malignancies

CD4+ CD56+ malignancies represent rare hematopoietic neoplasms *(201–203,205)*, which were recently linked to plasmacytoid dendritic cells or type 2 dendritic cells (DC2), in the absence of B-, T-, and myeloid lineage markers *(204,205)*. Although they are uncommon, the topic warrants special attention, because the CD4+ CD56+ malignancies display distinct clinical behavior, morphologic, and immunophenotypic characteristics, including specific immunophenotypic-prognostic associations. These lesions typically present as cutaneous nodules associated with lymphadenopathy and/or splenomegaly. Cytopenia is frequent, with circulating malignant cells often detected. Massive bone marrow involvement is seen in more than 80% of the cases studied *(205)*. According to the new WHO classification, these tumors are referred to as blastic natural killer (NK) lymphoma/leukemia *(44)*.

In addition to CD4 and CD56 expression, the neoplastic cells may also express CD36, CD38, CD45[low], CD45RA, CD68, CD123, and HLA-DR. They are negative for CD16, CD57, CD116, and CD117 *(205)*. The disease is rapidly fatal without chemotherapy. However, as indicated in a recent multicentric study *(205)*, complete remission was observed in 78% of patients after polychemotherapy, although most patients relapsed in less than 2 yr.

2.4.4. Minimal Residual Disease

Although current data support multiparametric immunophenotyping as a valuable tool in the evaluation of minimal residual disease (MRD) in acute leukemia patients, its clinical utility in evaluation of MRD in lymphoid malignancies has not been well defined. Several recent large studies have addressed this issue, by exploring phenotypic aberrancies and variables in chronic B-cell lymphoproliferative disorders, which has set up a preliminary basis for the design of multiparametric panels used in the MRD investigations *(206–209)*. The largest study series (467 patients) has indicated that the incidence of aberrant phenotypes ranges from 80–100% in B-cell chronic lymphoproliferative disorders, and most of the cases studied (90%) display four or more phenotypic aberrancies *(206)*. Using the dilutional method, this study demonstrated a sensitivity limit of 10^{-4} to 10^{-5} in MRD monitoring.

2.5. DNA Ploidy Analysis and Simultaneous S-Phase Assessment

2.5.1. Traditional Approach

Analysis of DNA content in malignant tissues is among the earliest clinical applications of flow cytometry. It contains DNA ploidy categorization and calculation of S-phase fraction (SPF) according to the standardized or generally accepted terminology. The practical utility of DNA content analysis relies on its prognostic relevance, which has been the subject of many large trial studies, as well as reviews in the past decade, and has been best addressed in breast, bladder, prostate, colorectal, and hematopoietic malignancies *(191,210–214)*.

The results from these large trial studies are inconsistent regarding the correlations between prognosis and DNA ploidy or SFP, which are reflections of suboptimal study design and more importantly, significant interlaboratory variability as demonstrated in a recent CAP proficiency survey *(215)*. The technical variable factors are demonstrated in specimen preparation, gating, plus software choices as well as debris and aggregation modeling.

2.5.2. Recent Developments

2.5.2.1. USE OF FLUOROCHROME-CONJUGATED TUMOR-SPECIFIC ANTIGENS

Recently, multiparametric analysis and software compensation have introduced combined use of multiple fluorochrome-conjugated tumor specific antigens (i.e., FITC-conjugated CK5, 6, 8, 17, and 18) with assessment of DNA ploidy that enables not only clear separation of tumor vs background cells, but also detection of intratumor heterogeneity *(216–219)*.

2.5.2.2. SIMULTANEOUS SPECIFIC ANTIGENS AND SPF ASSESSMENT IN LIVING CELLS: DRAQ5

The development of a novel DNA dye DRAQ5 has enabled rapid simultaneous detection of specific surface or nuclear antigens and SPF in both living and fixed cells *(220–222)*. DRAQ5 demonstrates a high affinity for DNA and a high capacity to rapidly enter living cells or stain fixed cells. It shows special characteristics of excitation, which include optimal excitation by red-light at 647 nm as well as suboptimal excitation at 488 nm, 568 nm, and 633 nm lines, and then yields a deep red emission spectrum with extension into the low infra-red region. Because of these spectral features, DRAQ5 can be used in combination with FITC- and PE-labeled markers without the need for compensation. This offers a clear advantage over the traditional DNA dye such as propidium iodide, beause DRAQ5 can greatly reduce emission overlap with ultraviolet (UV)-excitable and visible range fluorochromes if the optimal excitation 647 nm is used.

A recent investigation has identified a significant correlation between Ki67 staining and the SFP using simultaneous quantification of Ki67 MAb and DNA content analysis to evaluate the proliferative activity of breast cancer *(223)*. The unique characteristics of DRAQ5 in both living and fixed cells permit the incorporation of cellular DNA content analysis into a variety of multiparametric analyses including simultaneous evaluation of the SPF and cycle-specific proteins, proliferation markers, as well as various surface and nuclear antigens.

3. APPLICATIONS OF FLOW CYTOMETRY IN MONITORING CANCER BIOTHERAPY

Conventional cytotoxic therapy of malignant neoplasm is often associated with significant morbidity, mainly attributed by the lack of specificity to malignant cells and hence traumatic insult on the normal counterparts. In the past decade, enormous efforts have been undertaken to develop methods or strategies for more specific and targeted therapies of malignant diseases by not only using MAbs *(224,225)* directed against tumor cells, but also stimulating immunological rejection of tumors through antigen-specific immune responses *(226,227)*. Strategies of the latter including tumor vaccines, gene-modified tumors, tumor antigen-encoding viral vectors, protein and peptide antigen, as well as dendritic cell-loaded antigen, are currently being investigated in clinical trials. Multiparametric analysis by flow cytometry is of special value in monitoring both phenotypic and functional characteristics of the antigen-specific immune responses, as suggested in recent reviews and results of a workshop sponsored by the Society for Biological Therapy *(226–228)*.

3.1. Monoclonal Antibody Therapy of Hematological Malignancies

Because of the understanding of lineage-specific antigens in hematological malignancies and the relative accessibility of the malignant cells in blood and bone marrow, leukemias or lymphomas have provided successful testing grounds for the use of MAb therapy *(224)*. Recent technological advancements, especially the development of human or chimeric monoclonal antibodies, have significantly overcome the toxicities associated with host immune responses to rodent-derived MAbs. The first humanized MAb for the treatment of hematological malignancies, rituximab (anti-CD20 MAb) was approved about 6 yr ago, and has revolutionized the treatment of NHL *(229,230)*. Currently, a range of MAbs is available in clinical studies and therapies, including anti-CD22, anti-CD33, anti-CD45, anti-CD52, and anti-tyrosine kinase STI571. Furthermore, protein engineering to combine MAbs with other biological active molecules such as radioisotopes, toxins, chemotherapy, and cytokines, has enabled a new spectrum of agents for clinical activity *(224)*. As the antigen expression intensity in hematological malignancies becomes important for decision-making in relation to the MAb therapy, information obtained using flow cytometric analysis such as the number of antigen receptor sites per molecule is of special clinical utility *(231)*. Flow cytometric analysis functions as a critical tool in the monitoring of MAb therapy by providing qualitative as well as quantitative measures of targeted markers.

3.2. Measurement of In Vitro Antigen-Specific Immune Responses

3.2.1. Peptide Major Histocompatibility Complex Tetramers

By applying this emerging technology to multiparametric analysis, one can detect antigen-specific T cells that bind specifically, stably, and avidly, to soluble fluorochrome-labeled multimeric major histocompatability complex (MHC) peptide complexes, by gating on $CD8^+$ T-cells and looking for expression of antigen-specific TCRs (224,232). Several recent studies have demonstrated the utility of flow cytometric analysis using peptide MHC tetramers to quantify $CD8^+$ T cells that are specific for tumor antigens or control antigens used in immunotherapy protocols (233–235). Although the clinical relevance of tetramer-based analyses needs to be established by more large prospective trials, there is clear promise for the application of tetramers as a "front-line" clinical immune monitoring system (228).

3.2.2. Intracellar Cytokines

Evaluation of the T-cell immune status has evolved from enumeration of $CD4^+$ and $CD8^+$ T cells to identification of functional T-cell subsets, because the latter has become increasingly critical in the monitoring of immunotherapy. Previous studies using murine models (236) have set up the basis for accessing functional immune responses in humans by characterizing the cytokine secretion pattern of T cells in peripheral blood, lymph nodes, or other tissues. The understanding of the cytokine secretion pattern of a given T-cell subset, requires simultaneous collection of multidimensional data including soluble cytokines, cytokine-producing cells, surface receptors, and other functional parameters. Multiparametric analysis by flow cytometry provides a perfect setting for this type of multidimensional studies (237,238).

Recent studies with serial analysis of intracellular cytokine induction have demonstrated its correlation with clinical outcome. For example, Maraveyas et al. (239) suggested a possible association of the induction of intracellular IL-2 with improved survival in a study of stage IV malignant melanoma. In an anti-idiotype vaccine study in ovarian cancer patients by Reinartz et al. (240), the generation of antigen-specific antibodies and prolonged survival were found to correlate with an altered cytokine profile from secretion of IL-2 and IFN-α to T helper 2 type cytokines.

4. THE FUTURE

There is an emerging trend of combining flow cytometry with other techniques. The combination of flow cytometry and molecular biological techniques is particularly powerful, and can be considered two complementary cornerstones of the 21st-century diagnostic pathology. It offers the opportunity to study heterogeneous populations of cells with varying immunophenotypic and at the same time, genotypic features (241). This approach can be applied in a wide spectrum of analyses, including but not limited to gene products, TCR gene rearrangements, steroid hormone receptors, oncogene products, multidrug resistance gene products, minimal residual disease, gene therapy, cellular based FISH, and flow karyotyping.

As an example, the detection of TCR gene rearrangement by flow cytometry using MAbs directed against the TCR Vβ chain families is now possible in clinical practice, with a fast and easy approach owing to the availability of a commercial testing kit (Figs. 7 and 8). These reagents are useful indicators for the detection of possible clonal expansion of T cells in T-cell neoplasms, where no other markers of clonal expansion are currently available. Recent studies have established reference ranges for TCR Vβ repertoire in healthy controls (242), as

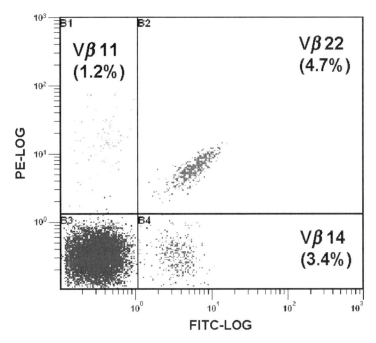

Fig. 7. Triple staining of TCR Vβ in whole blood with Vβ MAbs conjugated using only two fluorochromes (with permission and Courtesy of Beckman Coulter, INC.). In any given vial of the IO Test Beta Mark Kit (by Beckman Coulter, INC), there are three precalibrated and mixed Vβ MAbs, each of which is labeled using either FITC, or PE, or FITC + PE. As shown here, the mAb mixture in this vial includes Vβ14-FITC, Vβ11-PE, and Vβ22-FITC+PE. Simultaneous detection of the TCR Vβ and T-cell subset antigens can be achieved using multiparametric analysis.

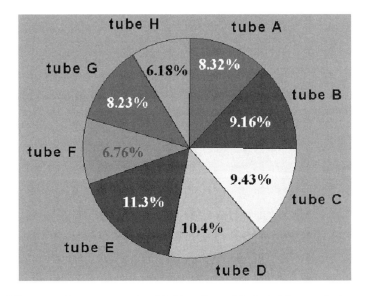

Fig. 8. TCR Vβ repertoire coverage by IO Test Beta Mark (with permission and Courtesy of Beckman Coulter, INC.). This diagram shows the mean percentage of the Vβ domains covered by the Vβ MAb mixture in each vial of the IO Test Beta Mark kit. About 70% of the T-cell repertoire is addressed using a total of 24 Vβ MAbs included in this kit.

well as validated the use of the Vβ antibody panel covering up to 70% of the Vβ domains in T-ALL samples and T-cell lines *(243)*.

Technological advances in the field of flow cytometry continue to provide opportunities for expansion of clinical applications in cancer diagnosis and therapy using multiparametric analysis. The commercial availability of high speed *(244)* and three laser machines, plus advanced reagents and software compensation programs, has marked an era of multi-multi-color immunophenotyping *(245)*, likely introduced in practice of routine clinical flow cytometry in the not too distant future. This future of "high-throughput flow cytometry" can be a successful practice, only if the emphasis on clinico-pathologic correlation continues to dominate the center stage of clinical flow cytometry.

REFERENCES

1. Orfao A, Schmitz G, Brando B, et al. 1999. Clinically useful information provided by the flow cytometric immunophenotyping of hematological malignancies: current status and future directions. Clin. Chem. 45:1708–1717.
2. Jennings CD and Foon KA. 1997. Recent advances in flow cytometry: application to the diagnosis of hematologic malignancy. Blood 90:2863–2892.
3. Orfao A, Ruiz-Arguelles A, Lacombe L, Ault K, Basso G, Danova M. 1995. Flow cytometry: its applications in hematology. Haematologica 80:69–81.
4. Basso G, Buldini B, De Zen L, Orfao A. 2001. New methodologic approaches for Immunophenotyping acute leukemias. Haematologica 86:675–698.
5. Bennett JM, Catovsky D, Daniel MT, et al. 1985. Proposed revised criteria for the classification of acute myeloid leukemia. A report of the French-American-British Cooperative Group. Ann. Intern. Med. 103:620–625.
6. Harris NL, Jaffe ES, Stein H, et al. 1994. A revised European-American Classification of lymphoid neoplasms: a proposal from the International Lymphoma Study Group. Blood 84:1361–1392.
7. Harris NL, Jaffe ES, Diebold J, et al. 1999. World Health Organization classification of neoplastic diseases of the hematopoietic and lymphoid tissues: report of the Clinical Advisory Committee meeting. J. Clin. Oncol. 17:3835–3849.
8. Harris NL, Jaffe ES, Diebold J, Flandrin G, Muller-Hermelink HK, Vardiman J. 2000. Lymphoma Classification—from controversy to consensus: the REAL and WHO Classification of lymphoid neoplasm. Ann. Oncol. 11(Suppl 1):503–510.
9. Jaffe ES, Sander CA, Flaig MJ. 2000. Cutaneous lymphomas: a proposal for a unified approach to classification using the REAL/WHO Classification. Ann. Oncol. 11(Suppl 1):517–521.
10. Isaacson PG. 2000. Review: the current status of lymphoma classification. Br. J. Haematol. 109:258–266.
11. McKenna RW. 2000. Multifaceted approach to the diagnosis and classification of acute leukemias. Clin. Chem. 46:1252–1259.
12. Krause JR. 2000. Morphology and classification of acute myeloid leukemias. Clin. Lab. Med. 20:1–16.
13. Bene MC, Castoldi G, Knapp W, et al. 1995. Proposals for the immunological classification of acute leukemias. European Group for the Immunological Characterization of Leukaemias. Leukemia 9:1783–1786.
14. Vardiman JW, Harris NL, Brunning RD. 2002. The World Health Organization (WHO) classification of the myeloid neoplasms. Blood 100:2292–2302.
15. Rothe G and Schmitz G. 1996. Consensus protocol for the flow cytometric Immunophenotyping of hematopoietic malignancies. Working Group on Flow Cytometry and Image Analysis. Leukemia 10:877–895.

16. Lanza F. 1996. Towards standardization in Immunophenotyping hematological malignancies. How can we improve the reproducibility and comparability of flow cytometric results? Working group for Leukemia Immunophenotyping. Eur. J. Histochem. 40(Suppl 1):7–14.

17. Davis BH, Foucar K, Szozarkowski W, et al. 1997. U.S.-Canadian consensus recommendations on the immunophenotypic analysis of hematologic neoplasia by flow cytometry: medical indications. Cytometry 30:249–263.

18. Braylan RC, Borowitz MJ, Davis BH, Stelzer GT, Stewart CC. 1997. U.S.-Canadian consensus recommendations on the immunophenotypic analysis of hematologic neoplasia by flow cytometry. Cytometry 30:213.

19. Ruiz Arguelles A, Duque RE, Orfao A. 1998. Report on the first Latin American consensus conference for flow cytometric Immunophenotyping of leukemia. Cytometry 34:39–42.

20. General Haematology Task Force of the British Committee for Standardization in Hematology. 1994 Immunophenotyping in the diagnosis of acute leukaemias. J. Clin. Pathol. 47:777–781.

21. General Haematology Task Force of the British Committee for Standardization in Hematology. 1994. Immunophenotyping in the diagnosis of chronic lymphoproliferative disorders. J. Clin. Pathol. 47:871–875.

22. Stelzer GT, Shults KE, Loken MR. 1993. CD45 gating for routine flow cytometric analysis of human bone marrow specimens. Ann. NY Acad. Sci. 677:265–280.

23. Borowitz MJ, Guenther KL, Shults KE, Stelzer GT. 1993. Immunophenotyping of acute leukemia by flow cytometric analysis. Use of CD45 and right-angle light scatter to gate on leukemic blasts in three-color analysis. Am. J. Clin. Pathol. 100:534.

24. Bagwell CB and Adams EG. 1993. Fluorescence spectral overlap compensation for any number of flow cytometry parameters. Ann. NY Acad. Sci. 677:167–184.

25. Henderson LO, Marti GE, Gaigalas A, et al. 1998. Terminology and nomenclature for standardization in quantitative fluorescence cytometry. Cytometry 33:97–105.

26. Schwartz A, Marti GE, Poon R, et al. 1998. Standardizing flow cytometry: a classification system of fluorescence standards used for flow cytometry. Cytometry 33:106–114.

27. Van Dilla MA, Dean PN, Laerum OD, et al. 1985. Flow Cytometry: Instrumentation and Data Analysis: Academic Press, Orlando, FL.

28. Shapiro HM. 1994. Practical Flow Cytometry, 3rd Ed. New York: Wiley-Liss, Inc.

29. Keren DF, McCoy JP Jr, Carey JL. 2001 Flow Cytometry in Clinical Diagnosis, 3rd ed. ASCP Press: Chicago.

30. Corver WE, Fleuren GJ, Cornelisse CJ. 2002. Software compensation improves the analysis of heterogeneous tumor samples stained for multiparameter DNA flow cytometry. J. Immunol. Methods 260:97–107.

31. Zhang YZ, Kemper C, Bakke A, Haugland RP. 1998. Novel flow cytometry compensation standards: internally stained fluorescent microspheres with matched emission spectra and long-term stability. Cytometry 33:244–248.

32. Stewart CC and Stewart SJ. 1999. Four color compensation. Cytometry 38:161–175.

33. Roederer M. 2001. Spectral compensation for flow cytometry: visualization artifacts, limitations, and caveats. Cytometry 45:194–205.

34. Roederer M. 2001. Compensation is not dependent on signal intensity or on number of parameters. Cytometry 46:357–359.

35. Gratama JW, Bolhuis RLH, van't Veer MB. 1999. Review: quality control of flow cytometric Immunophenotyping of haematological malignancies. Clin. Lab. Haem. 21:155–160.

36. Barnett D, Granger V, Reilly JT. 1994. The United Kingdom external quality assurance schemes (UK NEQAS) for leukaemia phenotyping. Br. J. Haematol. 86:83.

37. Reilly JT and Barnett D. 2001. UK NEQAS for leukocyte Immunophenotyping: the first 10 years. J. Clin. Pathol. 54:508–511.

38. Borowitz MJ, Bray R, Gascoyne R, et al. 1997. US-Canadian consensus recommendations on the immunophenotypic analysis of hematologic neoplasia by flow cytometry: data analysis and interpretation. Cytometry 30: 236–244.

39. Stelzer GT, Marti G, Hurley A, McCoy P Jr, Lovett EJ, Schwartz A. 1997. US-Canadian consensus recommendations on the immunophenotypic analysis of hematologic neoplasia by flow cytometry: standardization and validation of laboratory procedures. Cytometry 30:214–230.

40. Stewart CC, Behm FG, Carey JL, et al. 1997. US-Canadian consensus recommendations on the immunophenotypic analysis of hematologic neoplasia by flow cytometry: selection of antibody combinations. Cytometry 30:231–235.

41. Homburger HA, Rosenstock W, Paxton H, Paton ML, Landay AL. 1993. Assessment of interlaboratory variability of immunophenotyping: results of the College of American Pathologists Flow cytometry survey. Ann. NY Acad. Sci. 677:43–49.

42. Kluin-Nelemans JC, van Wering ER, van't Veer MB, et al. 1996. Pitfalls in the immunophenotyping of leukaemia and leukaemic lymphomas: survey of 9 years of quality control in The Netherlands. Br. J. Haematol. 95:692–699.

43. van't Veer MB, Kluin-Nelemans JC, van der Schoot CE, et al. 1992. Quality assessment of immunological marker analysis and the immunological diagnosis in leukaemia and lymphoma: multi-centre study. Br. J. Haematol. 80:458–465.

44. Jaffe ES, Harris NL, Stein H, Vardiman JW, eds. 2001. World Health Organization Classification of Tumors: Tumors of Haematopoietic and Lymphoid Tissues. IARC Press: Lyon, France.

45. Vardiman JW, Harris NL, Brunning RD. 2002. The World Heath Organization (WHO) classification of the myeloid neoplasms. Blood 100:2292–2302.

46. San Miguel JF, Martinex A, Macedo A, et al. 1997. Immunophenotyping investigation of minimal residual disease is a useful approach for predicting relapse in acute myeloid leukemia patients. Blood 90:2465–2470.

47. Ciudad J, San Miguel JF, Lopez-Berges MC, et al. 1998. Prognostic value of immunophenotypic detection of minimal residual disease in acute lymphoblastic leukemia. J. Clin. Oncol. 16:3774–3781.

48. San Miguel JF, Gonzalez M, Orfao A. 1998. Minimal residual disease in acute myeloid malignancies, in Textbook of malignant hematology, Degos L, Herman F, Linch D, Lowenberg B, eds, Martin Dunitz: London, pp. 871–891.

49. Ciudad J, San Miguel JF, Lopez-Berges MC, et al. 1999. Detection of abnormalities in B-cell differentiation pattern is a useful tool to predict relapse in precursor B-ALL. Br. J. Haematol. 104:695–705.

50. Lucio P, Parreira A, van dem Beemd MWM, van Lochem EG, et al. 1999. Flow cytometric analysis of normal B-cell differentiation: a frame of reference for the detection of minimal residual disease in precursor B-ALL. Leukemia 13:419–427.

51. Weir EG and Borowitz MJ. 2001. Flow cytometry in the diagnosis of acute leukemia. Semin. Hematol. 38:124–138.

52. Hrusak O and Porwit-MacDonald A. 2002. Antigen expression patterns reflecting genotype of acute leukemias. Leukemia 16:1233–1258.

53. Viswanatha DS, Foucar K, Berry B, et al. 2000. Blastic mantle cell leukemia: an unusual variant of blastic mantle cell lymphoma. Mod. Pathol. 13:825–833.

54. Pui C, Rubnitz J, Hancock M, et al. 1998. Reappraisal of the clinical and biologic significance of myeloid-associated antigen expression in childhood acute lymphoblastic leukemia. J. Clin. Oncol. 16:3768–3773.

55. Hann IM, Richards SM, Eden OB, et al. 1998. Analysis of the immunophenotype of children treated on the Medical Research Council United Kingdom ALL Trial X1 (MRCUK ALL X1). Leukemia 12:1249–1255.

56. Czuczman M, Dodge R, Stewart C, et al. 1999. Value of immunophenotype in intensively treated adult acute lymphoblastic leukemia: Cancer and Leukemia Group B Study 8364. Blood 93:3931–3939

57. Khalidi H, Chang K, Medeiros J, et al. 1999. Acute lymphoblastic leukemia survey of immunophenotype, French-American-British classification, frequency of myeloid antigen

expression, and karyotypic abnormalities in 210 pediatric and adult cases. Am. J. Clin. Pathol. 111:467–476.

58. Uckun FM, Sather HN, Gaynon PS, et al. 1997. Clinical features and treatment outcome of children with myeloid antigen positive acute lymphoblastic leukemia: a report from the Children's Cancer Group. Blood 90:28–35.

59. Putti MC, Rondelli R, Cocito MG, et al. 1998. Expression of myeloid markers lacks prognostic impact in children treated for acute lymphoblastic leukemia: Italian experience in AIEOP-ALL 88–91 studies. Blood 92:795–801.

60. Lauria F, Raspadori D, Martinelli G, et al. 1994. Increased expression of myeloid antigen markers in adult acute lymphoblastic leukaemia patients: diagnostic and prognostic implications. Br. J. Haematol. 87:286–292.

61. Borowitz MJ, Rubnitz J, Nash M, Pullen DJ, Camitta B. 1994. Surface antigen phenotype can predict TEL-AML1 rearrangement in childhood B-precursor ALL: a Pediatric Oncology Group study. Leukemia 12:1764–1770.

62. Trka J, Zuna J, Haskovec C, et al. 1999. Detection of BCR/ABL, MLL/AF4 and TEL/AML1 hybrid genes and monitoring of minimal residual disease in pediatric patient with acute lymphoblastic leukemia. Cas. Lek. Cesk. 138:12–17.

63. Maloney K, Mc Gavran L, Murphy J, et al. 1999. TEL-AML1 fusion identifies a subset of children with standard risk acute lymphoblastic leukemia who have an excellent prognosis when treated with therapy that includes a single delayed intensification. Leukemia 13:1708–1712.

64. Raynaud SD, Dastugue N, Zoccola D, et al. 1999. Cytogenetic abnormalities associated with t(12;21): a collaborative study of 169 children with t(12;21)-positive acute lymphoblastic leukemia. Leukemia 13:1325–1330.

65. De Zen L, Orfao A, Cazzanigo G, et al. 2000. Quantitative multiparametric immunophenotyping in acute lymphoblastic leukemia: correlation with specific genotype. 1. ETV6/AML1 ALLs identification. Leukemia 14:1225–1231.

66. Tabernero MD, Bortoluci AM, Alaejos I, et al. 2001. Adult precursor B-ALL with BCR/ABL gene rearrangement displays a unique immunophenotype based on the pattern of CD10, CD34, CD13, and CD38 expression. Leukemia 15:406–414.

67. Behm FG, Smith FO, Raimondi SC, Pui CH, Bernstein ID. 1996. Human homologue of the rat chondroitin sulfate proteoglycan, NG2, detected by monoclonal antibody 7.1, identifies childhood acute lymphoblastic leukemias with t(4;11) (q21;q23) or t(11;19) (q23;p13) and MLL gene rearrangements. Blood 87:1134–1139.

68. Smith FO, Rauch C, Williams DE, et al. 1996. The human homologue of rat NG2, a chondroitin sulfate proteoglycan, is not expressed on the cell surface of normal hematopoietic cells but is expressed by acute myeloid leukemia blasts from poor-prognosis patients with abnormalities of chromosome band 11q23. Blood 87:1123–1133.

69. Pui CH, Behm FG, Downing JR, et al. 1994 11q23/MLL rearrangement confers a poor prognosis in infants with acute lymphoblastic leukemia. J. Clin. Oncol. 12:909–915.

70. Forestier E, Johansson B, Gustafsson G, et al. 2000. Prognostic impact of karyotypic findings in childhood acute lymphoblastic leukaemia: a Nordic series comparing two treatment periods. For the Noric Society of Paediatric Haematology and Oncology (NOPHO) Leukaemia Cytogenetic Study Group. Br. J. Haematol. 110:147–153.

71. Madzo J, Zuna J, Muzikova K, et al. 2003. Slower molecular response to treatment predicts poor outcome in patients with TEL/AML1 positive acute lymphoblastic leukemia. Cancer 97:105–113.

72. Naeim F. 2001. Acute lymphoblastic leukemia. In: Naeim's Atlas of Bone Marrow and Blood Pathology, 1st ed. Philadelphia: W.B. Saunders, pp. 82–91.

73. Kita K, Miwa H, Nakase K, et al. 1993. Clinical importance of CD7 expression in acute myelocytic leukemia. The Japan Cooperative Group of Leukemia/Lymphoma. Blood 81:2399–2405.

74. Ferrando AA and Look AT. 2000. Clinical implications of recurring chromosomal and associated molecular abnormalities in acute lymphoblastic leukemia. Semin. Hematol. 37:381–395.

75. Uckun FM, Sensel MG, Sun L, et al. 1998. Biology and treatment of childhood T-lineage acute lymphoblastic leukemia. Blood 91:735–746.
76. Pullen J, Shuster JJ, Link M, et al. 1999. Significance of commonly used prognostic factors differs from children with T cell acute lymphocytic leukemia (ALL), as compared to those with B-precursor ALL. A Pediatric Oncology Group (POG) study. Leukemia 13:1696–1707.
77. Schneider NR, Carroll AJ, Shuster JJ, et al. 2000 New recurring cytogenetic abnormalities and association of blast cell karyotypes with prognosis in childhood T-cell acute lymphoblastic leukemia: a pediatric oncology group report of 343 cases. Blood 96:2543–2549.
78. Niehues T, Kapaun P, Harms DO, et al. 1999. A classification based on T cell selection-related phenotypes identifies a subgroup of childhood T-ALL with favorable outcome in the COALL studies. Leukemia 13:614–617.
79. Bernard OA, Busson-LeConiat M, Ballerini P, et al. 2001. A new recurrent and specific cryptic translocation, t(5;14)(q35;q32), is associated with expression of the Hox11L2 gene in T-acute lymphoblastic leukemia. Leukemia 15:1495–1504.
80. Reading CL, Estey EH, Huh YO, et al. 1993. Expression of unusual immunophenotype combinations in acute myelogenous leukemia. Blood 81:3083–3090.
81. Bene M, Bernier M, Casasnovas R, et al. 1998. The reliability and specificity of c-kit for the diagnosis of acute myeloid leukemias and undifferentiated leukemias. Blood 92:596–599.
82. Cascavilla N, Musto P, D'Arena G, et al. 1998. CD117 (c-kit) is a restricted antigen of acute myeloid leukemia and characterizes early differentiative levels of M5 FAB Subtype. Haematologica 83:392–397.
83. Nomdedeu J, Mateu R, Altes A, et al. 1999. Enhanced myeloid specificity of CD117 compared with CD13 and CD33. Leuk. Res. 23:341–347.
84. Macedo A, Orfao A, Gonzalez M, et al. 1995. Immunological detection of blast cell subpopulations in acute myeloblastic leukemia at diagnosis: implications for minimal residual disease studies. Leukemia 9:993–998.
85. San Miguel JF, Ciudad J, Vidriales MB, et al. 1999. Immunophenotypical detection of minimal residual disease in acute leukemia. Crit. Rev. Oncol. Hematol. 32:175–185.
86. Nisson PE, Watkins PC, Sacchi N. 1992. Transcriptionally active chimeric gene derived from the fusion of the AML1 gene and a novel gene on chromosome 8 in t(8;21) leukemic cells. Cancer Genet. Cytogenet. 63:81–88.
87. Baer MR, Stewart CC, Lawrence D, et al. 1997. Expression of the neural cell adhesion molecule CD56 is associated with short remission duration and survival in acute myeloid leukemia with t(8,21)(q22;q22). Blood 90:1643–1648.
88. Sainty D, Liso V, Cantu-Rajnoldi A, et al. 2000. A new morphologic classification system for acute promyelocytic leukemia distinguishes cases with underlying PLZF/RARa gene rearrangements. Group Francais de Cytogenetique Hematologique, UK Cancer Cytogenetics Group and BIOMED 1 European Community-Concerted Action "Molecular Cytogenetic Diagnosis in Haematological Malignancies." Blood 96:1287–1296.
89. Grimwade D, Biondi A, Mozziconacci MJ, et al. 2000 Characterization of acute promyelocytic leukemia cases lacking the classic t(15:17): results of the European Working Party. Groupe Francais de Cytogenetique Hematologique, Groupe de Fancais d'Hematologie Cellulaire, UK Cancer Cytogenetics Group and BIOMED 1 European Community-Concerted Action "Molecular Cytogenetic Diagnosis in Haematological Malignancies." Blood 96:1297–1308.
90. Paietta E, Andersen J, Racevskis J, et al. 1994. Significantly lower P-glycoprotein expression in acute promyelocytic leukemia than in to the types of acute myeloid leukemia: immunological, molecular and functional analyses. Leukemia 8:968–973.
91. Piedras J, Lopez-Karpovitch X, Cardenas R. 1998. Light scatter and immunophenotypic characteristics of blast cells in typical acute promyelocytic leukemia and its variant. Cytometry 32:286–290.
92. Erber WN, Asbahr H, Rule SA, Scott CS. 1994. Unique immunophenotype of acute promyelocytic leukaemia as defined by and CD68 antibodies. Br. J. Haematol. 88:101–104.

93. Orfao A, Chillon MC, Bortoluci AM, et al. 1999. The flow cytometric pattern of CD34, CD15, and CD13 expression in acute myeloblastic leukemia is highly characteristic of the presence of PML-RARalpha gene rearrangements. Haematologica 84:405–412.

94. Biondi A, Luciano A, Bassan R, et al. 1995. CD2 expression in acute promyelocytic leukemia is associated with microgranular morphology (FAB M3v) but not with any PML gene breakpoint. Leukemia 9:1461–1466.

95. Guglielmi C, Martelli MP, Diverio D, et al. 1998. Immunophenotype of adult and childhood acute promyelocytic leukaemia: correlation with morphology, type of PML gene breakpoint and clinical outcome. A cooperative Italian study on 196 cases. Br. J. Haematol. 102:1035–1041.

96. Di Bona E, Sartori R, Zambello R, et al. 2002. Prognostic significance of CD56 antigen expression in acute myeloid leukemia. Haematologica 87:250–256.

97. Casasnovas RO, Campos L, Mugneret F, et al. 1998. Immunophenotypic patterns and cytogenetic anomalies in acute non-lymphoblastic leukemia subtypes: a prospective study of 432 patients. Leukemia 12:34–43.

98. Schwartz S, Heinecke A, Zimmermann M, et al. 1999. Expression of the C-kit receptor (CD117) is a feature of almost all subtypes of de novo acute myeloblastic leukemia (AML), including cytogenetically good-risk AML, and lacks prognostic significance. Leuk. Lymphoma 34:85–94.

99. Adriaansen HJ, te Boekhorst PA, Hagemeijer AM, et al. 1993. Acute myeloid leukemia M4 with bone marrow eosinophilia (M4Eo) and inv(16) (p13q22)exhibits a specific immunophenotype with CD2 expression. Blood 81:3043–3051.

100. Paietta E, Wiernik PH, Andersen J, Bennett J, Yunis J. 1993. Acute myeloid leukemia M4 with inv(16) (p13q22) exhibits a specific immunophenotype with CD2 expression. Blood 82:2595.

101. Kornblau SM, Thall P, Huh YO, Estey E, Andreeff M. 1995. Analysis of CD7 expression in acute myelogenous leukemia: martingale residual plots combined with 'optimal' cutpoint analysis reveals absence of prognostic significance. Leukemia 9:1735–1741.

102. Sorensen PH, Chen CS, Smith FO, et al. 1994. Molecular rearrangements of the MLL gene are present in most cases of infant acute myeloid leukemia and are strongly correlated with normocytic or myelomonocytic phenotypes. J. Clin. Invest. 93:429–437.

103. Mann KP, DeCastro CM, Liu J, et al. 1997. Neural cell adhesion molecule (CD56)-positive acute myelogenous leukemia and myelodysplastic and myeloproliferative syndromes. Am. J. Clin. Pathol. 107:653–660.

104. Baer MR, Stewart CC, Lawrence D, et al. 1998. Acute myeloid leukemia with 11q23 translocations: myelomonocytic immunophenotype by multiparameter flow cytometry. Leukemia 12:317–325.

105. Kostler WJ, Brodowicz T, Hejna M, Wiltschke C, Zielinski CC. 2000. Detection of minimal residual disease in patients with cancer: a review of techniques, clinical implications, and emerging therapeutic consequences. Cancer Detect. Prev. 24:376–403.

106. San Miguel JF, Vidriales MB, Orfao A. 2002. Immunological evaluation of minimal residual disease (MRD) in acute myeloid leukaemia (AML). Best Pract. Res. Clin. Haematol. 15: 105–118.

107. Sievers EL and Radich JP. 2000. Detection of minimal residual disease in acute leukemia. Curr. Opin. Hematol. 7:212–216.

108. Cavé H, Van der Werff J, Bosch T, et al. 1998. Clinical significance of minimal residual disease in childhood acute lymphoblastic leukemia. N. Engl. J. Med. 339:591–598.

109. Coustan-Smith E, Behm FG, Sanchez J, et al. 1998. Immunological detection of minimal residual disease in children with acute lymphoblastic leukaemia. Lancet 351:550–554.

110. van Dongen JJ, Seriu T, Panzer-Grumayer ER, et al. 1998. Prognostic value of minimal residual disease in acute lymphoblastic leukemia in childhood: a prospective study of the international BFM study group. Lancet 352:1731–1738.

111. Campana D and Pui CH. 1995. Detection of minimal residual disease in acute myeloid leukemia: methodologic advances and clinical significance. Blood 85:1416–1434.

112. Campana D and Coustan-Smith. 1999. Detection of minimal residual disease in acute leukemia by flow cytometry. Cytometry 38:139–152.

113. Ciudad J, Orfao A, Vidriales B, et al. 1998. Immunophenotypic analysis of CD19+ precursors in normal human adult bone marrow: implications for minimal residual disease detection. Haematologica 83:1069–1075.

114. San Miguel JF, Vidriales MB, Lopez-Berges C, et al. 2001. Early immunophenotypical evaluation of minimal residual disease in acute myeloid leukemia identified different patient risk groups and may contribute to postinduction treatment stratification. Blood 98:1746–1751.

115. Baer MR. 2002. Detection of minimal residual disease in acute myeloid leukemia. Curr. Oncol. Rep. 4:398–402.

116. Sainati L, Spinelli M, Leszl A, et al. 1997. Combined cell sorting and FISH for detection of minimal residual disease in bone marrow of children with acute leukemia or solid tumors. Eur. J. Histochem. 41:167–168.

117. van Dongen JJ, Szczepanski T, de Bruijn MA, et al. 1996. Detection of minimal residual disease in acute leukemia patients. Cytokines Mol. Ther. 2:121–133.

118. Lavabre-Bertrand T, Janossy G, Ivory K, et al. 1994. Leukemia associated changes identified by quantitative flow cytometry. 1. CD10 expression. Cytometry 18:209–217.

119. Chucrallah AE, Stass SA, Huh YO, et al. 1995. Adults acute lymphoblastic leukemia at relapse. Cytogenetic, immunophenotipic, and molecular changes. Cancer 76:985–991.

120. van Wering ER, Beishuizen A, Roeffen ET, et al. 1995. Immunophenotypic changes between diagnosis and relapse in childhood acute lymphoblastic leukemia. Leukemia 9:1523–1533.

121. Guglielmi C, Cordone I, Boecklin F, et al. 1997. Immunophenotype of adult and childhood acute lymphoblastic leukemia: changes at first relapse and clinico-prognostic implications. Leukemia 11:1501–1507.

122. Macedo A, San Miguel JF, Vidriales MB, et al. 1996 Phenotypic changes in acute myeloid leukaemia: implications in the detection of minimal residual disease. J. Clin. Pathol. 49:15–18.

123. Baer MR, Stewart CC, Dodge RK, et al. 2001. High frequency of immunophenotype changes in acute myeloid leukemia at relapse: implications for residual disease detection. Blood 97:3574–3580.

124. Brunning RD, Bennett JM, Flandrin G, et al. 2001. Myelodysplastic syndromes. In Tumors of Haematopoietic and Lymphoid Tissues. Jaffe ES, Harris NL, Stein H, Vardiman JW, eds. IRAC Press, Lyon, France, pp. 61–74.

125. Greenberg P, Cox C, LeBeau MM, et al. 1997. International scoring system for evaluating prognosis in myelodysplastic syndromes. Blood 89:2079–2088.

126. Hensen IM and Hokland P. 1994 The proliferative activity of Myelopoiesis in myelodysplasia evaluated by multiparameter flow cytometry. Br. J. Haematol. 87:477–482.

127. Kanter-Lewensohn L, Hellstrom-Lindberg E, Kock Y, et al. 1996. Analysis of CD34 positive cells in bone marrow from patients with myelodysplastic syndrome and acute myeloid leukemia and in normal individuals: a comparison between FACS analysis and immunohistochemistry. Eur. J. Haematol. 56:124–129.

128. Kuiper-Kramer PA, Huisman CM, Van der Molen-Sinke J, Abbes A, Van Eijk HG. 1997. The expression of transferring receptors on erythroblasts in anemia of chronic disease, myelodysplastic syndromes and iron deficiency. Acta. Haematol. 97:127–131.

129. Bowen KL and Davis BH. 1997. Abnormal patterns of expression of CD16 (FcR-III) and CD11b (CRIII) antigens by developing neutrophils in the bone marrow patients with myelodysplastic syndrome. Lab. Hematol. 3:292–298.

130. Cermak J, Michalova K, Vitek A. 2002. Myelodysplastic syndrome-classification, prognosis and therapy. Cas. Lek. Cesk. 141(suppl):33–37.

131. Elghetany MT. 1998. Surface marker abnormalities in myelodysplastic syndromes. Haematologica 83:1104–1115.

132. Miller DT and Stelzer GT. 2001. Contributions of flow cytometry to the analysis of the myelodysplastic syndrome. Clin. Lab. Med. 21:811–828.

133. Stetler-Stevenson M, Arthur DC, Jabbour N, et al. 2001. Diagnostic utility of flow cytometric immunophenotyping in myelodysplastic syndrome. Blood 98:979–987.

134. Maynadié M, Picard F, Husson B, et al. 2002. Immunophenotypic clustering of myelodysplastic syndromes. Blood 100:2349–2356.

135. Catovsky D, Matutes E, Buccheri V, et al. 1991. A classification of acute leukemia for the 1990s. Ann. Hematol. 62:16–21.

136. Matutes E, Morilla R, Farahat N, et al. 1997. Definition of acute biphenotypic leukemia. Haematologica 82:64–66.

137. Rossi G, Pelizzari AM, Bellotti D, Tonelli M, Barlati S. 2000. Cytogenetic analogy between myelodysplastic syndrome and acute myeloid leukemia of elderly patients. Leukemia 14:636–641.

138. Weber M, Wenzel U, Thiel E, Knauf W. 2000. Chromosomal aberrations characteristic for sAML/sMDS are not detectable by random screening using FISH in peripheral blood-derived grafts used for autologous transplantation. J. Hematother. Stem Cell Res. 9:861–865.

139. Luna-Fineman S, Shannon KM, Lange BJ. 1995. Childhood monosomy 7: epidemiology, biology, and mechanistic implications. Blood 85:1985–1999.

140. Hasle H, Arico M, Basso G, et al. 1999. Myelodysplastic syndrome, juvenile myelomonocytic leukemia, and acute myeloid leukemia associated with complete or partial monosomy 7. European working group on MDS in Childhood (EWOG-MDS). Leukemia 13:376–385.

141. Borowitz MJ, Gockerman JP, Moore JO, et al. 1989. Clinicopathologic and cytogenic features of CD34 (My 10)-positive acute nonlymphocytic leukemia. Am. J. Clin. Pathol. 91:265–270.

142. Geller RB, Zahurak M, Hurwitz CA, et al. 1990. Prognostic importance of immunophenotyping in adults with acute myelocytic leukaemia: the significance of the stem-cell glycoprotein CD34 (My10) (see comments). Br. J. Haematol. 76:340–347.

143. Sperling C, Buchner T, Creutzig U, et al. 1995. Clinical, morphologic, cytogenetic and prognostic implications of CD34 expression in childhood and adult de novo AML. Leuk. Lymphoma 17:417–426.

144. Venditti A, Del Poeta G, Buccisano F, et al. 1998. Prognostic relevance of the expression of TdT and CD7 in 335 cases of acute myeloid leukemia. Leukemia 12:1056–1063.

145. Rowan RM, Bain BJ, England JM, et al. 1994. General Haematology Task Force of BCSH. Immunophenotyping in the diagnosis of chronic lymphoproliferative disorders. J. Clin. Pathol. 47:871–875.

146. Erber WN. 1996. Immunophenotypic analysis of haematological disorders. In Haematology: Proc. Inter. Soc. Haematol. 26th Congress. Singapore pp. 328–324.

147. Tbakhi A, Edinger M, Myles J, Pohlman B, Tubbs RR. 1996. Flow cytometric immunophenotyping of non-Hodgkin's lymphoma and related disorders. Cytometry 25:113–124.

148. Ichinohasama R. 2000. Immunophenotypic analysis in the diagnosis of malignant lymphoma. Nippon Rinsho. 58:591–597.

149. Ward MS. 1999. The use of flow cytometry in the diagnosis and monitoring of malignant hematological disorders. Pathology 31:382–392.

150. Dunphy CH. 2000. Contribution of flow cytometric immunophenotyping to the evaluation of tissues with suspected lymphoma? Cytometry 42:296–306.

151. Stetler-Stevenson M and Braylan RC. 2001. Flow cytometric analysis of lymphomas and lymphoproliferative disorders. Semin. Hematol. 38:111–123.

152. Weisberger J, Wu CD, Lui Z, et al. 2000. Differential diagnosis of malignant lymphomas and related disorders by specific pattern of expression of immunophenotypic markers revealed by multiparameter flow cytometry (review). Int. J. Oncol. 17:1165–1177.

152a. Bagg A and Kallakury BVS. 1999. Molecular pathology of leukemia and lymphoma. Am. J. Clin. Pathol. 112(Suppl 1):S76–S92.

153. Siebert JD, Mulvaney DA, Potter KL, et al. 1999. Relative frequencies and sites of presentation of lymphoid neoplasm in a community hospital according to the Revised European-American Classification. Am. J. Clin. Pathol. 111:379–386.

154. Dighiero G, Travade P, Chevret S, et al. 1991. B-cell chronic lymphocytic leukemia: present status and future directions (review). Blood 78:1901–1914.

155. Robbins BA, Ellison DJ, Spinosa JC, et al. 1993. Diagnostic application of two-color flow cytometry in 161 cases of hairy cell leukemia. Blood 82:1277–1287.

156. Picker L, Weiss LM, Medeiros LJ, et al. 1987. Immunophenotypic criteria for the diagnosis of non-Hodgkin's lymphoma. Am. J. Pathol. 128:181–201.

157. Geisler C, Larsen J, Hansen N, et al. 1991. Prognostic importance of flow cytometric immunophenotyping of 540 consecutive patients with B-cell chronic lymphocytic leukemia. Blood 78:1795–1802.

158. Tefferi A, Bartholmai BJ, Witzig TE, et al. 1996. Heterogeneity and clinical relevance of the intensity of CD20 and immunoglobulin light-chain expression in B-cell chronic lymphocytic leukemia. Am. J. Clin. Pathol. 106:457–461.

159. Huh YO, Pugh WC, Kantarjian HM, et al. 1994. Detection of subgroups of chronic B-cell leukemias by FMC7 monoclonal antibody. Am. J. Clin. Pathol. 101:283–289.

160. Molica S, Levato D, Dattilo A, et al. 1998. Clinico-prognostic relevance of quantitative immunophenotyping in B-cell chronic lymphocytic leukemia with emphasis on the expression of CD20 antigen and surface immunoglobulins. Eur. J. Haematol. 60:47–52.

161. Finn WG, Thangavelu M, Yelavarthi KK, et al. 1996. Karyotype correlates with peripheral blood morphology and immunophenotype in chronic lymphocytic leukemia. Am. J. Clin. Pathol. 105:458–467.

162. Matutes E, Oscier D, Garcia-Marco J, et al. 1996. Trisomy 12 defines a group of CLL with atypical morphology: correlation between cytogenetic, clinical and laboratory features in 544 patients. Br. J. Haematol. 92:382–388.

162a. Guarini A, Gardano G, Mauro FR, et al. 2003. Chronic lymphocytic leukemia patients with highly stable and indolent disease show distinctive phenotypic and genotypic features. Blood 102:1035–1041.

162b. Cerretini R, Chena C, Grere I, et al. 2003. Structural aberrations of chromosomes 17 and 12 in chronic B-cell disorders. Eur. J. Haematol 71:433–438.

162c. Goorha S, Glenn MJ, Drozd-Borysiuk E, et al. 2004. A set of commercially available fluorescent *in-situ* hybridization probes efficiently detects cytogenetic abnormalities in patients with chronic lymphocytic leukemia. Genet. Med. 6:48–53.

163. Damle RN, Wasil T, Fais F, et al. 1999 Ig V gene mutation status and CD38 expression as novel prognostic indicators in chronic lymphocytic leukemia. Blood 94:1840–1847.

164. Hamblin TJ, Davis Z, Gardiner A, et al. 1999. Unmutated *Ig Vh* genes are associated with a more aggressive form of chronic lymphocytic leukemia. Blood 94:1848.

164a. Rosenwald A. 2003. DNA microarrays in lymphoid malignancies. Oncology 17:1743–1748.

164b. Keating MJ, Chiorazzi N, Messmer B, et al. 2003. Biology and treatment of chronic lymphocytic leukemia. Hematology (Am Soc Hematol Educ Program):153–175.

165. Jaffe ES, Campo E, Raffeld M. 1999. Mantle cell lymphoma: biology and diagnosis, in Hematology 1999: The American Society of Hematology Education Program Book, Schecter GP, et al., eds. American Society of Hematology: New Orleans, LA, pp. 319–328.

166. Tworek JA, Singleton TP, Schnitzer B, et al. 1998. Flow cytometric and immunohistochemical analysis of small lymphocytic lymphoma, mantle cell lymphoma and plasmacytoid small lymphocytic lymphoma. Am. J. Clin. Pathol. 110:582–589.

167. Dorfman DM and Pinkus GS. 1994. Distinction between small lymphocytic and mantle cell lymphoma by immunoreactivity for CD23. Mod. Pathol. 7:326–331.

168. Kilo MN and Dorfman DM. 1996. The utility of flow cytometric immunophenotypic analysis in distinction of small lymphocytic lymphoma/chronic lymphocytic leukemia form mantle cell lymphoma. Am. J. Clin. Pathol. 105:451–457.

169. Ginaldi L, De Martinis M, Matutes E, et al. 1998. Levels of expression of CD19 and CD20 in chronic B cell leukaemias. J. Clin. Pathol. 51:364–369.

170. Dunphy CH, Wheaton SE, Perkins SL. 1997. CD23 expression in transformed small lympho-cytic lymphomas/chronic lymphocytic leukemias and blastic transformations of mantle cell lymphoma. Mod. Pathol. 10:818:822.

171. Weisenburger DD and Armitage JO. 1996 Mantle cell lymphoma—an entity comes of age. Blood 87:4483–4494.

172. Diaz D.L, Alkan S, Huang JC, et al. 1998. Usefulness of an immunohistochemical panel in paraffin-embedded tissues for the differentiation of B-cell non-Hodgkin's lymphomas of small lymphocytes. Mod. Pathol. 11:1046–1051.

173. Soslow RA, Zukerberg LR, Harris NL, et al. 1997. BCL-1 (PRAD-1/Cyclin D-1) over-expres-sion distinguishes the blastoid variant of mantle cell lymphoma from B-lineage lymphoblastic lymphoma. Mod. Pathol. 10:810–817.

174. Kurtin PJ, Hobday KS, Ziesmer S, et al. 1999. Demonstration of distinct antigenic profiles and small B-cell lymphomas by paraffin section immunohistochemistry. Am. J. Clin. Pathol. 112:319–329.

175. Jain P, Giustolisi GM, Atkinson S, et al. 2002. Detection of cyclin D1 in B cell lympho-proliferative disorders by flow cytometry. J. Clin. Pathol. 55:940–945.

176. Lai R, Arber DA, Chang KL, et al. 1998. Frequency of bcl-2 expression in non-Hodgkin's lymphoma: a study of 778 cases with comparison of marginal zone lymphoma and monocytoid B-cell hyperplasia. Mod. Pathol. 11:864–869.

177. Lai R, Weiss LM, Chang KL, et al. 1999. Frequency of CD43 expression in non-Hodgkin lymphoma: a survey of 742 cases and further characterization of rare CD43+ follicular lym-phomas. Am. J. Clin. Pathol. 111:488–494.

178. Ferry JA, Yang WI, Zukerberg LR, et al. 1996. CD5+ extranodal marginal zone B-cell (MALT) lymphoma: a low grade neoplasm with a propensity for bone marrow involvement and relapse. Am. J. Clin. Pathol. 105:31–37.

179. Tefferi A, Li CY, Phyliky R. 1988. Immunotyping in chronic lymphocytosis: review of the natural history of the condition in 145 adult patients. Mayo Clin. Proc. 63:801–806.

180. Matutes E, Meeus P, McLennan K, et al. 1997. The significance of minimal residual disease in hairy cell leukemia treated with deoxycoformycin: a long-term follow-up study. Br. J. Haematol. 98:375–383.

181. Matutes E. 1995. Contribution of immunophenotype in the diagnosis and classification of haemopoietic malignancies. J. Clin. Pathol. 48:194–197.

182. Anderson K, Boyd A, Fisher D, et al. 1985. Hairy cell leukemia: a tumor of pre-plasma cells. Blood 65:620–629.

183. Schwarting R, Stein H, Wang CY. 1985. The monoclonal antibodies S-HCL1 (leu-14) and S-HCL3 (Leu M5) allow the diagnosis of hairy cell leukemia. Blood. 65:974:983.

184. Lin CW, O'Brien S, Faber J, et al. 1999. De novo CD5+ Burkitt lymphoma, leukemia. Am J Clin Pathol 112:828–835.

185. Harada H, Kawano MM, Huang N, et al. 1993. Phenotypic difference of normal plasma cells from mature myeloma cells. Blood 81:2658–2663.

186. Rawstron AC, Owen RG, Davies FE, et al. 1997. Circulating plasma cells in multiple myeloma: characterization and correlation with disease stage. Br. J. Haematol. 46:55.

187. Ocqueteau M, Orfao A, Almeida J, et al. 1998. Immunophenotypic characterization of plasma cells from monoclonal gammopathy of undetermined significance patients: implications for the differential diagnosis between MGUS and multiple myeloma. Am. J. Pathol. 152: 1655–1665.

188. Almeida J, Orfao A, Ocqueteau M, et al. 1999. High-sensitive immunophenotyping and DNA ploidy studies for the investigation of minimal residual disease in multiple myeloma. Br. J. Haematol. 107:121–131.

189. Almeida J, Orfao A, Mateo G, et al. 1999. Immunophenotypic and DAN content characteris-tics of plasma cell in multiple myeloma and monoclonal gammopathy of undetermined signifi-cance. Pathol. Biol. 47:119–127.

190. San Miguel JF, Almeida J, Mateo G, et al. 2002. mmunophenotypic evaluation of the plasma cell compartment in multiple myeloma: a tool from comparing the efficacy of different treatment strategies and predicting outcome. Blood 99:1853–1856.

191. Lima M, Teixeira Mdos A, Fonseca S, et al. 2000. Immunophenotypic aberrations, DNA content, and cell cycle analysis of plasma cells in patients with myeloma and monoclonal gammopathies. Blood Cells Mol. Dis. 26:634–645.

192. Zandecki M, Facon T, Bernardi F, et al. 1995. CD19 and immunophenotype of marrow plasma cell in monoclonal gammopathy of undetermined significance. J. Clin. Pathol. 48:548–552.

193. Sebestyen A, Berczi L, Mihalik R, et al. 1999. Syndecan-1 (CD138) expression in human non-Hodgkin lymphoma. Br. J. Haematol. 104:412–419.

194. Gentile TC, Uner AH, Hutchison RE, et al. 1994. CD3+ CD56+ aggressive variant of large granular lymphocyte leukemia. Blood 84:2315–2321.

195. Gentile TC, Hadlock KG, Uner AH, et al. 1998. Large granular lymphocyte leukaemia occurring after renal transplantation. Br. J. Haematol. 101:507–512.

196. Hanson MN, Morrison VA, Peterson BA, et al. 1996. Post-transplant T-cell lymphoproliferative disorders: an aggressive late complication of solid organ transplantation. Blood 88:3626–3533.

197. Weiss L, Wood G, Warnke R. 1985. Immunophenotypic differences between dermatopathic lymphadenopathy and lymph node involvement in mycosis fungoides. Am. J. Pathol. 120:179–185.

198. van der Putte S, Toonstra J, van Wichen D, et al. 1988. Aberrant immunophenotypes in mycosis fungoides. Arch. Dermatol. 124:373–380.

199. Carey J, Maeda K, Douglas M, et al. 1989. Immunophenotypic analysis of the leukemic phase of mycosis fungoides. Lab. Invest. 57:14A.

200. Hanson CA, Kurtin PJ, Hoyer JD, et al. 1998. Aberrant T-cell immunophenotype in viral infections: a limitation in the immunophenotypic diagnosis of T-cell lymphoproliferative disorders. Mod. Pathol. 130A.

201. Brody JP, Allen S, Schulman P, et al. 1995. Acute agranular CD4-positive natural killer cell leukemia. Comprehensive clinicopathologic studies including virologic and in vitro culture with inducing agents. Cancer 75:2474–2483.

202. DiGiuseppe JA, Louise DC, Williams JE, et al. 1997. Blastic natural killer cell leukemia/lymphoma: a clinicopathologic study. Am. J. Surg. Pathol. 21:1223–1230.

203. Uchiyama N, Ito K, Kawai K, et al. 1998. CD2−, CD4+, CD56+ agranular natural killer cell lymphoma of the skin. Am. J. Dermatopathol. 20:513–517.

204. Chaperot L, Bendriss N, Manches O, et al. 2001. Identification of a leukemic counterpart of the plasmacytoid dendritic cells. Blood 97:3210–3217.

205. Feuillard J, Jacob MC, Valensi F, et al. 2002. Clinical and biologic features of CD4+CD56+ malignancies. Blood 99:1556–1563.

206. Sanchez ML, Almeida J, Vidriales B, et al. 2002. Incidence of phenotypic aberrations in a series of 467 patients with B chronic lymphoproliferative disorders: basis for the design of specific four-color stainings to be used for minimal residual disease investigation. Leukemia 16:1460–1469.

207. Inaba T, Shimazaki C, Sumikuma T, Nakagawa M. 2001. T-cell associated antigen-positive B-cell lymphoma. Leuk. Lymphoma 42:1161–1171.

208. Kingma DW, Imus P, Xie XY, et al. 2002. CD2 is expressed by a subpopulation of normal B cells and is frequently present in mature B-cell neoplasms. Cytometry 50:243–248.

209. Echeverri C, Fisher S, King D, Craig FE. 2002. Immunophenotypic variability of B-cell non-Hodgkin lymphoma: a retrospective study of cases analyzed by flow cytometry. Am. J. Clin. Pathol. 117:615–620.

210. Check I. 2001. Clinical Applications of DNA Content Analysis. In Flow Cytometry in Clinical Diagnosis, 3rd ed., Keren DF, McCoy JP Jr, Carey JL, eds. ASCP Press: Chicago, p. 71.

211. Witzig TE and Katzmann JA. 2001. Clinical utility of DNA ploidy and cell proliferation measurements by flow cytometry. In: Flow Cytometry in Clinical Diagnosis, 3rd ed., Keren DF, McCoy JP Jr, Carey JL, eds. ASCP Press: Chicago.

212. Ross JS. 1996. DNA ploidy and cell cycle analysis in cancer diagnosis and prognosis. Oncology (Huntingt.) 10:867–882.

213. Schipper DL, Wagenmans MJ, Peters WH, Wagener DJ. 1998. Significance of cell proliferation measurement in gastric cancer. Eur. J. Cancer 34:781–790.

214. Wenger CR and Clark GM. 1998 S-phase fraction and breast cancer—a decade of experience. Breast Cancer Res. Treat. 51:255–265.

215. Pathologists CoA. 1998. Flow Cytometry Survey Set FL-B. Northfield, IL: Collage of American Pathologists.

216. Corver WE, Koopman LA, van der Aa J, et al. 2000. Four-color multiparameter DNA flow cytometric method to study phenotypic intratumor heterogeneity in cervical cancer. Cytometry 39:96–107.

217. Oelschlaegel U, Freund D, Range U, Ehninger G, Nowak R. 2001. Flow cytometric DNA-quantification of three-color immunophenotyped cells for subpopulation specific determination of aneuploidy and proliferation. J. Immunol. Meth. 253:145–152.

218. Sanchez-Carbayo M, Ciudad J, Urrutia M, Navajo JA, Orfao A. 2001 Diagnostic performance of the urinary bladder carcinoma antigen ELISA test and multiparametric DNA/cytokeratin flow cytometry I urine voided samples from patients with bladder carcinoma. Cancer 92: 2811–2819.

219. Kimmig R, Wimberger P, Kapsner T, Hillemanns P. 2001. Flow cytometric DNA analysis using cytokeratin labeling for identification of tumor cells in carcinomas of breast and the female genital tract. Ana Cell Pathol. 22:165–178.

220. Smith PJ, Wiltshire M, Davies S, Patterson LH, Hoy T. 1999. A novel cell permeant and far red-fluorescing DNA probe, DRAQ5, for blood cell discrimination by flow cytometry. J. Immunol. Meth. 229:131–139.

221. Wiltshire M, Patterson LH, Smith PJ. 2000. A novel deep red/low infrared fluorescent flow cytometric probe, DRAQ5NO, for the discrimination of intact nucleated cells in apoptotic cell population. Cytometry 39:217–223.

222. Smith PJ, Blunt N, Wiltshire M, et al. 2000. Characteristics of a novel deep red/infrared fluorescent cell permeant DNA probe, DRAQ5, in intact human cells analyzed by flow cytometry, confocal and multiphoton microscopy. Cytometry 40:280–291.

223. Gorisse MC, Venteo L, Pluot M. 1999. A method for simultaneous quantification of monoclonal antibody Ki-67 and DNA content by flow cytometry. Application to breast carcinomas. Anal. Quant. Cytol. Histol. 21:8–16.

224. Dearden C. 2002 Monoclonal antibody therapy of haematological malignancies. BioDrugs 16:283–301.

225. Countouriotis A, Moore TB, Sakamoto KM. 2002. Cell surface antigen and molecular targeting in the treatment of hematologic malignancies. Stem Cells 20:215–229.

226. Clay TM, Hobeika AC, Mosca PJ, Lyerly HK, Morse MA. 2001. Assays for monitoring cellular immune responses to active immunotherapy of cancer. Clin. Cancer Res. 7:1127–1135.

227. Morse MA, Clay TM, Hobeika AC, Mosca PJ, Lyerly HK. 2001. Monitoring cellular immune responses to cancer immunotherapy. Curr. Opin. Mol. Ther. 3:45–52.

228. Keilholz U, Weber J, Finke JH, et al. 2002. Immunologic monitoring of cancer vaccine therapy: results of a workshop sponsored by the Society for Biological Therapy. J. Immunother. 25:97–138.

229. Grillo-Lopez AJ. 2002. AntiCD20 mAbs: modifying therapeutic strategies and outcomes in the treatment of lymphoma patients. Expert Rev. Anticancer Ther. 2:323–329.

230. Cheson BD. 2002. Hematologic malignancies: new developments and future treatments. Semin. Oncol. 29(Suppl 13):33–45.

231. Rossmann ED, Lundin J, Lenkei R, Mellstedt H, Osterborg A. 2001. Variability in B-cell antigen expression: implications for the treatment of B-cell lymphomas and leukemias with monoclonal antibodies. Hematol. J. 2:300–306.

232. Constantin CM, Bonney EE, Altman JD, Strickland OL. 2002. Major histocompatibility complex (MHC) tetramer technology: an evaluation. Biol. Res. Nurs. 4:115–127.

233. Romero P, Dunbar PR, Valmori D, et al. 1998. Ex vivo staining of metastatic lymph nodes by class I major histocompatibility complex tetramers reveals high numbers of antigen-experienced tumor-specific cytolytic T lymphocytes. J. Exp. Med. 188:1641–1650.

234. Lee KH, Wang E, Nielsen MB, et al. 1999. Increased vaccine-specific T cell frequency after peptide-based vaccination correlates with increased susceptibility to in vitro stimulation but does not lead to tumor regression. J. Immunol. 163:6292–6300.

235. Dhodapkar MV, Steinman RM, Sapp M, et al. 1999. Rapid generation of broad T-cell immunity in humans after a single injection of mature dendritic cells. J. Clin. Investig. 104:173–180.

236. Paul WE and Seder RA. 1994. Lymphocytes responses and cytokines. Cell 76:241–251.

237. Maino VC and Picker LJ. 1998. Identification of functional subsets by flow cytometry: intracellular detection of cytokine expression. Cytometry 34:207–215.

238. Moore JS and Zaki MH. 2001 Clinical cytokine network cytometry. Clin. Lab. Med. 21:795–809.

239. Maraveyas A, Baban B, Kennard D, et al. 1999. Possible improved survival of patients with stage IV AJCC melanoma receiving SRL 172 immunotherapy: correlation with induction of increased intracellular interleukin-2 in peripheral blood lymphocytes. Ann. Oncol. 10:817–824.

240. Reinartz S, Boerner H, Koehler S, et al. 1999. Evaluation of immunological responses in patients with ovarian cancer treated with the anti-idiotype vaccine ACA 125 by determination of intercellular cytokines–a preliminary report. Hybridoma. 18:41–45. 71.

241. McCoy JP Jr and Goolsby C. 2001. Clinical Molecular Cytometry: Merging Flow Cytometry with Molecular Biology in Laboratory Medicine, In: Flow Cytometry in Clinical Diagnosis, 3rd ed., Keren DF, McCoy JP Jr, Carey JL, eds. ASCP Press: Chicago.

242. van den Beemd R, Boor PP, van Lochem EG, et al. 2000. Flow cytometric analysis of the Vbrepertoire in healthy controls. Cytometry 40:336–345.

243. Langerak AW, van den Beemd R, Wolvers-Tettero IL, et al. 2001. Molecular and flow cytometric analysis of the Vβ repertoire for clonality assessment in mature TCRαβ T-cell proliferations. Blood 98:165–173.

244. Ashcroft RG and Lopez PA. 2000. Commercial high speed machines open new opportunities in high throughput flow cytometry (HTFC). J. Immunol. Meth. 243:13–24.

245. Bigos M, Baumgarth N, Jager GC, et al. 1999. Nine color eleven parameter immunophenotyping using three laser flow cytometry. Cytometry 36:36–45.

12

Molecular Diagnostics in Neoplastic Hematopathology

Daniel A. Arber

1. INTRODUCTION

Neoplastic hematopathology was one of the first areas of medicine to use genetic-related testing for diagnostic purposes. The discovery and characterization of the Philadelphia chromosome in chronic myelogenous leukemia *(1,2)* is viewed by many as the beginning of the diagnostic era of cytogenetics and became a defining feature in the evaluation of patients with chronic myeloproliferative disorders. The discovery of rearrangements of immunoglobulin genes in lymphocytes and their use as clonal markers in lymphoid proliferations introduced the molecular genetic tool of Southern blot analysis to lymphoma diagnosis *(3,4)*.

Since these early discoveries, many other genetic changes have been associated with hematologic malignancies. The detection of these recurring abnormalities, and the characterization of the molecular events involved, have resulted in revised disease classifications and therapies directed against genetically defined disease groups. In addition to the expansion of knowledge of genetic abnormalities, the methodology to detect these changes has rapidly advanced. Currently, Southern blot analysis is less commonly performed, being replaced by the polymerase chain reaction (PCR), reverse-transcriptase PCR (RT-PCR), "real-time" quantitative PCR, and fluorescence *in situ* hybridization (FISH). This chapter will review the major molecular genetic changes of leukemia and lymphoma, as well as the various issues related to methodology and testing.

2. ROLE OF CYTOGENETICS AND MOLECULAR DIAGNOSTICS IN THE CLASSIFICATION OF LYMPHOMA AND LEUKEMIA

The applications of molecular genetic studies in neoplastic hematopathology include determination of clonality, identification of abnormalities associated with a specific disease subtype, determination of changes of prognostic significance, and detection of residual disease. The routine evaluation of samples for lymphoma does not usually include karyotype analysis and most lymphoma cases are diagnosed without molecular genetic testing. Such testing may be performed when the differential diagnosis of reactive vs neoplastic cannot be resolved by morphologic or immunophenotypic studies, or when the question of subtyping of lymphoma cannot be resolved by more commonly used methods. Molecular studies are more often performed to monitor for minimal residual disease in lymphoma patients.

In chronic leukemias, molecular studies are helpful in confirming a neoplastic over a reactive process and in subclassifying the process. These studies are not usually necessary to make a diagnosis of acute leukemia, but add significant information about prognosis in acute

From: *Cancer Diagnostics: Current and Future Trends*
Edited by: R. M. Nakamura, W. W. Grody, J. T. Wu, and R. B. Nagle © Humana Press Inc., Totowa, NJ

leukemia. For this reason, karyotype analysis, supplemented by appropriate molecular testing, is recommended for acute leukemias. Some of these methods are also useful in the monitoring of residual disease.

3. GENERAL DIAGNOSTIC APPROACHES

3.1. Primary Diagnosis

In the primary diagnosis of acute leukemia, the molecular genetic alterations of the leukemia are primarily of prognostic importance, and karyotype analysis is usually an acceptable first line of testing. However, some karyotype abnormalities may be cryptic and will be missed by standard karyotype analysis. In addition, the detection of some abnormalities will result in different leukemia therapy and require more rapid detection. When cryptic or therapeutically significant abnormalities are suspected, RT-PCR or FISH based assays are commonly employed. When a chronic myeloproliferative disorder is suspected, detection of the Philadelphia chromosome has both diagnostic and therapeutic implications. Although this abnormality is usually detected by karyotype analysis, a cryptic t(9;22) may only be detectable by RT-PCR or FISH assays.

In the primary diagnosis of malignant lymphoma, karyotype analysis is not usually performed, and molecular studies are not necessary in the majority of cases. Molecular genetic studies are useful in two settings in the diagnosis of lymphoma. First, when the differential diagnosis is between a reactive condition, malignant lymphoma and another neoplasm, B-cell and/or T-cell-associated gene rearrangement studies are useful. Detection of a disease-associated gene fusion product by PCR or FISH may be helpful, but is not necessary to confirm the presence of a clonal lymphoid neoplasm. Possible exceptions in follicular lymphomas and plasma cell disorders will be discussed in more detail below. The second major use of molecular studies in lymphoma is in subclassification, especially the lymphomas of small B-lymphocytes. The molecular detection of tumor cell infection by specific viruses is helpful in the classification of a small group of malignant lymphomas.

3.2. Residual Disease Testing

Molecular diagnostic testing is commonly used to monitor patients for disease recurrence. Although Southern blot and standard karyotype analyses can detect only 5% or more cells, some PCR-based tests can detect tumor burdens as low as 0.001%. Such a detection level is associated with disease relapse in some malignancies, but others require higher levels of molecular abnormalities associated with relapse. FISH analysis is less sensitive in the detection of residual disease, because many tests will not reliably detect a tumor burden below 5%. However, recently described FISH methods have reported detection levels that rival PCR-based tests (5).

For minimal residual disease testing, there are marked differences in the level of detection based on the PCR methodology utilized. For leukemias, most PCR testing uses RT-PCR directed against a specific fusion product and low levels of this fusion can be detected. Because some of these methods may be too sensitive for clinical use, quantitative PCR (Q-PCR) methods are used to quantify the level of the fusion product. Q-PCR methods have been proven clinically useful in early studies. For many leukemias without balanced cytogenetic abnormalities, however, PCR-based testing cannot be performed, and less sensitive FISH methods are used to monitor for residual disease.

Balanced translocations also occur in certain malignant lymphomas and can be monitored similar to leukemias. However, the only molecular markers available for most malignant lymphomas are T- or B-cell gene rearrangements. This is also true for some acute lymphoblastic leukemias. Southern blot analysis for these gene rearrangements is not sufficiently sensitive for residual disease testing, and PCR testing is typically performed. Most PCR-based B- and T-cell gene rearrangement studies, however, use relatively nonspecific primers, termed consensus primers, that weaken the level of detection of these assays to levels of 0.1–1%. To increase the detection of B- or T-cell gene rearrangements, some investigators have developed more sensitive PCR primers based on the exact sequence of a given patient's gene rearrangement *(6,7)*. Although these methods detect low levels of residual disease, as low as 0.001%, they are not routinely offered in most diagnostic laboratories. Less labor intensive and patient specific methods have been reported that may allow for the sensitive detection of low-level disease in patients with lymphoid malignancies. These methods may become available in the future *(8)*.

4. MOLECULAR DIAGNOSTICS OF LEUKEMIA

A large number of recurring balanced and unbalanced cytogenetic abnormalities occur in leukemia. Many of these are unique to specific disease types, and several categories of molecular abnormalities are now recognized. The detection of these genetic changes in leukemia is required for the diagnosis of some diseases, particularly chronic myelogenous leukemia and provides significant prognostic information for the acute leukemias. Detailed recent reviews of the biology and clinical significance of some of these abnormalities have been recently published *(9–11)*.

4.1. Acute Myeloid Leukemia

The recently published World Health Organization (WHO) classification of acute myeloid leukemia (AML) includes four categories with recurring cytogenetic abnormalities *(12)*. The detection of these abnormalities by karyotype or molecular genetic analysis is required for diagnosis of these disease types, and cases with these abnormalities are considered as acute leukemias without regard to the blast cell count. These include acute promyelocytic leukemia with t(15;17)(q22;q21) or *PML/RARα* and variants; AML with t(8;21)(q22;q22) or *AML1/ETO*; AML with inv (16) (p13q22)/t(16;16)(p13;q22) or *CBFβ/MYH11* and AML with 11q23 *(MLL)* abnormalities. These are some of the most common recurring genetic abnormalities, but other genetic changes of significance may also be present in AML and myelodysplasia (Table 1). The genetic changes of leukemia result in a variety of mechanisms related to the development of disease, and some of the basic mechanisms will be discussed. Figure 1 provides a simplified overview of how some fusion products affect hematopoiesis.

4.1.1. Acute Promyelocytic Leukemia

Acute promyelocytic leukemia results from abnormalities of the *RARα* gene, located on chromosome 17q21 *(13)*. *RARα* is a nuclear hormone receptor that binds to specific DNA sequences referred to as retinoic acid responsive elements in a heterodimeric complex with retinoid-X receptors *(RXRα)*. The *RARα/RXRα* complexes can repress transcription through a variety of mechanisms, but normal physiologic concentrations of retinoic acid in the body control this activity, allowing for normal activation of gene transcription. In most cases of

Table 1
Some of the Common Cytogenetic/Molecular Genetic Abnormalities
in Acute Myeloid Leukemia and Myelodysplasia

Translocation	Involved genes	Most common disease type
inv(3)/t(3;3)(q21;q26)	Ribophorin 1/EVI1	Myelodysplasia
t(3;21)(q26;q22)	*EVI1, EAP* or *MDS1/AML1*	Myelodysplasia
t(3;5)(q25;q34)	*NPM/MLF1*	Myelodysplasia, M2, M6
t(8;21)(q22;q22)	*AML1/ETO*	M2
t(6;9)(p23;q34)	*DEK/CAN*	M1,M2,M4
t(7;11)(p15;p15)	*NUP98/HOXA9*	M2,M4
t(15;17)(q22;q21)	*PML/RARα*	M3
t(11;17)(q23;q21)	*PLZF/RARα*	M3
t(11;17)(q13;q21)	*NuMA/RARα*	M3
t(5;17)(q31;q21)	*NPM/RARα*	M3
inv(16)/t(16;16)(p13;q22)	*CBFβ/MYH11*	M4Eo
t(9;11)(P22;q23)	*AF9/MLL*	M5
Other 11q23 abnormalities	*MLL*	M4,M5
t(1;22)(p13;q13)	*OTT/MAL*	M7

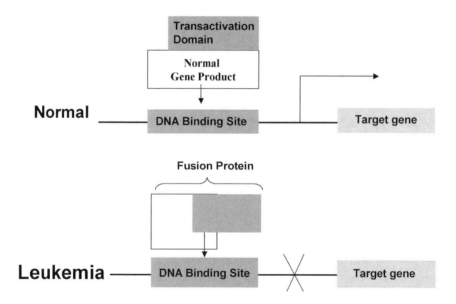

Fig. 1. Overview of how some acute leukemia fusion products affect normal hematopoiesis. In many cases, the normal gene products bind specific areas of DNA. Once bound, the normal transactivation domains cause transcription of adjacent target genes involved in hematopoiesis. Abnormal fusion products may alter this process by many mechanisms, including altering DNA binding and loss of the normal transactivation domain. Color image available for viewing at **www.humanapress.com**.

acute promyelocytic leukemia, the *RARα* gene fuses with the *PML* gene on chromosome 15q22. As a result of this fusion, physiologic levels of retinoic acid are no longer sufficient to control the effects of *RARα* and gene transcription is blocked. Therapeutic strategies that include all-*trans* retinoic acid (ATRA) provide pharmacologic concentrations of retinoic acid allowing for the return of normal transcription. Acute promyelocytic leukemia has a generally good prognosis.

The t(15;17) is usually detectable by karyotype analysis at diagnosis. Molecular detection of *PML/RARα* is usually performed by RT-PCR or FISH analysis. Three different isoforms of the fusion may occur and RT-PCR assays should be designed to detect them all. They vary by differences in breakpoints within the *PML* gene. Breaks in intron 6 are termed bcr-1, long, or L forms; breaks in exon 6 are termed bcr-2, variable, or V-forms; and breaks in intron 3 are termed bcr-3, short, or S-forms. Some differences in clinical presentation occur with the different forms, including an association between the microgranular variant and the S-form, and V-form disease may have a lower disease-free survival *(14)*. However, most laboratories do not distinguish between the different breakpoint types.

The *PML/RARα* RT-PCR test has been shown useful in early detection of residual disease in acute promyelocytic leukemia, and as a predictor of relapse of that disease *(15)*. Most assays for *PML/RARα* detect one translocated cell in 10,000–100,000 cells. However, this test appears less useful when more sensitive assays detecting one abnormal cell in one million are used. This ultra-sensitive test will be positive in patients that are in long term remission and do not appear clinically relevant *(16)*. This suggests that serial quantitative assays may be useful to follow patients with very low levels of disease.

Although *PML/RARα* is the most common fusion in this disease, other translocations of *RARα* on chromosome 17 with *PLZF* at 11q23, *NuMA* at 11q13, *NPM* at 5q35 and *STAT 5b* at 17q11 may occur *(17)*. Cases that lack an *RARα* translocation or have a translocation involving *PLZF* or *STAT 5b*, do not respond to all-*trans*-retinoic acid and require a different therapeutic approach *(13,18)*.

4.1.2. CBF Leukemias

The disruption of normal transcription factor activity is a common event in abnormalities associated with acute leukemias. The core binding factor (CBF) is a complex that includes elements encoded by the *AML1* (aka *RUNX1* or *CBFα2*) gene on chromosome 21q22 and the *CBFβ* gene at 16q22. Recurring translocations of these genes are some of the most common in acute leukemia *(19,20)*. The CBF is critical in normal hematopoietic development and translocations involving these genes result in disruption of hematopoiesis by a variety of mechanisms.

The t(8;21)(q22;q22) results in an *AML1/ETO* (aka *AML1/MTG8*) fusion that eliminates the transcriptional activating domain of the CBF *(21,22)*. This abnormality is associated with a distinct type of AML that represents a subgroup of M2 AMLs in the French-American-British (FAB) classification and a specific type of AML in the WHO classification. Another distinct type of AML that commonly has admixed abnormal eosinophils, termed M4Eo in the FAB classification, is associated with inv(16)(p13q22)/t(16;16)(p13;q22). These abnormalities result in a fusion of the *CBFβ* and *MYH11* genes of chromosome 16 *(23)*. The *MYH11* gene encodes the smooth muscle myosin heavy chain (SMMHC). Although this fusion does not effect the transcriptional activating domain of the CBF, it still acts as a suppressor of *AML1* function and may sequester *AML1* from transcriptionally active sites. Both of these leukemia types respond well to high-dose chemotherapy.

The CBF is also involved in other leukemias. The *AML1* gene is associated with chromosome 3 translocations that involve the *EVI1* and *MDS1* genes, in association with myelodysplasia and blast transformation of chronic myelogenous leukemia. In addition, *AML1* is disrupted in the t(12;21)(p13;q22) of pediatric acute lymphoblastic leukemia. This results in a fusion with the *TEL* gene (*see* Section 4.2.2.).

Most of the translocations that involve the CBF proteins can be detected by karyotype analysis, but the inv(16) of *CBFβ/MYH11* may be missed and the t(12;21) of *TEL/AML1* is not usually detectable by routine karyotype. For these abnormalities, molecular studies are often needed at the time of the original diagnosis. RT-PCR and FISH assays are most commonly performed. For residual disease detection, RT-PCR for *AML1/ETO* and *CBFβ/MYH11* must be interpreted with caution. It appears that other genetic aberrations, which may not be detectable by karyotype analysis, are necessary for these types of leukemia to develop *(24)*. In patients that have been treated for AML with t(8;21) or AML with inv(16)/t(16;16), standard qualitative PCR testing may detect low levels of these fusions during remission that may not correlate with relapse of the disease *(25,26)*. These PCR tests suggest that the fusion products may persist indefinitely and that qualitative PCR for *AML1/ETO* and *CBFβ/MYH11* is not clinically useful for residual disease testing. It is assumed, however, that new methods for quantitative PCR will be of clinical significance, by showing that an increasing number of cells with *AML1/ETO* or *CBFβ/MYH11* over time correlates with relapse of disease.

4.1.3. MLL *Leukemias*

AML with 11q23 (*MLL*) abnormalities is a specific subtype of AML in the WHO classification confering a generally poor prognosis. However, this category represents a heterogenous group of diseases with as many as 40 different translocation partners reported with the *MLL* gene. In addition, abnormalities that are not associated with balanced translocations may occur with *MLL*.

MLL is a large, 90 kb gene that contains 36 exons and codes for a 431 kDa protein *(27,28)*. The protein contains AT-hooks, which are known to regulate transcription by inducing changes in DNA conformation permitting the association of transcription factors with regulatory regions of DNA. These AT-hooks recognize specific DNA structures. Other regions of *MLL* are capable of repressing transcription from reporter constructs, mediate homodimerization, mediate interactions with nuclear proteins, contain transcriptional activating activity, and are involved with ATP-dependent chromatin remodeling.

Although there are numerous translocation partners with *MLL*, the most common in AML are chromosomes 6q27 (*AF6* gene), 9p22 (*AF9*), 19p13.3 (*ENL*), 19p13.1 (*ELL*), 19p13.3 (*EEN*), 16p13 (*CBP*) and 22q13 (*p300*). The t(4;11), involving the *AF4* gene, is more common in infant acute lymphoblastic leukemia (ALL) and adult therapy-related ALL. *MLL* abnormalities are also common in therapy-related AML, particularly after therapy with topoisomerase II inhibitors. Partial tandem duplications of *MLL* also occur in AML and are more common in patients with normal karyotypes *(29,30)*. In general, the presence of *MLL* translocations and partial tandem duplications indicates an unfavorable prognosis, but the t(9;11) in childhood AML has been shown to confer a good prognosis *(31)*.

Karyotype analysis may not detect abnormalities of 11q23, and this method cannot detect the partial tandem duplications of the *MLL* gene. Because of the multitude of potential *MLL* translocation partners, the PCR-based tests are of limited value. Most laboratories use FISH-based testing for *MLL* translocations, but this method will not detect the internal tandem duplications. RT-PCR for *MLL* internal tandem duplications is not performed in most laboratories, and reports of such duplications in healthy donors *(32)* suggests that only a quantitative assay for this abnormality would be useful as a diagnostic test.

4.1.4. Nucleoporin Protein Fusions

Nucleoporins represent one of several components of nuclear pore complexes; structures that allow macromolecules to move in and out of the cell nuclear. A number of chromosomal rearrangements in *de novo* AML, therapy-related AML, and myelodysplasia involve nucleoporins *(11)*. The most commonly involved genes are *NUP98*, on chromosome 11p15, and *CAN* (aka *NUP214*) on chromosome 9q34. It appears that nucleoporin fusion proteins act as aberrant transcription factors as well as altering nuclear transport by binding to soluble transport factors. *NUP98* usually fuses with homeobox genes, including *HOXA9* (on chromosome 7p15), *PMX1* (1q24), and *HOXD13* (2q31) but other gene fusions have been described. *CAN* commonly fuses with the *DEK* gene in t(6;9)(p23;q34) a *de novo* AML type associated with erythroid hyperplasia, dysplasia and bone marrow basophilia *(33)*. Although RT-PCR or FISH can be performed to test for all of these abnormalities, such testing is not offered in most molecular diagnostic laboratories.

4.1.5. Receptor Tyrosine Kinase Abnormalities

The receptor tyrosine kinases are cell surface transmembrane enzymes that are involved in ligand binding and signal transduction *(34)*. Genes that encode receptor tyrosine kinases include *c-kit*, *PDGFRβ*, *c-fms*, and *FLT-3*. Mutations, internal duplications, and tyrosine kinase fusion proteins involving these genes occur in several different leukemia types. One tyrosine kinase gene of possible interest is *c-kit*, because c-kit protein is often expressed in AML. This gene is mutated in gastrointestinal stromal tumors and mast cell disease, but is infrequently mutated in AML. *FLT-3* (aka *STK1* and *flk2*), however, is another tyrosine kinase gene that frequently undergoes length mutations of the juxtamembrane or point mutations in the second tyrosine kinase domain *(35,36)*. The FLT-3 protein is expressed in early hematopoietic progenitor cells and is involved in early stem cell survival and myeloid differentiation. Internal length or point mutations occur in 20–27% of adult AMLs and are most common in AMLs with normal cytogenetics. These mutations are associated with decreased disease free survival in adult AML. Because of the relatively high frequency and clinical significance of these mutations in AML, *FLT-3* mutation testing will become more common in the future *(37)*.

4.2. Acute Lymphoblastic Leukemia

Similar to AML, a wide variety of genetic abnormalities occur in acute lymphoblastic leukemia (ALL). The most common abnormalities will be described and some of the more common aberrations are listed in Table 2.

4.2.1. ALL With t(9;22)

The Philadelphia chromosome (Ph), or t(9;22)(q34;q11), is a member of the nonreceptor protein tyrosine kinase family that results from a fusion of the *ABL* gene on chromosome 9 and the *BCR* gene on chromosome 22.

Three *BCR/ABL* variants may occur *(38–40)*, but the p190 (aka p185) variant is most commonly associated with ALL. These leukemias are usually of precursor B-cell lineage, but they also usually show aberrant expression of the myeloid-associated antigens CD13 and CD33. Ph+ ALL represents less than 5% of pediatric ALLs and 20–25% of adult ALLs. A number of adult Ph+ ALL cases will demonstrate the p210 variant, rather than p190, and both types of Ph+ ALL in adults are generally considered to have a poor prognosis. Details of the various t(9;22) fusions and their detection methods are discussed below for chronic myelogenous leukemia.

Table 2
Some of the Common Cytogenetic/Molecular Genetic
Abnormalities in Acute Lymphoblastic Leukemia

	Translocation	Involved genes
Precursor B ALL (L1/L2)		
	t(9;22)(q34;q11)	*BCR/ABL*
	t(12;21)(p13;q22)	*TEL/AML1*
	t(1;19)(q23;p13)	*E2A/PBX*
	t(17;19)(q22;p13)	*E2A/HLF*
	t(4;11)(q21;q23)	*AF4/MLL*
	Other 11q23 abnormalities	*MLL*
B ALL (L3)		
	t(8;14)(q24;q32)	*IgH/MYC*
	t(2;8)(p12;q24)	*Igκ/MYC*
	t(8;22)(q24;q11)	*Igλ/MYC*
T ALL (L1/L2)		
	1q32 abnormalities	*TAL1*
	t(8;14)(q24;q11)	*TCRα/MYC*
	t(11;14)(p15;q11)	*TCRδ/RBTN1*
	t(11;14)(p13;q11)	*TCRδ/RBTN2*
	t(10;14)(q24;q11)	*TCRδ/HOX11*
	del 9(p21)	*p16 and p15*
	t(1;7)(p34;q34)	*TCRβ/LCK*

4.2.2. ALL With t(12;21)

The t(12;21)(p13;q22) results from a fusion of the CBF gene *AML1* on chromosome 21 and the *TEL* (aka *ETV6*) gene on chromosome 12 *(41,42)*. *TEL* is normally a transcriptional repressor and the *TEL/AML1* fusion redirects this repressor function to *AML1* targets. This genetic abnormality is the most common recurring defect in pediatric ALL, present in 20–25% of cases *(43)*, but is uncommon in adult ALL. The defect was only recently identified, because it is not easily detected by routine karyotype analysis, and requires molecular studies. This type of ALL is considered to have a good prognosis, but very late relapses may occur. Both FISH and RT-PCR methods can detect this abnormality *(44)* and several reports using quantitative PCR have shown that this is a reliable method of following patients for residual disease *(45,46)*.

4.2.3. ALL With E2A Translocations

Several translocations involving the *E2A* gene on chromosome 19q23 occur in ALL. Although these are more common in childhood leukemia (5–6% of pediatric ALLs), they may occur at any age *(47)*. These translocations commonly occur in cytoplasmic μ-positive, pre-B ALL and are associated with a poor prognosis. *E2A* is a helix–loop–helix protein coding gene involved in B-cell development *(48,49)* and commonly fuses with the *PBX1* gene on chromosome 1q23, which is a homeodomain-containing HOX cofactor. This fusion encodes a chimeric transcription factor that causes inappropriate expression of genes critical for cell growth and differentiation. *E2A* less commonly fuses with the *HLF* gene on chromosome 17q21–22, and this fusion activates antiapoptotic pathways *(50)*. Karyotype, FISH, or RT-PCR can detect both abnormalities, but these molecular studies are often not offered by diagnostic laboratories.

4.2.4. ALL With MLL *Translocations*

MLL translocations in ALL are most common in cases of infant ALL and therapy-related ALL, and usually show a unique pro-B (CD10-negative) immunophenotype with aberrant expression of the myeloid-associated antigens CD15 and CD65 *(27,51)*. The majority of *MLL*-associated ALLs demonstrate the t(4;11), involving the *AF4* gene.

4.2.5. Other Abnormalities in ALL

The mature B-cell ALLs (FAB L3) are also termed Burkitt cell leukemia because they are leukemic presentations of Burkitt or Burkitt-like lymphoma. They are associated with translocations that involve the *c-myc* gene on chromosome 8q24. The features of this disease are described below with other lymphomas.

T-cell ALL is less common than precursor and mature B-cell ALL, but many recurring genetic abnormalities have been reported. The more common of these abnormalities are listed in Table 2. These abnormalities are not routinely tested in most molecular diagnostic laboratories.

4.3. Chronic Myeloproliferative Disorders

4.3.1. Chronic Myelogenous Leukemia

The detection of the Philadelphia chromosome is considered definitional for chronic myelogenous leukemia, and is useful in the exclusion of other chronic myeloproliferative disorders and reactive hyperplasias. The *BCR/ABL* fusion of t(9;22)(q34;q11), may result in three different sized variants *(38–40)*. The p190 (aka p185) results from what is termed an e1a2 junction, and is commonly associated with precursor B-cell ALL, as discussed above. The p210 variant is typically formed from a splicing of b2a2, b3a2, or a mixture of the two, and is often associated with chronic myelogenous leukemia. A less common variant, p230, is formed from an e19a2 junction and is associated with a rare neutrophilic type of chronic myelogenous leukemia. The *BCR/ABL* fusion product results in unregulated tyrosine kinase activity and activates a number of pathways including, but not limited to, Ras, Jun-kinase, and PI-3. This results in an increase in cell proliferation and a decrease in apoptosis. A recently introduced tyrosine kinase inhibitor originally identified as STI571 and now marketed as Gleevec (Novartis, Hanover, NJ) blocks the tyrosine kinase activity of this fusion. This drug results in hematologic and morphologic remissions in many patients and a cytogenetic remission in some patients.

Although karyotype analysis remains the first line test for identification of the Philadelphia chromosome, a small subset of cases will have cryptic translocations that cannot be detected without FISH or RT-PCR. In addition, karyotype analysis may be suboptimal for evaluation of residual disease after bone marrow transplantation or Gleevec therapy. Because low levels of *BCR/ABL* may remain in terminally differentiated cells after therapy, qualitative RT-PCR assays are also of limited value. For this reason, many laboratories now offer quantitative RT-PCR for *BCR/ABL*. These tests commonly detect the p190 and p210 variants, and many laboratories do not offer testing for the less common p230 variant.

4.3.2. Other Chronic Myeloproliferative Disorders

The majority of other chronic myeloproliferative disorders do not have recurring balanced cytogenetic abnormalities, but the lack of detection of *BCR/ABL* is often needed for the diagnosis of these diseases by excluding chronic myelogenous leukemia. A recurring balanced translocation occurs in a rare subtype of chronic myelomonocytic leukemia associated with an increase in eosinophils *(52,53)*. The t(5;12)(q31;p12) results in a *TEL/PDGFβR* fusion with tyrosine kinase activity similar to chronic myelogenous leukemia. Testing for this translocation is not offered in most molecular diagnostic laboratories.

5. MOLECULAR DIAGNOSTICS OF LYMPHOMA

Gene rearrangements and recurring translocations may be studied in lymphoma. Although these tests are not needed for most cases, they can be useful in the diagnosis of clonality as well as disease subclassification. These studies are usually not performed until after evaluation of the tissue morphology and immunophenotyping *(54)*, and those results usually direct which molecular studies are appropriate. The most common aberrations in lymphoma are listed in Table 3.

5.1. B-Cell Lymphoma

5.1.1. Immunoglobulin Heavy- and Light-Chain Gene Rearrangements

The detection of B-cell associated gene rearrangements is the most global means of detecting clonality in B-cell proliferations. The majority of malignant lymphomas are B-cell neoplasms. Rearrangement of the *IgH* gene on chromosome region 14q32 occurs in all normal developing B lymphocytes *(55–57)*. This chromosomal region contains over 100 variable (V) regions, 30 diversity (D), and 6 joining (J) regions (Fig. 2). When the B cell undergoes *IgH* gene rearrangement, one V, one D, and one J region move into close proximity of each other, with a wide diversity of possible VDJ combinations. Additional diversity is created by the random addition of so-called N-nucleotides between V, D, and J segments by terminal deoxynucleotidyl transferase. Because each normal B cell undergoes a relatively unique rearrangement, differences among each cell indicate a polyclonal B-cell population. Following rearrangement of the IgH gene, the immunoglobulin κ-light chain region of chromosome 2p11 rearranges in a similar fashion with the exception that it does not contain diversity (D) regions. If this rearrangement is not productive in either allele (approximately one-third of cases), the κ-light-chain constant region locus is deleted and the immunoglobulin λ-light-chain region on chromosome 22q11 undergoes rearrangement. Because mature B-cell lymphomas are clonal neoplasms, IgH and κ-light- chain gene rearrangements are detectable in essentially all cases. The precursor B-cell malignancies (lymphoblastic lymphomas, and leukemia), however, do not undergo the complete lymphocyte maturation process and may not undergo κ-light chain gene rearrangement. Because λ-light-chain rearrangements do not always occur, and when present, occur later in B-cell development, this region is not usually evaluated as a diagnostic test for clonality.

Immunoglobulin heavy and κ-light-chain gene rearrangements are detected by Southern blot analysis or by use of PCR, with most laboratories now using PCR as the primary method. The use of PCR for the detection of *IgH* gene rearrangements allows for the use of smaller

Table 3
Common Molecular Genetic Abnormalities Associated
With Non-Hodgkin's Lymphoma

Gene studied	Chromosomal site	Most common disease associations
Immunoglobulin heavy-Chain (*IgH*) rearrangements	14q32	B-cell neoplasms
Immunoglobulin light κ-chain (*Igκ*) rearrangements	2p11	B-cell neoplasms
JH/BCL-1	t(11;14)(q13;q32)	Mantle cell lymphoma
JH/BCL-2	t(14;18)(q32;q21)	Follicular lymphoma, some diffuse large B-cell lymphomas
PAX-5/IgH	t(9;14)(p13;q32)	Lymphoplasmacytic lymphoma
API2/MLT	t(11;18)(q21;q21)	Extranodal marginal zone lymphoma
BCL-6 translocations	t(3;n)(q27;n)	Some diffuse large B-cell lymphomas
C-MYC translocations	t(8;n)(q24;n)	Burkitt's lymphoma
T-cell receptor α-chain (TCRα) rearrangements	14q11	T-cell neoplasms
T-cell receptor γ-chain (TCRγ) rearrangements	7q15	T-cell neoplasms
NPM/ALK	t(2;5)(p23;q35)	Anaplastic large cell lymphoma

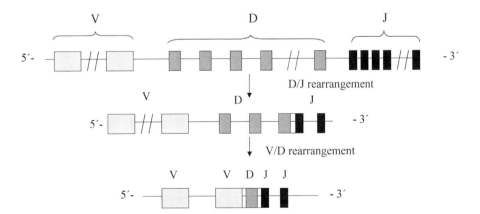

Fig. 2. Overview of the events of B- and T-cell associated gene rearrangements. Various variable (V), diversity (D) (if present) and joining (J) regions rearrange to form a specific VDJ or VJ segment for each lymphoid cell. Detection of the same VDJ or VJ rearrangement in a large population of cells is one means of determining monoclonality of a lymphoid proliferation. Color image available for viewing at **www.humanapress.com**.

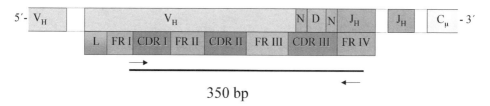

350 bp

Fig. 3. The VDJ rearrangement of the immunoglobulin heavy-chain gene (IgH) is the target of IgH PCR testing. The variable regions of each rearranged gene can be divided into three framework (FR) regions. PCR testing with primers directed against FRIII and the J_H (FRIV) regions give the smallest product and are the single most reliable test for this gene rearrangement. Assays directed against the FRI region are more likely to detect a higher percentage of IgH rearrangements, but the size of the PCR product and the large number of FRI primers needed for this assay limit its diagnostic use. Color image available for viewing at **www.humanapress.com**.

amounts of DNA and DNA from paraffin-embedded tissue. This method uses *consensus* primer pairs that anneal to the V and J regions of the rearranged chromosome 14 *(58)*. Certain nucleotide sequences are similar among the different V and J regions, and the consensus primers are made to anneal to these sequences even if they are not a perfect match. Because different, polyclonal rearrangements result in slightly different sized PCR products, a smear or ladder is observed on the gel in polyclonal specimens and one or two discrete bands are observed with a clonal proliferation. Capillary electrophoresis instruments are useful for DNA separation and replaced the use of gels in the evaluation of PCR products in many laboratories. Using this instrumentation, amplification products can be separated at the one base pair level, and polyclonal samples may show a range of peaks with no single dominate peak, compared to a dominate peak when a clonal population is present.

The primers with the highest detection rate for the *IgH* gene rearrangements are directed against a region termed framework (FR) III of the various V_H genes (Fig. 3). FRIII directed primers detect 60–70% of clonal B-cell malignancies *(59)*. The addition of other framework regions, particularly FRII primers, increase the detection rate of this test. Framework I is composed of multiple families of regions that require multiple PCR reactions to detect reliably. Based on the location of FRI, a combination of primers should detect the highest percentage of B-cell clones, but the products are often too large to reliably detect in paraffin-embedded tissues. Therefore, a combination of primers is more suitable for all specimen types and will detect 70–90% of B-cell neoplasms, depending on the type of disease.

Somatic mutations of the *IgH* gene of some mature B disorders, especially follicular lymphomas and plasma cell malignancies, alter the sequence of the region amplified by the primers so that primer hybridization is suboptimal or does not occur, resulting in false negative PCR results *(58)*. Because of these frequent somatic mutations, a negative IgH PCR result does not exclude the presence of a monoclonal B cell proliferation. In addition, consensus primers are not a perfect match to the sequence being amplified and result in less efficient amplification. This results in lower sensitivity of detection, and impacts on the use of consensus IgH primers in the detection of minimal residual disease. Most tests that employ consensus primers for *IgH* gene rearrangements can detect only down to a level of one clonal cell in 100 polyclonal cells.

PCR tests directed against rearrangement of the κ-light-chain gene (*Igκ*) or the κ deleting segment are also useful in the detection of B-cell clonality in mature B-cell proliferations, and are reported to successfully detect clonality in up to 50% of B-cell lymphomas *(60,61)*. Although this method does not detect as many B-cell neoplasms as the IgH PCR test, *Igκ* PCR is useful as a second-line test. *Igκ* PCR testing also uses consensus primers and this test suffers from the same minimal residual disease detection limitations of the standard IgH test.

Several studies have cloned and sequenced the specific gene rearrangements in B-cell lymphomas and created primers specific for the individual patient's disease *(6,7)*. Although this approach is time consuming and expensive, it allows for detection of very low levels of disease (in the range of 1 abnormal cell in 100,000 cells), which would presumably result in earlier treatment of the disease. However, this approach has limitations because patient specific primers cannot be developed in all cases, some tumors have more than one clone, and all clones may not be detectable by the very specific primers developed.

5.1.2. Specific Disease Types

Specific cytogenetic translocations are also associated with some types of malignant lymphoma. Unlike the translocations of acute leukemia, many of the more common lymphoma translocations do not involve large introns and are reliably amplified at the DNA level. Therefore, PCR tests for these are performed on paraffin-embedded tissues.

5.1.2.1. B-Cell Small Lymphocytic Lymphoma/ Chronic Lymphocytic Leukemia

Molecular studies are not always necessary for the diagnosis of B-cell small lymphocytic lymphoma/chronic lymphocytic leukemia (CLL), although all cases show *IgH* gene rearrangements, and they are usually detectable by PCR analysis. Characteristic cytogenetic abnormalities in CLL include deletions of 13q14, 11q22-23, 17p13 and 6q21, and trisomy 12, with 13q deletions having the best prognosis and 17p deletions the worst *(62)*. Trisomy 12, originally thought common in CLL, is more often associated with atypical features or cases undergoing transformation to a higher-grade process. Because the genetic abnormalities in CLL do not represent recurring balanced translocations, they cannot be routinely diagnosed using PCR. Deletions and trisomies are often evaluated by FISH analysis.

Recently, there has been interest in dividing cases of CLL into two groups based on IgH variable region gene mutations. Lack of mutation of this gene is associated with more aggressive disease in CLL *(63,64)*. Despite its clinical significance, IgH variable region gene mutation analysis is not offered in many diagnostic laboratories owing to its complexity. This test requires PCR amplification of the *IgH* gene rearrangement, usually requiring use of FRI directed primers. From this PCR product, the variable region of the monoclonal population is sequenced and the degree of mutation in the sequence is compared to a database. FISH analysis may become available in additional laboratories in the future.

5.1.2.2. Lymphoplasmacytic Lymphoma

The t(9;14)(p13;q32) was originally reported to be detected in approximately half of lymphoplasmacytic lymphomas *(65)* but is probably much less frequent than originally thought. This translocation involves the *PAX-5* gene on chromosome 9 and the *IgH* gene on chromosome 14. The site of the translocation on chromosome 14 differs from the region involved in the *JH/BCL-1* and *JH/BCL-2* translocations, occurring 3' to the constant region of the IgH locus in the switch μ region. *PAX-5* normally encodes a B-cell specific transcription factor known as B-cell-specific activator protein (BSAP) that is involved in the control of B-cell proliferation and differentiation *(66)*. Involvement of this gene may result in the plasmacytoid differentiation of these tumors. *PAX-5/IgH* translocations have also been reported in rare cases of marginal zone lymphoma and diffuse large B-cell lymphoma *(65,67)*. Southern blot analysis, RT-PCR, or FISH may be used to detect *PAX-5* rearrangements. However, this lymphoma type is less common than other types with recurring translocations and these methods are not offered in most diagnostic laboratories at this time.

5.1.2.3. MARGINAL ZONE LYMPHOMAS

The t(11;18)(q21;q21) is detected in approximately one-third of marginal zone lymphomas by classic karyotype analysis *(68,69)*. Recently, this translocation has been shown to involve the apoptosis inhibitor gene (*API2*) on chromosome 11 and the *MLT* gene (also known as *MALT1*) on chromosome 18 *(70)*. *API2/MLT* translocations appear specific for only the nonsplenic, extranodal marginal zone lymphomas, occurring in approx 40% of gastric and lung marginal zone lymphomas, but not detected in splenic marginal zone lymphomas and the primary nodal marginal zone lymphomas previously termed monocytoid B-cell lymphomas *(71–74)*. In addition, the extranodal marginal zone lymphomas with increased large cells or evidence of large cell transformation do not demonstrate this translocation, even in the accompanying low-grade component. The presence of t(11;18) in gastric marginal zone lymphoma is associated with a lack of response to *Helicobacter pylori* therapy *(75)*.

Multiple breakpoint sites are described for *API2/MLT*, and RT-PCR or FISH analyses are usually needed to detect this abnormality. Because most of these tumors are now diagnosed based on small tissue biopsies without saved frozen tissue, FISH analysis on paraffin embedded tissue may be the most optimal means of detecting this translocation.

In addition to the relatively common *API2/MLT* translocation and the less common *PAX-5/IgH* translocation in marginal zone lymphoma, trisomy 3 and t(1;14)(q21–22;q32) have been reported. The t(1;14) results in a fusion or the *BCL-10* gene and the *IgH* gene. Although this abnormality appears to occur in less than 10% of marginal zone lymphomas, overexpression of nuclear BCL-10 protein is associated with both t(1;14) and t(11;18)-positive marginal zone lymphomas.

5.1.2.4. FOLLICULAR LYMPHOMA

As a result of somatic hypermutation of the *IgH* gene in follicular center cells, only 35–50% of follicular lymphomas will have a detectable *IgH* rearrangement by PCR analysis using a single primer set *(59,76,77)*. Because these mutations do not affect the overall gene rearrangement, virtually all follicular lymphomas will show a rearrangement by Southern blot analysis. Despite the relatively high false-negative rate for *IgH* gene rearrangement by PCR analysis, most (70–80%) follicular lymphomas will demonstrate t(14;18)(q32;q21) involving the *IgH* gene on chromosome 14 and the *BCL-2* gene on chromosome 18 (Fig. 4) *(78)*, and 70–90% of these translocations are detectable by PCR analysis *(79,80)*. Over expression of bcl-2 protein, which results from this translocation, is associated with a loss of apoptosis. This translocation is detectable by either Southern blot or by PCR (*JH/BCL-2*) analysis *(79)*. Most translocations involve the major breakpoint region (MBR) of *BCL-2*, but 5–10% involve a minor cluster region (MCR) that requires the use of different PCR primers and Southern blot probes to detect *(80–82)*. More recently described minor translocation clusters (including 3'BCL2 and 5'MCR) appear to be involved in most of the remaining cases, but are not routinely tested *(83)*. Although most *JH/BCL-2* translocations can be detected from paraffin-embedded tissues, some breakpoints result in PCR products that are very large and may not be detectable after fixation *(84)*.

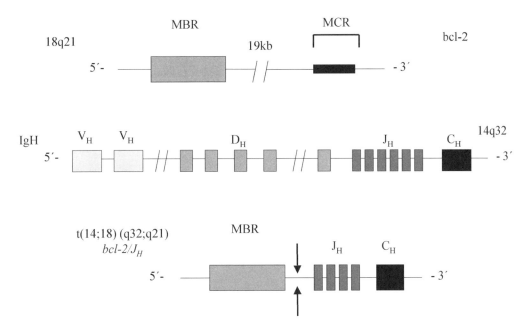

Fig. 4. The t(14;18) of follicular lymphoma most commonly results in a 5' juxtaposition of the major breakpoint region (MBR) of the BCL-2 gene on chromosome 18 to a position adjacent to the joining (J) region of the immunoglobulin heavy chain (IgH) gene on chromosome 14. Color image available for viewing at **www.humanapress.com**.

The t(14;18) has also been reported to be detected by *JH/BCL-2* PCR analysis in normal peripheral blood and in reactive lymph nodes *(85–87)*. These reports suggest that this translocation can occur in small numbers of cells without the development of malignant lymphoma. Nonnested PCR tests for *JH/BCL-2* that do not amplify over 45 cycles do not usually produce these "false positive" results *(88)*. Detection of t(14;18) by molecular methods is not necessary for the diagnosis of most cases of follicular lymphoma. However, such testing may be valuable in the detection of minimal residual disease, such as in bone marrow aspirate material following chemotherapy, or bone marrow transplantation for follicular lymphoma.

5.1.2.5. MANTLE CELL LYMPHOMA

The t(11;14)(q13;q32), which involves the *IgH* gene of chromosome 14 and the *BCL-1/PRAD1* gene of chromosome 11, is present in the majority of mantle cell lymphoma cases *(89,90)*. The *BCL-1* gene encodes a cell cycle protein (termed cyclin D1, PRAD1 or BCL-1) and overexpression is associated with the aggressive behavior of this tumor. Detection of such overexpression has been useful in further defining this disease. The major translocation cluster (MTC) region is involved in 40–50% of cases, but the remaining translocations involve a multitude of different sites that are not easily detectable by PCR analysis *(91)*. Methods for detection of BCL-1 mRNA are described that detected over 95% of cases of mantle cell lymphoma, and the mRNA expression presumably occurs with translocations that involve the MTC as well as other breakpoints *(92,93)*. This method requires a quantitative reverse transcriptase PCR procedure that is not readily available in most laboratories. Mantle cell lymphomas also demonstrate nuclear overexpression of BCL-1/cyclin D1 protein, related to the translocation involving *BCL-1/PRAD1*. Detection of cyclin D1 by immunohistochemistry is a more sensitive test for mantle cell lymphoma than direct PCR *(94)*. Weak expression of BCL-1 protein has been described in other lymphoid tumors, including hairy cell leukemia *(95)*. FISH detection of t(11;14) is performed by some laboratories and is a more sensitive method for the detection of this abnormality than the direct PCR test performed in most laboratories *(96)*.

5.1.2.6. Diffuse Large B-Cell Lymphoma

The t(14;18)(q32;q21), identical to the translocations of follicular lymphomas, is identified in 17–38% of diffuse large B-cell lymphoma with detection methods identical to those described above *(59,97–99)*. A number of studies have suggested that the presence of t(14;18) in large cell lymphoma is a poor prognostic indicator *(98,99)*, which appears to contradict the findings of gene array studies *(see* below). In both follicular lymphomas and diffuse large B-cell lymphomas, detection of this translocation does not correlate with BCL-2 protein expression.

Many diffuse large B-cell lymphomas, including some with t(14;18), have abnormalities involving the *BCL-6/LAZ3*gene on chromosome region 3q27 *(100–104)*. Translocations involving *BCL-6* involve the *IgH* region of 14q32, the κ-light chain region of 2p11, or the λ-light chain region of 22q11. Translocations involving chromosomes 1, 9, 11,, and 12 have also been reported with *BCL-6* in diffuse large B-cell lymphoma. Rearrangements of *BCL-6* have also been reported to occur in other types of B-cell lymphoma, particularly follicular lymphomas, and marginal zone lymphomas. The clinical significance of the detection of *BCL-6* rearrangements in large cell lymphoma is controversial *(98,105)*. PCR based detection methods are limited by the large number of translocations that occur with this gene, the high frequency of somatic mutations of the gene, and because the translocations usually occur within an intron adjacent to the coding exons of the gene *(104,106)*. As a result, long range PCR, RT-PCR or FISH methods are needed. Most methods require fresh or frozen tissue, but FISH analysis may be performed on paraffin-embedded tissue. Recently, the quantitative detection of *BCL-6* RNA has been shown to have prognostic significance, and may become more common in the future *(107)*.

Although BCL-6 expression and t(14;18) are both markers of a possible germinal center cell origin in diffuse large B-cell lymphoma, gene array studies are better suited for identifying germinal center cell phenotypes than a single molecular or immunohistochemical assay *(108,109)*. These methods have identified three gene-expression subgroups of diffuse large B-cell lymphoma. The germinal center B-cell-like lymphomas express genes characteristic of normal germinal centers. Detection of *c-rel* amplification and t(14;18) are the most specific abnormalities in the germinal center B-cell-like group, but in contrast to previous studies on the prognostic significance of t(14;18), this lymphoma group is reported to be associated with a more favorable prognosis. The activated B-cell-like group expresses genes characteristic of mitogenically activated peripheral blood B cells, and are associated with a worse prognosis. Type 3 lymphomas do not express either germinal center or activated B-cell genes at a high level. Although these subgroups are prognostically significant, gene array methods are not currently available for diagnostic use.

5.1.2.7. Burkitt/Burkitt-Lymphoma

Burkitt's lymphoma is usually associated with translocations involving the *c-MYC* gene of chromosome region 8q24, particularly the t(8;14)(q24;q32) identified in approx 80% of cases *(110,111)*. The remaining cases demonstrate t(8;22)(q24;q11) or t(2;8)(p11;q24). The site of translocation differs between endemic and sporadic Burkitt's lymphoma *(112–115)*. In endemic disease, the t(8;14) occurs up to 300 kb 5' from the coding region of the *c-myc* gene, although sporadic Burkitt's characteristically involves a translocation within the actual *c-myc* gene. These translocations may also occur in the Burkitt-like lymphomas and in a small number of diffuse large B-cell lymphomas. Variations in these translocations, including translocations involving the constant regions rather than joining regions of 14q32, make them poor targets for detection by routine PCR. Southern blot analysis for *c-myc* is the most commonly used method of detecting this abnormality. FISH studies may also be performed and can be used on paraffin-embedded tissues.

5.2. T-Cell Lymphoma

5.2.1. T-Cell Receptor Gene Rearrangements

The T-cell receptor (*TCR*) genes undergo VDJ or VJ rearrangements similar to the immunoglobulin heavy and κ-light chain genes in the sequential order of TCRδ (chromosome 14q11), TCRγ (7q15), TCRβ (7q34) and TCRα (14q11) *(56,116,117)*. Approximately 95% of circulating T cells are of the α/β type, but a small population of γ/δ T cells do not undergo *TCRβ* and *TCRα* rearrangements. Southern blot analysis of the *TCRβ* chains will detect over 90% of T-cell malignancies but may not detect gene rearrangements in malignancies of γ/δ T cells or natural killer cells. The DNA may be hybridized with probes directed against the *TCRβ* constant region (Cβ) or with a cocktail of probes directed against *TCRβ* joining regions 1 and 2 (Jβ1 and 2).

PCR-based assays for T-cell clonality are usually directed against either *TCRβ* or *TCRγ*. Because of the complexity of the TCRβ locus, PCR for these rearrangements requires a large number of primers *(118)*. The TCRγ region is less complex with only four V region families containing 11 genes and five J region genes. Because the TCRγ locus is consistently rearranged prior to the TCRβ locus, PCR analysis with primers directed against the Vγ1–8, Vγ9, Vγ10 and Vγ11, coupled with a multiplex of J region primers will detect over 90% of clonal T cell neoplasms *(119–121)*. Because it is a PCR based test directed against genomic DNA, *TCRγ* PCR can be performed on paraffin-embedded tissue. In addition, TCRγ rearrangements can be detected in lymphomas of γ/δ T cells, that may not demonstrate evidence of clonality on Southern blotting for *TCRβ*. In contrast to the PCR for *IgH* gene rearrangements, if all of the TCRγ variable and joining regions sequences are covered by the PCR reactions, this test will result in very few false negative reactions when compared to Southern blot analysis.

5.2.2. Specific Disease Types

The t(2;5)(p23;q35) is the only recurring translocation that is routinely tested in mature T-cell lymphomas. It is the most common cytogenetic abnormality in noncutaneous forms of anaplastic large cell lymphoma. Anaplastic large cell lymphoma, as it is defined in the REAL and WHO classifications, is a T-cell or null-cell lymphoma *(12,122)*. The t(2;5)(p23;q35) results in a fusion transcript of the nucleolar phosphoprotein (*NPM*) gene of chromosome 5 and the anaplastic lymphoma kinase (*ALK*) gene of chromosome 2 *(123,124)*. Other reported *ALK* gene fusion partners are *TPM3* at 1q21, *TFG* at 3q21, *ATIC* at 2q35, *CTLC* at 17q23, and *MSN* at Xq11-12 *(125,126)*. The t(2;5) fusion product can be detected by reverse transcriptase PCR by amplifying a fairly small cDNA fragment *(127)*. Because the fusion product is small, it may also be detected in paraffin sections. The abnormality may also be detected by FISH analysis, which is a more sensitive test than RT-PCR *(128)*. This translocation results in expression of the ALK protein, which is not normally expressed in lymphoid cells. ALK expression can be detected by immunohistochemistry *(129)*, and in the right morphologic setting, ALK expression correlates well with FISH or other detection of t(2;5) *(128)*. ALK expression has been shown to correlate with improved survival in this disease, compared to ALK-negative anaplastic large cell lymphoma *(128,130)*. ALK expression may be nuclear, cytoplasmic, or both, and translocations involving the *ALK* gene, other than t(2;5), that are described in anaplastic large cell lymphoma are also associated with ALK-immunoreactivity *(131,132)*. The improved survival of ALK-positive lymphomas is independent of the translocation partner *(132)*. Because all ALK translocations, including many *NPM/ALK* translocations, are not detectable by RT-PCR analysis and the protein expression has such clinical relevance, ALK immunohistochemistry is the preferred test for this disease. The RT-PCR test may still have utility in monitoring for minimal residual disease.

T-cell prolymphocytic leukemia is associated with cytogenetic abnormalities of chromosome regions 14q, 8q, and 11q. The most common abnormality is inv (14)(q11q32). Chromosome 8 abnormalities include iso(8q) or trisomy 8 *(133)*. Chromosome 11 abnormalities include 11q23 abnormalities that do not appear to involve the *MLL* gene. Several reports have identified the combined cytogenetic abnormality of isochromosome 7q and trisomy 8 in hepatosplenic γδ T cell lymphoma *(134)*. None of these abnormalities are routinely screened for diagnostic purposes, and FISH analysis is the best method for detecting many of the changes.

5.3. Viruses in Lymphoma

Several lymphoma types are associated with clonal viral integration of the lymphoma cells. Detection of the associated virus is often helpful in the classification of the neoplastic process.

5.3.1. B-Cell Lymphomas

The Epstein–Barr virus (EBV) is associated with Burkitt's lymphoma and the large B cells of lymphomatoid granulomatosis *(135,136)*. Molecular detection of EBV RNA is seen in 90% of endemic cases of Burkitt's lymphoma compared to a frequency of 20–30% in sporadic cases. EBV-positive Burkitt's lymphoma, however, is usually negative for EBV latent membrane protein (LMP) by immunohistochemistry and the *in situ* hybridization test for EBER is the preferred method for detecting EBV in this disease.

Hepatitis C is reported to be associated with a variety of types of B-cell lymphomas *(137)*. Most of the reported cases occur in patients with mixed cryoglobulinemia, a disease with a known association with lymphoplasmacytic lymphoma. Because most studies of this virus in lymphoma use serologic or PCR methodologies, definite infection of the lymphoma cells with the virus has not been demonstrated for most cases.

Infection with Kaposi sarcoma herpes virus/human herpes virus-8 (KSHV/HHV-8) is associated with primary effusion lymphomas, plasmablastic lymphoma, and multicentric Castleman's disease *(138)*. KSHV/HHV-8 is usually detected by direct PCR, but recently described antibodies directed against the latent nuclear antigen of KSHV, are suitable for use in paraffin section and may offer an alternative to the PCR test. Detection of KSHV/HHV8 is particularly useful in the rare primary effusion lymphomas, a disease with pleomorphic cells that do not usually immunoreact with T- or B-cell antibodies.

5.3.2. T-Cell Lymphomas

There is a strong association between HTLV-1 infection and adult T-cell leukemia/lymphoma (ATLL) *(139)*. Clonal integration of the virus occurs in almost all ATLL patients, but *in situ* hybridization studies for this virus are difficult to perform and not routinely offered. The virus may be detectable by serologic studies or PCR analysis.

Nasal type NK/T cell lymphoma has a high association with clonal EBV in the tumor cells *(135)*. *In situ* hybridization detection of the virus in cells may be diagnostically useful in the small biopsy specimens obtained to evaluate for this disease. Because many of these cases are true NK neoplasms, they will not demonstrate T-cell receptor gene rearrangements, and the detection of EBV by *in situ* hybridization in the tumor cells is often the only diagnostic molecular test that is helpful. These tumors will usually not express EBV LMP by immunohistochemistry.

5.3.3. Classical Hodgkin's Disease

The Epstein–Barr virus is detectable in the neoplastic cells of approx 40% of cases of classical Hodgkin's disease *(135)*. The virus is commonly detected in cases of the mixed cellularity type, and may be detected by either *in situ* hybridization or EBV-LMP-1 immunohistochemistry.

6. FUTURE DIRECTIONS IN MOLECULAR DIAGNOSTICS OF HEMATOPOIETIC NEOPLASMS

The rapid expansion in new technologies for molecular analysis creates an overwhelming potential for future testing *(140)*. Only some of these potential methods will be summarized.

6.1. Protein Expression

The overexpression of some proteins resulting from molecular genetic gene fusions can be detected by immunohistochemistry *(141)*. Several examples of the use of aberrant protein expression have been described and include cyclin D1 protein in mantle cell lymphoma and ALK protein in anaplastic large cell lymphoma. These immunohistochemical tests are cost-effective and reliable surrogates for molecular events, and more examples of clinically useful immunohistochemical markers will become clear in the future. One example is the expression of TAL-1 protein as a marker of T-cell lymphoblastic leukemia and lymphoma.

6.2. Karyotype Analysis and FISH

Advances in FISH analysis should allow for the detection of lower levels of genetic abnormalities. In addition, spectral karyotyping (SKY), a method of specifically labeling all chromosomes in 24 colors for analysis, should increase the ability to identify translocations and other cryptic aberrations *(142)*.

Comparative genomic hybridization (CGH) is a research tool that evaluates the binding of tumor DNA to normal chromosomes to determine loss or gains of genetic material *(143)*. A similar technology employs CGH methods on DNA arrays. These methods allow for the evaluation of all areas of the genome, in contrast to only specific regions studied by PCR. The diagnostic applications of CGH are still unclear.

6.3. Gene Array Technology

Gene array analysis offers the ability to identify biologic disease subtypes that may correlate with prognosis and even response to specific chemotherapeutic agents. As mentioned previously, the early work using gene arrays in diffuse large B-cell lymphoma has identified prognostically significant subgroups *(108,109)* and there are similar studies using this methodology in acute leukemia *(144,145)*. The role of this methodology in diagnosis remains unclear, but these methods appear more suited to compliment existing diagnostic methods, rather than to replace them. The large amount of data that can be generated from these arrays also limits their use, and smaller, more specific arrays that are more disease specific may be needed before they come into routine use.

6.4. Quantitative PCR and RT-PCR

Because a variety of tumor-associated molecular genetic changes may remain at low levels after treatment without clinical relevance, the serial quantification of these signals may be of prognostic importance. Therefore, the various methods of "real-time," quantitative PCR are of interest *(146)*. This methodology is rapidly entering the diagnostic laboratory. One issue that relates to quantitative PCR that still needs to be resolved is consistency in reporting quantitative values between laboratories. In addition, clinical studies are needed for most diseases to determine the optimal timetable for residual disease testing as well as guidelines for the level of molecular disease that constitutes a significant risk for relapse. Such levels may vary by disease type. Such studies are underway and many of these questions should be resolved in the near future.

REFERENCES

1. Nowell PC. Hungerford DA. 1960. Minute chromosome in human chronic granulocytic leukemia. Science 132:1497.
2. Rowley JD. 1973. New consistent chromosomal abnormality in chronic myelogenous leukemia identified by quinacrine fluorescence and giemsa staining. Nature 243:290–293.
3. Seidman JG and Leder P. 1978. Arrangement and rearrangement of antibody genes. Nature 276:790–795.
4. Arnold A, Cossman J, Bakhshi A, Jaffe ES, Waldmann TA, Korsmeyer SJ. 1983. Immunoglobulin-gene rearrangements as unique clonal markers in human lymphoid neoplasms. N. Engl. J. Med. 309:1593–1599.
5. Pelz AF, Kroning H, Franke A, Wieacker P, Stumm M. 2002. High reliability and sensitivity of the BCR/ABL1 D-FISH test for the detection of BCR/ABL rearrangements. Ann. Hematol. 81:147–153.
6. Kurokawa T, Kinoshita T, Murate T, et al. 1997. Complementarity determining region-III is a useful molecular marker for the evaluation of minimal residual disease in mantle cell lymphoma. Br. J. Haematol. 98:408–412.
7. van Belzen N, Hupkes PE, Doekharan D, Hoogeveen-Westerveld M, Dorssers LCJ, van't Veer MB. 1997. Detection of minimal disease using rearranged immunoglobulin heavy chain genes from intermediate- and high-grade malignant B cell non-Hodgkin's lymphoma. Leukemia 11:1742–1752.
8. Donovan JW, Ladetto M, Zou G, et al. 2000. Immunoglobulin heavy-chain consensus probes for real-time PCR quantification of residual disease in acute lymphoblastic leukemia. Blood 95:2651–2658.
9. Harrison CJ. 2000. The management of patients with leukaemia: The role of cytogenetics in this molecular era. Br. J. Haematol. 108:19–30.
10. Crans HN and Sakamoto KM. 2001. Transcription factors and translocations in lymphoid and myeloid leukemia. Leukemia 15:313–331.
11. Scandura JM, Boccuni P, Cammenga J, Nimer SD. 2002. Transcription factor fusions in acute leukemia: variations on a theme. Oncogene 21:3422–3444.

12. Jaffe ES, Harris NL, Stein H, Vardiman JW. 2001. World Health Organization classification of tumours. Pathology and genetics of tumours of haematopoietic and lymphoid tissues. IARC Press: Lyon.

13. Grimwade D. 1999. The pathogenesis of acute promyelocytic leukaemia: evaluation of the role of molecular diagnosis and monitoring in the management of the disease. Br. J. Haematol. 106:591–613.

14. Gonzalez M, Barragan E, Bolufer P, et al, 2001. Pretreatment characteristics and clinical outcome of acute promyelocytic leukaemia patients according to the PML-RAR alpha isoforms: a study of the PETHEMA group. Br. J. Haematol. 114:99–103.

15. Miller WH, Levine K, DeBlasio A, Frankel SR, Dmitrovsky E, Warrell RP. 1993. Detection of minimal residual disease in acute promyelocytic leukemia by a reverse transcription polymerase chain reaction assay for the PML/RAR-alpha fusion mRNA. Blood 82:1689–1694.

16. Tobal K and Liu Yin JA. 1998. RT-PCR method with increased sensitivity shows persistence of PML-RARA fusion transcripts in patients in long-term remission of APL. Leukemia 12:1349–1354.

17. Zelent A, Guidez F, Melnick A, Waxman S, Licht JD. 2001.Translocations of the RAR alpha gene in acute promyelocytic leukemia. Oncogene 20:7186–7203.

18. Melnick A and Licht JD. 1999. Deconstructing a disease: RARa, its fusion partners, and their roles in the pathogenesis of acute promyelocytic leukemia. Blood 93:3167–3215.

19. Friedman AD. 1999. Leukemogenesis by CBF oncoproteins. Leukemia 13:1932–1942.

20. Dann EJ, Fears S, Arad-Dann H, Nucifora G, Rowley JD. 2000. Lineage specificity of CBFA2 fusion transcripts. Leuk. Res. 24:11–17.

21. Downing JR. 1999. The AML1-ETO chimaeric transcription factor in acute myeloid leukaemia: biology and clinical significance. Br. J. Haematol. 106:296–308.

22. Licht JD. 2001. AML1 and the AML1-ETO fusion protein in the pathogenesis of t(8;21) AML. Oncogene 20:5660–5679.

23. Liu PP, Hajra A, Wijmenga C, Collins FS. 1995. Molecular pathogenesis of the chromosome 16 inversion in th M4Eo subtype of acute myeloid leukemia. Blood 85: 2289–2302.

24. Higuchi M, O'Brien D, Kumaravelu P, Lenny N, Yeoh EJ, Downing JR. 2002. Expression of a conditional AML1-ETO oncogene bypasses embryonic lethality and establishes a murine model of human t(8;21) acute myeloid leukemia. Cancer Cell 1:63–74.

25. Jurlander J, Caligiuri MA, Ruutu T, et al. 1996. Persistence of the AML1/ETO fusion transcript in patients treated with allogeneic bone marrow transplantation for t(8;21) leukemia. Blood 88:2183–2191.

26. Tobal K, Johnson PR. Saunders MJ, Harrison CJ, Liu Yin JA. 1995. Detection of CBFB/MYH11 transcripts in patients with inversion and other abnormalities of chromosome 16 at presentation and remission. Br. J. Haematol. 91:104–108.

27. DiMartino JF and Cleary ML. 1999. MLL rearrangements in haematological malignancies: lessons from clincal and biological studies. Br. J. Haematol. 106:614–624.

28. Ayton PM and Cleary ML. 2001. Molecular mechanisms of leukemogenesis mediated by MLL fusion proteins. Oncogene 20:5695–5707.

29. Schnittger S, Kinkelin U, Schoch C, et al. 2000. Screening for MLL tandem duplication in 387 unselected patients with AML identify a prognostically unfavorable subset of AML. Leukemia 44:796–804.

30. Dohner K, Tobis K, Ulrich R, et al. 2002. Prognostic significance of partial tandem duplications of the MLL gene in adult patients 16 to 60 years old with acute myeloid leukemia and normal cytogenetics: A study of the acute myeloid leukemia study group Ulm. J. Clin. Oncol. 20: 3254–3261.

31. Rubnitz JE, Raimondi SC, Tong X, et al. 2002. Favorable impact of the t(9;11) in childhood acute myeloid leukemia. J. Clin. Oncol. 20:2302–2309.

32. Schnittger S, Wörmann B, Hiddemann W, Griesinger F. 1998. Partial tandem duplications of the MLL gene are detectable in peripheral blood and bone marrow of nearly all healthy donors. Blood 92:1728–1734.

33. Alsabeh R, Brynes RK, Slovak ML, Arber DA. 1997. Acute myeloid leukemia with t(6;9) (p23;q34). Association with myelodysplasia, basophilia, and initial CD34 negative immunophenotype. Am. J. Clin. Pathol. 107:430–437.

34. Gupta R, Knight CL, Bain BJ. 2002. Receptor tyrosine kinase mutations in myeloid neoplasms. Br. J. Haematol. 117:489–508.

35. Schnittger S, Schoch C, Dugas M, et al. 2002. Analysis of FLT3 length mutations in 1003 patients with acute myeloid leukemia: correlation to cytogenetics, FAB subtype, and prognosis in the AMLCG study and usefulness as a marker for the detection of minimal residual disease. Blood 100:59–66.

36. Kottaridis PD, Gale RE, Frew ME, et al. 2001. The presence of a FLT3 internal tandem duplication in patients with acute myeloid leukemia (AML) adds important prognostic information to cytogenetic risk group and response to the first cycle of chemotherapy: analysis of 854 patients from the United Kingdom Medical Research Council AML 10 and 12 trials. Blood 98: 1752–1759.

37. Stirewalt DL, Willman CL, Radich JP. 2001. Quantitative, real-time polymerase chain reactions for FLT3 internal tandem duplications are highly sensitive and specific. Leuk. Res. 25:1085–1088.

38. Melo JA. 1997. BCR-ABL gene variants. Baillieres Clin. Haematol. 10:203–222.

39. Advani AS and Pendergast AM. 2002. Bcr-Abl variants: biological and clinical aspects. Leuk. Res. 26:713–720.

40. Holyoake TL. 2001. Recent advances in the molecular and cellular biology of chronic myeloid leukaemia: lessons to be learned from the laboratory. Br. J. Haematol. 113:11–23.

41. Golub TR, Barker GF, Bohlander SK, et al. 1995. Fusion of the TEL gene on 12p13 to the AML1 gene on 21q22 in acute lymphoblastic leukemia. Proc. Natl. Acad. Sci. USA 92: 4917–4921.

42. Romana SP, Mauchauffe M, Le Coniat M, et al. 1995. The t(12;21) of acute lymphoblastic leukemia results in a tel-AML1 gene fusion. Blood 85:3662–3670.

43. Borkhardt A, Cazzaniga G, Viehmann S, et al. 1997. Incidence and clinical relevance of TEL/AML1 fusion genes in children with acute lymphoblastic leukemia enrolled in the German and Italian multicenter therapy trials. Blood 90:571–577.

44. Kempski H, Chalker J, Chessells J, et al. 1999. An investigation of the t(12;21) rearrangement in children with B-precursor acute lymphoblastic leukaemia using cytogenetic and molecular methods. Br. J. Haematol. 105:684–689.

45. Drunat S, Olivi M, Brunie G, et al. 2001. Quantification of TEL-AML1 transcript for minimal residual disease assessment in childhood acute lymphoblastic leukaemia. Br. J. Haematol. 114:281–289.

46. de Haas V, Breunis WB, Dee R, et al. 2002. The TEL-AML1 real-time quantitative polymerase chain reaction (PCR) might replace the antigen receptor-based genomic PCR in clinical minimal residual disease studies in children with acute lymphoblastic leukaemia. Br. J. Haematol. 116:87–93.

47. Khalidi HS, O'Donnell MR, Slovak ML, Arber DA. 1999. Adult precursor-B acute lymphoblastic leukemia with translocations involving chromosme band 19p13 is associated with poor prognosis. Cancer Genet. Cytogenet. 109:58–65.

48. Kee BL, Quong MW, Murre C. 2000. E2A proteins: essential regulators at multiple stages of B-cell development. Immunol. Rev. 175:138–149.

49. Aspland SE, Bendall HH, Murre C. 2001. The role of E2A-PBX1 in leukemogenesis. Oncogene 20:5708–5717.

50. Seidel MG and Look AT. 2001. E2A-HLF usurps control of evolutionarily conserved survival pathways. Oncogene 20:5718–5725.

51. Ishizawa S, Slovak ML, Popplewell L, et al. 2003. High frequency of pro-B acute lymphoblastic leukemia in adults with secondary leukemia with 11q23 abnormalities. Leukemia 6: 1091–1095.

52. Baranger L, Szapiro N, Gardais J, et al. 1994. Translocation t(5;12)(q31-q33;p12-p13): a non-random translocation associated with a myeloid disorder with eosinophilia. Br. J. Haematol. 88:343–347.

53. Golub TR, Barker GF, Lovett M, Gilliland DG. 1994. Fusion of PDGF receptor b to a novel ets-like gene, tel, in chronic myelomonocytic leukemia with t(5;12) chromosomal translocation. Cell 77:307–316.

54. Arber DA. 2000. Molecular diagnostic approach to non-Hodgkin's lymphoma. J. Mol. Diag. 2:178–190.

55. Korsmeyer SJ, Hieter PA, Revetch JV, Poplack DG, Waldmann TA, Leder P. 1981. Developmental hierarchy of immunoglobulin gene rearrangements in human leukemic pre-B-cells. Proc. Natl. Acad. Sci. USA 78:7096–7100.

56. Cossman J, Uppenkamp M, Sundeen J, Coupland R, Raffeld M. 1988. Molecular genetics and the diagnosis of lymphoma. Arch. Pathol. Lab. Med. 112:117–127.

57. Pascual V and Capra JD. 1991. Human immunoglobulin heavy-chain variable region genes: organization, polymorphism, and expression. Adv. Immunol. 49:1–74.

58. Segal GH, Jorgensen T, Masih AS, Braylan, RC. 1994. Optimal primer selection for clonality assessment by polymerase chain reaction analysis: I. Low grade B-cell lymphoproliferative disorders of nonfollicular center cell type. Hum. Pathol. 25:1269–1275.

59. Abdel-Reheim FA, Edwards E, Arber DA. 1996. Utility of a rapid polymerase chain reaction panel for the detection of molecular changes in B-cell lymphoma. Arch. Pathol. Lab. Med. 120:357–363.

60. Gong JZ, Zheng S, Chiarle R, et al. 1999. Detection of immnoglobulin k light chain rearrangements by polymerase chain reaction. An improved method for detecting clonal B-cell lymphoproliferative disorders. Am. J. Pathol. 155:355–363.

61. Seriu T, Hansen-Hagge TE, Stark Y, Bartram CR. 2000. Immunoglobulin k gene rearrangements between the k deleting element and Jk recombination signal sequences in acute lymphoblastic leukemia and normal hematopoiesis. Leukemia 14:671–674.

62. Dohner H. Stilgenbauer S, Benner A, et al. 2000. Genomic aberrations and survival in chronic lymphocytic leukemia. N. Engl. J. Med. 343:1910–1916.

63. Damle RN, Wasil T, Fais F, et al. 1999. Ig V gene mutation status and CD38 expression as novel prognostic indicators in chronic lymphocytic leukemia. Blood 94:1840–1847.

64. Hamblin TJ, Davis Z, Gardiner A, Oscier DG, Stevenson FK. 1999. Unmutated Ig V_H genes are associated with a more aggressive form of chronic lymphocytic leukemia. Blood 94:1848–1854.

65. Iida S, Rao PH, Nallasivam P, et al. 1996. The t(9;14)(p13;q32) chromosomal translocation associated with lymphoplasmacytoid lymphoma involves the *PAX-5* gene. Blood 88:4110–4117.

66. Hagman J, Wheat W, Fitzsimmons D, Hodsdon W, Negri J, Dizon F. 2000. Pax-5/BSAP: regulator of specific gene expression and differentiation in B lymphocytes. Curr. Top. Microbiol. Immunol. 245:169–194.

67. Morrison AM, Chott A, Schebesta M, Haas OA, Busslinger M. 1998. Deregulated *PAX-5* transcription from a translocated *IgH*promoter in marginal zone lymphoma. Blood 92:3865–3878.

68. Griffin CA, Zehnbauer BA, Beschorner WE, Ambinder R, Mann R. 1992. t(11;18)(q21;q21) is a recurrent chromosome abnormality in small lymphocytic lymphoma. Genes Chromosom. Cancer 4:153–157.

69. Auer IA, Gascoyne RD, Conners JM, et al. 1997. t(11;18)(q21;q21) is the most common translocation in MALT lymphomas. Ann. Oncol. 8:979–985.

70. Dierlamm J, Baens M, Wlodarska I, et al. 1999. The apoptosis inhibitor gene *API2* and a novel 18q gene, *MLT*, are recurrently rearranged in the t(11;18)(q21;q21) associated with mucosa-associated lymphoid tissue lymphomas. Blood 93:3601–3609.

71. Rosenwald A, Ott G, Stilgenbauer S, et al. 1999. Exclusive detection of the t(11;18)(q21;q21) in extranodal marginal zone B cell lymphomas (MZBL) of MALT type in contrast to other MZBL and extranodal large B cell lymphomas. Am. J. Pathol. 155:1817–1821.

72. Motegi M, Yonezumi M, Suzuki H, et al. 2000. API2-MALT1 chimeric transcripts involved in mucosa-associated lymphoid tissue type lymphoma predict heterogeneous products. Am. J. Pathol. 156:807–812.

73. Remstein ED, James CD, Kurtin PJ. 2000. Incidence and subtype specificity of *API2-MALT1* fusion translocations in extranodal, nodal, and splenic marginal zone lymphomas. Am. J. Pathol. 156:1183–1188.

74. Baens M, Maes B, Steyls A, Geboes K, Marynen P, De Wolf-Peeters C. 2000. The product of the t(11;18), an API2-MLT fusion, marks nearly half of gastric MALT type lymphomas without large cell proliferation. Am. J. Pathol. 156:1433–1439.

75. Du MQ, Dogan A, Liu H, et al. 2001. MALT lymphoma with t(11;18)(q21; q21) expresses nuclear bcl10 and fails to respond to *H. pylori* eradicaton therapy. Mod. Pathol. 14:161A.

76. Segal GH, Jorgensen T, Scott M, Braylan RC. 1994. Optimal primer selection for clonality assessment by polymerase chain reaction analysis: II. Follicular lymphomas. Hum. Pathol. 25:1276–1282.

77. Ashton-Key M, Diss TC, Isaacson PG, Smith MEF. 1995. A comparative study of the value of immunohistochemistry and the polymerase chain reaction in the diagnosis of follicular lymphoma. Histopathology 27:501–508.

78. Weiss LM, Warnke RA, Sklar J, Cleary ML. 1987. Molecular analysis of the t(14;18) chromosomal translocation in malignant lymphomas. N. Engl. J. Med. 317:1185–1189.

79. Turner GE, Ross FM, Krajewski AS. 1995. Detection of t(14;18) in British follicular lymphoma using cytogenetics, Southern blotting and polymerase chain reaction. Br. J. Haematol. 89:223–225.

80. Ladanyi M and Wang S. 1992. Detection of rearrangements of the BCL2 major breakpoint region in follicular lymphomas. Correlation of polymerase chain reaction results with Southern blot analysis. Diagn. Mol. Pathol. 1:31–35.

81. Ngan BY, Nourse J, Cleary ML. 1989. Detection of chromosomal translocation t(14;18) within the minor cluster region of *bcl-2* by polymerase chain reaction and direct genomic sequencing of the enzymatically amplified DNA in follicular lymphomas. Blood 7:1759–1762.

82. Liu J, Johnson RM, Traweek ST. 1993. Rearrangement of the BCL-2 gene in follicular lymphoma. Detection by PCR in both fresh and fixed tissue samples. Diagn. Mol. Pathol. 2:241–247.

83. Buchonnet G, Jardin F, Jean N, et al. 2002. Distribution of BCL2 breakpoints in follicular lymphoma and correlation with clinical features: specific subtypes or same disease? Leukemia 16:1852–1856.

84. Wang YL, Addya K, Edwards RH, et al. 1998. Novel *bcl-2* breakpoints in patients with follicular lymphoma. Diagn. Mol. Pathol. 7:85–89.

85. Limpens J, de Jong D, van Krieken JHJM, et al. 1991. *Bcl-2/JH* rearrangements in benign lymphoid tissues with follicular hyperplasia. Oncogene 6:2271–2276.

86. Ohshima K., Masahiro K, Kobari S, Masuda Y, Eguchi F, Kimura N. 1993. Amplified bcl-2/JH rearrangements in reactive lymphadenopathy. Virchows Arch. B 63:197–198.

87. Limpens J, Stad R. Vos C, et al. 1995. Lymphoma-assocaited translocation t(14;18) in blood B cells of normal individuals. Blood 85:2528–2536.

88. Segal GH, Scott M, Jorgensen T, and Braylan RC. 1994. Standard polymerase chain reaction analysis does not detect t(14;18) in reactive lymphoid hyperplasia. Arch. Pathol. Lab. Med 118:791–794.

89. Rosenberg CL, Wong E, Petty EM, et al. 1991. *PRAD1*, a candidate *BCL1* oncogene: mapping and expression in centrocytic lymphoma. Proc. Natl. Acad. Sci. USA 88:9638–9642.

90. Rimokh R, Berger F, Delsol G, et al. 1994. Detection of the chromosomal translocation t(11;14) by polymerase chain reaction in mantle cell lymphomas. Blood 83:1871–1875.

91. Raynaud SD, Bekri S, Leroux D, et al. 1993. Expanded range of 11q23 breakpoints with differeng patterns of cyclin D1 expression in B-cell malignancies. Genes Chromosom. Cancer 8:80–87.

92. de Boer CJ, van Krieken JHJM, Kluin-Nelemans HC, Kluin PM, Schuuring E. 1995. Cyclin D1 messenger RNA overexpression as a marker of mantle cell lymphoma. Oncogene 10: 1833–1840.

93. Ives Aguilera NS, Bijwaard KE, Duncan B, et al. 1998. Differential expression of cyclin D1 in mantle cell lymphoma and other non-Hodgkin's lymphomas. Am. J. Pathol. 153:1969–1976.

94. Bosch F, Jares P, Campo E, Lopez-Guillermo A, Piris MA, Villamor N, et al. 1994. *PRAD-1/ cyclin D1* gene overexpression in chronic lymphoproliferative disorders: a highly specific marker of mantle cell lymphoma. Blood 84:2726–2732.

95. Bosch F, Campo E, Jares P, et al. 1995. Increased expression of the *PRAD-1/CCND1* gene in hairy cell leukaemia. Br. J. Haematol. 91:1025–1030.

96. Li JY, Gaillard F, Moreau A, et al. 1999. Detection of translocation t(11;14)(q13;q32) in mantle cell lymphoma by fluorescence *in situ* hybridization. Am. J. Pathol. 154:1449–1452.

97. Lipford E, Wright JJ, Urba W, et al. 1987. Refinement of lymphoma cytogenetics by the chromosme 18q21 major breakpoint region. Blood 70:1816–1823.

98. Yunis JJ, Mayer MG, Arnesen MA, Aeppli DP, Oken, MM, Frizzera, G. 1989. *bcl-2* and other genomic alterations in the prognosis of large-cell lymphoma. N. Engl. J. Med. 320:1047–1054.

99. Hill ME, MacLennan KA, Cunningham DC, et al. 1996. Prognostic significance of BCL-2 expression and BCL-2 major breakpoint region rearrangement in diffuse large cell non-Hodgkin's lymphoma: a British National Lymphoma Investigation study. Blood 88:1046–1051.

100. Bastard C, Tilly H, Lenormand B, et al. 1992. Translocations involving band 3q27 and Ig gene regions in non-Hodgkin's lymphoma. Blood 79:2527–2531.

101. Ye BH, Lista F, Lo Coco F, et al. 1993. Alterations of a zinc finger-encoding gene, *BCL-6*, in diffuse large-cell lymphoma. Science 262:747–750.

102. Lo Coco F, Ye BH, Lista, F, et al. 1994. Rearrangements fo the *BCL6* gene in diffues large cell non-Hodgkin's lymphoma. Blood 83:1757–1759.

103. Muramatsu M, Akasaka T, Kadowaki N, et al. 1996. Rearrangement of the *BCL6* gene in B-cell lymphoid neoplasms: comparison with lymphomas associated with *BCL2* rearrangement. Br. J. Haematol. 93:911–920.

104. Kawamata N, Nakamura Y, Miki T, et al. 1998. Detection of chimaeric transcripts of the IgH and BCL6 genes by reverse-transcriptase polymerase chain reaction in B-cell non-Hodgkin's lymphomas. Br. J. Haematol. 100:484–489.

105. Bastard C, Deweindt C, Kerckaert JP, et al. 1994. *LAZ3* rearrangements in non-Hodgkin 's lymphoma: correlation with histology, immunophenotype, karyotype, and clinical outcome in 217 patients. Blood 83:2423–2427.

106. Peng HZ, Du MQ, Koulis A, et al. 1999. Nonimmunoglobulin gene hypermutation in germinal center B cells. Blood 93:2167–2172.

107. Lossos IS, Jones CD, Warnke R, et al. 2001. Expression of a single gene, BCL-6, strongly predicts survival in patients with diffuse large B-cell lymphoma. Blood 98:945–951.

108. Alizadeh AA, Eisen MB, Davis RE, et al. 2000. Distinct types of diffuse large B-cell lymphoma identified by gene expression profiling. Nature 403:503–511.

109. Rosenwald A, Wright G, Chan WC, et al. 2002. The use of molecular profiling to predict survival after chemotherapy for diffuse large-B-cell lymphoma. N. Engl. J. Med. 346:1937–1947.

110. Dalla-Favera R, Bregni M, Erikson J, Patterson D, Gallo RC, Croce CM. 1982. Human *c-myc onc* gene is located on the region of chromosome 8 that is translcoated in Burkitt lymphoma cells. Proc. Natl. Acad. Sci. USA 79:7824–7827.

111. Yano T, van Krieken JHJM, Magrath IT, Longo DL, Jaffe ES, Raffeld M. 1992. Histogenetic correlations between subcategories of small noncleaved cell lymphomas. Blood 79:1282–1290.

112. Battey J, Moulding C, Taub R, et al. 1983. The human *c-myc* oncogene: structural consequences of translocation into the *IgH* locus in Burkitt lymphoma. Cell 34:779–787.

113. Pelicci PG, Knowles DM, Magrath I, Dalla-Favera R. 1986. Chromosomal breakpoints and structural alterations of the *c-myc* locus differ in endemic and sporadic forms of Burkitt lymphoma. Proc. Natl. Acad. Sci. USA 83:2984–2988.

114. Neri A, Barriga F, Knowles DM, Magrath IT, Dalla-Favera R. 1988. Different regions of the immunoglobulin heavy-chain locus are involved in chromosomal translocations in distinct pathogenetic forms of Burkitt lymphoma. Proc. Natl. Acad. Sci. USA 85:2748–2752.

115. Joos S, Falk MH, Lichter P, et al. 1992. Variable breakpoints in Burkitt lymphoma cells with chromosmal t(8;14) translocation separate *c-myc* and the *IgH* locus up to several hundred kb. Hum. Mol. Genet. 1:625–632.

116. de Villartay JP, Hockett RD, Coran D, Korsmeyer SJ, Cohen DI. 1988. Deletion of the human T-cell receptor d-gene by a site-specific recombination. Nature 335:170–174.

117. de Villartay JP, Pullman AB, Andrade R, et al. 1989. g/d lineage relationship within a consecutive series of human precursor T-cell neoplasms. Blood 74:2508–2518.

118. Zemlin M, Hummel M, Anagnostopoulos I, Stein H. 1998. Improved polymerase chain reaction detection of clonally rearranged T-cell receptor b chain genes. Diagn. Mol. Pathol. 7:138–145.

119. Greiner TC, RaffeldM, Lutz C, Dick F, Jaffe ES. 1995. Analysis of T cell receptor-g gene rearrangements by denaturing gradient gel electrophoresis of GC-clamped polymerase chain reaction products. Correlation with tumor-specific sequences. Am. J. Pathol. 146:46–55.

120. Theodorou J, Bigorgne C, Delfau MH, et al. 1996. VJ rearrangements of the TCRg locus in peripheral T-cell lymphomas: analysis by polymerase chain reaction and denaturing gradient gel electrophoresis. J. Pathol. 178:303–310.

121. Greiner TC and Rubocki RJ. 2002. Effectiveness of capillary electrophoresis using fluorescent-labeled primers in detecting T-cell receptor gamma gene rearrangements. J. Mol. Diagn. 4: 137–143.

122. Harris NL, Jaffe ES, Stein H, et al. 1994. A revised European-American classification of lymphoid neoplasms: a proposal from the International Lymphoma Study Group. Blood 84:1361–1392.

123. Le Beau MM, Bitter MA, Larson RA, et al. 1989. The t(2;5)(p23;q35): a recurring chromosomal abnormality in Ki-1 positive anaplastic large cell lymphoma. Leukemia 3:866–870.

124. Morris SW, Kirstein MN, Valentine MB, et al. 1994. Fusion of a kinase gene, *ALK,* to a nucleolar protein gene, *NPM,* in non-Hodgkin's lymphoma. Science 263:1281–1284.

125. Drexler HG, Gignac SM, von Wasielewski R, Werner M, Dirks WG. 2000. Pathobiology of NPM-ALK and variant fusion genes in anaplastic large cell lymphoma and other lymphomas. Leukemia 14:1533–1559.

126. Kutok JL and Aster JC. 2002. Molecular biology of anaplastic lymphoma kinase-positive anaplastic large-cell lymphoma. J. Clin. Oncol. 20:3691–3702.

127. Ladanyi M, Cavalchire G, Morris SW, Downing J, Filippa DA. 1994. Reverse transcriptase polymerase chain reaction for the Ki-1 anaplastic large cell lymphoma-associated t(2;5) translocation in Hodgkin's disease. Am. J. Pathol. 145:1296–1300.

128. Cataldo KA, Jalal SM, Law ME, et al. 1999. Detection of t(2;5) in anaplastic large cell lymphoma: comparison of immunohistochemical studies, FISH, and RT-PCR in paraffin-embedded tissue. Am. J. Surg. Pathol. 23:1386–1392.

129. Pulford K, Lamant L, Morris SW, et al. 1997. Detection of anaplastic lymphoma kinase (ALK) and nucleolar protein nucleophosmin (NPM)-ALK in normal and neoplastic cells with the nonclonal antibody ALK1. Blood 89:1394–1404.

130. Gascoyne RD, Aoun P, Wu D, et al. 1999. Prognostic significance of anaplastic lymphoma kinase (ALK) protein expression in adults with anaplastic large cell lymphoma. Blood 93: 3913–3921.

131. Rosenwald A, Ott G, Pulford K, et al. 1999. t(1;2)(q21;p23) and t(2;3)(p23;q21): two novel variant translocations of the t(2;5)(p23;q35) in anaplastic large cell lymphoma. Blood 94: 362–364.

132. Falini B, Pulford K, Pucciarini A, et al. 1999. Lymphomas expressing ALK fusion protein(s) other than NPM-ALK. Blood 94:3509–3515.

133. Brito-Babapulle V, Pomfret M, Matutes E, Catovsky, D. 1987. Cytogenetic studies on prolymphocytic leukemia. II. T cell prolymphocytic leukemia. Blood 70:926–931.

134. Jonveaux P, Daniel MT, Martel V, Maarek O, Berger R. 1996. Isochromosome 7q and trisomy 8 are consistent primary, non-random chromosomal abnormalities associated with hepatosplenic T y/d lymphoma. Leukemia 10:1453–1455.

135. Weiss LM and Chang KL. 1996. Association of the Epstein-Barr virus with hematolymphoid neoplasia. Adv. Anatom. Pathol. 3:1–15.

136. Cohen JI. 2000. Epstein-Barr virus infection. N. Engl. J. Med. 7:481–492.

137. Lai R and Weiss LM. 1998. Hepatitis C virus and non-Hodgkin's lymphoma. Am. J. Clin. Pathol. 109:508–510.

138. Dupin N, Fisher A, Kellam P, et al. 1999. Distribution of human herpesvirus-8 latently infected cells in Kaposi's sarcoma, multicentric Castleman's disease, and primary effusion lymphoma. Proc. Natl. Acad. Sci. USA 96:4546–4551.

139. Minamoto GY, Gold JWM, Scheinberg DA, et al. 1988. Infection with human T-cell leukemia virus type I in patients with leukemia. N. Engl. J. Med. 318:219–222.

140. Going JJ and Gusterson BA. 1999. Molecular pathology and future developments. Eur. J. Cancer 35:1895–1904.

141. Falini B and Mason DY. 2002. Proteins encoded by genes involved in chromosomal alterations in lymphoma and leukemia: clinical value of their detection by immunocytochemistry. Blood 99:409–426.

142. Bayani JM and Squire JA. 2002. Applications of SKY in cancer cytogenetics. Cancer Investigation 20:373–386.

143. Zitzelsberger H, Lehmann L, Werner M, Bauchinger M. 1997. Comparative genomic hybridisation for the analysis of chromosomal imbalances in solid tumours and haematological malignancies. Histochem. Cell Biol. 108:403–417.

144. Yeoh EJ, Ross ME, Shurtleff SA, et al. 2002. Classification, subtype discovery, and prediction of outcome in pediatric acute lymphoblastic leukemia by gene expression profiling. Cancer Cell 1:133–143.

145. Ferrando AA, Neuberg DS, Staunton J, et al. 2002. Gene expression signatures define novel oncogenic pathways in T cell acute lymphoblastic leukemia. Cancer Cell 1:75–87.

146. Bernard PS and Wittwer CT. 2002. Real-time PCR technology for cancer diagnostics. Clin. Chem. 48:1178–1185.

13

HER2 and Topoisomerase IIα in Breast Carcinoma

Kenneth J. Bloom

1. INTRODUCTION

In order for the human breast to develop and function appropriately, the cells of the breast must communicate with each other in a precise and coordinated fashion. A major mechanism of communication is signal transduction; a process where external signaling molecules, or ligands, alter the behavior of a cell by affecting the transcription of various genes. Behavior of the cell is modified primarily by phosphorylating or dephosphorylating a series of transmembrane, intracellular, and adaptor proteins possessing enzymatic activity. The enzymatic activity of one protein turns on the enzymatic activity of the next protein in the pathway resulting in signal propagation *(1)*. Not all proteins are capable of interacting directly with each other, therefore adaptor proteins may be necessary to serve as a bridge. Signal transduction molecules include Shk adaptor proteins, which when phosphorylated, create docking sites for SH-2 domain containing molecules, such as, Grb2, PLC-γ, STAT, and focal adhesion kinases.

When the amino acid tyrosine serves as the substrate for phosphorylation, the resulting protein is known as a tyrosine kinase. There are approx 100 known protein tyrosine kinase genes, 58 of which encode transmembrane receptors (RTK) *(2,3)*. All RTKs have a common structure consisting of an extracellular binding domain, a transmembrane α-helix and an intracellular domain, which possesses intrinsic tyrosine kinase activity. RTKs show diversity, predominantly in their external binding domains and can be categorized into 20 subfamilies. One of these families, the epidermal growth factor receptor (EGFR) family, is composed of EGFR, human epidermal growth factor receptor 2 (HER2), HER3, and HER4 *(4,5)*.

1.1. HER2 Signaling

Three things are necessary to elicit a signal from the EGFR family of receptors: a ligand, a receptor, and a dimerization partner *(6,7)*. Ligands of the EGFR family include EGF, TGF-α, and amphiregulin, which are specific for EGFR, heparin-binding EGF, epiregulin, and betacellulin, binding EGFR and HER4, and the neuregulins, which bind HER3 and HER4 *(8)*. There are no known ligands for HER2. After a ligand binds to a receptor, that receptor must dimerize with another member of the EGFR family to trigger phosphorylation. It may dimerize with a like member of the family, which is known as homodimerization, or it may dimerize with a different member of the family, which is known as heterodimerization *(9,10)*.

From: *Cancer Diagnostics: Current and Future Trends*
Edited by: R. M. Nakamura, W. W. Grody, J. T. Wu, and R. B. Nagle © Humana Press Inc., Totowa, NJ

When HER2 is available, it is the preferred dimerization partner of the other family members *(11)*. Moreover, HER2 heterodimers are stable and their signals are more potent than other receptor combinations *(1,7)*. The specific tyrosine residue on the intracellular portion of the phosphorylated receptor depends on the combination of ligand and dimer pair *(12)*. Because there are four family members, ten dimer pair combinations are possible. Significant intracellular crosstalk with other signaling pathways and the variety of different ligands allow for significant diversity in signaling. Major pathways activated include the Ras/MAPK pathway, PI3K/Akt pathway, STAT pathway and PLC-γ pathway *(13–15)*. The end result is induction of the activated cell to proliferate, survive, gain increased motility, and induce growth of new blood vessels.

Factors that influence the ability of a signal to induce changes in a target cell include the strength and length of time the signal stays activated before it is turned off. Not all ligand–dimer pair combinations show the same ability to propagate an intracellular signal. For example, the signaling strength of a HER2/HER3 dimer activated by heregulin is significantly stronger than that activated by EGF *(16)*. Signaling is eventually inactivated by endocytosis *(17)*. The receptor remains transiently activated after endocytosis, although the specific pathway activated may change once the receptor loses its association with the membrane. The process of endocytosis varies depending on the ligand, dimerization pair, and cellular pH. EGF occupied homodimers are rapidly endocytosed and undergo lysosomal degradation, thus terminating the signal. In contrast, EGF heterodimers containing HER2 show enhanced signaling as EGF is dissociated from the receptor in the early endosomes, allowing the receptor to recycle back to the cell surface.

1.2. HER2 Distribution

The 185 KD HER2 protein is encoded by the HER2 gene located on chromosome 17q *(4,18)*. This gene shares homology to the rat gene *neu* and is thus sometimes referred to as HER-2/neu *(19)*. In breast carcinoma, there is a tight association between the number of copies of the HER2 gene, the amount of HER2 mRNA and the number of HER2 receptors *(20–23)*. Occasional tumors may show an increased number of receptors with a normal complement of HER2 genes, the purported single copy over-expressers. It has been suggested that many of these tumors represent stromal rich carcinomas and that the stromal elements dilute the determination of the HER2 gene copy number. Although this may be true for determinations performed by Southern Blot, it should not be a factor in the determination of gene copy number by fluorescent *in situ* hybridization (FISH) analysis.

Limited studies have looked at the distribution of the EGFR family and few have specifically addressed the distribution of HER2 protein. Scanning laser microscopy has shown that HER2 protein is randomly distributed along the cell membrane, although there is a preference towards the basal and lateral portions of the cell. The HER2 molecules cluster in groups of approx 1000 receptors that increase in size as protein synthesis is upregulated *(24)*. Eventually, these clusters coalesce and give the appearance of complete membrane staining with an anti-HER2 antibody. There are approx 20,000 HER2 receptors expressed on the surface of benign breast epithelial cells, but the absolute number varies with age and menstrual status as well as a number of less well-defined factors *(25)*. Most breast carcinomas express more receptors than benign breast epithelial cells *(26)*. HER2 protein is synthesized and transported in the cytoplasm and after activation, is degraded through a process of endocytosis. Therefore, it is not unusual to find evidence of HER2 in the cytoplasm of tumor cells.

2. TESTING METHODS

2.1. Protein Overexpression

Robertson et al. attempted to define the range of HER2 expression in breast tissue by evaluating expression as a continuous variable in 123 invasive breast carcinomas utilizing radioimmunohistochemistry (rIHC) *(27)*. BT474 cells, which express 730,000 receptors, were also radiolabeled and used as a control along with nine reduction mammoplasty specimens. The staining intensity of cells obtained from the reduction mammoplasty specimens ranged from 1.4% to 4.2% (10,220–30,600 receptors) of the BT474 control cell line, with a mean of 2.7% (17,520 receptors). Ninety-one percent of the carcinomas overexpressed HER2 protein relative to the mammoplasty specimens and showed a bimodal distribution, with one peak ranging up to 332,880 receptors and the second peak beginning at 770,880 receptors. Five percent of the cases underexpressed HER2 protein.

Eppenberger-Castori et al. evaluated the expression of HER2 protein as a continuous variable in 3208 fresh/frozen invasive breast carcinomas by enzyme immunoassay using cytosol preparations. A bimodal distribution pattern was observed, although significant overlap was present between the two peaks *(28)*.

Bloom et al. evaluated the immunohistochemical expression of HER2 protein as a continuous variable in 500 consecutive cases of invasive breast cancer utilizing the HercepTest™ kit and image analysis *(29)*. The intensity of HER2 expression was determined from immunostained slides by assessing six distinct regions of tumor and then calculating the average staining intensity. When plotted as a continuous variable the average staining intensity revealed a bimodal distribution with all tumors in the second peak revealing amplification of the HER2 gene. The consistency of this bimodal distribution pattern can be used to validate assays that assess HER2 protein expression.

2.1.1. Biology of HER2 Overexpression

Differences in the definition of HER2 overexpression have plagued the literature. When overexpression is defined as an increased number of HER2 receptors compared to normal breast epithelial cells, most breast carcinomas are classified as showing overexpression. In practice, overexpression has been assessed by immunohistochemistry. The large variety of antibodies, fixation methods, antigen retrieval techniques, and scoring systems have all contributed to the lack of a standardized definition of HER overexpression. The advent of trastuzumab necessitated the development of a standardized assay so that patients could enroll in clinical trials. Preclinical data had suggested that only tumor cells expressing more than several hundred thousand HER2 receptors respond to trastuzumab.

The number of HER2 receptors on a cell's surface is dependent on the balance of protein synthesis vs destruction. Gene amplification is the most common mechanism of increased protein synthesis in breast carcinomas but other mechanisms, including posttranscriptional events, reduced destruction of receptors, increased recycling of receptors to the cell surface, and receptor mutations are possible. Unlike EGFR, in which constitutively activated mutations are common, no known mutations of HER2 exist in humans *(5)*. Data on posttranscriptional factors is limited. Tubbs et al. studied a series of 144 formalin-fixed paraffin-embedded (FFPE) invasive breast carcinomas and could not identify increased mRNA in tumors showing significant overexpression by IHC without amplification of the HER2 gene *(30)*. Slamon et al. also assessed the relationship between HER2 gene amplification, mRNA expression, and protein expression on a series of invasive breast carcinomas *(22)*. All testing was performed on well-preserved frozen tumor samples in which DNA, mRNA, and protein were all optimally preserved. Approximately 97% of the cases demonstrated a direct relationship between the level of HER2 gene amplification (assessed by Southern blot), the expression of HER2 mRNA (assessed by Northern blot) and the expression of HER2 protein (assessed by Western blot and immunohistochemistry). However, 3% of the tumors showed markedly increased expression of HER2 mRNA and protein despite a normal complement of HER2 genes. The difference between these two studies may be related to the use of FFPE rather than frozen tissue, or the determination of gene amplification by FISH analysis rather than Southern blot.

2.1.2. Immunohistochemistry

Most immunohistochemical stains routinely performed in clinical practice are qualitative, meaning they are performed to detect the presence or absence of a specific protein. Because the goal is merely detection, it is common to vary the conditions of the assay, such as the concentration of antibody, time of incubation, and antigen retrieval method, in order to enhance staining. HER2 is expressed on all breast carcinoma cells, therefore a qualitative HER2 assay is unwarranted. Instead, a quantitative assay that correlates the pattern and intensity of immunostaining with the number of HER2 receptors is required. To achieve this goal, a standardized assay in terms of tissue handling, antibody, reagents, conditions, antigen retrieval method, and scoring was developed.

2.1.2.1. STANDARDIZING THE IHC ASSAY

The original trastuzumab clinical trials used an IHC method to screen a large number of FFPE tissue blocks to select appropriate patients. This assay, known as the clinical trial assay (CTA), was a labor-intensive IHC assay that initially used an antibody directed against the same extracellular domain epitope as trastuzumab, known as 4D5. However, the antibody was switched during the study to CB11, which is directed against an epitope on the intracellular domain of HER2. The CTA also defined a scoring system to semiquantitatively assess the immunohistochemical stain that ranged from 0 to 3+, and only patients whose tumors were scored as 2+ or 3+ were enrolled in the clinical trials. Cell-line data helped define the relationship between the number of HER2 receptors and the IHC staining pattern (Table 1). Although all of the samples in the original clinical trials were paraffin-embedded, the specific fixative used length of fixation. Storage condition of the tissue blocks was largely unknown.

The results of the clinical trials allowed trastuzumab to receive FDA approval; however, the FDA required that prior to treatment, the patient's tumor be tested for overexpression of HER2 protein. A commercial standardized immunohistochemical assay known as HercepTest™ was approved explicitly for this purpose. The intent of the HercepTest™ kit was to create a reproducible, easy to perform assay that would mirror the CTA. Standardization is the key attribute of the HercepTest™ kit. The assay specifies pre-analytic issues such as the fixative, the length of fixation, the antigen retrieval method, a predilute polyclonal antibody with all of its epitopes located on the intracellular domain of HER2, and the scoring method.

The HercepTest™ scoring system is identical to that created to assign eligibility for the trastuzumab clinical trials (Fig. 1). It looks at the completeness and intensity of the membrane stain. A score of zero shows no appreciable membrane staining or light partial staining in less than 10% of the cells; a score of 1+ shows light partial membrane staining in more

Table 1
Correlation of HER-2 Receptors and Amplification Status

IHC score	Assessment	Cell line	Pattern	Number of receptors	Gene copies
0	Neg	MDA-231	No staining or membrane staining in less than 10% of the tumor cells	21,600 ± 6,700	2.4 ± 0.2
1	Neg	MDA-175	Faint or barely perceptible partial membrane staining in more than 10% of tumor cells	92,400 ± 12,000	3.0 ± 0.4
2	Pos	MDA-361	Weak to moderate complete membrane staining in more than 10% of tumor cells	500,000 ± 100,000	
3	Pos	SK-BR-3	Strong complete membrane staining in more than 10% of tumor cells	2,390,000 ± 130,000	15.3 ± 3.9

than 10% of the cells. Complete membrane staining, if present, is not seen in more than 10% of the cells; a score of 2+ shows light to moderate complete membrane staining in more than 10% of the cells and a score of 3+ shows strong complete membrane staining in more than 10% of the tumor cells.

Initially, the HercepTest™ kit created a lot of controversy with reports stating that the kit was too sensitive or not sensitive enough *(31)*. Unfortunately, the majority of these studies changed the conditions specified in the kit, most commonly by changing the fixative and/or the antigen retrieval method *(32)*. Use of alcohol based fixatives or microwave-antigen retrieval have both been associated with significantly amplifying the strength of the HER2 immunostain leading to frequent false positive results. In a study of different HER2 antibodies, Press et al. reported a significant variation in detection rates by IHC using a large tissue block containing multiple breast tumors *(33)*.

Data from the NSABP B31 study highlights some of the problems in clinical practice *(34)*. The B31 trial is comparing adjuvant chemotherapy versus adjuvant chemotherapy plus trastuzumab in patients whose tumor showed 3+ overexpression of HER2 by IHC or amplification of the HER2 gene. Review of the first 104 specimens enrolled in the trial revealed significant discrepancies between the assessment at the submitting laboratory and reanalysis at the central NSABP laboratory. Large volume laboratories that used the HercepTest™ kit showed 96% concordance; smaller laboratories, however, achieved only 81% concordance

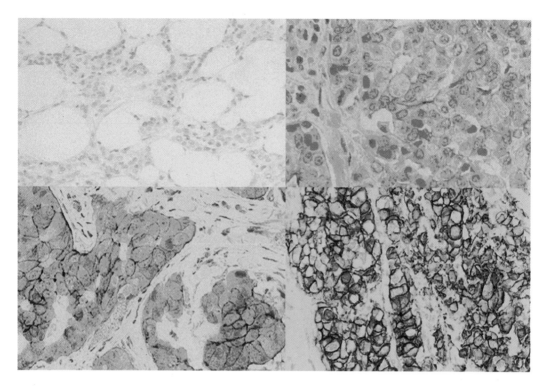

Fig. 1. Examples of breast carcinomas stained with the HercepTest™ kit. *Top left*, 0+; no appreciable membrane staining is seen. *Top right*, 1+; partial membrane staining is seen in more than 10% of the invasive tumor cells. No complete membrane staining is noted. *Bottom left*, 2+; moderate membrane staining is seen with complete membrane staining in more than 10% of the invasive tumor cells. Note the visible nucleoli. *Bottom left*, 3+; strong complete membrane staining is seen in almost all of the invasive tumor cells.

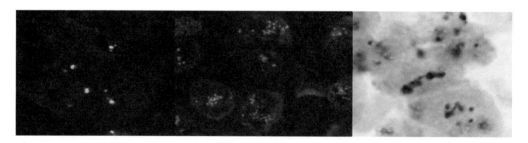

Fig. 2. Examples of *in situ* hybridization. The image on the left shows a breast carcinoma without evidence of HER2 gene amplification. The red signal represents the HER2 gene and the green signal represents a centromere probe to chromosome 17. There are equal numbers of HER2 and chromosome 17 signals. The middle image reveals numerous red signals representing amplification of the HER2 gene. Two copies of chromosome 17 (green signals) are seen in most cells. The image on the right is an example of chromogenic *in situ* hybridization. The increase number of signals represents amplification of the HER2 gene.

and those laboratories not using HercepTest™ or CB11 showed only 50% concordance. Following these results, the NSABP required that submitted blocks be tested in certified laboratories, either large volume laboratories, or laboratories showing strong concordance between their IHC results and FISH results. Additional testing of 240 blocks at the certified laboratories revealed 98% concordance. Most of the certified laboratories were reference laboratories that cannot control tissue fixation or storage, it has therefore been suggested that preanalytical issues may not be a major cause of interlaboratory variability (at least in cases assessed as 3+). Results from the United Kingdom National External Quality Assessment Scheme for Immunohistochemistry (UK NEQAS-ICC) also suggested that the lack of reproducibility of HER2 scoring between laboratories is likely not the result of tumor heterogeneity or preanalytic issues but rather the result of how the scoring system is applied *(35)*.

Although tumors assessed as 3+ by an experienced laboratory will likely have amplification of the HER2 gene, it is less clear that tumors assessed as 0 or 1+ will lack gene amplification. Mass et al. analyzed a subset of 0 and 1+ tumors for the presence of HER2 gene amplification and found that 7 of 207 (3%) tumors assessed as 0+ and 2 of 28 (7%) tumors assessed as 1+ were amplified by FISH *(36)*. How this relates to current IHC testing is unclear, because the CTA is no longer used and all testing was performed on archival specimens with unknown fixation and storage conditions. Bloom et al., prospectively studied 175 consecutive invasive breast carcinomas scored as 0 or 1+ with the HercepTest™ kit and showed that 4 of the 175 (2.4%) tumors showed amplification of the HER2 gene *(37)*. However, all four cases showed only borderline amplification and three of the four cases were assessed as 1+/2+ showing moderate to strong immunostaining in the majority of the tumor cells but failed to show complete membrane staining in more than 10% of cells. LeBeau showed 0 of 22 (0%); Couturier, 1 of 88 (1.1%); Jimenez, 0 of 21 (0%); Ridolfi, 1 of 56 (1.8%); and Tsuda, 0 of 165 (0%) tumors scored as 0 or 1+ with the HercepTest™ kit when amplified by FISH *(38–42)*.

2.1.2.2. IHC Scoring Methods

Initially, the HercepTest™ scoring system seems straightforward but many of the terms are ambiguous and have caused confusion. The assessment of signal strength as weak to moderate, or strong is the only difference between a 2+ and 3+ score. Similarly, determining if circumferential staining is present in 10% of the tumor cells is subject to observer variation. HER2 expression, when present, is preferentially located to the basal and lateral aspect of the cell, therefore if a cell is cut tangentially it may give the appearance of circumferential staining. To achieve better correlation with gene amplification, most pathologists now require strong, complete membrane staining in the majority of the invasive tumor cells before scoring an IHC stain as 3+.

2.1.2.3. Pathologists' Interpretation

Before assessing a HER2 immunostain, the pathologist should perform a standard checklist including:

1. Are the pre-analytical conditions of the assay met?
2. Is a validated assay used?
3. Is the positive control positive?
4. Is the negative control negative?
5. Is there no significant staining in normal ductal or lobular units?

Table 2
Correlation Between IHC and FISH Based on Method of IHC Scoring

Path	1	2	3	4	5	6	7	8	9	10
Manual	42%	61%	59%	83%	64%	65%	92%	76%	88%	83%
Image	94%	91%	90%	94%	95%	91%	95%	95%	94%	92%

Note: Correlation between IHC and FISH determined manually and with the aid of computerized image analysis in each of 10 pathologists.

Although these seem obvious, they are frequently ignored. For example, the use of an alcohol-based fixative invalidates the HercepTest™. This does not mean that the IHC assay will not produce a clean immunostain, it means the relationship between the staining pattern, and intensity and receptor copy number will be unknown. Another common problem is over-fixation. Laboratories that formalin fix breast specimens from the time they are received on Friday afternoon until the tissue is processed early Monday morning violate the specifications in the HercepTest™ guidelines and may lead to false negative results. Similarly, storing unstained slides at room temperature may diminish HER2 immunoreactivity *(43)*.

Even if the positive and negative controls stain as expected, careful review of the patient's slide must be performed. If staining is observed in benign epithelial elements, the stain should be repeated. The pathologist should also have knowledge of HER2 expression in various grades and types of breast cancer. Only 1–2% of well differentiated infiltrating ductal carcinomas and classic lobular carcinomas will overexpress HER2 as opposed to approx 30% of metastatic breast carcinomas and 20% of high grade infiltrating carcinomas *(44)*. An immunostain assessed as 3+ in a tubular carcinoma should be repeated and if positive should be verified with another methodology, such as FISH. There are several artifacts that may cause false positive staining and must be avoided, including edge artifact, crush artifact, and tissue retraction. Because all three of these artifacts are present in core-needle biopsies, great caution must be used when interpreting these specimens.

The assessment of a HER2 immunostain begins with the selection of a well preserved tissue block which minimizes known artifacts and contains a rim of normal breast tissue. The presence of normal breast tissue allows the observer to make sure significant staining is not present in benign elements. Review of the slide should begin with the ×4 or ×10 objective to assess the uniformity and intensity of the stain. A uniform staining pattern with a distinct membranous pattern giving a "chicken-wire" appearance, should be assessed as 3+. If a chicken-wire pattern is not clearly present, the observer should move up to the ×20 and ×40 objectives. These objectives can serve as an aid to define weak, moderate, and strong staining. A chicken-wire pattern visible on ×4 or ×10 equates to strong staining, on ×20, moderate staining and on ×40 weak staining. To avoid tangential sectioning, a nucleolus should be visible in any cell assessed as showing circumferential staining. This is possible because virtually all breast carcinomas that overexpress HER2 have visible nucleoli. A strong 1+ immunostain typically reveals a partial membrane stain with an intense granular appearance. The slide may look brown on lower power examination but a true chicken-wire pattern will not be present. Although interobserver variability is relatively low with tumors assessed as 0 and 3+, it may be significant in 2+ tumors.

2.1.2.4. USE OF IMAGE ANALYSIS

Although the human eye is excellent at distinguishing morphological characteristics, it is not adept at distinguishing shades of color. The immunohistochemical assessment of HER2 is largely dependent on the intensity of the stain, therefore image analysis may be a valuable tool to minimize interpathologist interpretation. Bloom et al. compared agreement among 10 pathologists in the assessment of 130 HER2 stained slides *(45)* (Table 2). Each pathologist scored the slides utilizing standard light microscopy according to the HercepTest™ guidelines with the aid of an image analyzer. The results were compared to the gene amplification status as assessed by FISH analysis. Although the experience of the pathologists varied, the concordance ranged from as low as 42% to as high as 92% on routine assessment. All of the pathologists achieved similar concordance, ranging from 90 to 95%, and even the most experienced pathologist showed improvement with the aid of the image analyzer. When the receiver operating characteristic (ROC) curves with conventional microscopy were analyzed for each of the ten pathologists, they had significantly different shapes, arguing that the variability was not just owing to differences in applying intensity thresholds but was related to something more fundamental in how the cases were scored. The ROC curves generated for each of the pathologists when using image analysis appeared similar. Other studies, using a variety of different image analysis systems, have also shown improved and more consistent HER2 scoring *(46,47)*.

2.2. HER2 Gene

There is a direct correlation between high levels of HER2 overexpression and amplification of the HER2 gene in carcinomas of the breast. The HER2 gene is located on chromosome 17 at 17q12. Several techniques have been employed to assess the HER2 gene including Southern Blotting techniques, FISH, chromogenic *in situ* hybridization (CISH), and polymerase chain reaction (PCR) techniques. Chromosome 17 frequently shows polysomy in breast carcinomas, therefore many of these assays include a reference probe for chromosome 17 so observers can differentiate between amplification of the gene and aneusomy of chromosome 17.

2.2.1. HER2 Amplicon

Amplification of the HER2 gene is not specific to HER2. The region of the chromosome that is amplified, known as the amplicon, is variable and usually involves other genes as well. The variability of the HER2-containing amplicon has been demonstrated in breast cancer cells lines as well as patient samples *(48)*. In addition to HER2, the minimal amplicon also includes GRB7, a signaling protein involved in migration and invasion, MLN64 (thought to be involved in cholesterol transport), NEUROD2, PNMT, ZNFN1A3, and EST 48582.

Additional genes may occasionally be coamplified with HER2 but it is unclear if these genes are located on the same amplicon. These include genes like THRα, RARα, topoisomerase II-α, MLN50, MLN51, and TRAF4. The increased responsiveness of HER2-amplified tumors to anthracycline therapy may be limited to those tumors in which the topoisomerase II-α gene, which is located telomeric to HER2, is co-amplified *(49,50)*. The variably sized amplicon has implications in probe design as well in assessing the prognostic and predictive significance of the FISH result.

2.2.2. FISH

Similar to IHC, FISH testing can be performed on FFPE tissue samples *(51)*, but since DNA is less subject to tissue fixation and processing than protein, FISH has been advocated as a more robust testing method to assess HER2 status. The process of FISH testing utilizes protease digestion to isolate the tumor nuclei, which are then heated to uncoil the DNA, flooded with a digoxigenin labeled probe, and cooled to allow the HER2 probe to anneal with the specific region of DNA. Following hybridization, the probe is visualized by applying fluorescent-labeled antibodies directed against the digoxigenin. In an optimally prepared specimen, detection of gene amplification is straight forward, although there is no accepted standard for evaluating a slide. Some scoring systems count only the HER2 signals, whereas others report the ratio of HER2 signals to a centromeric signal for chromosome 17 (Fig. 2). Since the HER2 gene is located on chromosome 17, the ratio allows the pathologist to differentiate aneusomy of chromosome 17 from true gene amplification. Studies comparing the two methods are highly correlative *(52)*. Slides prepared from FFPE blocks are generally between four and six microns in thickness, and thus do not represent complete nuclei. Initial reports in the literature suggested enumerating 60 cells, 15 cells from four different areas of the tumor would accurately detect gene amplification. Other reports suggested that enumerating as few as 20 cells will give identical results *(53)*.

One of the main advantages of FISH is that the pathologist knows when the assay has failed, because signals will not be detected; however, FISH, like any staining technique, is subject to variations in fixation, processing, storage, and detection. Even when hybridization is achieved, the intensity of the signals may be weak and the pathologist may underestimate the number of gene copies present. Furthermore, as the pathologist screens the slide, the intensity of the signal weakens as the slide is fluoresced.

FISH is an excellent technique but has two main difficulties in clinical practice. The most important limitation is the difficulty in guaranteeing that the invasive tumor cells have been observed. Identifying the invasive tumor on a 4',6-diamidino-2-phenylindole (DAPI) stained section can be challenging if the section is not completely composed of tumor. In many institutions this is complicated by assigning a cytogenetic technician to evaluate the FISH slides, who may not be qualified to evaluate if a DAPI stained cell is carcinoma or invasive. Although matching the hematoxylin and eosin (H&E) stained section to the FISH slide is essential prior to evaluation, occasionally the sections are not similar, especially with needle core biopsies. In many institutions, the tumor is identified on the originally reviewed H&E section and the FISH slide is later cut with sections for ER, PR, KI-67, and ploidy, once the diagnosis of invasive carcinoma is established. In these cases, the section removed for FISH analysis may be up to 200 μ away from the original H&E slide, and the circled area may not be representative of the tumor in the deeper section. Care must be taken to ensure that the H&E section used to select the invasive tumor and the FISH slide are step sections. A second limitation is background fluorescence, which is usually the result of either incomplete protease digestion or over-digestion. To the untrained pathologist, this fluorescence may look similar to coalescence of HER2 gene signals seen in tumors with amplification. However, in tumors showing real amplification, the individual nature of the signals can be observed on fine focus.

2.3. Other Tests Including CISH, PCR, ELISA, and SERUM

Southern and slot blotting were the first gene-based HER2 detection methods used in breast cancer specimens. These methods require fresh or frozen tissue but can be significantly hampered when the amount of tumor relative to the adjacent benign breast tissue and inflammatory cells is low, causing dilution of the tumor DNA. Chromogenic *in situ* hybridization or CISH has all of the advantages of IHC (routine microscope, lower cost, familiarity) and FISH (built-in internal control, subjective scoring, more robust DNA target), but is not FDA approved for selecting patients for trastuzumab therapy. The probes are identical for both CISH and FISH, however the HER2 gene is detected using a conventional peroxidase reaction, which is less sensitive than the fluorescence detection used in FISH *(54)*. Tanner et al. studied 157 invasive breast carcinomas by CISH and identified 27 tumors with amplification of the HER2 gene, all of which were also amplified by FISH *(55)*. Ten additional cases displayed HER2 gene amplification by FISH but not by CISH. This raised concern that CISH may not be able to detect tumors showing borderline amplification, although it is unknown if this subset of patients would respond to trastuzumab therapy. Tubbs et al., have reported excellent results with an alternative bright field testing method called gold-facilitated autometallographic *in situ* hybridization or GOLDFISH *(56)*. This technique is being developed but has shown excellent interpathologist reproducibility. PCR techniques, including differential, competitive, and real-time PCR, have predominantly been used to detect HER2 mRNA in peripheral blood and bone marrow samples *(30,57,58)*. Although it has correlated better with gene amplification status than IHC levels, it failed to predict survival in a study of 365 breast cancer patients *(59)*. The advent of laser capture microscopy and the acceptance of real-time PCR as a routine and reproducible laboratory technique, may increase the use of real time PCR to assess HER2 status.

ELISA-based measurements of HER2 protein in tumor cytosols, uniformly correlate with disease outcome *(28,60–64)*. The ELISA technique is made from fresh tissue samples to avoid the potential antigen damage associated with fixation, embedding, and uncontrolled storage. However, tumors are being discovered at a smaller size, precluding ELISA testing because insufficient tumor tissue is available to produce a cytosol.

Serum HER2 testing is a simple ELISA test that measures the extracellular domain (ECD) of the HER2 protein circulating in the serum. The ECD is a 100–110 protein released into the serum by specific metalloproteinases *(65)*. The level of detectable ECD protein correlates more to tumor burden than to the overexpression of HER2 in the tumor. As such, it is not surprising that many studies have failed to find a correlation between ECD levels and HER2 status as determined by FISH or IHC. The ease of a serum measurement is attractive and studies assessing how to best utilize the ECD protein measurement are ongoing. At this time however, ELISA is not recommended for selecting patients for trastuzumab therapy, although ELISA testing is an FDA approved method for the follow-up and monitoring of patient with metastatic breast carcinoma.

3. SIGNIFICANCE OF HER2 ALTERATIONS

3.1. HER2 as a Prognostic Factor

HER2 is an important prognostic factor in both node negative and node positive breast carcinomas. The prognostic significance of HER2 has been evaluated in more than 25,000 patients, encompassing 80 studies *(28,59,60,66–100)*. Endpoints have included metastasis free survival, disease free survival, and overall survival rates. All of the studies assessing gene amplification were predictive of outcome by univariate analysis although 10% of the studies utilizing IHC were not. By multivariate analysis, 71% of the studies revealed that HER2 status was independent of all other prognostic variables, including tumor size, grade, lymph nodes status, ER status, and vascular invasion in predicting an adverse prognostic significance. After analyzing the eight negative studies, five used immunohistochemistry (IHC) on FFPE tissues, two used Southern analysis, and one used a real time PCR technique.

3.2. HER2 as a Predictive Factor of Response to Therapy

Since its launch in 1998, trastuzumab, a monoclonal IgG1 class humanized murine antibody has become a major therapeutic option for patients with HER2 positive metastatic breast cancer and is currently being evaluated for use in the adjuvant and neo-adjuvant setting *(101–104)*. Developed by Genentech Corporation (South San Francisco, CA, USA), trastuzumab received FDA approval based on the results of the phase III pivot trial which showed that the addition of trastuzumab to chemotherapy (anthracycline plus cyclophosphamide or taxane) was associated with a longer time to disease progression (median, 7.4 vs 4.6 mo; $p < 0.001$), a higher rate of objective response (50 vs 32%; $p < 0.001$), a longer duration of response (median 9.1 vs 6.1 mo; $p < 0.001$), a lower rate of death at 1 yr (22 vs 33%; $p = 0.008$), longer survival (median survival 25.1 vs 20.3 mo; $p = 0.01$), and a 20% reduction in the risk of death *(105)*. Despite its dramatic benefits, significant cardiac dysfunction occurred more frequently in patients treated with anthracycline and cyclophosphamide plus trastuzumab compared to patients treated with anthracycline and cyclophosphamide alone (27 vs 8%). Cardiac toxicity still remains a limiting factor of trastuzumab use *(106)*.

The best method to identify patients who will respond to trastuzumab therapy has been a source of controversy. It has been suggested that FISH is more predictive of response than IHC but this is based on results of FISH testing performed retrospectively in patients that were already screened as either 2+ or 3+ by IHC. FISH assessment has not been tested prospectively and FISH results do not appear to outperform IHC when 3+ and 2+ tumors are evaluated independently. In the phase III clinical trial, the relative risk reduction of both time to progression and overall survival was similar, with virtually identical confidence intervals, in patients assessed as 3+ by IHC and assessed as amplified by FISH (Tables 3 and 4). In this series, FISH testing did not identify a subset of 2+ patients that benefited from trastuzumab therapy; however the number of patients treated was too small to achieve statistical significance. In a trial where trastuzumab was used as a first line single agent, the response rate in 111 patients with 3+ IHC staining was 35% while the response rate for 2+ tumors was 0%; the response rate in patients with and without HER2 gene amplification was 34% and 7% respectively *(107)*. When trastuzumab was used in advanced metastatic breast cancer patients as a third or fourth line therapy, the response rate in 222 patients with 3+ staining was 18% and the response rate for 2+ patients was 6%; the response rate in patients with and without HER2 gene amplification was 19% and 0%, respectively *(108)*. As seen by the above response rates, HER2 testing is best suited to identifying patients who are unlikely to respond to therapy rather than identifying those patients that will respond. Although the superiority of FISH over IHC remains controversial, most pathology laboratories are currently either screening all breast carcinomas with IHC and triaging selected tumors for FISH testing or using FISH as the only method for HER2 testing.

Besides predicting response to trastuzumab, HER2 status is also predictive of response to hormonal therapy *(109–113)*. Preclinical data shows that transfection of the HER-2 gene into HER2 negative, estrogen dependent cell lines leads to estrogen independence. Many studies have shown an inverse relationship between HER2 status and hormonal status in breast carcinoma *(72,91,94,114,115)*. These studies were limited by the assessment of HER2

Table 3
Trastuzumab + Chemo vs Chemo: Time to Progression

Subgroup	Relative risk	95% CI	No. of patients
IHC 3+	0.42	0.33–0.55	349
IHC 2+	0.82	0.54–1.24	120
FISH +	0.44	0.34–0.57	325
FISH–	0.66	0.45–0.99	126

Note: Data from the phase III clinical trial showing identical relative risk reduction and confidence intervals (CI) for both 3+ and FISH+ patients.

Table 4
Trastuzumab + Chemo vs Chemo: Overall Survival

Subgroup	Relative risk	95% CI	No. of patients
IHC 3+	0.70	0.54–0.92	349
IHC 2+	1.09	0.71–1.58	120
FISH +	0.69	0.53–0.91	325
FISH –	1.07	0.70–1.63	126

Note: Data from the phase III clinical trial showing identical relative risk reduction and confidence intervals (CI) for both 3+ and FISH+ patients.

and hormonal status as dichotomous variables, but a recent study assessed HER2 and hormonal status as continuous variables and confirmed that HER2-positive tumors are more often associated with a negative hormonal status than HER2-negative tumors. Furthermore, even in hormone receptor positive tumors, the expression of HER2 appears to be inversely related to the expression of ER and PR *(116)*. Many studies have shown that HER2-positive tumors are specifically resistant to tamoxifen therapy and some have suggested that HER2 expression may actually have an adverse effect on outcome in tamoxifen treated patients compared to untreated patients *(60,95,98,99,117)*. Other studies, including large intergroup studies in the United States have not confirmed this finding *(118)*. In postmenopausal women, there is a suggestion that aromatase inhibitors may be able to overcome the tamoxifen resistance seen in ER-positive HER2-positive tumors *(119)*.

HER2 protein overexpression has also been linked to resistance in patients treated with cytoxan, methotrexate, 5-fluorouracil (CMF) adjuvant chemotherapy, as well as taxane and cisplatin-based regimens *(86,120–122)*. Menard et al., however, showed that CMF chemotherapy overcomes the poor outcome ascribed to HER2 overexpressing tumors treated by radical mastectomy alone *(123)*. Cell lines expressing HER2 show increased resistance to paclitaxel, and clinical data suggests that HER2-positive patients receiving paclitaxel containing regimens without concomitant trastuzumab have a reduced response rate and a shorter duration of response than HER2 negative patients *(122)*. Other studies suggest that taxanes may provide sensitivity to HER2 overexpressing tumors. When the HER2 gene is transfected into MCF-7 cells, they acquire resistance to cisplatin *(124)*. However, when combined with trastuzumab in HER2-positive patients, both paclitaxel and cisplatin show significant activity. Pegram et al. showed a 24% response rate and a 48% clinical benefit in chemoresistant patients treated with trastuzumab and cisplatin *(125)*. Several studies have shown a 50–60% objective response rate in patients treated with a combination of trastuzumab and taxanes *(105)*.

HER2 overexpression has also been associated with enhanced response rates to anthracycline-containing chemotherapy regimens in some, but not all studies. Retrospective analysis of the data generated from the CALGB 8541 study provided evidence that HER2 overexpression was associated with increased responsiveness to high dose CAF chemotherapy *(87)*. In this study, lymph node positive patients were randomized to receive one of three doses of CAF. At 3-yr follow-up, significant improvements in disease free and overall survival were seen in HER2-positive patients receiving high-dose CAF therapy. The NSAPB B-11 trial also provided evidence that HER2-positive patients benefit from anthracyline based therapy *(126)*. Node-positive, ER/PR-negative patients were randomized to receive melphalan, doxorubicin and 5-fluorouracil or melphalan, and 5-fluorouracil alone. Patients whose tumors overexpressed HER2 showed significant improvements in disease-free survival with the anthracycline containing regimens. The SWOG study S8814 compared tamoxifen alone vs tamoxifen plus CAF chemotherapy in ER positive patients *(127)*. In contrast to HER2-negative patients, those patients whose tumor overexpressed HER2 protein showed significantly improved benefit from chemoendocrine therapy. In summary, although strong trends have been presented in published studies; including resistance to tamoxifen and sensitivity to anthracycline regimens for HER2-positive tumors, more studies are needed using appropriate control arms to confirm these important associations.

4. TOPOISOMERASE IIα

Topoisomerase IIα is a key enzyme in DNA replication and is the target of anthracycline chemotherapy. Although there appears to be an association between HER2 overexpression and benefit from anthracycline chemotherapy, it is not clear if this benefit is restricted to those patients with a concurrent topoisomerase IIα amplification. The relationship between HER2 amplification and topoisomerase IIα amplification; including whether they are part of the same amplicon, is currently the subject of investigation. Unlike HER2, there is not a tight correlation between gene amplification and protein expression.

4.1. Topoisomerase IIα Amplicon

The topoisomerase IIα gene is located on chromosome 17, telomeric to HER2. In theory, if HER2 and topoisomerase IIα were part of the same amplicon, the copy number of both genes should be identical, but this is frequently not the case. To date, all tumors showing amplification of the topoisomerase IIα gene have also shown amplification of the HER2 gene, but the converse is not true. Topoisomerase IIα amplification is evident in 40–45% of breast carcinomas with HER2 amplification but 30–40% show topoisomerase IIα deletion by FISH. Some of the discrepancies may be explained by the design and relative size of the FISH probes used to assess the genes. Mapping of the HER2-containing amplicon, using a series of overlapping FISH probes, reveals occasional skip areas possibly explaining the differences in HER2 and topoisomerase IIα copy numbers. There have been relatively few studies attempting to determine if topoisomerase IIα and HER2 are part of the same amplicon. Jarvinen et al. utilized fiber FISH to address this problem *(128)*. Fiber FISH is a technique used to map closely located genes, usually in normal DNA, but in this case the DNA fibers were prepared from malignant cells. HER2-topoisomerase IIα tandem repeats were expected to be seen if the two genes were indeed part of the same amplicon; but instead HER2–HER2–HER2 and topoisomerase IIα–topoisomerase IIα–topoisomerase IIα repeats were seen in separate DNA fibers, arguing that HER2 and topoisomerase IIα are part of different amplicons. To explain this finding, it has been suggested that the HER2 amplicon is created first and its telomeric end occurs at a breakpoint located between the HER2 and topoisomerase IIα genes. This breakpoint then serves as a starting point for a secondary amplicon housing the topoisomerase IIα gene. It is unclear how HER2 amplification leads to an interstitial deletion but it is likely to involve the DNA repair process *(129,130)*. The same phenomenon of interstitial deletions occurs following other amplifications such as cyclin D1 amplification *(131,132)*. Heterogeneity in topoisomerase IIα gene expression has been identified in breast carcinomas with some cells showing amplification and adjacent cells showing deletion. This coupled with the fact that all breast carcinomas with topoisomerase IIα amplification also reveal HER2 amplification, implies that the HER2 amplification takes place before or concurrent with the topoisomerase IIα aberration and supports the hypothesis that the chromosomal breakpoint of the HER2 amplicon is located between the HER2 and topoisomerase IIα genes.

4.2. Topoisomerase IIα and Response to Therapy

There are several arguments that HER2 by itself does not predict responsiveness to anthracycline therapy. First, there is no known interaction between topoisomerase IIα inhibitors and either the extracellular or intracellular domains of the HER2 protein. Pegram et al. induced HER2 protein overexpression in both mouse and human cells in vitro and did not see any alterations in the cell's responsiveness to topoisomerase IIα inhibitors. *(133,134)*. Jarvinen et al. showed that topoisomerase IIα amplified cell lines were associated with increased topoisomerase IIα protein expression and a significantly increased sensitivity to doxorubicin therapy, whereas cell lines with topoisomerase IIα gene deletion revealed decreased protein expression and decreased sensitivity to doxorubicin therapy. Other in vitro studies also demonstrated that the sensitivity of topoisomerase IIα inhibitors is directly related to the level of topoisomerase IIα protein *(135–138)*. Harris et al. found that topoisomerase IIα activity may be related to the expression level of HER2 even when gene amplification is not present *(139)*. Topoisomerase IIα levels were increased in unamplified cell lines when HER2 was activated by transfection of a chimeric receptor. The addition of trastuzumab downregulated both the HER2 and topoisomerase IIα activity levels in these cells.

In summary, there is a close interaction between HER2 and topoisomerase IIα expression levels in breast cancer. In approx 40% of breast carcinomas, HER2 gene amplification is associated with topoisomerase IIα amplification. However, even without gene amplification, HER2 activity appears to influence topoisomerase IIα expression and enhance responsiveness to anthracycline therapy.

5. CONCLUSION

HER2 is an important protein in breast carcinoma serving as prognostic marker in both node positive and node negative patients and as a predictive marker to trastuzumab therapy. Several options are available to assess HER2 status including IHC, FISH, CISH, and quantitative PCR. Currently, IHC and FISH are the only FDA approved methods and are the most widely used techniques for assessing HER2 status. Both techniques provide excellent results when performed in skilled laboratories according to the manufacturer's guidelines. Should further studies confirm the associations between HER2 and hormonal and/or anthracyline therapy it would seem likely that HER2 testing, which achieved standard of care status in the American Society of Clinical Oncology breast cancer clinical practice guidelines in 2001 would be of even greater value in the management of breast cancer patients.

REFERENCES

1. Karunagaran D, Tzahar E, Beerli RR, et al. 1996. ErbB-2 is a common auxiliary subunit of NDF and EGF receptors: implications for breast cancer. EMBO J. 15:254–264.
2. Hubbard SR. 1999. Structural analysis of receptor tyrosine kinases. Prog. Biophys. Mol. Biol. 71:343–358.
3. Hubbard SR and Till JH. 2000. Protein tyrosine kinase structure and function. Annu. Rev. Biochem. 69:373–398.
4. Coussens L, Yang-Feng TL, Liao YC, et al. 1985. Tyrosine kinase receptor with extensive homology to EGF receptor shares chromosomal location with neu oncogene. Science 230: 1132–1139.
5. Hynes NE and Stern DF. 1994. The biology of erbB-2/neu/HER-2 and its role in cancer. Biochim. Biophys. Acta. 1198:165–184.
6. Yarden Y and Sliwkowski MX. 2001. Untangling the ErbB signalling network. Nat. Rev. Mol. Cell. Biol. 2:127–137.
7. Tzahar E, Waterman H, Chen X, et al. 1996. A hierarchical network of interreceptor interactions determines signal transduction by Neu differentiation factor/neuregulin and epidermal growth factor. Mol. Cell. Biol. 16:5276–5287.
8. Pinkas-Kramarski R, Eilam R, Alroy I, Levkowitz G, Lonai P, Yarden Y. 1997. Differential expression of NDF/neuregulin receptors ErbB-3 and ErbB-4 and involvement in inhibition of neuronal differentiation. Oncogene 15:2803–2815.
9. Alroy Iand Yarden Y. 1997. The ErbB signaling network in embryogenesis and oncogene sis: signal diversification through combinatorial ligand-receptor interactions. FEBS Lett. 410:83–86.
10. Lemmon MA and Schlessinger J. 1994. Regulation of signal transduction and signal diversity by receptor oligomerization. Trends Biochem. Sci. 19:459–463.
11. Graus-Porta D, Beerli RR, Daly JM, Hynes NE. 1997. ErbB-2, the preferred heterodimerization partner of all ErbB receptors, is a mediator of lateral signaling. EMBO J. 16:1647–1655.
12. Olayioye MA, Neve RM, Lane HA, Hynes NE. 2000. The ErbB signaling network: receptor heterodimerization in development and cancer. EMBO J. 19:3159–3167.
13. Mansour SJ, Matten WT, Hermann AS, et al. 1994. Transformation of mammalian cells by constitutively active MAP kinase kinase. Science 265:966–970.
14. Carraway KL III, Soltoff SP, Diamonti AJ, Cantley LC. 1995. Heregulin stimulates mitogenesis and phosphatidylinositol 3-kinase in mouse fibroblasts transfected with erbB2/neu and erbB3. J. Biol. Chem. 270:7111–7116.
15. Muthuswamy SK, Siegel PM, Dankort D, Webster MA, Muller WJ. 1994. Mammary tumors expressing the neu proto-oncogene possess elevated c-Src tyrosine kinase activity. Mol. Cell. Biol. 14:735–743.
16. Tzahar E and Yarden Y. 1998. The ErbB-2/HER2 oncogenic receptor of adenocarcinomas: from orphanhood to multiple stromal ligands. Biochim. Biophys. Acta. 1377:M25–M37.
17. Waterman H, Sabanai I, Geiger B, Yarden Y. 1998. Alternative intracellular routing of ErbB receptors may determine signaling potency. J. Biol. Chem. 273:13819–13827.
18. Popescu NC, King CR, Kraus MH. 1989. Localization of the human erbB-2 gene on normal and rearranged chromosomes 17 to bands q12-21.32. Genomics 4:362–366.
19. Padhy LC, Shih C, Cowing D, Finkelstein R, Weinberg RA. 1982. Identification of a phosphoprotein specifically induced by the transforming DNA of rat neuroblastomas. Cell 28:865–871.
20. Ross JS and Fletcher JA. 1999. HER-2/neu (c-erb-B2. gene and protein in breast cancer. Am. J. Clin. Pathol. 112:S53–S67.

21. Schnitt SJ and Jacobs TW. 2001. Current status of HER2 testing: caught between a rock and a hard place. Am. J. Clin. Pathol. 116:806–810.

22. Slamon DJ Godolphin W, Jones LA, et al. 1989. Studies of the HER-2/neu proto-oncogene in human breast and ovarian cancer. Science 244:707–712.

23. Pauletti G, Dandekar S, Rong H, et al. 2000. Assessment of methods for tissue-based detection of the HER-2/neu alteration in human breast cancer: a direct comparison of fluorescence in situ hybridization and immunohistochemistry. J. Clin. Oncol. 18:3651–3664.

24. Nagy P, Jenei A, Kirsch AK, Szollosi J, Damjanovich S, Jovin TM. 1999. Activation-dependent clustering of the erbB2 receptor tyrosine kinase detected by scanning near-field optical microscopy. J. Cell Sci. 112:1733–1741.

25. Balsari A, Casalini P, Tagliabue E, et al. 1999. Fluctuation of HER2 expression in breast carcinomas during the menstrual cycle. Am. J. Pathol. 155:1543–1547.

26. Cooke T, Reeves J, Lannigan A, Stanton P. 2001. The value of the human epidermal growth factor receptor-2 (HER2) as a prognostic marker. Eur. J. Cancer 37:3–10.

27. Robertson KW, Reeves JR, Smith G, et al. 1996. Quantitative estimation of epidermal growth factor receptor and c-erbB- 2 in human breast cancer. Cancer Res. 56:3823–3830.

28. Eppenberger-Castori S, Kueng W, Benz C, et al. 2001. Prognostic and predictive significance of ErbB-2 breast tumor levels measured by enzyme immunoassay. J. Clin. Oncol. 19:645–656.

29. Bloom KJ and Assad L. 2002. Optimizing the immunohistochemical assessment of HER-2 expression to predict HER-2 gene amplification with the HercepTest kit. Mod. Pathol. 15:28A.

30. Tubbs RR, Pettay JD, Roche PC, Stoler MH, Jenkins RB, Grogan TM. 2001. Discrepancies in clinical laboratory testing of eligibility for trastuzumab therapy: apparent immunohistochemical false-positives do not get the message. J. Clin. Oncol. 19:2714–2721.

31. Roche PC and Ingle JN. 1999. Increased HER2 with U.S. Food and Drug Administration-approved antibody. J. Clin. Oncol. 17:434.

32. Jacobs TW, Gown AM, Yaziji H, Barnes MJ, Schnitt SJ. 1999. Comparison of fluorescence in situ hybridization and immunohistochemistry for the evaluation of HER-2/neu in breast cancer. J. Clin. Oncol. 17:1974–1982.

33. Press MF, Hung G, Godolphin W, Slamon DJ. 1994. Sensitivity of HER-2/neu antibodies in archival tissue samples: potential source of error in immunohistochemical studies of oncogene expression. Cancer Res. 54:2771–2777.

34. Paik S, Bryant J, Tan-Chiu E, et al. 2002. Real-world performance of HER2 testing—National Surgical Adjuvant Breast and Bowel Project experience. J. Natl. Cancer Inst. 94:852–854.

35. Rhodes A, Jasani B, Anderson E, Dodson AR, Balaton AJ. 2002. Evaluation of HER-2/neu immunohistochemical assay sensitivity and scoring on formalin-fixed and paraffin-processed cell lines and breast tumors: a comparative study involving results from laboratories in 21 countries. Am. J. Clin. Pathol. 118:408–417.

36. Mass RD. 2003. The concordance between the clinical trials assay (CTA) and fluorescence in situ hybridization (FISH) in the Herceptin pivotal trials. Proc. Am. Soc. Clin. Oncol. 19:75a.

37. Bloom KJ. 2001. A prospective analysis of HercepTest versus FISH in 202 consecutive primary invasive breast carcinomas. Mod. Pathol. 14:22A.

38. Lebeau A, Deimling D, Kaltz C, et al. 2001. Her-2/neu analysis in archival tissue samples of human breast cancer: comparison of immunohistochemistry and fluorescence in situ hybridization. J. Clin. Oncol. 19:354–363.

39. Couturier J, Vincent-Salomon A, Nicolas A, et al. 2000. Strong correlation between results of fluorescent in situ hybridization and immunohistochemistry for the assessment of the ERBB2 (HER-2/neu) gene status in breast carcinoma. Mod. Pathol. 13:1238–1243.

40. Jimenez RE, Wallis T, Tabasczka P, Visscher DW. 2000. Determination of Her-2/Neu status in breast carcinoma: comparative analysis of immunohistochemistry and fluorescent in situ hybridization. Mod. Pathol. 13:37–45.

41. Ridolfi RL, Jamehdor MR, Arber JM. 2000. HER-2/neu testing in breast carcinoma: a combined immunohistochemical and fluorescence in situ hybridization approach. Mod. Pathol. 13:866–873.

42. Tsuda H, Akiyama F, Terasaki H, et al. 2001. Detection of HER-2/neu (c-erb B-2) DNA amplification in primary breast carcinoma. Interobserver reproducibility and correlation with immunohistochemical HER-2 overexpression. Cancer 92:2965–2974.

43. Jacobs TW, Prioleau JE, Stillman IE, Schnitt SJ. 1996. Loss of tumor marker-immunostaining intensity on stored paraffin slides of breast cancer. J. Natl. Cancer Inst. 88:1054–1059.

44. Hoff ER, Tubbs RR, Myles JL, Procop GW. 2002. HER2/neu amplification in breast cancer: stratification by tumor type and grade. Am. J. Clin. Pathol. 117:916–921.

45. Bloom K J, Torre-Bueno J, Press M, Gown A, Bauer K, Harrington D. 2000. Comparison of HER-2/neu analysis using FISH and IHC when HercepTest is scored using conventional microscopy and image analysis. Comparison of HER-2/neu analysis using FISH and IHC when HercepTest is scored using conventional microscopy and image analysis. Breast Cancer Res. Treat. 64:99.

46. Wang S, Saboorian MH, Frenkel EP, et al. 2001. Assessment of HER-2/neu status in breast cancer. Automated Cellular Imaging System (ACIS)-assisted quantitation of immunohistochemical assay achieves high accuracy in comparison with fluorescence in situ hybridization assay as the standard. Am. J. Clin. Pathol. 116:495–503.

47. Lehr HA, Jacobs TW, Yaziji H, Schnitt SJ, Gown AM. 2001. Quantitative evaluation of HER-2/neu status in breast cancer by fluorescence *in situ* hybridization and by immunohistochemistry with image analysis. Am. J. Clin. Pathol. 115:814–822.

48. Kauraniemi P, Barlund M, Monni O, Kallioniemi A. 2001. New amplified and highly expressed genes discovered in the ERBB2 amplicon in breast cancer by cDNA microarrays. Cancer Res. 61:8235–8240.

49. Di Leo A, Gancberg D, Larsimont D, et al. 2002. HER-2 Amplification and Topoisomerase IIalpha Gene Aberrations as Predictive Markers in Node-positive Breast Cancer Patients Randomly Treated Either with an Anthracycline-based Therapy or with Cyclophosphamide, Methotrexate, and 5-Fluorouracil. Clin. Cancer Res. 8:1107–1116.

50. Jarvinen TA, Tanner M, Rantanen V, et al. 2000. Amplification and deletion of topoisomerase IIalpha associate with ErbB-2 amplification and affect sensitivity to topoisomerase II inhibitor doxorubicin in breast cancer. Am. J. Pathol. 156:839–847.

51. Pauletti G, Godolphin W, Press MF, Slamon DJ. 1996. Detection and quantitation of HER-2/neu gene amplification in human breast cancer archival material using fluorescence in situ hybridization. Oncogene 13:63–72.

52. Wang S, Saboorian MH, Frenkel E, Hynan L, Gokaslan ST, Ashfaq R. 2000. Laboratory assessment of the status of Her-2/neu protein and oncogene in breast cancer specimens: comparison of immunohistochemistry assay with fluorescence in situ hybridisation assays. J. Clin. Pathol. 53:374–381.

53. Persons DL, Bui MM, Lowery MC, et al. 2000. Fluorescence *in situ* hybridization (FISH) for detection of HER-2/neu amplification in breast cancer: a multicenter portability study. Ann. Clin. Lab. Sci. 30:41–48.

54. Zhao J, Wu R, Au A, Marquez A, Yu Y, Shi Z. 2002. Determination of HER2 Gene Amplification by Chromogenic In Situ Hybridization (CISH) in Archival Breast Carcinoma. Mod. Pathol. 15:657–665.

55. Tanner M, Gancberg D, Di Leo A, et al. 2000. Chromogenic in situ hybridization: a practical alternative for fluorescence in situ hybridization to detect HER-2/neu oncogene amplification in archival breast cancer samples. Am. J. Pathol. 157:1467–1472.

56. Tubbs R, Skacel M, Pettay J, et al. 2002. Interobserver interpretative reproducibility of GOLD-FISH, a first generation gold-facilitated autometallographic bright field in situ hybridization assay for HER-2/neu amplification in invasive mammary carcinoma. Am. J. Surg. Pathol. 26:908–913.

57. Pawlowski V, Revillion F, Hornez L, Peyrat JP. 2000. A real-time one-step reverse transcriptase-polymerase chain reaction method to quantify c-erbB-2 expression in human breast cancer. Cancer Detect. Prev. 24:212–223.

58. Bieche I, Onody P, Laurendeau I, et al. 1999. Real-time reverse transcription-PCR assay for future management of ERBB2-based clinical applications. Clin. Chem. 45:1148–1156.
59. Volpi A, De Paola F, Nanni O, et al. 2000. Prognostic significance of biologic markers in node-negative breast cancer patients: a prospective study. Breast Cancer Res. Treat. 63:181–192.
60. Ferrero-Pous M, Hacene K, Bouchet C, Le DV, Tubiana-Hulin M, and Spyratos F. 2000. Relationship between c-erbB-2 and other tumor characteristics in breast cancer prognosis. Clin. Cancer Res. 6:4745–4754.
61. Eissa S, Khalifa A, el Gharib A, Salah N, Mohamed MK. 1997. Multivariate analysis of DNA ploidy, p53, c-erbB-2 proteins, EGFR, and steroid hormone receptors for short-term prognosis in breast cancer. Anti Cancer Res. 17:3091–3097.
62. Dittadi R, Brazzale A, Pappagallo G, et al. 1997. ErbB2 assay in breast cancer: possibly improved clinical information using a quantitative method. Anti Cancer Res. 17:1245–1247.
63. Gaci Z, Bouin-Pineau MH, Gaci M, Daban A, Ingrand P, Metaye T. 2001. Prognostic impact of cathepsin D and c-erbB-2 oncoprotein in a subgroup of node-negative breast cancer patients with low histological grade tumors. Int. J. Oncol. 18:793–800.
64. el Ahmady O, el Salahy E, Mahmoud M, Wahab MA, Eissa S, Khalifa A. 2002. Multivariate analysis of bcl-2, apoptosis, P53 and HER-2/neu in breast cancer: a short-term follow-up. Anti Cancer Res. 22:2493–2499.
65. Codony-Servat J, Albanell J, Lopez-Talavera JC, Arribas J, Baselga J. 1999. Cleavage of the HER2 ectodomain is a pervanadate-activable process that is inhibited by the tissue inhibitor of metalloproteases-1 in breast cancer cells. Cancer Res. 59:1196–1201.
66. Slamon DJ, Clark GM, Wong SG, Levin WJ, Ullrich A, McGuire WL. 1987. Human breast cancer: correlation of relapse and survival with amplification of the HER-2/neu oncogene. Science 235:177–182.
67. Berger MS, Locher GW, Saurer S, et al. 1988. Correlation of c-erbB-2 gene amplification and protein expression in human breast carcinoma with nodal status and nuclear grading. Cancer Res. 48:1238–1243.
68. van de Vijver MJ, Peterse JL, Mooi WJ, et al. 1988. Neu-protein overexpression in breast cancer. Association with comedo- type ductal carcinoma in situ and limited prognostic value in stage II breast cancer. N. Engl. J. Med. 319:1239–1245.
69. Heintz NH, Leslie KO, Rogers LA, Howard PL. 1990. Amplification of the c-erb B-2 oncogene and prognosis of breast adenocarcinoma. Arch. Pathol. Lab. Med. 114:160–163.
70. Wright C, Angus B, Nicholson S, et al. 1989. Expression of c-erbB-2 oncoprotein: a prognostic indicator in human breast cancer. Cancer Res. 49:2087–2090.
71. Tsuda H, Hirohashi S, Shimosato Y, et al. 1990. Correlation between histologic grade of malignancy and copy number of c- erbB-2 gene in breast carcinoma. A retrospective analysis of 176 cases. Cancer 65:1794–1800.
72. Borg A, Tandon AK, Sigurdsson H, et al. 1990. HER-2/neu amplification predicts poor survival in node-positive breast cancer. Cancer Res. 50:4332–4337.
73. Paik S, Hazan R, Fisher ER, et al. 1990. Pathologic findings from the National Surgical Adjuvant Breast and Bowel Project: prognostic significance of erbB-2 protein overexpression in primary breast cancer. J. Clin. Oncol. 8:103–112.
74. Gullick WJ, Love SB, Wright C, et al. 1991. c-erbB-2 protein overexpression in breast cancer is a risk factor in patients with involved and uninvolved lymph nodes. Br. J. Cancer 63:434–438.
75. McCann AH, Dervan PA, O'Regan M, et al. 1991. Prognostic significance of c-erbB-2 and estrogen receptor status in human breast cancer. Cancer Res. 51:3296–3303.
76. Dykins R, Corbett IP, Henry JA, et al. 1991. Long-term survival in breast cancer related to overexpression of the c-erbB-2 oncoprotein: an immunohistochemical study using monoclonal antibody NCL-CB11. J. Pathol. 163:105–110.
77. Rilke F, Colnaghi MI, Cascinelli N, et al. 1991. Prognostic significance of HER-2/neu expression in breast cancer and its relationship to other prognostic factors. Int. J. Cancer 49:44–49.

78. Winstanley J, Cooke T, Murray GD, et al. 1991. The long term prognostic significance of c-erbB-2 in primary breast cancer. Br. J. Cancer 63:447–450.

79. Paterson MC, Dietrich KD, Danyluk J, et al. 1991. Correlation between c-erbB-2 amplification and risk of recurrent disease in node-negative breast cancer. Cancer Res. 51:556–567.

80. Toikkanen S, Helin H, Isola J, Joensuu H. 1992. Prognostic significance of HER-2 oncoprotein expression in breast cancer: a 30-year follow-up. J. Clin. Oncol. 10:1044–1048.

81. Allred DC, Clark GM, Tandon AK, et al. 1992. HER-2/neu in node-negative breast cancer: prognostic significance of overexpression influenced by the presence of in situ carcinoma. J. Clin. Oncol. 10:599–605.

82. Tiwari RK, Borgen PI, Wong GY, Cordon-Cardo C, Osborne MP. 1992. HER-2/neu amplification and overexpression in primary human breast cancer is associated with early metastasis. Anti Cancer Res. 12:419–425.

83. Bianchi S, Paglierani M, Zampi G, et al. 1993. Prognostic significance of c-erbB-2 expression in node negative breast cancer. Br. J. Cancer 67:625–629.

84. Press MF, Pike MC, Chazin, VR, et al. 1993. Her-2/neu expression in node-negative breast cancer: direct tissue quantitation by computerized image analysis and association of overexpression with increased risk of recurrent disease. Cancer Res. 53:4960–4970.

85. Descotes F, Pavy JJ, Adessi GL. 1993. Human breast cancer: correlation study between HER-2/neu amplification and prognostic factors in an unselected population. Anti Cancer Res. 13:119–124.

86. Giai M, Roagna R, Ponzone R, De Bortoli M, Dati C, Sismondi P. 1994. Prognostic and predictive relevance of c-erbB-2 and ras expression in node positive and negative breast cancer. Anti Cancer Res. 14:1441–1450.

87. Muss HB, Thor AD, Berry DA, et al. 1994. c-erbB-2 expression and response to adjuvant therapy in women with node- positive early breast cancer. N. Engl. J. Med. 330:1260–1266.

88. Tetu B and Brisson J. 1994. Prognostic significance of HER-2/neu oncoprotein expression in node-positive breast cancer. The influence of the pattern of immunostaining and adjuvant therapy. Cancer 73:2359–2365.

89. Hartmann LC, Ingle JN, Wold LE, et al. 1994. Prognostic value of c-erbB2 overexpression in axillary lymph node positive breast cancer. Results from a randomized adjuvant treatment protocol. Cancer 74:2956–2963.

90. Marks JR, Humphrey PA, Wu K, et al. 1994. Overexpression of p53 and HER-2/neu proteins as prognostic markers in early stage breast cancer. Ann. Surg. 219:332–341.

91. Quenel N, Wafflart J, Bonichon F, et al. 1995. The prognostic value of c-erbB2 in primary breast carcinomas: a study on 942 cases. Breast Cancer Res. Treat 35:283–291.

92. Charpin C, Garcia S, Bouvier C, et al. 1997. c-erbB-2 oncoprotein detected by automated quantitative immunocytochemistry in breast carcinomas correlates with patients' overall and disease-free survival. Br. J. Cancer 75:1667–1673.

93. Press MF, Bernstein L, Thomas PA, et al. 1997. HER-2/neu gene amplification characterized by fluorescence in situ hybridization: poor prognosis in node-negative breast carcinomas. J. Clin. Oncol. 15:2894–2904.

94. Andrulis IL, Bull SB, Blackstein ME, et al. 1998. neu/erbB-2 amplification identifies a poor-prognosis group of women with node-negative breast cancer. Toronto Breast Cancer Study Group. J. Clin. Oncol. 16:1340–1349.

95. Sjogren S, Inganas M, Lindgren A, Holmberg L, Bergh J. 1998. Prognostic and predictive value of c-erbB-2 overexpression in primary breast cancer, alone and in combination with other prognostic markers. J. Clin. Oncol. 16:462–469.

96. Harbeck N, Ross JS, Yurdseven S, et al. 1999. HER-2/neu gene amplification by fluorescence in situ hybridization allows risk-group assessment in node-negative breast cancer. Int. J. Oncol. 14:663–671.

97. Kakar S, Puangsuvan N, Stevens JM, et al. 2000. HER-2/neu assessment in breast cancer by immunohistochemistry and fluorescence in situ hybridization: comparison of results and correlation with survival. Mol. Diagn. 5:199–207.

98. Jukkola A, Bloigu R, Soini Y, Savolainen ER, Holli K, and Blanco G. 2001. c-erbB-2 positivity is a factor for poor prognosis in breast cancer and poor response to hormonal or chemotherapy treatment in advanced disease. Eur. J. Cancer 37:347–354.

99. Pinto AE, Andre S, Pereira T, Nobrega S, Soares J. 2001. C-erbB-2 oncoprotein overexpression identifies a subgroup of estrogen receptor positive (ER+) breast cancer patients with poor prognosis. Ann. Oncol. 12:525–533.

100. Tsutsui S, Ohno S, Murakami S, Hachitanda Y, Oda, S. 2002. Prognostic value of c-erbB2 expression in breast cancer. J. Surg. Oncol. 79:216–223.

101. Hortobagyi GN. 2001. Overview of treatment results with trastuzumab (Herceptin) in metastatic breast cancer. Semin. Oncol. 28:43–47.

102. McKeage K and Perry CM. 2002. Trastuzumab: a review of its use in the treatment of metastatic breast cancer overexpressing HER2. Drugs 62:209–243.

103. Shawver LK, Slamon D, Ullrich A. 2002. Smart drugs: tyrosine kinase inhibitors in cancer therapy. Cancer Cell 1:117–123.

104. Ligibel JA and Winer EP. 2002. Trastuzumab/chemotherapy combinations in metastatic breast cancer. Semin. Oncol. 29:38–43.

105. Slamon DJ, Leyland-Jones B, Shak S, et al. 2001. Use of chemotherapy plus a monoclonal antibody against HER2 for metastatic breast cancer that overexpresses HER2. N. Engl. J. Med. 344:783–792.

106. Schneider JW, Chang AY, Garratt A. 2002. Trastuzumab cardiotoxicity: Speculations regarding pathophysiology and targets for further study. Semin. Oncol. 29:22–28.

107. Vogel CL, Cobleigh MA, Tripathy D, et al. 2002. Efficacy and safety of trastuzumab as a single agent in first-line treatment of HER2-overexpressing metastatic breast cancer. J. Clin. Oncol. 20:719–726.

108. Cobleigh MA, Vogel CL, Tripathy D, et al. 1999. Multinational study of the efficacy and safety of humanized anti-HER2 monoclonal antibody in women who have HER2-overexpressing metastatic breast cancer that has progressed after chemotherapy for metastatic disease. J. Clin. Oncol. 17:2639–2648.

109. Piccart M, Lohrisch C, Di Leo A, Larsimont D. 2001. The predictive value of HER2 in breast cancer. Oncology 2:73–82.

110. Dowsett M. 2001. Overexpression of HER-2 as a resistance mechanism to hormonal therapy for breast cancer. Endocr. Relat. Cancer 8:191–195.

111. Muss HB. 2001. Role of adjuvant endocrine therapy in early-stage breast cancer. Semin. Oncol. 28:313–321.

112. Schmid P, Wischnewsky MB, Sezer O, Bohm R, Possinger K. 2002. Prediction of response to hormonal treatment in metastatic breast cancer. Oncology 63:309–316.

113. Nunes RA and Harris LN. 2002. The HER2 extracellular domain as a prognostic and predictive factor in breast cancer. Clin. Breast Cancer 3:125–135.

114. Marsigliante S, Muscella A, Ciardo V, et al. 1993. Enzyme-linked immunosorbent assay of HER-2/neu gene product (p185) in breast cancer: its correlation with sex steroid receptors, cathepsin D and histologic grades. Cancer Lett. 75:195–206.

115. Zeillinger R, Kury F, Czerwenka K, et al. 1989. HER-2 amplification, steroid receptors and epidermal growth factor receptor in primary breast cancer. Oncogene 4:109–114.

116. Konecny G, Pauletti G, Pegram M, et al. 2003. Quantitative association between HER-2/neu and steroid hormone receptors in hormone receptor-positive primary breast cancer. J. Natl. Cancer Inst. 95:142–153.

117. Carlomagno C, Perrone F, Gallo C, et al. 1996. c-erb B2 overexpression decreases the benefit of adjuvant tamoxifen in early-stage breast cancer without axillary lymph node metastases. J. Clin. Oncol. 14:2702–2708.

118. Elledge RM, Green S, Ciocca D, et al. 1998. HER-2 expression and response to tamoxifen in estrogen receptor-positive breast cancer: a Southwest Oncology Group Study. Clin. Cancer Res. 4:7–12.

119. Ellis MJ, Coop A, Singh B, et al. 2001. Letrozole is more effective neoadjuvant endocrine therapy than tamoxifen for ErbB-1- and/or ErbB-2-positive, estrogen receptor-positive primary breast cancer: evidence from a phase III randomized trial. J. Clin. Oncol. 19:3808–3816.

120. Berns EM, Foekens JA, van Staveren IL, et al. 1995. Oncogene amplification and prognosis in breast cancer: relationship with systemic treatment. Gene 159:11–18.

121. Sparano JA. 2000. Taxanes for breast cancer: an evidence-based review of randomized phase II and phase III trials. Clin. Breast Cancer 1:32–40.

122. Yu D. 2001. Mechanisms of ErbB2-mediated paclitaxel resistance and trastuzumab- mediated paclitaxel sensitization in ErbB2-overexpressing breast cancers. Semin. Oncol. 28:12–17.

123. Menard S, Valagussa P, Pilotti S, 2001. Response to cyclophosphamide, methotrexate, and fluorouracil in lymph node-positive breast cancer according to HER2 overexpression and other tumor biologic variables. J. Clin. Oncol. 19:329–335.

124. Benz CC, Scott GK, Sarup JC, et al. 1993. Estrogen-dependent, tamoxifen-resistant tumorigenic growth of MCF-7 cells transfected with HER2/neu. Breast Cancer Res. Treat. 2:85–95.

125. Pegram MD, Lipton A, Hayes DF, et al. 1998. Phase II study of receptor-enhanced chemosensitivity using recombinant humanized anti-p185HER2/neu monoclonal antibody plus cisplatin in patients with HER2/neu-overexpressing metastatic breast cancer refractory to chemotherapy treatment. J. Clin. Oncol. 16:2659–2671.

126. Paik S, Bryant J, Park C, et al. 1998. erbB-2 and response to doxorubicin in patients with axillary lymph node- positive, hormone receptor-negative breast cancer. J. Natl. Cancer Inst. 90:1361–1370.

127. Ravdin PM, Green S, Albain V. 1998. Initial report of the SWOG biological correlative study of c-erbB-2 expression as a predictor of outcome in a trial comparing adjuvant CAF T with tamoxifin (T) alone. Proc. Am. Soc. Clin. Oncol. 17:97a.

128. Jarvinen TA, Tanner M, Barlund M, Borg A, Isola J. 1999. Characterization of topoisomerase II alpha gene amplification and deletion in breast cancer. Genes Chromosomes Cancer 26: 142–150.

129. Pipiras E, Coquelle A, Bieth A, Debatisse M. 1998. Interstitial deletions and intrachromosomal amplification initiated from a double-strand break targeted to a mammalian chromosome. EMBO J. 17:325–333.

130. Liang F, Han M, Romanienko PJ, Jasin M. 1998. Homology-directed repair is a major double-strand break repair pathway in mammalian cells. Proc. Natl. Acad. Sci. USA 95:5172–5177.

131. Jin Y, Hoglund M, Jin C, et al. 1998. FISH characterization of head and neck carcinomas reveals that amplification of band 11q13 is associated with deletion of distal 11q. Genes Chromosomes Cancer 22:312–320.

132. Tanner MM, Karhu RA, Nupponen NN, et al. 1998. Genetic aberrations in hypodiploid breast cancer: frequent loss of chromosome 4 and amplification of cyclin D1 oncogene. Am. J. Pathol. 153:191–199.

133. Pegram MD, Pauletti G, Slamon DJ. 1998. HER-2/neu as a predictive marker of response to breast cancer therapy. Breast Cancer Res. Treat. 52:65–77.

134. Pegram MD, Finn RS, Arzoo K, Beryt M, Pietras RJ, Slamon DJ. 1997. The effect of HER-2/neu overexpression on chemotherapeutic drug sensitivity in human breast and ovarian cancer cells. Oncogene 15:537–547.

135. Gudkov AV, Zelnick CR, Kazarov AR, et al. 1993. Isolation of genetic suppressor elements, inducing resistance to topoisomerase II-interactive cytotoxic drugs, from human topoisomerase II cDNA. Proc. Natl. Acad. Sci. USA 90:3231–3235.

136. Asano T, An T, Mayes J, Zwelling LA, Kleinerman ES. 1996. Transfection of human topoisomerase II alpha into etoposide-resistant cells: transient increase in sensitivity followed by down-regulation of the endogenous gene. Biochem. J. 319:307–313.

137. Withoff S, Keith WN, Knol AJ, et al. 1996. Selection of a subpopulation with fewer DNA topoisomerase II alpha gene copies in a doxorubicin-resistant cell line panel. Br. J. Cancer 74:502–507.

138. Zhou Z, Zwelling LA, Kawakami Y, An T, Kobayashi K, Herzog C, Kleinerman ES. 1999. Adenovirus-mediated human topoisomerase IIalpha gene transfer increases the sensitivity of etoposide-resistant human breast cancer cells. Cancer Res. 59:4618–4624.
139. Harris LN, Yang L, Liotcheva V, et al. 2001. Induction of topoisomerase II activity after ErbB2 activation is associated with a differential response to breast cancer chemotherapy. Clin. Cancer Res. 7:1497–1504.

14

Study of Sentinel Lymph Nodes in the Staging of Malignant Neoplasms

Alice A. Roberts and Alistair J. Cochran

1. INTRODUCTION

Surgeons have long appreciated the significance of lymph node metastases to cancer prognosis. As far back as the 6th century, Actus of Amida observed that "malignant phlegmons" develop in the armpits of advanced breast cancer patients *(1)*. The importance of lymph node metastases was recognized early on, and this naturally led to investigations of the underlying physiology. In 1622, Aselius demonstrated lymphatic drainage into lacteals of a postprandial dog, thus laying the groundwork for centuries of attempts to map lymphatic pathways. The most common approach was to inject dye into peripheral sites and dissect adjacent tissues looking for colored lymphatics. Various dyes, including India ink and mercury, were utilized to map lymphatic drainage in human cadavers and research animals. In the mid-20th century, radioisotopes were employed as markers of lymph drainage; some early experiments in humans employed radioactive colloid gold *(2)*, and later the less active technetium-99 (TC-99) came into use *(3)*. Peritumoral injections of radiocolloid are now used in sentinel node biopsy to visualize draining nodes preoperatively by lymphoscintigraphy and intraoperatively using a handheld Geiger counter. The presence of lymph node metastases overrides all other prognostic factors for solid tumors and the surgical approach is usually altered by the presence of metastatic tumor in a lymph node. Staging for most solid tumors depends on knowing the tumor status of the draining lymph nodes. As the surgeon Moynihan aptly stated, "surgery of malignant disease is not the surgery of organs; it is the anatomy of the lymphatic system" *(4)*.

2. REGIONAL NODE DISSECTION

Many patients with solid tumors are staged by screening regional lymph nodes, such as the ipsilateral axillary nodes in breast cancer. The role of tumor-positive lymph nodes in the staging of solid neoplasms is widely accepted; however, the therapeutic value of complete excision of draining lymph nodes remains somewhat controversial. Some contend that there is no therapeutic value in treating such patients because nodal involvement reflects aggressive disease that has already spread beyond local nodes *(5)*. Regional lymphadenectomy is not likely to alter cancer progression in individuals with aggressive tumors that have already metastasized extensively and systematically nor will it benefit individuals with node-negative disease. It is clear that the only likely survival benefit of regional node dissection is to patients with metastases that are absolutely or substantially limited to the primary drain-

From: *Cancer Diagnostics: Current and Future Trends*
Edited by: R. M. Nakamura, W. W. Grody, J. T. Wu, and R. B. Nagle © Humana Press Inc., Totowa, NJ

ing lymph node group, for example, individuals who are node-positive but do not have substantial distant metastatic deposits (there is evidence that distant micrometastases may lie dormant for many years). These patients typically have moderate grade malignancies and no clinically detectable tumor metastases.

Regional node dissection may be associated with significant side effects and financial costs. Patients have had debilitating, even fatal, complications stemming from inadequate lymphatic drainage after regional node dissections *(6)*. One way to reduce both morbidity and cost of node dissection is to remove only the one to several nodes that are most likely to contain metastatic tumor. These nodes can be subjected to close pathologic scrutiny by evaluating multiple tissue levels for hematoxylin and eosin (H&E) staining and ancillary tests, such as immunohistochemistry and molecular analyses.

3. SENTINEL LYMPH NODE DISSECTION

The idea of a primary draining node or "sentinel lymph node" (SLN) has occurred to a range of investigators. Cabanas, for example, used the term "sentinel" to describe a lymph node at the superficial epigastric venous plexus that received primary lymphatic drainage from the penis *(7)*. Cabanas conceived of the SLN as an anatomically fixed lymph node that was the primary drainage node and thus the first site of tumor metastases. Other investigators had difficulty confirming Cabanas' anatomically designated SLN, and some individuals with bilateral negative anatomically defined SLN developed subsequent metastatic penile carcinoma *(8)*. Morton and Cochran et al. at UCLA took the SLN concept a critical step further by reasoning that because lymphatic anatomy and drainage patterns differ between individuals, the SLN is unlikely to be anatomically fixed. The Morton–Cochran concept of the SLN is physiologic rather than anatomic, thus the SLN must be identified individually for each patient. SLN dissection (SLND) was subsequently developed using perioperative lymphatic mapping as a means to identify the regional lymph node(s), the primary draining nodes with the highest probability of early metastasis. The SLND technique involves peritumoral injection of radioisotope and/or dye markers that drain into the lymphatics. In cases using radioisotope, the most radioactive lymph node is visualized by lymphoscintigraphy and localized intraoperatively by a hand-held Geiger counter. If peritumoral dye injections are done, the surgeon traces the lymphatics by dissection looking for blue-colored nodes. By this method, the earliest draining node(s) or SLN, considered "high risk" lymph nodes for metastases, can be selectively removed and subjected to extensive pathologic analysis (beyond what is feasible for an entire regional node dissection).

Morton et al. initially developed a feline model to demonstrate the feasibility of intraoperative lymphatic mapping *(9)*, and then conducted trials to evaluate the extent that SLN tumor status predicts for the tumor status of the remaining regional nodes in patients with *thick* melanomas *(3)*. Initially, intraoperative frozen sections were subjected to rapid immunohistochemical analysis to evaluate the tumor status of the SLN. It was thought that once the technique was validated, the decision to perform a completion node dissection would be based on the results of the intraoperative frozen section. In the earliest cases, the intraoperative SLN biopsy was followed by complete regional lymphadenectomy until it became clear that SLN tumor status reliably predicts the tumor status of the entire node bed *(10)*. This first study of the "physiologic" SLN in humans demonstrated clearly that absence of tumor in the non-SLN was reliably predicted by a tumor-free SLN, thus raising the possibility of sparing node-negative patients the potentially harmful side effects of regional node dissection. Oncologists and surgeons have now developed an interest in the oncologic and surgical implications of tumor-draining SLN in a wide range of different malignancies.

4. CLINICAL SIGNIFICANCE OF SENTINEL LYMPH NODE METASTASES

SLND is a minimally invasive staging technique established for staging and management of clinically node-negative melanoma patients with primaries of up to intermediate thickness, viewed by many as the standard of care for these patients *(11)*. SLND spares clinically node-negative cancer patients with tumor-free SLN the more invasive and morbid technique of regional lymph node dissection. Breast cancer staging also increasingly relies on SLND, sparing these patients a full axillary node dissection. SLND remains an investigative staging technique for other solid neoplasms. The development of ancillary techniques, such as immunohistochemistry and molecular analysis, has increased the frequency of detection of "positive" SLN resulting from the detection of smaller tumor deposits and singly dispersed tumor cells. The clinical significance of such minute tumor deposits and single tumor cells in SLN is an area of intense investigation, and the results are critical to interpreting the results of SLND.

4.1. Melanoma

Tumor involvement of the SLN is the most significant negative predictive factor for a patient with apparently localized melanoma, and is associated with a 40% decrease in 5-yr survival. Melanoma is more difficult to manage when regional nodes contain tumor, and 20–30% of patients with clinically negative nodes have occult metastases on microscopic examination. The likelihood of SLN metastases increases with increasing thickness and ulceration of the primary melanoma; however, SLN status is the most important predictor of outcome in clinically node-negative melanoma patients, and nodal metastases outweigh all other risk factors. Melanoma thickness and ulceration are important prognosticators for SLN-negative patients but are much less predictive in SLN-positive patients *(10,12)*. SLND is thus a highly useful staging and prognostic technique for clinically node-negative melanomas and has dramatically fewer side effects than more extensive regional lymph node dissection.

4.2. Breast Cancer

The lymphatics that drain from the breast to the lymph nodes of the ipsilateral axilla are the primary route for breast cancer metastasis, and axillary lymph node status is the most important predictor of recurrence and survival in breast cancer. Internal mammary nodes are harder to access surgically and are less frequently the site of metastases. These nodes are utilized less for staging breast cancer. Axillary SLNs have been localized by isosulfan blue dye mapping *(13,14)*, by radioisotope localization *(15)*, and by a combination of both approaches, which is generally considered to be the superior method *(13–16)*. Mapping using combined blue dye and radioisotope is accurate, the rate of detection of metastases comparing favorably to complete axillary lymph node dissection (ALND) *(17–21)*. Prospective studies have shown that most breast cancer patients remain disease free as long as three years after a negative SLN biopsy, indicating a low false-negative rate for axillary SLND *(22)*. A meta-analysis by Miltenburg et al. determined that SLN biopsy is as effective as ALND for staging axillary lymph nodes in breast cancers *(23)*.

Some authors have questioned the value of lymphoscintigraphy in breast SLND, maintaining that it does not increase the detection rate of axillary sentinel nodes and that a negative scan does not preclude identification of an axillary sentinel node intraoperatively *(24)*. Although axillary SLND may have prognostic power, it may be critically lacking in sensitivity if the localization technique excludes the internal mammary SLN. The prognostic significance of axillary and internal mammary nodes is similar and taken together the different node groups provide information that is cumulative, suggesting that there is utility in assessing internal mammary SLN (IMSLN) *(25)*. However, in most series, the incidence of isolated breast cancer metastases to IMSLN has been very low, and IMSLN sampling by the traditional surgical method has been associated with increased mortality, supporting the view that IMSLN sampling has no additive value to axillary SLN staging and may actually harm the patient *(26)*. In a series of 700 breast cancer cases from the H. Lee Moffitt Cancer Center at UCLA, no cases of isolated metastases to IMSLN were identified *(17)*. Likewise, in a multicenter validation study by Krag et al., only 1 of 443 patients (0.3%) had isolated drainage to an IMSLN *(15)*. Using a different approach, Ogawa et al. performed lymphatic mapping by lymphoscintigraphy and thoracoscopy on 49 breast cancer patients and found SLN among the internal mammary nodes in 15 cases (31%) *(27)*. Of 11 patients who underwent thoracoscopic biopsies, 2 had tumor metastases, only one of which was limited to the IMSLN, an incidence of 1% *(27)*. The thoroscopic approach may address some concerns regarding increased morbidity in IMSLN biopsy, making this approach more clinically viable. If the internal mammary pathway harbors tumor-draining SLN, additional surgery may be necessary to biopsy these nodes, though many believe that tumor in the internal mammary nodes is controllable by customary radiotherapy. Furthermore, the therapeutic value of both complete axillary dissection (and axillary SLND) has not been established, and axillary lymphatic staging may be sufficient to predict prognosis for most patients. At present, IMSLN biopsy remains a controversial and investigational procedure.

5. A TEAM APPROACH TO SENTINEL LYMPH NODE DETECTION

Successful outcome in SLND for melanoma and breast cancers depends on an effective collaboration between surgeon, nuclear medicine specialist, and pathologist, all of whom have worked together to master the technique *(28,29)*. During the surgical learning phase, completion dissection of the entire node basin must be performed (regardless of the tumor status of the SLN until all participants demonstrate acceptable performance of the technique. Diagnostic accuracy in SLND depends on optimal site, type, timing, and dosage of marker injection, as well as good pre-operative lymphoscintographic imaging and interpretation. The surgeon carefully dissects the lymph node bed identified by lymphoscintigraphy. Following the signpost offered by the blue colored afferent lymphatic(s), the bluest and most radioactive (by Geiger counter) lymph node(s) are identified, carefully dissected out, and removed. It should be remembered that often, only a part of the SLN may be blue colored. Many patients may have more than one SLN, and 98% of positive axillary SLN are found by removing nodes with enhanced radioactivity although this may be only 10% of the hottest lymph node identified *(30)*. SLN radioactivity may be relatively limited, especially in the presence of a relatively high tumor burden that can limit radioisotope uptake. In fact, if the SLN is replaced by tumor, lymph flow will be deviated and another node (that may be tumor-free) may appear to be the SLN. Great caution is required in managing lymph node groups where there is relatively abundant tumor present. In fact, the SLND technique is not intended for this class of patients.

The radioisotope used for SLND must be short-lived with limited tissue penetration, as is Technetium-99m ($t_{1/2}$ = 6 h). Trained early-read assessment of the preoperative lymphoscintogram by a radiologist is critical. If a lymphoscintogram is performed hours before surgery, a second peritumoral injection of radioisotope will usually not be required. The surgeon uses the lymphoscintogram to select an optimal skin incision site and dissects into the underlying soft tissue looking for blue colored lymphatics and node(s). At UCLA, the SLN is identified as the most radioactive node by hand-held Geiger counter and is secondarily assessed for visible blue coloration. However, if a second, blue lymph node is seen, it will also be removed and analyzed as a SLN.

6. PATHOLOGIC PROCESSING OF SENTINEL LYMPH NODES

Although Morton et al. initially developed the SLN approach using intraoperative frozen sections, identification of small metastatic foci and single tumor cells is more accurate in permanent sections owing to superior fixation and staining, and higher certainty of complete nodal sections *(10)*. Facing of the frozen section block and subsequent refacing of the formalin-fixed, paraffin-embedded material can result in loss of diagnostic tissue. Instead, the pathologist may do intraoperative touch imprints of the cut face of the bisected SLN. A recent report supports the utility of intraoperative touch imprints of SLN for detection of breast cancer metastases *(31)*, although others are less enthusiastic about this approach. SLN are processed somewhat differently for melanoma and breast cancer cases owing to differences in the kinetics of extension of these two tumors within the lymph node. In both types of cases, the SLN specimen is handled with care. If an intact rim of perinodal fat is present around each dissected node, it may be possible to detect tumor emboli within afferent lymphatics and assess extra-nodal spread.

6.1. Melanoma

Melanoma SLND is usually performed at the time of wide local resection of cutaneous melanoma. Surgeons submit each SLN in an individual container of 10% formalin and label it with the node color and level of radioactivity (cpm). The pathologist records the number and dimensions of the SLN(s) and notes the surgeon's description—color (blue) and counts (cpm)—of each node. If there is more than one node, and one is blue-colored and selectively radioactive, this is noted, and the node is submitted separately for SLN workup. In melanoma cases, additional nodes that are neither blue nor more radioactive than the background are considered *incidental nonsentinel nodes*; however, these nodes are also submitted individually for SLN workup.

Because melanomas typically metastasize to the subcapsular space first, particularly along the longest meridian of the node, the pathologist bisects the SLN through its longest circumference and evaluates both cut surfaces for tumor (using a hand lens or dissecting microscope), as well as foci of blue coloration *(32)*. Node halves are placed cut face down into cassettes and formalin-fixed for 24–48 h. After processing, paraffin-embedded blocks are sectioned at 2 to 4 µ*M* intervals with minimal preparatory facing off of the block. Ten sections are cut from each half of the node (a total of 20 sections and used for H&E staining and immunohistochemical staining with antibodies to S-100, HMB-45, and Melan-A/MART-1;

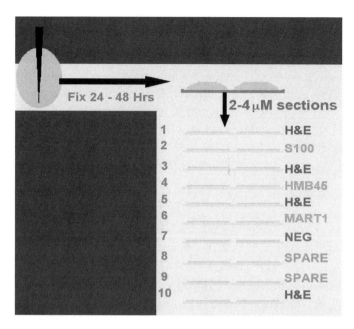

Fig. 1. Histopathologic analysis of melanoma sentinel lymph nodes. SLN are bisected, then formalin-fixed for 24 to 48 h, processed by histology, and ultimately embedded in paraffin. The tissue blocks are sectioned at 2–4 µM intervals, including 10 sections from each half of the SLN for hematoxylin and eosin (H&E) staining, as well as immunohistochemical staining with antibodies to S100, HMB45, and MART1/MelanA. Color image available for viewing at **www.humanapress.com**.

Fig. 1). It is critical that the lymph node capsule is present in its entirety on sections or the entire sentinel node package may need to be repeated.

6.2. Breast Cancer

There are several approaches to the pathologic examination of SLN draining breast cancers. The College of American Pathologists' Surgical Pathology Committee, recommends submission of the entire (bisected) SLN for preparation of serial sections that will be alternately used for three H&E stained slides and three cytokeratin immunostained slides *(33)*. Examination of at least three levels of a bisected or multi-sectioned SLN (50 to 100 µM intervals) can detect between 70 and 90% of SLN *(34)*. Turner et al. of the John Wayne Cancer Institute (Santa Monica) have recommended cytokeratin immunostaining of two levels of the paraffin block to detect breast cancer metastases *(35)*.

At UCLA, breast surgeons typically send the pathologist fibroadipose tissue that contains from one to three lymph nodes. The pathologist dissects all lymph nodes from the breast SLN specimen and records their individual dimensions and color in the surgical pathology report. Serial-sections of the SLN are cut at 2-mm intervals along the long axis and the entire node is submitted. If there is more than one SLN, they are submitted in separate cassettes for SLN workup. Six serial histologic sections are prepared for H&E stains (serial no. 1, 3, and 5) and for possible cytokeratin staining (serial no. 2, 4, and 6). The three H&E sections are examined first, and if no diagnostic cancer is detected on the H&E sections, pan-cytokeratin (kerAE1,3) immunostaining is done on serial sections no. 2 and 4. Serial section no. 6 is used for an immunostaining negative control.

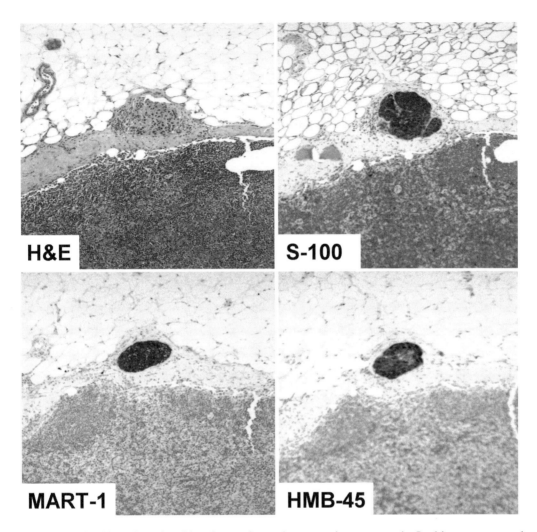

Fig. 2. Sentinel lymph node with subcapsular melanoma micrometastasis. In this case, a capsular lymphatic micrometastasis from a cutaneous nevoid melanoma is visible on the H&E stain and on immunostaining for S100, MART1, and HMB45 markers. There is also strong immunostaining of metastatic melanoma with HMB45 in addition to the other immunomarkers. The strong HMB45 positivity is consistent with the malignant nature of the melanocytic cells. Color image available for viewing at **www.humanapress.com**.

7. MICROSCOPIC ANALYSIS OF SENTINEL LYMPH NODES

7.1. Melanoma

There is no doubt that histopathologic analysis of SLN is an acquired skill, and melanoma metastases, other than large multicellular colonies, may be difficult to see on H&E staining. Small melanoma metastases and micrometastases are typically found within the subcapsular sinus (Fig. 2), although they have on occasion been identified primarily in the internal nodal sinuses. As the metastases grow, they may expand into the lymph node parenchyma and/or through the capsule. The pathologist first scans the H&E slide at low power (×40–100) and assesses the different nodal compartments with particular focus on the subcapsular sinus.

Lymphatics within the perilymphatic tissue are also evaluated. Sequential high power (×400) fields are then scanned for single or clustered atypical cells that are suspicious for tumor cells. The entire node is carefully examined because melanoma metastases can occasionally be confined to the lymphoid parenchyma and/or the central nodal sinuses. Extracapsular invasion by tumor worsens the prognosis and is recorded if present *(36)*. If metastases are detected, the pathologist records the number of tumor foci and the dimension of the largest focus, using image analysis or a micrometer *(37)*.

7.2. Breast Cancer

H&E slides from breast SLN are examined at both low and high power, analogous to the approach for melanoma SLN. Breast cancer metastases frequent the intranodal sinuses (more than the subcapsular sinus), although large metastases may displace part or all of the node. H&E staining alone is insufficient to detect metastases from lobular carcinomas, which may present as scattered small cells within the lymph node parenchyma. SLND is sometimes performed for ductal-carcinoma-*in situ* (DCIS), and 10–15% of patients with DCIS may have undetected, associated microinvasive DCIS and regional lymph nodes metastases *(38, 39)*. We have observed that SLN metastases in patients with DCIS do occur and may be quite large with areas that recapitulate the DCIS morphology seen in the breast.

8. IMMUNOHISTOCHEMICAL ANALYSIS OF SLN

8.1. Melanoma

Scattered, single tumor cells inapparent on H&E stained sections may be visualized using immunohistochemistry targeting melanoma markers, such as S100, HMB45, or MelanA/MART1. The immunoreactive single tumor cells may be seen clustering near a metastatic colony of melanoma cells first detected on the H&E stained slide. Immunohistochemistry plays a crucial role in the detection of micrometastases by highlighting individual cells and small clusters of melanoma cells, thereby improving the sensitivity of SLN analysis. When a node metastasis is first observed in immunostained sections, the pathologist should review the H&E sections with guidance from the immunostained sections and try to retrospectively identify the tumor cells. The proportion of SLN in which tumor is identified initially in the H&E sections increases with experience, but immunohistochemical analysis is still required to maximize the sensitivity for micrometastases and to confirm the diagnosis of melanoma as the primary.

In addition to S100, HMB45, and MelanA/MART1, antibodies to tyrosinase and glyco-protein-100 may be used as markers for melanoma *(40,41)*, as well as combined antibody cocktails. S100 stains 100% of melanomas, whereas the other epitopes are absent from 5–15% of melanomas. However, S100 also stains cells in the node that are not melanocytic, including dendritic leukocytes of the paracortex. Separation of dendritic cells with reduced dendrites from small (nevocytic) melanoma cells can be difficult. It is therefore essential to use a combination of single immunomarkers, such as S100, HMB45, and MelanA/MART1.

8.2. Breast Cancer

Cytokeratin immunostaining is helpful for detecting micrometastases and discriminating "atypical" but benign cells, such as activated histiocytes or reactive endothelial cells, from true metastases. If metastatic breast cancer is first observed on cytokeratin stains, morpho-

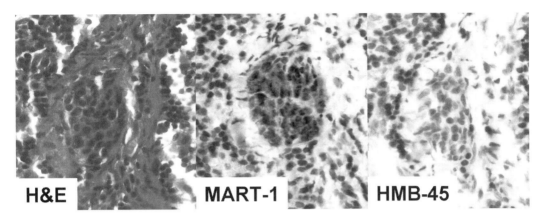

Fig. 3. Sentinel lymph node with trabecular nevus. In this case, a trabecular nevus is visible on an H&E stain and on immunostaining for MART1 and HMB45 markers (S100 not shown). There is positive immunostaining of metastatic melanoma with MART1. Weak to absent staining with HMB45, as is characteristic for benign capsular nevi. Color image available for viewing at **www.humanapress.com**.

logic comparison is made to corresponding cells in the H&E sections of the SLN and to the cytology of the primary tumor.

9. PITFALLS IN THE MICROSCOPIC DIAGNOSIS OF SENTINEL LYMPH NODES

The major pitfalls in the microscopic evaluation of sentinel nodes for melanoma occur from errors in reading immunostained sections. Discrimination of the pigment in melanophages from immunopositive cells is aided by antibody visualization with aminoethylcarbazole (red) rather than diaminobenzidine (brown). Additional potential S100-positive distractors include reactive dendritic cells, (Fig. 2B) capsular and capsular or trabecular nevi (Fig. 3), histiocytes, intranodal and perinodal nerves, and ganglion cells. Nonspecific HMB-45 immunostaining of calcified trabeculae in inguinal or pelvic lymph nodes may be recognized by its acellular chunky appearance.

Discrimination of benign cells from metastatic melanoma requires consideration of nodal architecture and cytologic features of the cells of interest. Nevocytes within lymph nodes are typically found in a different compartment (intracapsular and intratrabecular) from metastatic melanoma cells (initially subcapsular, later subcapsular, and intraparenchymal). Benign nevocytes commonly appear as layered small polygonal or spindled cells around capsular vessels or within trabeculae (Fig. 3), as opposed to usually larger melanoma cells that occur individually and in small aggregates within the subcapsular sinus (Fig. 2). Capsular/trabecular nevocytes have a low nuclear to cytoplasmic ratio and lack prominent nucleoli. Histiocytes and macrophages have small, kidney bean-shaped nuclei with small nucleoli, although reactive histiocytes and endothelial cells may have a more alarming cytologic appearance. Paracortical dendritic cells characteristically have elongated cell processes, although these may be reduced in frequency, complexity, and length as a result of tumor-released immune suppressive factors *(42–44)*. Suspicious features for melanoma cells include large size, high nuclear to cytoplasmic ratio, prominent nucleoli, mitotic figures, and the presence of fine punctate melanin granules (as opposed to the coarse granules of melanin seen in melanophages).

False positive interpretations of SLN removed for breast cancer can result from weak cytokeratin staining of fibroblastic reticular cells, particularly when antibodies directed at low-molecular keratins are used. The reticular cells may be distinguished by their mesh-like arrangement and benign cytologic features *(45)*. In comparison to the multiple markers used for melanoma, cytokeratin immunostaining is not as specific for breast cancer, and metastatic carcinoma from other primaries may need to be excluded.

10. APPLICATION OF THE SENTINEL LYMPH NODE APPROACH TO OTHER SOLID MALIGNANCIES

10.1. Gastric Cancer

Lymphatic mapping for gastric carcinoma is of interest in countries such as Japan where the incidence of this disease is relatively high. The use of SLND for gastric tumors has potential advantages for identifying nodal metastases, because diagnostic imaging is usually insufficient to detect lymph node metastases of gastric cancers. The complex nature of the gastrointestinal lymphatics raises the concern that selective SLND might miss skip metastases, reportedly common in gastric cancers. Because of these concerns, the SLND approach to gastric cancer is still in its validation stage, although the results are promising enough to warrant larger trials *(46)*. On average, two to four SLN are identified in surgeries where lymphatic mapping is done for gastric cancers *(47)*.

Hiratsuka et al. performed intraoperative SLN biopsy in gastric cancer patients by administering intraoperative, peritumoral injections of green dye, followed by gastrectomy, and extensive lymphadenectomy *(48)*. In all but 1 of 74 patients, they were able to detect a SLN (an average of 2.6 SLN per patient), and the SLN tumor status predicted overall lymph node status in 90% of cases. In a different approach, Ichikura et al. performed intra-operative lymphatic mapping in 62 patients via endoscopic dye injection into the gastric submucosa adjacent to the tumor *(49)*. In most cases, green-stained lymph nodes were identified within 5 min, occasionally localized in the contralateral side from the primary tumor and even outside the perigastric area *(49)*. The unpredictable drainage of some gastric carcinomas highlights the complexity of the gastric lymphatics and the importance of functional lymphatic mapping in identifying the nodes that truly drain a gastric carcinoma. At present, the goal is increased detection of lymph node metastases from gastric cancer rather than minimization of the area of lymph node dissection *(47)*. Lymphatic mapping may assist in the staging of gastric cancer by increasing the rate of lymph node detection and by identifying a subset of draining lymph nodes that warrant close pathologic scrutiny rather than a single sentinel node. Given the complex lymphatic drainage of the stomach, all dye-colored nodes detected may not be "sentinel" nodes by conventional standards.

10.2. Colorectal Cancer

Regional nodal metastasis is the most significant risk factor for local and distant metastases from colorectal cancer *(50)*. Although 55% of patients with colorectal cancer present with node-negative localized disease, up to 30% develop metastases following colectomy *(50)*. Special pathologic procedures, such as pinning and stretching of the resected bowel and the application of fat dissolving chemicals are undertaken to increase the number of nodes identified in colectomy specimens. SLN analysis of colorectal cancers has been controversial, reflecting concerns regarding the possibility of "skip metastases," metastases in second or third echelon nodes with apparent sparing of first echelon nodes. However, reliance on anatomical considerations, such as physical proximity to tumor, has been proven unreliable by lymphoscintographic studies.

The most common approach to intraoperative SLN mapping for colorectal cancer has been to inject isosulfan blue subserosally around the tumor. Saha et al. report a multicenter trial of SLND on 203 patients with colorectal cancer to determine accuracy, upstaging, skip metastasis, and aberrant drainage *(51)*. Blue dye was injected subserosally around the tumor and one to four blue staining nodes were marked as SLN for detailed histological analysis *(51)*. SLN mapping was successful in 98% of patients with an average of 1.7 SLN per patient; 37% of the patients had positive SLN, 63% were negative, and skip metastases were seen in only 8 (4%) of the patients *(51)*. Occult micrometastases not visible on H&E staining, but detected by immunohistochemistry, were found in 14% of patients. In 5% of the patients, unusual lymphatic drainage resulted in a change in the extent of the lymphadenectomy *(51)*.

In an alternative approach, Wong et al. performed ex vivo mapping of colorectal carcinoma in 26 patients following resection of a bowel segment containing a primary tumor *(52)*. Within 30 min of removal, the specimens were delivered to pathology, grossly evaluated, and opened longitudinally on the antimesenteric border. Isosulfan blue was injected submucosally around the primary tumor. The injection site was massaged for a few minutes, and the mesenteric fat dissected to look for blue-stained (sentinel) nodes *(52)*. One to six blue-stained nodes were identified as SLN in 24 of 26 specimens, and of 14 specimens with negative SLN, one had metastases in other dissected nodes; four patients with negative mesenteric nodes on H&E staining were upstaged by cytokeratin immunohistochemistry *(52)*.

Focused analysis of SLN with multiple serial sections for H&E and immunohistochemistry can detect nodal metastases missed on conventional H&E screening, as well as identify SLN in unexpected locations. For example, Wood et al. successfully removed intraoperatively identified SLN from 97 of 100 consecutive patients undergoing colectomy, and the SLN accurately reflected the status of the nodal basin in 92 (95%) of them *(53)*. Unexpected lymphatic drainage that altered the operative approach was found in eight patients, and 18 patients were upstaged by identification of occult nodal micrometastases missed on routine H&E staining but detected on multiple sections or by cytokeratin immunostaining *(53)*. The results indicate that increased sensitivity for detecting lymphatic metastases is provided by the SLND technique. In another study of 55 patients, the SLN was successfully identified intraoperatively in 45 cases (82%) and the SLN status correctly predicted regional nodal status in 44 (98%) cases *(54)*. Cytokeratin immunohistochemistry was critical to diagnosing tumor deposits in 6 of 14 positive SLN, and there was a 3% false-negative rate because of one case that had a negative SLN and a small pericolonic non-SLN replaced by tumor that was likely the true SLN *(54)*.

SLND for colorectal cancer permits selection of high-risk lymph nodes for ancillary studies such as immunohistochemistry and molecular analysis that would not be feasible on the large number of nodes typically obtained from a colectomy specimen. Bilchik et al. injected isosulfan blue peritumorally during 100 colectomies, and SLN were identified in 97% of cases *(55)*. All mesenteric nodes identified were examined by H&E staining; however, multiple serial sections of SLN were prepared for H&E staining and cytokeratin immunostaining, and in some cases RT-PCR analysis was done. Metastases were found in 26% of patients by H&E staining and immunohistochemistry and the remaining 74% had occult nodal micrometastases detected by immunohistochemistry or RT-PCR analysis *(55)*. In eight cases, aberrant lymphatic drainage was discovered that required changes in the operative approach. Cytokeratin mRNA was detected in 12 of 26 patients (46%) that were negative on H&E and cytokeratin immunostaining *(55)*. Focused examination of SLN with the use of immunohistochemistry and RT-PCR analysis identified or raised the possibility of micrometastatic colon cancer in a significant number of patients that would have been node-negative on conventional lymph node analysis by H&E staining alone.

10.3. Gynecologic Cancers

Lymph node metastases constitute the most important prognostic factor in squamous cell carcinoma (SCC) of the vulva *(56,57)*. The standard of care for SCC of the vulva with greater than 1 mm invasion has long been bilateral ilioinguinal node dissection, a procedure associated with high morbidity and frequent recurrences *(58)*. Efforts to limit morbidity have included more superficial inguinal resections; however, deep inguinal or femoral node metastases have been reported in cases with negative superficial nodes *(59)*. Intraoperative lymphatic mapping has been done with isosulfan blue dye *(60)*, radioisotope *(61)*, and a combination of both *(62)*. These attempts have been moderately successful at localizing the SLN draining vulvar carcinoma, and preliminary studies have had very low false-negative rates for metastases *(60)*.

Pilot studies of SLND for cervical carcinoma have also yielded preliminary but promising results. The lymphatic drainage from the cervix is not always readily predictable, suggesting a role for dynamic lymphatic mapping in improving the detection rate of lymph node metastases. Medl et al. performed paracervical injections of isosulfan blue in three patients and identified disease-positive SLN either at the iliac artery or in the obturator space; all other pelvic lymph nodes removed were negative *(63)*. Verheijen et al. reported localization of SLN as far as the common iliac level in 6 of 10 patients with early stage cervical cancer by a combined radioisotope and blue dye labeling technique *(64)*. O'Boyle et al. identified SLN in 12 of 20 patients with cervical cancer by the use of isosulfan blue, and reported more reliable detection where the tumor was <4 cm in greatest dimension *(65)*.

Burke et al. attempted lymphatic mapping for advanced endometrial cancers by intraoperative injection of isosulfan blue dye into the subserosal myometrium at three distinct sites *(66)*. After 10 min, blue lymph nodes were observed in paraaortic, common iliac and pelvic sites, underscoring the complexity of uterine lymphatic drainage. Holub et al. have reported successful detection (83.3%) of SLN in early stage endometrial cancer based on intraoperative application of blue dye to several points on the uterine serosal surface *(67)*.

10.4. Genitourinary Cancers

SLN mapping has been investigated for the staging of prostate cancer. Wawroschek et al. localized SLN in 11 cases of prostate cancer via transrectal prostatic injection of technetium-99m colloid 1 d prior to pelvic lymphadenectomy *(68)*. SLN were identified by lymphoscintigraphy and intraoperative use of a Geiger counter. Three of four patients had metastases in SLN only, two had positive SLN outside of the standard pelvic lymphadenectomy area, and one had positive non-SLN associated with negative SLN *(68)*. In a larger study, Vogt et al. used lymphoscintigraphy and intraoperative probe measurement for the identification of SLN in 117 patients with prostate cancer. SLN were detected in 114 of 117 cases with an average of four SLN per patient, 25 of 28 patients with lymph node metastases had positive SLN, and 15 of these 25 had metastases limited to the SLN *(69)*.

Cabanas *(7)* and Fowler *(70)* used anatomic landmarks to identify SLN draining penile cancer; however, several subsequent studies of this anatomy-dependent approach had unacceptable false-negative rates *(71,72)*. Larger series have had more success with intraoperative lymphatic mapping for penile carcinoma. For example, Valdes-Olmos et al. reported a sensitivity of 89% and a negative predictive value of 96% for detection of SLN metastases by combined lymphoscintigraphy and blue dye technique; bilateral inguinal drainage was identified in 81% of cases *(73)*. In another study, combined radioisotope and dye was used to detect SLN metastases with a reported sensitivity of 80%, although on clinical follow-up the false-negative rate was unacceptably high (22%) *(74)*.

Lymphatic mapping of bladder cancers may be facilitated by the tentatively easy accessibility of the bladder mucosa via cystoscopy. In one study, 13 patients with bladder cancer received preoperative, peritumoral injections of radioisotope and dye (via cystoscopy), localizing SLN in 11 of the patients *(75)*. Four of the patients had positive SLN and no other positive lymph nodes, and three of the positive SLN were located outside the obturator fossa *(75)*.

11. REVERSE TRANSCRIPTASE-POLYMERASE CHAIN REACTION ANALYSIS OF SENTINEL LYMPH NODES

11.1. Melanoma

Reverse transcriptase-polymerase chain reaction (RT-PCR) is an extremely sensitive method for amplifying small amounts of mRNA that can detect one positive cell in a background of 10^6 or 10^7 negative cells. It is potentially a more sensitive, but less specific technique than immunohistochemistry for detecting SLN metastases. The RT-PCR technique requires sacrifice of tissue that will be unavailable for histologic analysis. The lower specificity is the result of the limited specificity of tumor markers. In the absence of morphologic data, it cannot be determined that the mRNA signal derives from malignant cells.

The application of the RT-PCR technique to the analysis of melanoma SLN is the subject of much ongoing study. In a recent report, Boi et al. describe the analysis of 88 melanoma SLN from 74 patients by RT-PCR to detect tyrosinase mRNA in fresh tissue: 40 were positive by tyrosinase RT-PCR, 28 of which were negative by H&E staining and by immunostaining for S100, HMB-45, and tyrosinase *(76)*. The frequency of detection of occult metastases by tyrosinase PCR alone was relatively high in this study (31%), therefore at least some of the tyrosine RT-PCR-positive SLN may have contained true metastases, but it is not clear how to distinguish these from false-positives.

To estimate the false positive rate for SLN RT-PCR studies, Gutzmer et al. compared the results of tyrosinase and HMB45 RT-PCR studies on SLN from melanoma patients to control studies on lymph nodes from nonmelanoma patients *(77)*. All nodes were initially analyzed by preparation of multiple sections for H&E staining and immunostaining for HMB45 and MART1 *(77)*. Fourteen of 39 melanoma SLN were positive on tyrosinase RT-PCR; only 8 of the 14 were positive on H&E and/or immunostaining, and HMB-45 PCR was positive in only 3 of the 14, indicating suboptimal sensitivity with this primer *(77)*. Analyses of 29 nonmelanoma lymph nodes yielded four positive on tyrosinase-RT-PCR and negative on all other measures, indicating that tyrosinase-PCR may have insufficient specificity for determining tumor status of the SLN *(77)*. The false positive rate for tyrosinase-RT-PCR may be underestimated because two melanoma SLN-containing nevi were excluded from PCR analysis, presumably because a positive RT-PCR signal would be difficult to interpret in those cases.

Bostick et al. tested multiple markers (MAGE3, MART1, and tyrosinase mRNAs) in RT-PCR analysis of SLN from 72 melanoma patients in parallel with H&E staining and immunohistochemistry, for melanoma metastases *(78)*. Sixteen of 17 patients with H&E-and/or IHC-positive SLN expressed two or more mRNA markers by RT-PCR; however, 20 of 55 patients with histopathologically negative SLN also expressed two or more mRNA markers *(78)*. Patients with histopathologically melanoma-free SLN who were RT-PCR-positive by multiple markers had increased risk of recurrence compared to individuals who were positive for one or none of the mRNA markers *(78)*. These results suggest that H&E staining and immunohistochemistry alone may fail to detect a subgroup of clinically significant melanoma micrometastases positive for multiple melanoma markers on RT-PCR analysis.

In another study, Bonin et al. investigated multiple RT-PCR targets for melanoma SLN, including MAGE1, MAGE3, melanocyte inhibitory antigen (MIA), and MelanA/MART1 mRNAs *(79)*. They used a sensitive RT-PCR method to amplify mRNAs from a central, longitudinal cut of archived formalin-fixed, paraffin-embedded SLN specimens, and stained additional sections with H&E and antibodies for S100 and HMB45 proteins *(79)*. From 47 SLN, 10 were positive on H&E and immunostaining, as well as by tyrosinase RT-PCR, and, of the remaining 37, only 2 were negative on H&E and immunostaining but positive on tyrosinase RT-PCR *(79)*. A higher proportion of the SLN that were negative on H&E and immunohistochemical stains were PCR-positive for MART-1 (76%) and MIA (62%), than for MAGE1 (38%), MAGE3 (19%) mRNAs, or tyrosinase (5%), suggesting that the former targets might yield a greater number of false-positive results *(79)*. In this study, overall results showed no correlation between tumor stage and positivity for a particular marker mRNA or the number of positive marker mRNAs *(79)*.

In a larger study, an Italian group performed tyrosinase RT-PCR on 448 SLN from 308 patients, and the results were positive in 149 (48%) of these cases, in comparison to only 58 cases (17%) exhibiting SLN metastases revealed histologically (H&E and/or immunostaining) *(80)*. The RT-PCR results correlated strongly with tumor thickness of primary melanoma and with the clinical stage *(80)*. However, 18 of the 149 RT-PCR-positive cases had intracapsular aggregates of nevus cells, and are therefore possible false-positives. Both nodal nevi and schwann cells associated with nodal nerves are potential sources of a nonspecific tyrosinase mRNA signal that may yield a false-positive result. Indeed, nodal melanocytic nevi have been shown to occur at a higher rate in melanoma patients than in patients with breast cancer *(81)*, indicating an increased potential for false-positive results from melanoma SLN assessed by tyrosinase PCR.

Analyses of SLN by RT-PCR are difficult to validate because the RT-PCR technique requires wholesale RNA isolation from a piece of tissue and thus precludes morphologic assessment of that tissue. This problem can be partially addressed by taking alternate sections for RT-PCR and immunohistologic analysis, but there may still be no morphologic correlate for positive in vitro RT-PCR results, and *in situ* hybridization techniques are not sufficiently sensitive. *In situ* RT-PCR is an alternative approach that offers simultaneous mRNA detection and morphologic detail. The *in situ* RT-PCR technique for tyrosinase has been successfully applied to melanoma tissue cultures *(82)*. However, *in situ* RT-PCR for melanoma markers on formalin-fixed, paraffin-embedded SLN specimens have yielded lower, (and less consistent) signals *(83)*.

11.2. Breast Cancer

RT-PCR has been applied to the analysis of axillary SLN draining breast cancers with mixed results. Several previous studies report a higher incidence of positive SLN detected by RT-PCR for cytokeratin or other markers, as compared to routine histologic and/or immunohistochemical analyses *(84–86)*. However, several of these studies have shown poor concordance between positive immunostaining results and RT-PCR, in part because of false-negative RT-PCR results *(84,86)*. The use of multiple markers may eliminate some of these false-negative RT-PCR results. Indeed, one study demonstrated a significantly higher sensitivity for detection of metastases in RT-PCR studies that targeted multiple breast tumor markers (95.6%) than in individual studies with any single marker (78.8–83.6%) *(85)*. The expression of at least two of three markers (maspin, cytokeratin 19, or mammaglobin I) resulted in the highest concordance with positivity on H&E stains or cytokeratin-19 immunostains *(85)*.

12. CLINICAL SIGNIFICANCE OF LYMPH NODE MICROMETASTASES

With the advent of sensitive screening techniques, including SLND and molecular analyses, for detecting lymph node metastases, a need for clinical data establishing the prognostic relevance of small tumor deposits or micrometastases has been recognized The RT-PCR technique offers an increased sensitivity for detecting SLN metastases, which successfully distinguishes true metastases from false positives. The appropriate therapy for patients with SLN that are PCR-positive only has not been clearly established. In order to understand the prognostic implications of micrometastases, accurate information regarding size and numbers of micrometastases must be combined with long-term clinical follow-up data.

12.1. Melanoma

The recent American Joint Committee on Cancer (AJCC) Cancer Staging Manual (6th ed.) defines nodal micrometastases as those detectable only by microscopy and not clinically or radiographically, i.e., occult metastases *(87,88)*. According to the AJCC guidelines, metastatic tumor to a local node constitutes stage III. Subclassifications within this category are largely based on the number of positive nodes and whether they are clinically detected. Some classification schemes for melanoma have taken into account the percent of the node cross-section involved by tumor (Cochran et al., unpublished data), whereas others are based on the micrometer diameter of nodal metastases, which has been linked to prognosis in some studies *(37)*. In contrast to prior editions, size of individual melanoma metastases is not a consideration in the new AJCC staging guidelines for melanoma; although, the AJCC recommends that extent of tumor involvement in SLN be measured and recorded in the pathology report *(88)*.

Currently, there is ongoing investigation into the clinical significance of patients with occult micrometastatic melanoma in locoregional nodes, sentinel and non-sentinel, detected by serial H&E stained sections, immunohistochemistry and/or RT-PCR. The available evidence indicates that these techniques identify occult (clinically and radiographically unapparent) nodal metastases with increased frequency over conventional screening. Although the impact of these occult melanoma metastases on disease progression is still under investigation, their presence has been linked to other negative prognostic factors, and some investigators have found evidence that micrometastases detected by RT-PCR may be clinically relevant.

Gershenwald et al., of the MD Anderson Cancer Center (University of Texas), have observed that 8 of 10 archived SLN-negative melanoma cases with later nodal recurrences had micrometastases that were retrospectively identified by additional serial sectioning or immunohistochemistry *(89)*. Similarly, Blaheta et al. have reported nodal recurrences in 6 of 20 patients who were positive by tyrosinase RT-PCR (but negative on serial H&E sections and immunohistochemistry for HMB-45 or S100) during a median follow-up of 34 mo *(90)*. Blaheta et al. have also reported significantly higher tumor thickness in melanoma patients with nodal micrometastases identified exclusively by RT-PCR as compared to patients with negative results by RT-PCR *(91)*.

In an ongoing investigation with a large series of melanoma patients, Li et al. found that H&E staining combined with S100 immunostaining-detected metastatic disease in 52 of 233 (22%) of patients tested; whereas, 114 of 181 (63%) of patients with immunohistologically negative nodes had positive tyrosinase RT-PCR results *(82)*. Importantly, PCR-positive and PCR-negative patient groups differed significantly in Breslow thickness, Clark level, and the presence of ulceration of the primary tumor; all of which are factors that have been shown to correlate with recurrence and survival *(82)*. Hochberg et al. report that tyrosinase and MIA expression were sensitive indicators of melanoma SLN micrometastases that were negative on routine histopathologic examination and that positive MART-1 PCR in SLN was negatively correlated with overall survival *(92)*.

The above results imply that micrometastases identified by PCR alone could have clinical relevance, but long-term follow-up is necessary to establish real differences in recurrence and overall survival. The ongoing national, multicenter Sunbelt Melanoma Trial is investigating the utility of lymph node dissection and interferon therapy for patients who have SLN metastases detected only by PCR *(93)*.

12.2. Breast Cancer

In the case of breast cancer nodal micrometastases, data indicate a lack of clinical significance for tumor deposits under 2 mm *(94)*. However, the prognostic significance of small tumor deposits in lymph nodes remains controversial. Some authors have suggested that tumor cell colonies of any size are clinically significant, whereas single cell tumor metastases are not *(95)*. The tumor-node-metastasis (TNM) staging guidelines from the Union International Contra la Cancrum (UICC) define "isolated tumor cells" as single tumor cells or cell clusters under 0.2 mm in size *(96)*. The 2002 AJCC guidelines have also adopted the "0.2 mm or less" size cutoff for "isolated tumor cells" and classifies them as pN0(itc) *(97)*. Breast tumor metastases that measure between 0.2 mm and 2.0 mm are considered "micrometastases" and are classified as pN1 (mcm) *(97)*. The AJCC recommends that the prognostic relevance of isolated tumor cells become validated before adjuvant therapy is given to patients classified as pN0 (itc) with otherwise good prognostic factors *(97)*.

The measurement of the micrometer diameter of nodal metastases has prognostic significance *(37)* but may be confounded by variety in lymph node size and nodal enlargement resulting from factors other than tumor *(98)*. The College of American Pathologists has taken the position that the prognostic and predictive value of micrometastases identified using immunohistochemistry in SLN is still unproven; they do not recommend basing therapeutic decisions for breast cancer on such findings until their clinical significance has been demonstrated *(99)*.

Immunohistochemical analysis is critical for detecting occult micrometastases. The median size of micrometastases detected on cytokeratin immunohistochemistry is approx 0.1 mm, compared to 1.0 mm for H&E staining *(45)*. Based on an analysis of 120 patients (from a series of 1680 primary operable breast cancers) who had metastatic breast cancer to a single node, de Mascarel et al. determined that nodal metastases detected on serial H&E sectioning predict both recurrence and survival; whereas, immunohistochemically detected micrometastases predicted only recurrence for infiltrating ductal carcinomas and had no prognostic significance for infiltrating lobular carcinomas *(100)*. However, a recent review of the literature by Dowlatshahi et al. identified survival differences in breast cancer patients with micrometastases in studies involving relatively large patient populations (ranging from 147 to 921) and a follow-up of at least 6 yr *(95)*. The literature review suggested that occult metastases detected by immunohistochemistry do have important prognostic implications, although they noted differences between authors in size parameters defining micrometastases, indicating a need to follow standard criteria *(95)*.

The prognostic significance of SLN micrometastases may depend upon factors other than their size, such as the extent of down-regulation of the immune system by the primary tumor. Sentinel nodes in particular may exhibit features of immune suppression, such as reduction in dendritic cell number and arborization. For example, Cochran et al. have demonstrated significant reductions in total paracortical area of melanoma draining SLN, and in the density of paracortical interdigitating dendritic cells, of which almost all lacked the complex dendrites associated with active antigen presentation *(42,43)*. These morphologic changes may reflect the action of tumor generated immunosuppressive factors released by the primary melanoma and may act against immune surveillance, facilitating expansion of the primary tumor and the establishment of early metastases.

13. CONCLUSION

The past 10 yr have seen the technique of sentinel lymph node analysis validated as a low morbidity alternative to regional node dissection for staging in cases of melanoma and breast cancer. The SLND technique has worked well for detecting early melanoma metastases in clinically node-negative patients, particularly those with tumors of intermediate thickness. Likewise, in breast cancer studies of axillary SLN biopsies show excellent correlation with the status of the remaining axillary node bed. Two factors have contributed to the success of the SLND technique; the ability to identify the primary tumor-draining node(s) (SLN) using dynamic lymphoscintigraphy and radio-guided surgery and intensive, focused pathologic examination of SLN by multiple levels and immunohistochemistry. In particular, immunohistochemical markers permit detection of nodal metastases easily missed on routine H&E slides, thereby increasing the sensitivity for detection of micrometastatic disease.

The development of sensitive ancillary techniques for tumor detection, such as RT-PCR, has given us the capacity to detect smaller and smaller metastatic deposits in SLN. The use of molecular techniques in SLN analysis is still investigative, and the establishment of protocols with adequate sensitivity and specificity for the detection of tumor metastases is challenging. It is, however, likely that these techniques will become an important part of the assessment of SLN in the near future. At present, immunohistochemical stains provide the advantage of a morphologic reference to weed out false positives, whereas RT-PCR does not. The use of *in situ* PCR has theoretic potential; however, the procedure is technically demanding and may not be commercially viable in its present form.

The clinical significance of single tumor deposits less than 0.2 cm in SLN is undetermined, and some authors distinguish between "single tumor cells" or clusters less than 0.02 cm and "micrometastases" considered as those clusters between 0.02 cm and 0.2 cm. Basic tumor biology, however, suggests that the presence of any tumor cells in a tissue is a significant finding and that the biological significance of the finding increases as tumor size and organization increase. Once a tumor deposit is recognized, it necessitates a clinical decision, therefore distinctions between metastases that are clinically significant and those that are too small to warrant additional treatment must be based on data from clinical trials. Ultimately, the surgeon has to decide whether a completion node dissection is necessary, and the oncologist has to decide whether adjuvant chemotherapy and/or radiation therapy are indicated. Before the clinical data are in, one possible approach may be to incorporate characteristics of the primary tumor that are known to affect prognosis, such as tumor size, depth of invasion, and/or ulceration, into treatment decisions for cancer patients with SLN that contain very small tumor deposits or are positive by PCR alone.

REFERENCES

1. Osbourne M and Smith SR. 2002. The historical background of lymphatic mapping, in: Sentinel Lymph Node Biopsy, H.S.C. III, Editor. Martin Dunitz: New York, NY, pp. 1–10.
2. Fee H, Robinson DS, Sample WF, Graham LS, Holmes EC, Morton DL. 1978. The determination of lymph shed by colloidal gold scanning in patients with malignant melanoma: a preliminary study. Surgery 84:626–632.
3. Morton DL, Wen DR, Wong JH, et al. 1992. Technical details of intraoperative lymphatic mapping for early stage melanoma. Arch. Surg. 127:392–399.
4. Moynihan B. 1908. The surgical treatment of cancer of the sigmoid flexure and rectum. Surg. Gynecol. Obstet. 6:463–466.
5. Fife K and Thompson JF. 2001. Lymph-node metastases in patients with melanoma: what is the optimum management? Lancet Oncol. 2:614–621.
6. Harris MN, Shapiro RL, Roses DF. 1995. Malignant melanoma. Primary surgical management (excision and node dissection) based on pathology and staging. Cancer 75:715–725.
7. Cabanas RM. 1977. An approach for the treatment of penile carcinoma. Cancer 39:456–466.
8. Wespes E, Simon J, Schulman CC. 1986. Cabanas approach: is sentinel node biopsy reliable for staging penile carcinoma? Urology 28:278–279.
9. Wong JH, Cagle LA, Morton DL. 1991. Lymphatic drainage of skin to a sentinel lymph node in a feline model. Ann. Surg. 214(5):637–641.
10. Cochran AJ, Essner R, Rose DM, Glass EC. 2000. Principles of sentinel lymph node identification: background and clinical implications. Langenbecks Arch. Surg. 385:252–260.
11. Edwards MJ, Martin KD, McMasters KM. 1998. Lymphatic mapping and sentinel lymph node biopsy in the staging of melanoma. Surg. Oncol. 7:51–57.
12. Reintgen D, Balch CM, Kirkwood J, Ross M. 1997. Recent advances in the care of the patient with malignant melanoma. Ann. Surg. 225:1–14.
13. Giuliano A, Kirgan DM, Guenther M, Morton DL. 1994. Lymphatic mapping and sentinel lymphadenectomy for breast cancer. Ann. Surg. 220:391–401.
14. Giuliano AE, Dale PS, Turner RR, Morton DL, Evans SW, Krasne DL. 1995. Improved axillary staging of breast cancer with sentinel lymphadenectomy. Ann. Surg. 222:394–399.
15. Krag D, Weaver D, Ashikaga T, et al. 1998. The sentinel node in breast cancer—a multicenter validation study. N. Engl. J. Med. 339:941–946.

16. Cody H 3rd. 2002. Current surgical management of breast cancer. Curr. Opin. Obstet. Gynecol. 14:45–52.
17. Bass S, Cox C, Ku N. 1999. The role of sentinel lymph node biopsy in breast cancer. J. Am. Coll. Surg. 189:183–194.
18. Cox CE, Haddad F, Bass S, et al. 1998. Lymphatic mapping in the treatment of breast cancer. Oncology 12:1283–1292.
19. Albertini JJ, Lyman GH, Cox C, et al. 1996. Lymphatic mapping and sentinel node biopsy in the patient with breast cancer. J. Am. Med. Assoc. 276:1818–1822.
20. Nwariaku FE, Euhus DM, Beitsch PD, et al. 1998. Sentinel lymph node biopsy, an alternative to elective axillary dissection for breast cancer. Am. J. Surg. 176:529–531.
21. Offodile R, Hoh C, Barsky SH, et al. 1998. Minimally invasive breast carcinoma staging using lymphatic mapping with radiolabeled dextran. Cancer 82:1704–1708.
22. Haigh PI and Giuliano AE. 2000. Sentinel lymphadenectomy in node negative breastcancer. Cancer Treat. Res. 103:25–37.
23. Miltenburg DM, Miller C, Karamlou TB, Brunicardi FC. 1999. Meta-analysis of sentinel lymph node biopsy in breast cancer. J. Surg. Res. 84:138–142.
24. Upponi S, McIntosh SA, Wishart GC, Balan KK, Purushotham AD. 2002. Sentinel lymph node biopsy in breast cancer—is lymphoscintigraphy really necessary? Eur. J. Surg. Oncol. 28:479–480.
25. Noguchi M. 2002. Relevance and practicability of internal mammary sentinel node biopsy for breast cancer. Breast Cancer 9:329–336.
26. Kern K. 2002. A rational approach to internal mammary node biopsy in the era of lymphatic mapping for breast cancer. J. Surg. Oncol. 79:5–9.
27. Ogawa YIT, Sawada T, Chung SH, et al. 2003. Thoracoscopic internal mammary sentinel node biopsy for breast cancer. Surg. Endosc. 17:315–319.
28. Cox CE, Bass SS, Boulware D, Ku NK, Berman C, Reintgen DS. 1999. Implementation of new surgical technology: outcome measures for lymphatic mapping of breast carcinoma. Ann. Surg. Oncol. 6:553–561.
29. Tafra L. 2001. The learning curve and sentinel node biopsy. Am. J. Surg. 182:347–350.
30. Carlson G, Murray DR, Thourani V, Hestley A, Cohen C. 2002. The definition of the sentinel lymph node in melanoma based on radioactive counts. Curr. Opin. Obstet. Gynecol. 14:45–52.
31. Lee A, Krishnamurthy S, Sahin A, Symmans WF, Hunt K, Sneige, N. 2002. Intraoperative touch imprint of sentinel lymph nodes in breast carcinoma patients. Cancer 96:225–231.
32. Cochran AJ, Robert ME, Wen DR. 1994. Pathology of the lymph nodes in patients with malignant melanoma. Pathology 2:385–400.
33. Cibull ML. 1999. Handling sentinel lymph node biopsy specimens.A work in progress. Arch. Pathol. Lab. Med. 123:620–621.
34. Treseler PA and Tauchi PS. 2000. Pathologic analysis of the sentinel lymph node. Surg. Clin. North Am. 80:1695–1719.
35. Turner RR, Ollila DW, Stern S, Giuliano AE. 1999. Optimal histopathologic examination of the sentinel lymph node for breast carcinoma staging. Am. J. Surg. Pathol. 23:263–267.
36. Singletary S, Byers RM, Shallenberger R. 1986. Prognostic factors in patients with regional cervical nodal metastases from cutaneous malignant melanoma. Am. J. Surg. 152:371–375.
37. Starz H, Balda BR, Kramer KU, Buchels H, Wang H. 2001. A micromorphometry-based concept for routine classification of sentinel lymph node metastases and its clinical relevance for patients with melanoma. Cancer 91:2110–2121.
38. Klauber-DeMore N, Tan LK, Liberman L. et al. 2000. Sentinel lymph node biopsy: is it indicated in patients with high-risk ductal carcinoma-in-situ and ductal carcinoma-in-situ with microinvasion? Ann. Surg. Oncol. 7:636–642.
39. Pendas S, Dauway E, Giuliano R, Ku N, Cox CE, Reintgen DS. 2000. Sentinel node biopsy in ductal carcinoma in situ patients. Ann. Surg. Oncol. 7:15–20.
40. Slominski A, Coming of age of melanogenesis-related proteins. 2002. Arch. Pathol. Lab. Med. 126:775–777.

41. Boyle JL, Haupt HM, Stern JB, Multhaupt HA. 2002. Tyrosinase expression in malignant melanoma, desmoplastic melanoma, and peripheral nerve tumors. PG - 816-22. Arch. Pathol. Lab. Med. 126:816–822.

42. Huang RR, Wen DR, Gu J, et al. 2000. Selective Modulation of Paracortical Dendritic Cells and T-Lymphocytes in Breast Cancer Sentinel Lymph Nodes. Breast J. 6:225–232.

43. Cochran AJ, Morton DL, Stern S, Lana AM, Essner R, Wen DR. 2001. Sentinel lymph nodes show profound downregulation of antigen-presenting cells of the paracortex: implications for tumor biology and treatment. Mod. Pathol. 14:604–608.

44. Cochran AJ, Pihl E, Wen DR, Hoon DSB, Korn EL. 1987. Zoned immune suppression of lymph nodes draining malignant melanoma: Histologic and immunohistologic studies. J. Nat. Cancer Inst. 78:399–405.

45. Turner R. 2002. Sentinel Lymph Node Biopsy for Breast Cancer: Pathologic Aspects, in Sentinel Lymph Node Biopsy, H.S.C. III, Editor. Martin Dunitz: New York, NY, pp. 191–208.

46. Kitagawa Y, Kubota T, Otani Y, et al. 2001. Clinical significance of sentinel node navigation surgery in the treatment of early gastric cancer. Nippon Geka Gakkai Zasshi 102:753–757.

47. Maruyama K, Sasako M, Kinoshita T, Sano T, Katai H. 1999. Can sentinel node biopsy indicate rational extent of lymphadenectomy in gastric cancer surgery? Fundamental and new information on lymph-node dissection. Langenbecks Arch. Surg. 384:149–157.

48. Hiratsuka M, Miyashiro I, Ishikawa O, et al. 2001. Application of sentinel node biopsy to gastric cancer surgery. Surgery 129:335–340.

49. Ichikura T, Morita D, Uchida T, et al. 2002. Sentinel node concept in gastric carcinoma. World J. Surg. 26:318–322.

50. Saha S, Nora D, Wong JH, Weise D. 2000. Sentinel lymph node mapping in colorectal cancer—a review. Surg. Clin. North Am. 80:1811–1819.

51. Saha S, Bilchik A, Wiese D, et al. 2001. Ultrastaging of colorectal cancer by sentinel lymph node mapping technique—a multicenter trial. Ann. Surg. Oncol. 8:94S–98S.

52. Wong JH, Steineman S, Calderia C, Bowles J, Namiki T. 2001. Ex vivo sentinel node mapping in carcinoma of the colon and rectum. Ann. Surg. 233:515–521.

53. Wood TF, Nora DT, Morton DL, et al. 2002. One hundred consecutive cases of sentinel lymph node mapping in early colorectal carcinoma: detection of missed micrometastases. J. Gastrointest. Surg. 6:322–329.

54. Paramo JC, Summerall J, Poppiti R, Mesko TW. 2002. Validation of sentinel node mapping in patients with colon cancer. Ann. Surg. Oncol. 9:550–554.

55. Bilchik AJ, Tollenaar RA, van de Velde CJ, et al. 2002. Ultrastaging of early colon cancer using lymphatic mapping and molecular analysis. Eur. J. Cancer 38:977–985.

56. Makar AP, Scheistroen M, van den Weyngaert D, Trope CG. 2001. Surgical management of stage I and II vulvar cancer: the role of the sentinel node biopsy. Review of literature. Int. J. Gynecol. Cancer. 11:255–262.

57. Morgan MA and Mikuta JJ. 1999. Surgical management of vulvar cancer. Semin. Surg. Oncol. 17:168–172.

58. Terada KY, Shimizu DM, Wong JH. 2000. Sentinel node dissection and ultrastaging in squamous cell cancer of the vulva. Gynecol. Oncol. 76:40–44.

59. Ghurani GB and Penalver MA. 2001. An update on vulvar cancer. Am. J. Obstet. Gynecol. 185:294–299.

60. Levenback C. 2000. Intraoperative lymphatic mapping and sentinel node identification: gynecologic applications. Recent Results Cancer Res. 157:150–158.

61. Decesare SL, Fiorica JV, Roberts WS. et al. 1997. A pilot study utilizing intraoperative lymphoscintigraphy for identification of the sentinel lymph nodes in vulvar cancer. Gynecol. Oncol. 66:425–428.

62. Terada KY, Coel MN, Ko P, Wong JH. 1998. Combined use of intraoperative lymphatic mapping and lymphoscintigraphy in the management of squamous cell cancer of the vulva. Gynecol. Oncol. 70:65–69.

63. Medl M, Peters-Engl C, Schutz P, Vesely M, Sevelda P. 2000. First report of lymphatic mapping with isosulfan blue dye and sentinel node biopsy in cervical cancer. Anticancer Res. 20:1133–1134.

64. Verheijen RH, Pijpers R, van Diest PJ, Burger CW, Buist MR, Kenemans P. 2000. Sentinel node detection in cervical cancer. Obstet. Gynecol. 96:135–138.

65. O'Boyle JD, Bernstein SG, Lifshitz S, Muller CY, Miller DS. 2000. Intraoperative lymphatic mapping in cervix cancer patients undergoing radical hysterectomy: A pilot study. Gynecol. Oncol. 79:238–243.

66. Burke TW, Levenback C, Tornos C, Morris M, Wharton JT, Gershenson DM. 1996. Intraabdominal lymphatic mapping to direct selective pelvic and paraaortic lymphadenectomy in women with high-risk endometrial cancer: results of a pilot study. Gynecol. Oncol. 62: 169–173.

67. Holub Z, Kliment L, Lukac J, Voracek J. 2001. Laparoscopically-assisted intraoperative lymphatic mapping in endometrial cancer: preliminary results. Eur. J. Gynaecol.Oncol. 22: 118–121.

68. Wawroschek F, Vogt H, Weckermann D, Wagner T, Harzmann R. 1999. The sentinel lymph node concept in prostate cancer—first results of gamma probe-guided sentinel lymph node identification. Eur. Urol. 36:595–600.

69. Vogt H, Wawroschek F, Wengenmair H, et al. 2002. Sentinel lymph node diagnosis in prostatic carcinoma: I: Method and clinical evaluation. Nuklearmedizin 41:95–101.

70. Fowler JE Jr. 1984. Sentinel lymph node biopsy for staging penile cancer. Urology 23:352–353.

71. Pettaway CA, Pisters LL, Dinney CP, et al. 1995. Sentinel lymph node dissection for penile carcinoma: the M. D. Anderson Cancer Center experience. J. Urol. 154:1999–2003.

72. Bouchot O, Bouvier S, Bochereau G, Jeddi M. 1993. Cancer of the penis: the value of systematic biopsy of the superficial inguinal lymph nodes in clinical NO stage patients. Prog. Urol. 3:228–233.

73. Valdes Olmos RA, Tanis PJ, Hoefnagel CA, et al. 2001. Penile lymphoscintigraphy for sentinel node identification. Eur. J. Nucl. Med. 28:581–585.

74. Tanis PJ, Lont AP, Meinhardt W, Olmos RA, Nieweg OE, Horenblas S. 2002. Dynamic Sentinel Node Biopsy for Penile Cancer: Reliability of a Staging Technique. J. Urol. 168:76–80.

75. Sherif A, De La Torre M, Malmstrom PU, Thorn M. 2001. Lymphatic mapping and detection of sentinel nodes in patients with bladder cancer. J. Urol. 166:812–815.

76. Boi S, Cristofolini P, Togni R, et al. 2002. Detection of nodal micrometastases using immunohistochemistry and PCR in melanoma of the arm and trunk. Melanoma Res. 12:147–153.

77. Gutzmer R, Kaspari M, Brodersen JP, et al. 2002. Specificity of tyrosinase and HMB45 PCR in the detection of melanoma metastases in sentinel lymph node biopsies. Histopathology 41: 510–518.

78. Bostick P, Morton DL Turner RR, et al. 1999. Prognostic significance of occult metastases detected by sentinel lymphadenectomy and reverse transcriptase-polymerase chain reaction in early-stage melanoma patients. J. Clin. Oncol. 17:3238–3244.

79. Bonin S, Niccolini B, Calacione R. 2002. Molecular analyses of sentinel lymph nodes: an open question. J. Eur. Acad. Dermatol. Venereol. 16:34–39.

80. Riccioni L, Farabegoli P, Nanni O, et al. 2002. The sentinel lymph node in melanoma: utilization of molecular biology (RT-PCR) to detect occult metastases. Pathologica 94:190–195.

81. Carson K, Wen DR, Li PX, et al. 1996. Nodal nevi and cutaneous melanomas. Am. J. Surg. Pathol. 20:834–840.

82. Li W, Stall A, Shivers SC, et al. 2000. Clinical relevance of molecular staging for melanoma: comparison of RT-PCR and immunohistochemistry staining in sentinel lymph nodes of patients with melanoma. Int. J. Biomarkers 231:81–88.

83. Guo J, Cheng L, Wen DR, Huang RR, Cochran AJ. 1998. Detection of tyrosinase mRNA in formalin-fixed, paraffin-embedded archival sections of melanoma, using the reverse transcriptase in situ polymerase chain reaction. Diagn. Mol. Pathol. 7:10–15.

84. Branagan G, Hughes D, Jeffrey M, Crane-Robinson C, Perry PM. 2002. Detection of micrometastases in lymph nodes from patients with breast cancer. Br. J. Surg. 89:86–89.

85. Manzotti M, Dell'Orto P, Maisonneuve P, Zurrida S, Mazzarol G, Viale G. 2001. Reverse transcription-polymerase chain reaction assay for multiple mRNA markers in the detection of breast cancer metastases in sentinel lymph nodes. Int. J. Cancer 95:307–312.

86. Peley G, Toth J, Csuka O, Sinkovics I, Farkas E, Koves I. 2001. Immunohistochemistry and reverse transcriptase polymerase chain reaction on sentinel lymph nodes can improve the accuracy of nodal staging in breast cancer patients. Int. J. Biol. Markers 16:227–232.

87. McNeil C. 2000. Micrometastases matter in new melanoma staging system. J. Natl. Cancer Inst. 92:1370–1371.

88. Balch CM, Buzaid AC, Soong SJ, et al. 2001. Final version of the American Joint Committee on Cancer staging system for cutaneous melanoma. J. Clin. Oncol. 19:3635–3648.

89. Gershenwald J, Colome MI, Lee JE, et al. 1998. Patterns of recurrence following a negative sentinel lymph node biopsy in 243 patients with stage I or II melanoma. J. Clin. Oncol. 16: 2253–2260.

90. Blaheta H, Sotlar K, Breuninger H, et al. 2001. Does intensive histopathological workup by serial sectioning increase the detection of lymph node micrometastasis in patients with primary cutaneous melanoma? Melanoma Res. 11:57–63.

91. Blaheta H, Paul T, Sotlar K, et al. 2001. Detection of melanoma cells in sentinel lymph nodes, bone marrow and peripheral blood by a reverse transcription-polymerase chain reaction assay in patients with primary cutaneous melanoma: association with Breslow's tumour thickness. Br. J. Dermatol. 145:195–202.

92. Hochberg M, Lotem M, Gimon Z, Shiloni E, Enk CD. 2002. Expression of tyrosinase, MIA and MART-1 in sentinel lymph nodes of patients with malignant melanoma. Br. J. Dermatol. 146:244–249.

93. Shivers S, Li W, Lin J, et al. 2001. The clinical relevance of molecular staging for melanoma. Recent Results Cancer Res. 158:187–199.

94. Dowlatshahi K, Fan M, Bloom KJ, Spitz DJ, Patel S, Snider HC Jr. 1999. Occult metastases in the sentinel lymph nodes of patients with early stage breast carcinoma: A preliminary study. Cancer 86:990–996.

95. Dowlatshahi K, Fan M, Snider HC, Habib FA. 1997. Lymph node micrometastases from breast carcinoma: reviewing the dilemma. Cancer 80:1188–1197.

96. Sobin LH, Wittekind CW (eds). 2002. TNM classification of malignant tumors, 6th ed. Lawrence, Erlbaum, and Associates.

97. Tjan-Heijnen VC. 2001. Micro-metastases in axillary lymph nodes: an increasing classification and treatment dilemma in breast cancer due to the introduction of the sentinel lymph node procedure. Breast Cancer Res. Treat. 70:81–88.

98. Noguchi M. 2002. Therapeutic relevance of breast cancer micrometastases in sentinel lymph nodes. Br. J. Surg. 89:1505–1515.

99. Hammond M, Fitzgibbons PL, Compton CC, et al. 2000. College of American Pathologists Conference XXXV: solid tumor prognostic factors-which, how and so what? Summary document and recommendations for implementation. Cancer Committee and Conference Participants. Arch. Pathol. Lab. Med. 124:958–965.

100. de Mascarel I, Bonichon F, Coindre JM, Trojani M. 1992. Prognostic significance of breast cancer axillary lymph node micrometastases assessed by two special techniques: reevaluation with longer follow-up. Br. J. Cancer 66:523–527.

15

A Marker for Early Diagnosis of Lung Cancer

The Heterogeneous Nuclear Ribonucleoprotein A2/B1 (hnRNP A2/B1)

Jordi Tauler, Alfredo Martínez, and James L. Mulshine

1. INTRODUCTION

Lung cancer is the most important leading cause of cancer death. In the United States alone, 169,000 new cases were identified in 2002 *(1)* and lung cancer is responsible for more than 1 million deaths worldwide *(2)*. Lung cancer has a lower incidence than other types of cancer (breast, colon, prostate, and cervical) but is more lethal. Throughout most of the world, 5-yr survival is less than 10%. Even with smoking cessation, the risk of lung cancer remains elevated because the injury in the airway tissue cannot be reversed *(3)*. One of the reasons for such high mortality is the late detection of lung cancer, which in most cases occurs after metastatic dissemination. In those cases, the benefits of chemotherapy are modest. The classical diagnostic imaging technology, chest X-ray, is not sensitive enough to provide a reliable early diagnosis of lung cancer. One approach to improve early detection is looking for specific molecular markers that may be tools for a better understanding of the initial steps of carcinogenesis.

1.1. The Link Between Cancer and hnRNP A2/B1

To find specific markers, we developed a panel of monoclonal antibodies against whole-cell lysates of a nonsmall-cell lung carcinoma (NSCLC) cell line. These antibodies were used to screen a sputum specimen archive collected at the Johns Hopkins University. The archive contains sputum samples from a high-risk cohort, obtained on a yearly basis. Follow-up was established in order to determine the development of lung cancer for up to 8 yr. The screening, by immunocytochemical analysis, was focused on the bronchial epithelial exfoliated cells recovered in sputum samples. One of the mouse monoclonal antibodies, 703D4, was able to predict with a 90% accuracy (20 of 22 detected true positive cases) those individuals who would progress to invasive tumors within 2 yr *(4)*. The antigen recognized by 703D4 antibody was characterized by a combination of high-performance liquid chromatography (HPLC) and immunoprecipitation techniques. A single 31 kDa protein was obtained and identified as heterogeneous nuclear ribonucleoprotein (hnRNP) A2/B1 *(5)*.

Additional independent clinical trials have been performed with 703D4. In 1997, two prospective studies were conducted: a multicenter collaboration by the Lung Cancer Early Detection Working Group (LCEDWG) in stage I resected, disease-free patients, and a Chinese industrial mining population, Yunnan Tin Corp. These two studies predicted patient outcome with an accuracy of 67 and 69%, respectivley, in the first year of follow-up *(6)*.

From: *Cancer Diagnostics: Current and Future Trends*
Edited by: R. M. Nakamura, W. W. Grody, J. T. Wu, and R. B. Nagle © Humana Press Inc., Totowa, NJ

Analyzing bronchial lavages from patients with metaplastic bronchial epithelial cells or tumor cells, it has been shown that 95% of the specimens had overexpression of hnRNP A2/B1. Moreover, in 80 specimens reported as morphologically normal, 41 revealed hnRNP A2/B1 overexpression. In 33 of those cases, a lung cancer was found within 1 yr *(7)*. In the five clinical trials reported, after analyzing from high risk cohorts, totaling about 800 individuals, the overall sensitivity and specificity were both around 80%.

A previously reported randomized chemoprevention trial using retinoid acid, utilized archival bronchial biopsy specimens from chronic smokers and were analyzed with 703D4. In both normal and abnormal bronchial epithelium, hnRNP A2/B1 overexpression was reported in 40% of the samples. No significant correlation between retinoid treatment and hnRNP A2/B1 overexpression was found but a frequent overexpression of hnRNP A2/B1 in central airways of chronic smokers was reported. This pattern of expression was comparable to a previous study showing overexpression of hnRNP A2/B1 in the morphologically normal airways surrounding a primary lung cancer *(8,9)*. The results from the prospective studies suggest a strong association between overexpression of hnRNP A2/B1 and the development of lung cancer. This association has been confirmed with studies of bronchial lavages showing that hnRNP A2/B1 overexpression is a common feature in established lung tumors *(7)*.

The study of the correlation between hnRNP A2/B1 overexpression and molecular alterations has demonstrated that morphologically normal cells with hnRNP A2/B1 overexpression show the same pattern of genetic alterations in microsatellite alterations (MA) and loss of heterozygosity (LOH) than similarly positive dysplastic or metaplastic cells. This observation suggests that these cells could be clonally derived and that hnRNP A2/B1 status is more informative than morphological criteria alone. Moreover, subcellular localization of hnRNP A2/B1 overexpression is also informative; cells with cytoplasmic hnRNP A2/B1 overexpression appear to present a higher number of genetic alterations. The subcellular localization varied in different cell clusters of the same case as shown in Fig. 1 *(10)*. Another study reported similar results, looking for the association between neoplastic clonal expansion in NSCLC and overexpression of hnRNP A2/B1. The conclusion was that lung cancer cells undergoing clonal expansion frequently upregulate hnRNP A2/B1 *(11)*. These phenotypically normal cells with upregulation of hnRNP A2/B1 could be interpreted as precursors of a future tumor. This result is important because it shows the potential origin of the clonal expansion and could be detected early by monitoring hnRNP A2/B1 overexpression.

During mammalian lung development, hnRNP A2/B1 expression is found in the earliest lung buds. As lung development progresses, the pattern of expression changes with detected expression now noted in cuboidal epithelial cells of the distal primitive alveoli. At this stage in lung development, hnRNP A2/B1 expression in the proximal conducting airways decreases and disappears completely in the adult organ. Overexpression of hnRNP A2/B1 at critical periods of lung development was comparable to the expression levels found in lung cancers and preneoplastic lesions. Thus, these data were consistent with the hypothesis that hnRNP A2/B1 is an oncodevelopmental protein *(12)*.

The expression of hnRNP A2/B1 was also analyzed in breast cancer by immunohistochemistry. Overexpression was detected in 56.5% of primary invasive breast cancers, whereas it was only expressed in 9.7% specimens of normal breast tissue. By Northern analy-

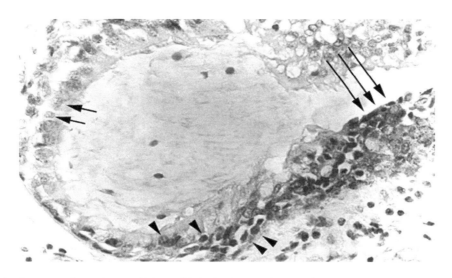

Fig. 1. Cross-section of a small bronchiole in human lung stained for hnRNP A2/B1. Normal-appearing bronchial epithelial cells (short arrows) are devoid of hnRNP A2/B1 expression, whereas the hyperplastic cells (long arrows) show cytoplasmic hnRNP A2/B1 immunoreactivity. Some of the cells located between the normal and hyperplastic cells display nuclear localization of hnRNP A2/B1 (arrowheads). Reproduced with permission from ref. *10*. Color figure available for viewing at **www.humanapress.com**.

sis, a higher level of hnRNP A2/B1 was found on breast cancer cells compared to normal cells. Interestingly, exposure of breast cancer cells to retinoids may reduce hnRNP A2/B1 expression, and regulate the translocation of hnRNP A2/B1 from the nucleus to the cytoplasm as shown in Fig. 2 *(13)*. This retinoid-related translocation of hnRNP A2/B1 could be significant given the strong correlation between subcellular localization and malignity as previously described by Man et al. *(10)*. Overexpression of hnRNP A2/B1 has been detected in pancreatic tissue from smokers and in pancreatic tumor cells *(14)*. Moreover, comparing the gene-expression profiles between adenocarcinoma metastases of multiple tumor types and unmatched primary adenocarcinomas, eight genes were up-regulated in metastasis. Four of the genes were components of the translation machinery and hnRNP A/B was included in this group *(15)*, establishing yet another link between this protein family and cancer progression.

There is strong evidence supporting hnRNP A2/B1 overexpression as an early marker for lung cancer, and with less data for cancers of other organs such as breast and pancreas. Despite these promising results, the molecular mechanism linking this overexpression and cancer remains largely unknown.

2. hnRNPS: TRANSMITTING THE INFORMATION

There has been an explosion of information in biological literature recently regarding the role of hnRNP A2/B1 and related family members in a host of functions from splice regulation, transcriptional regulation to shuttling dynamics. Much of this work has been performed in other nonneoplastic disease conditions. To understand the potential link between hnRNP and tumor biology, we will review hnRNP biology.

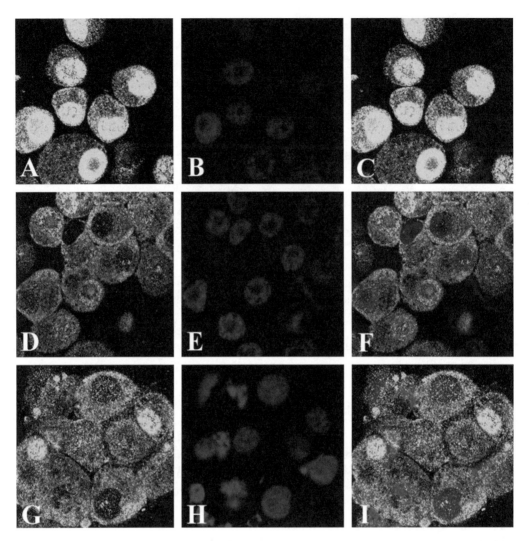

Fig. 2. Confocal microscopy of breast cancer cell line MDA-MB-231 stained for hnRNP A2/B1 (green, A,D,G) and counterstained with DAPI (blue B,E,H). Untreated cells (**A–C**) show intense nuclear expression. After 24 h of retinoid (13cRA) exposure (**D–F**), hnRNP A2/B1 has been translocated from the nucleus to the cytoplasm. Treatment with HPR resulted in a partial translocation of hnRNP A2/B1 expression (**G–I**). Reproduced with permission from ref. *13*. Color figure available for viewing at **www.humanapress.com**.

2.1. The World of hnRNP Proteins

Over the past few years, it has become evident that properly translating an mRNA into a specific protein requires more information than the coding sequence alone. This information should cover other aspects, such as nuclear export, subcellular localization, translation and stability, and could be provided through specific RNA-binding proteins.

The hnRNPs were initially described as an important group of chromatin-associated RNA-binding proteins, but they play a major role in the interpretation and transmission of this information as well. The hnRNPs are a complex group of proteins with 20 major proteins

Table 1
Structure and Possible Functions of hnRNP Proteins

hnRNP proteins	kDa	Domain structure	Possible functions	References
A1	34	2xRBD, RGG	mRNA splicing, mRNA export, Telomere biogenesis	*(47,66–68)* *(69)* *(70)*
A2/B1	36/38	2xRBD, RGG	mRNA splicing, mRNA localization, mRNA stability Telomere biogenesis	*(50,56,60)* *(37,39)* *(33)* *(42,43)*
C1/C2	41/43	1xRBD	mRNA splicing, mRNA stability	*(16)* *(71)*
D (AUF-1)	44–48	2xRBD, RGG	Telomere biogenesis, mRNA stability Recombination	*(72)* *(73)* *(74)*
E1/E2	38–39	3xKH	mRNA stability, Translational control	*(75)* *(71,76)*
F	53	3xRBD	mRNA splicing	*(76)*
H/H'(DSEF-1)	56	3xRBD	mRNA splicing, Polyadenylation	*(77,78)* *(79)*
I (PTB)	59	4xRBD	mRNA splicing, Polyadenylation mRNA localization,	*(80, 81)* *(82)* *(83)*
K	62	3xKH, RGG	Transcription, Translational regulation	*(84,85)* *(86–88)*
L	68	4xRBD	mRNA export, mRNA stability	*(89)* *(90)*
Q	55–70	3xRBD, RGG	mRNA splicing	*(91)*
U	120	RGG	Nuclear retention	*(16)*

Abbr: RBD, RNA-binding domain; RGG; arginine-glycine-glycine-rich domain

identified and many of them having several isoforms. In addition, some less abundant proteins have also been classified as hnRNPs. The more abundant hnRNP proteins and their functions are summarized in Table 1.

The hnRNP proteins play a role in a wide range of functions such as mRNA splicing, mRNA export, mRNA subcellular localization, telomere biogenesis, mRNA stability, translational control, transcription, polyadenylation, and nuclear retention. Most hnRNP proteins contain one or more RNA-binding motifs and have RNA-binding specificity, but can also recognize DNA.

Many of the most abundant hnRNP proteins are localized in the nucleus but they shuttle between the nucleus and the cytoplasm. There is no evidence for an established and defined composition of the hnRNPs associated with pre-mRNAs. Most likely, there is a unique combination of hnRNPs for each pre-mRNA. This unique combination is not stable during the RNA maturation process and changes through the export of the pre-mRNA from the nucleus to the cytoplasm. HnRNP proteins are part of the pathway of gene expression, involved with transcription complex formation through the final mature mRNA found in the cytoplasm *(16,17)*.

2.2. Structure and Function of hnRNP A2/B1

The hnRNP A2/B1 protein is the most abundant major hnRNP protein that binds to pre-mRNA and is involved in biogenesis of mRNA. HnRNP A2/B1 is a member of the hnRNP A/B family which has three different genes: *A1, A2/B1,* and *A3 (18,19)*. A common origin for the *A1* and *A2* genes by duplication from an ancestral gene that could also be shared for A3 has been suggested. The hnRNP *A2/B1* gene is divided in 12 exons and 11 introns. HnRNP A2 is the more abundant isoform and results from an alternative splicing that eliminates exon 2; hnRNP B1 contains the 12 exons but it accounts only for 2–5% of total A2/B1 transcripts *(20)*. An additional isoform, less abundant than B1 and known as B0 is generated by the elimination of exon 9. The hnRNP A2/B1 protein has a molecular mass of 31 kDa. The three genes (*A1, A2/B1,* and *A3*) are alternatively spliced and generate different isoforms that share a common modular structure with a highly conserved N-terminal domain, and a more divergent, glycine-rich C-terminal domain, also known as arginine-glycine-glycine (RGG) domain. The N-terminal domain has two RNA-binding domains (RBD), arranged in tandem, also named RNA recognition motif (RRM). This modular structure has been referred to as 2xRBD-Gly (Fig. 3).

The RBD domains are responsible for RNA-binding interactions but some cooperation of the RGG domain has also been reported *(21)*. The RGG domain has other important functions such as protein–protein interactions and the ability to promote RNA annealing. Methylated residues are found only in the RGG domain. Inhibition of the methylation of these residues results in a shift from nuclear to cytoplasmatic localization, as shown by immunoblotting and immunocytochemistry *(22)*. A 29 amino acid sequence, called M9, in the RGG domain mediates rapid shuttling between nucleus and cytoplasm. This particular sequence acts both as nuclear localization determinant and as nuclear export sequence *(23)*. It is likely that promoters of hnRNP A1 and hnRNP A2/B1 are coregulated to ensure the observed coordinate expression of these products in different cell types and tissues *(24)*. We will describe the most relevant functions reported for hnRNP A2/B1 and focus on the relationships of these functions and potential links with growth regulation and carcinogenesis.

The nature of the regulation of hnRNP A2/B1 is poorly understood. The hnRNP A1 has a short 5'UTR that starts with a pyrimidine tract similar to the one found in mRNAs encoded by *terminal oligo-pyrimidine (TOP)* genes. These genes code for ribosomal proteins and other proteins related in the production and function of translational machinery. Analyzing the structural features of this pyrimidine tract and the translation behavior of hnRNP A1, this hnRNP could be included in the class of *TOP* genes, suggesting a role for hnRNP A1. This motif may also apply to hnRNP I but it does not appear relevant to hnRNP A2/B1 and hnRNP C1/C2. Despite the important similarities between hnRNP A1 and hnRNP A2/B1, it seems that there are important differences to their translational regulation *(25)*. A recent study

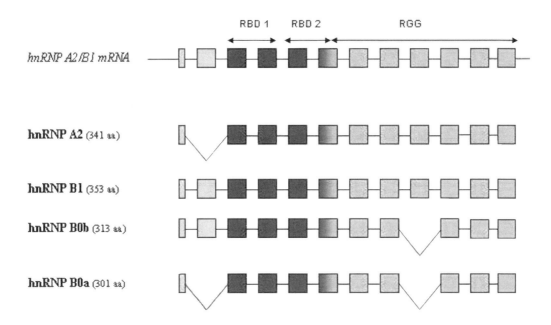

Fig. 3. The coding sequence of hnRNP A2/B1 is divided into 12 exons. A very short first exon, 2 aa. is present in all isoforms. Exon 2, a 12 aa mini-exon, is spliced in the most abundant isoform, hnRNP A2, and also in the rare isoform, hnRNP B0a. Exon 9 is spliced in isoforms hnRNP B0a and hnRNP B0b. RNA-binding domains (RBD) expand from exon 3 to exon 6: RBD1 in exon 3 and 4; RBD2 in exon 5 and part of exon 6. Arginine-glycine-glycine (RGG) domain, expand along the N-terminal domain, from exon 6 to exon 12. hnRNP A2 is the most abundant isoform (80–98%), however, the relative expression of the different isoforms vary with age and tissue types *(92–94)*. Color image available for viewing at **www.humanapress.com**.

reported that Sam68, a nuclear RNA-binding protein, binds a specific nucleotide motif, UAAA, in hnRNP A2/B1 suggesting a possible role of Sam68 in the posttranscriptional regulation of these genes *(26)*. Sam68 is a substrate for *Src*-family tyrosine kinases during mitosis and is a member of the signal transduction and activation of RNA metabolism (STAR) family. This family comprises mediator proteins connecting RNA metabolism with signal transduction pathways *(27–29)*.

A previous result suggested that nuclear DEAF-1-related (NUDR), a nuclear *Drosophila* Deformed epidermal autoregulatory factor (DEAF-1) -related protein, may regulate the expression in vivo of hnRNP A2/B1, acting as a transcriptional repressor. Thus, the down regulation of NUDR could explain the overexpression of hnRNP A2/B1 in some cancers *(30)*. However, other studies showed a down-regulation of hnRNP A2/B1 in human lung and breast carcinoma cells under hypoxic conditions as shown in Fig. 4. This down-regulation of hnRNP A2/B1 is not mediated by the transcription factor hypoxia inducible factor 1, HIF-1 *(31)*. Moreover, in brain tumors, the binding of hnRNP A2/B1 with the 3'UTR of glucose transporter 1 (Glut 1) mRNA in a region called AU-rich response element (AURE) has been demonstrated. That interaction of hnRNP A2/B1, which also forms a complex with hnRNP L in vivo, with the AURE of Glut 1 mRNA is critical for the regulation of Glut 1 expression. Hypoxia and hypoglycemia decrease polysomal levels of hnRNP A2 and hnRNP L resulting in an increase of Glut 1 mRNA stability *(32,33)*. Nevertheless, some recent data suggest that

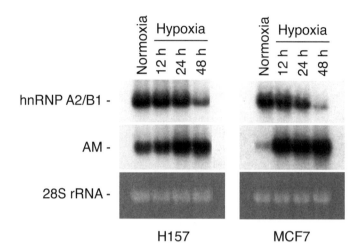

Fig. 4. Down-regulation of hnRNP A2/B1 under hypoxic conditions in H157 (lung cancer cell line) and MCF 7 (breast cancer cell line). hnRNP A2/B1 expression levels were maintained after 24 h but an important decrease was revealed after 48 h of treatment. Northern blots were probed with hnRNP A2/B1 and, subsequently, with adrenomedullin, a previously reported hypoxia-inducible gene. Adrenomedullin levels were elevated in both cell lines after 24 h. Ethidium bromide staining of 28S RNA was used to assess for equal loading and RNA integrity *(95)*. Reproduced with permission from ref. *31*.

pVHL, a tumor-supressor gene, down-regulates hnRNP A2/B1 expression in renal clear cell carcinomas, through a mechanism involving ubiquitination and targeting to proteasome degradation *(34)*. *pVHL* regulates protein turnover of HIF-1, a transcription factor for hypoxia-inducible genes. The absence of *pVHL* in renal clear cells is associated with a hypoxic phenotype with cells expressing increased levels of vascular endothelial growth factor (VEGF) and Glut 1 *(35,36)*. This suggests increased levels of both Glut 1 and hnRNP A2/B1 in renal clear cells, associated with reduced levels of the tumor suppressor gene, *pVHL*. In contrast, in brain tumors, the relation between Glut 1 and hnRNP A2/B1 is inversely related under hypoxic conditions. The reports of Garayoa et al. and Hamilton et al. suggest the down regulation of hnRNP A2/B1 under hypoxia conditions, in lung, breast, and brain tumors. Because hypoxia is an inherent condition in solid tumors it seems likely that hnRNP A2/B1 downregulation could play an important role in the survival of these tumors, mainly by allowing expression of tumor-survival genes. If this hypothesis proves true, we could envision hnRNP A2/B1 as a tumor-suppressor gene product. The up-regulation observed in tumors may reflect an adaptive response from the cell attempting to counteract the carcinogenesis process.

Another function of hnRNP A2/B1 is the regulation of cytoplasmatic mRNA transport. A 21 nucleotide segment called hnRNP A2 response element (A2RE) has been defined in the myelin basic protein mRNA. This sequence, recognized by hnRNP A2/B1, is necessary and sufficient for cytoplasmatic transport of the mRNA of this protein. Mutations in the A2RE abolish binding of hnRNP A2/B1 and block the transport of myelin basic protein mRNA to the cytoplasm *(37)*. The A2RE can interact with either of the two RRM domains of hnRNP A2/B1 acting in *cis*. This A2RE might be present in a variety of different mRNAs transported by hnRNP A2/B1 *(38)*. However, the distribution of the cytoplasmatic pool of hnRNP

A2 is microtubule dependent. The M9 domain drives the translocation to the nucleus, but in the absence of M9 domain and in the presence of intact microtubules, proteins containing the second of the RRMs were concentrated in the distal processes of oligodendrocytes *(39)*. There is strong evidence supporting the shifting of hnRNP A2/B1 from nucleus to cytoplasm, suggesting the involvement of hnRNP A2/B1 in mRNA transport. Recently, it has been suggested that hnRNP A2/B1 interaction with actin may be central to the mechanism for transferring pre-mRNA from the nucleus to the cytoplasm *(40)*.

hnRNP A2/B1 also binds single stranded telomeric repeats (TTAGGG)n found at the end of the chromosome. This interaction protects the telomeres from nuclease degradation and sustains telomerase activity *(41)*. The hnRNP B1 and hnRNP B0b bind telomeric repeats in a tandem fashion with more affinity, in vitro, than hnRNP A2 *(42)*. A model has been proposed in which telomerase binding to hnRNPs would promote telomere access *(43)*. If hnRNP A2/B1 is playing an important role in the regulation of the changes in telomere length its expression might alter the balance of telomere length regulation. Given the importance of telomere length regulation in controlling cell division *(44,45)*, changes in the expression of hnRNP A2/B1 might also influence cell life span or even immortality of cancer cells.

Alternative splicing of pre-mRNAs from a single gene is predicted to occur in the majority of human genes *(46)*. Like other hnRNP proteins, hnRNP A2/B1 is involved in regulation of alternative splicing and in mRNA transport. A seminal study demonstrating how hnRNP A2/B1 could regulate 5' splice-site selection was one of the early observations suggesting the importance of this class of molecules *(20)*. Increased levels of serine/arginine-rich proteins (SR proteins) results in the selection of intron-proximal 5' sites when a pre-mRNA contains two or more 5' alternative splicing sites, but increased levels of hnRNP A2/B1 promotes the selection of intron-distal 5' sites. hnRNP A1 binds pre-mRNA more strongly than hnRNP A2/B1. In contrast, hnRNP A2/B1 has an order of magnitude stronger splice-site switching activity than hnRNP A1, but this regulation is not specific of target sequence *(47,48)*.

Although there are a significant number of papers showing the important role of hnRNP A1 in alternative splicing, this function had not been extensively studied for hnRNP A2/B1. However, recent reports have changed this situation. First, hnRNP A2/B1 may control alternative splicing of hnRNP A1 mRNA. Different intronic regions, or control elements, flanking the alternative exon 7b have been implicated in production of the A1 and A1B mRNA splice isoforms. These regions are; CE1a and CE1d, which are downstream of exon 7 and CE4m and CE4p located downstream of exon 7b respectively. Different hnRNP A/B binding sites are present in these regions. Some of them match the consensus for hnRNP A1, UAGRR(A/U), which is similar to the sequence of the telomere repeats (TTAGGG) recognized by hnRNP A2/B1 as previously described. These control elements promoting alternative splicing in the hnRNP A1 pre-mRNA are organized in groups adjacent to A/B binding sites. CE1a and CE4 may be bound by hnRNP A1 to promote skipping of exon 7b in vivo and distal 5' splice site selection in vitro *(47,49)*. However, the distal 5' splice selection is conserved in an extract prepared from mouse cells that are severely deficient in hnRNP A1 proteins. It has been shown that hnRNP A2 compensates the hnRNP A1 deficiency and controls, the alternative splicing of hnRNP A1 *(50)*. hnRNP A1 also plays an important role in alternative splicing of several proteins such as CD44 *(51)*. If hnRNP A2/B1 potentially regulates alternative splicing of hnRNP A1, hnRNP A2/B1 may indirectly and potentially influence the alternative splicing of CD44. Because splice variants of CD44 have been implicated in tumorigenesis and tumor progression *(52,53)*, a link between hnRNP A2/B1 and regulation of tumor progression could be established by this pathway.

Second, the alternative splicing of protein 4.1R in exon 16 (E16) is required during erythropoiesis for the establishment of proper mechanical integrity of the erythrocyte membrane *(54,55)*. A highly conserved 42-nucleotide exonic element (CE[16]) has been characterized in exon E16. This element interacts with hnRNP A/B proteins and regulates the alternative splicing of exon E16. Binding of hnRNP A/B to CE[16] skips E16 in early erthyroid progenitors. If hnRNP A/B proteins are depleted from nuclear extracts, E16 inclusion increases significantly, whereas repletion with recombinant hnRNP A/B restores E16 silencing. Moreover, downregulation of hnRNP A/B expression temporally correlates with the inclusion of E16 during erythropoiesis, suggesting that it could be the functional switch for E16 expression *(56)*. A similar mechanism has been reported in the human immunodeficiency virus type 1 (HIV-1). The splicing of HIV-1 mRNA is a complex process and it could be repressed by exonic splicing silencers (ESS). Interaction of hnRNP proteins with ESS could regulate HIV-1 pre-mRNA splicing *(57,58)*.

Hou and colleagues have recently shown the relationship between changes in expression levels of hnRNP A2/B1 and developmental processes *(56)*. This could be linked to previously described results regarding the role of hnRNP A2/B1 as an oncodevelopmental protein *(12)*. If hnRNP A2/B1 expression is altered, developmental pathways could potentially be activated in differentiated cells by a modified alternative splicing. These changes might be related to tumorigenesis.

Third, hnRNP A1 and A2 show a decreased expression in senescent fibroblasts *(59)*. The constitutive decrease of the ratio hnRNP A1 or A2 to SF2/ASF is accompanied by an increase of one of the INK4a mRNA isoforms, *p16INK4a*, whereas overexpression of hnRNP A1 or A2 appears to increase the steady state mRNA levels of both isoforms: *p14ARF* and *p16INK4a*. If the ratio hnRNP A1 or A2 to SF2/ASF increases, the isoform *p14ARF* is preferentially chosen *(60)*. These proteins, *p14ARF* and *p16INK4a*, are both cell growth inhibitors. *p14ARF* participates in stabilizing *p53* protein levels and *p16INK4a* is involved in the pRb pathway *(61,62)*. Given the role of *p14ARF* and *p16INK4a* in the control of cell proliferation, changes in the expression of *p14ARF* and *p16INK4a* modulated by changes in the expression of hnRNP A2/B1 could modify pathways of cell proliferation control.

Since the characterization of hnRNP A2/B1, its strong correlation with lung cancer has been widely reported. A role as a marker for this disease seems to be clearly characterized. However, analyzing the structure and function of hnRNP A2/B1 there is not a definitive link between hnRNP A2/B1 and cancer promotion and progression. The search for such a mechanism could be exceedingly complex but still may lead to a fundamental contribution in understanding the nature of the cancer process.

3. FUTURE DIRECTIONS

Spiral computed tomography (CT) is highly sensitive and has been very promising in pilot clinical trials screening high-risk populations in which very small primary lung cancers (less than 1 cm in diameter) are frequently detected *(63)*. Because spiral CT services are so widely available and cost of these exams are becoming so affordable, this technology is likely to supercede biomarker-based early lung cancer detection. However, biomarkers such as hnRNP A2/B1 provide superb tools to evaluate the mechanistic complexity of lung cancer. In these cases, the small size of the tumor may allow different approaches to manage the disease, ranging from less invasive surgical interventions to targeted drug delivery *(64,65)*. In addition, these biomarkers may inform the downstream clinical management of CT-detected lung cancer. The integrated development of these techniques to detect and manage early lung cancer may contribute to the eventual reduction in lung cancer mortality.

REFERENCES

1. Jemal A, Thomas A, Murray T, et al. 2002. Cancer statistics. CA Cancer J. Clin. 52:23–47.
2. Carney DN. 2002. Lung cancer-time to move on from chemotherapy. N. Engl. J. Med. 346:126–128.
3. Gaffney M and Altshuler B. 1988. Examination of the role of cigarette smoke in lung carcinogenesis using multistage models. J. Natl. Cancer. Inst. 80:925–931.
4. Tockman MS, Gupta PK, Myers JD, et al. 1988. Sensitive and specific monoclonal antibody recognition of human lung cancer antigen on preserved sputum cells: a new approach to early lung cancer detection. J. Clin. Oncol. 6:1685–1693.
5. Zhou J, Mulshine JL, Unsworth EJ, et al. 1996. Purification and characterization of a protein that permits early detection of lung cancer. Identification of heterogeneous nuclear ribonucleoprotein-A2/B1 as the antigen for monoclonal antibody 703D4. J. Biol. Chem. 271:10760–10766.
6. Tockman MS, Mulshine JL, Piantadosi S, et al. 1997. Prospective detection of preclinical lung cancer: results from two studies of heterogeneous nuclear ribonucleoprotein A2/B1 overexpression. Clin. Cancer Res. 3:2237–2246.
7. Fielding P, Turnbull L, Prime W, et al. 1999. Heterogeneous nuclear ribonucleoprotein A2/B1 up-regulation in bronchial lavage specimens: a clinical marker of early lung cancer detection. Clin. Cancer Res. 5:4048–4052.
8. Zhou J, Mulshine JL, Ro JY, et al. 1998. Expression of heterogeneous nuclear ribonucleoprotein A2/B1 in bronchial epithelium of chronic smokers. Clin. Cancer Res. 4:1631–1640.
9. Zhou J, Jensen SM, Steinberg SM, et al. 1996. Expression of early lung cancer detection marker p31 in neoplastic and non-neoplastic respiratory epithelium. Lung Cancer 14:85–97.
10. Man YG, Martinez A, Avis IM, et al. 2000. Phenotypically different cells with heterogeneous nuclear ribonucleoprotein A2/B1 overexpression show similar genetic alterations. Am. J. Respir. Cell. Mol. Biol. 23:636–645.
11. Zhou J, Nong L, Wloch M, et al. 2001. Expression of early lung cancer detection marker: hnRNP-A2/B1 and its relation to microsatellite alteration in non-small cell lung cancer. Lung Cancer 34:341–350.
12. Montuenga LM, Zhou J, Avis I, et al. 1998. Expression of heterogeneous nuclear ribonucleoprotein A2/B1 changes with critical stages of mammalian lung development. Am. J. Respir. Cell. Mol. Biol. 19:554–562.
13. Zhou J, Allred DC, Avis I, et al. 2001. Differential expression of the early lung cancer detection marker, heterogeneous nuclear ribonucleoprotein-A2/B1 (hnRNP-A2/B1) in normal breast and neoplastic breast cancer. Breast Cancer Res. Treat. 66:217–224.
14. Yan-Sanders Y, Hammons GJ, Lyn-Cook BD. 2002. Increased expression of heterogeneous nuclear ribonucleoprotein A2/B1 (hnRNP) in pancreatic tissue from smokers and pancreatic tumor cells. Cancer Lett. 183:215–220.
15. Ramaswamy S, Ross KN, Lander ES, et al. 2003. A molecular signature of metastasis in primary solid tumors. Nat. Genet. 33:49–54.
16. Krecic AM and Swanson MS. 1999. hnRNP complexes: composition, structure, and function. Curr. Opin. Cell Biol. 11:363–371.
17. Dreyfuss G, Kim VN, Kataoka N. 2002. Messenger-RNA-binding proteins and the messages they carry. Nat. Rev. Mol. Cell. Biol. 3:195–205.
18. Plomaritoglou A, Choli-Papadopoulou T, and Guialis A. 2000 Molecular characterization of a murine, major A/B type hnRNP protein: mBx. Biochimica. et Biophysica. Acta. 1490:54–62.
19. Ma AS, Moran-Jones K, Shan J, et al. 2002. Heterogeneous nuclear ribonucleoprotein A3, a novel RNA trafficking response element-binding protein. J. Biol. Chem. 277:18010–18020.

20. Mayeda A, Munroe SH, Caceres JF, et al. 1994. Function of conserved domains of hnRNP A1 and other hnRNP A/B proteins. EMBO J. 13:5483–5495.

21. Biamonti G, Ruggiu M, Saccone S, et al. 1994. Two homologous genes, originated by duplication, encode the human hnRNP proteins A2 and A1. Nucleic Acids Res. 22:1996–2002.

22. Nichols RC, Wang XW, Tang J, et al. 2000. The RGG domain in hnRNP A2 affects subcellular localization. Exp. Cell. Res. 256:522–532.

23. Pollard VW, Michael WM, Nakielny S, et al. 1996. A novel receptor-mediated nuclear protein import pathway. Cell. 86:985–994.

24. Biamonti G, Bassi MT, Cartegni L, et al. 1993. Human hnRNP protein A1 gene expression. Structural and functional characterization of the promoter. J. Mol. Biol. 230:77–89.

25. Camacho-Vanegas O, Weighardt F, Ghigna C, et al. 1997. Growth-dependent and growth-independent translation of messengers for heterogeneous nuclear ribonucleoproteins. Nucleic Acids Res. 25:3950–3954.

26. Itoh M, Haga I, Li QH, et al. 2002. Identification of cellular mRNA targets for RNA-binding protein Sam68. Nucleic Acids Res. 30:5452–5464.

27. Fumagalli S, Totty NF, Hsuan JJ, et al. 1994. A target for Src in mitosis. Nature 368:871–874.

28. Taylor SJ and Shalloway D. 1994. An RNA-binding protein associated with Src through its SH2 and SH3 domains in mitosis. Nature 368:867–871.

29. Vernet C and Artzt K. 1997. STAR, a gene family involved in signal transduction and activation of RNA. Trends Genet. 13:479–484.

30. Michelson RJ, Collard MW, Ziemba AJ, et al. 1999. Nuclear DEAF-1-related (NUDR) protein contains a novel DNA binding domain and represses transcription of the heterogeneous nuclear ribonucleoprotein A2/B1 promoter. J. Biol. Chem. 274:30510–30519.

31. Garayoa M, Man YG, Martinez A, et al. 2003. Downregulation of hnRNP A2/B1 Expression in Tumor Cells under Prolonged Hypoxia. Am. J. Respir. Cell. Mol. Biol. 28:80–85.

32. Tsukamoto H, Boado RJ, Pardridge WM. 1996. Differential expression in glioblastoma multiforme and cerebral hemangioblastoma of cytoplasmic proteins that bind two different domains within the 3'-untranslated region of the human glucose transporter 1 (GLUT1) messenger RNA. J. Clin. Invest. 97:2823–2832.

33. Hamilton BJ, Nichols RC, Tsukamoto H, et al. 1999. hnRNP A2 and hnRNP L bind the 3'UTR of glucose transporter 1 mRNA and exist as a complex in vivo. Biochem. Biophys. Res. Comm. 261:646–651.

34. Pioli PA and Rigby WF. 2001. The von Hippel-Lindau protein interacts with heteronuclear ribonucleoprotein a2 and regulates its expression. J. Biol. Chem. 276:40346–40352.

35. Iliopoulos O, Levy AP, Jiang C, et al. 1996. Negative regulation of hypoxia-inducible genes by the von Hippel-Lindau protein. Proc. Natl. Acad. Sci. USA 93:10595–10599.

36. Gnarra JR, Zhou S, Merrill MJ, et al. 1996. Posttranscriptional regulation of vascular endothelial growth factor mRNA by the product of the VHL tumor suppressor gene. Proc. Natl. Acad. Sci. USA 93:10589–10594.

37. Munro TP, Magee RJ, Kidd GJ, et al. 1999. Mutational analysis of a heterogeneous nuclear ribonucleoprotein A2 response element for RNA trafficking. J. Biol. Chem. 274:34389–34395.

38. Shan J, Moran-Jones K, Munro TP, et al. 2000. Binding of an RNA trafficking response element to heterogeneous nuclear ribonucleoproteins A1 and A2. J. Biol. Chem. 275:38286–38295.

39. Brumwell C, Antolik C, Carson JH, et al. 2002. Intracellular trafficking of hnRNP A2 in oligodendrocytes. Exp. Cell. Res. 279:310–320.

40. Percipalle P, Jonsson A, Nashchekin D, et al. 2002. Nuclear actin is associated with a specific subset of hnRNP A/B-type proteins. Nucleic Acids Res. 30:1725–1734.

41. McKay SJ and Cooke H. 1992. hnRNP A2/B1 binds specifically to single stranded vertebrate telomeric repeat TTAGGGn. Nucleic Acids Res. 20:6461–6464.

42. Kamma H, Fujimoto M, Fujiwara M, et al. 2001. Interaction of hnRNP A2/B1 isoforms with telomeric ssDNA and the in vitro function. Biochem. Biophys. Res. Comm. 280:625–630.

43. Ford LP, Wright WE, Shay JW. 2002. A model for heterogeneous nuclear ribonucleoproteins in telomere and telomerase regulation. Oncogene 21:580–583.

44. Levy MZ, Allsopp RC, Futcher AB, et al. 1992. Telomere end-replication problem and cell aging. J. Mol. Biol. 225:951–960.

45. Harley CB, Vaziri H, Counter CM, et al. 1992. The telomere hypothesis of cellular aging. Exp. Gerontol. 27:375–382.

46. Lander ES, Linton LM, Birren B, et al. 2001. Initial sequencing and analysis of the human genome. Nature 409:860–921.

47. Chabot B, Blanchette M, Lapierre I, et al. 1997. An intron element modulating 5' splice site selection in the hnRNP A1 pre-mRNA interacts with hnRNP A1. Mol. Cell. Biol. 17:1776–1786.

48. Eperon IC, Makarova OV, Mayeda A, et al. 2000. Selection of alternative 5' splice sites: role of U1 snRNP and models for the antagonistic effects of SF2/ASF and hnRNP A1. Mol. Cell. Biol. 20:8303–8318.

49. Blanchette M and Chabot B. 1999. Modulation of exon skipping by high-affinity hnRNP A1-binding sites and by intron elements that repress splice site utilization. EMBO J. 18:1939–1952.

50. Hutchison S, LeBel C, Blanchette M, et al. 2002. Distinct sets of adjacent heterogeneous nuclear ribonucleoprotein (hnRNP) A1/A2 binding sites control 5' splice site selection in the hnRNP A1 mRNA precursor. J. Biol. Chem. 277:29,745–29,752.

51. Matter N, Marx M, Weg-Remers S, et al. 2000. Heterogeneous ribonucleoprotein A1 is part of an exon-specific splice-silencing complex controlled by oncogenic signaling pathways. J. Biol. Chem. 275:35353–35360.

52. Cooper DL and Dougherty GJ. 1995. To metastasize or not? Selection of CD44 splice sites. Nat. Med. 1:635–637.

53. Sherman L, Sleeman J, Dall P, et al. 1996. The CD44 proteins in embryonic development and in cancer. Curr. Top. Microbiol. Immunol. 213:249–269.

54. Conboy J. 1999. The role of alternative pre-mRNA splicing in regulating the structure and function of skeletal protein 4.1. Proc. Soc. Exp. Biol. Med. 220:73–78.

55. Chasis JA, Coulombel L, Conboy J, et al. 1993. Differentiation-associated switches in protein 4.1 expression. Synthesis of multiple structural isoforms during normal human erythropoiesis. J. Clin. Invest. 91:329–338.

56. Hou VC, Lersch R, Gee SL, et al. 2002. Decrease in hnRNP A/B expression during erythropoiesis mediates a pre-mRNA splicing switch. EMBO J. 21:6195–6204.

57. Bilodeau PS, Domsic JK, Mayeda A, et al. 2001. RNA splicing at human immunodeficiency virus type 1 3' splice site A2 is regulated by binding of hnRNP A/B proteins to an exonic splicing silencer element. J. Virol. 75:8487–8497.

58. Caputi M, Mayeda A, Krainer AR, et al. 1999. hnRNP A/B proteins are required for inhibition of HIV-1 pre-mRNA splicing. EMBO J. 18:4060–4067.

59. Hubbard K, Dhanaraj SN, Sethi KA, et al. 1995. Alteration of DNA and RNA binding activity of human telomere binding proteins occurs during cellular senescence. Exp. Cell. Res. 218:241–247.

60. Zhu D, Xu G, Ghandhi S, et al. 2002. Modulation of the expression of p16INK4a and p14ARF by hnRNP A1 and A2 RNA binding proteins: implications for cellular senescence. J. Cell. Physiol. 193:19–25.

61. Sherr CJ. 1998. Tumor surveillance via the ARF-p53 pathway. Genes Dev. 12:2984–2991.

62. Ruas M and Peters G. 1998. The p16INK4a/CDKN2A tumor suppressor and its relatives. Biochim. Biophys. Acta. 1378:F115–F177.

63. Mulshine JL. 2003. Opinion: Screening for lung cancer: in pursuit of pre-metastatic disease. Nat. Rev. Cancer 3:65–73.

64. Wattenberg LW, Wiedmann TS, Estensen RD, et al. 2000. Chemoprevention of pulmonary carcinogenesis by brief exposures to aerosolized budesonide or beclomethasone dipropionate and by the combination of aerosolized budesonide and dietary myo-inositol. Carcinogenesis 21:179–182.

65. Dahl AR, Grossi IM, Houchens DP, et al. 2000. Inhaled isotretinoin (13-*cis* retinoic acid) is an effective lung cancer chemopreventive agent in A/J mice at low doses: a pilot study. Clin. Cancer Res. 6:3015–3024.

66. van der Houven van Oordt W, Diaz-Meco MT, Lozano J, et al. 2000. The MKK(3/6)-p38-signaling cascade alters the subcellular distribution of hnRNP A1 and modulates alternative splicing regulation. J. Cell. Biol. 149:307–316.

67. Mayeda A and Krainer AR. 1992. Regulation of alternative pre-mRNA splicing by hnRNP A1 and splicing factor SF2. Cell. 68:365–375.

68. Tange TO, Damgaard CK, Guth S, et al. 2001. The hnRNP A1 protein regulates HIV-1 tat splicing via a novel intron silencer element. EMBO J. 20:5748–5758.

69. Izaurralde E, Jarmolowski A, Beisel C, et al. 1997. A role for the M9 transport signal of hnRNP A1 in mRNA nuclear export. J. Cell. Biol. 137:27–35.

70. Fiset S and Chabot B. 2001. hnRNP A1 may interact simultaneously with telomeric DNA and the human telomerase RNA in vitro. Nucleic Acids Res. 29:2268–2275.

71. Rajagopalan LE, Westmark CJ, Jarzembowski JA, et al. 1998. hnRNP C increases amyloid precursor protein (APP) production by stabilizing APP mRNA. Nucleic Acids Res. 26:3418–3423.

72. Eversole A and Maizels N. 2000. In vitro properties of the conserved mammalian protein hnRNP D suggest a role in telomere maintenance. Mol. Cell. Biol. 20:5425–5432.

73. Xu N, Chen CY, Shyu AB. 2001. Versatile role for hnRNP D isoforms in the differential regulation of cytoplasmic mRNA turnover. Mol. Cell. Biol. 21:6960–6971.

74. Dempsey LA, Sun H, Hanakahi LA, et al. 1999. G4 DNA binding by LR1 and its subunits, nucleolin and hnRNP D, A role for G-G pairing in immunoglobulin switch recombination. J. Biol. Chem. 274:1066–1071.

75. Chkheidze AN, Lyakhov DL, Makeyev AV, et al. 1999. Assembly of the alpha-globin mRNA stability complex reflects binary interaction between the pyrimidine-rich 3' untranslated region determinant and poly(C) binding protein alphaCP. Mol. Cell. Biol. 19:4572–4581.

76. Min H, Chan RC, Black DL. 1995. The generally expressed hnRNP F is involved in a neural-specific pre-mRNA splicing event. Genes Devel. 9:2659–2671.

77. Chou MY, Rooke N, Turck CW, et al. 1999. hnRNP H is a component of a splicing enhancer complex that activates a c-src alternative exon in neuronal cells. Mol. Cell. Biol. 19:69–77.

78. Chen CD, Kobayashi R, Helfman DM. 1999. Binding of hnRNP H to an exonic splicing silencer is involved in the regulation of alternative splicing of the rat beta-tropomyosin gene. Genes Dev. 13:593–606.

79. Bagga PS, Arhin GK, Wilusz J. 1998. DSEF-1 is a member of the hnRNP H family of RNA-binding proteins and stimulates pre-mRNA cleavage and polyadenylation in vitro. Nucleic Acids Res. 26:5343–5350.

80. Chan RC and Black DL. 1997. The polypyrimidine tract binding protein binds upstream of neural cell-specific c-src exon N1 to repress the splicing of the intron downstream. Mol. Cell. Biol. 17:4667–4676.

81. Ashiya M and Grabowski PJ. 1997. A neuron-specific splicing switch mediated by an array of pre-mRNA repressor sites: evidence of a regulatory role for the polypyrimidine tract binding protein and a brain-specific PTB counterpart. Rna-A Pub. RNA Soc. 3:996–1015.

82. Cote CA, Gautreau D, Denegre JM, et al. 1999. A Xenopus protein related to hnRNP I has a role in cytoplasmic RNA localization. Mol. Cell. 4:431–437.

83. Moreira A, Takagaki Y, Brackenridge S, et al. 1998. The upstream sequence element of the C2 complement poly(A) signal activates mRNA 3' end formation by two distinct mechanisms. Genes Dev. 12:2522–2534.

84. Du Q, Melnikova IN, Gardner PD. 1998. Differential effects of heterogeneous nuclear ribonucleoprotein K on Sp1- and Sp3-mediated transcriptional activation of a neuronal nicotinic acetylcholine receptor promoter. J. Biol. Chem. 273:19,877–19,883.

85. Miau LH, Chang CJ, Shen BJ, et al. 1998. Identification of heterogeneous nuclear ribonucle-oprotein K (hnRNP K) as a repressor of C/EBPbeta-mediated gene activation. J. Biol. Chem. 273:10784–10791.
86. Habelhah H, Shah K, Huang L, et al. 2001. ERK phosphorylation drives cytoplasmic accumulation of hnRNP-K and inhibition of mRNA translation. Nature Cell. Biol. 3:325–330.
87. Ostareck DH, Ostareck-Lederer A, Wilm M, et al. 1997. mRNA silencing in erythroid differentiation: hnRNP K and hnRNP E1 regulate 15-lipoxygenase translation from the 3' end. Cell 89:597–606.
88. Ostareck DH, Ostareck-Lederer A, Shatsky IN, et al. 2001. Lipoxygenase mRNA silencing in erythroid differentiation: The 3'UTR regulatory complex controls 60S ribosomal subunit joining. Cell 104:281–290.
89. Pinol-Roma S, Swanson MS, Gall JG, et al. 1989. A novel heterogeneous nuclear RNP protein with a unique distribution on nascent transcripts. J. Cell. Biol. 109:2575–2587.
90. Liu X and Mertz JE. 1995. HnRNP L binds a cis-acting RNA sequence element that enables intron-dependent gene expression. Genes Dev. 9:1766–1780.
91. Mourelatos Z, Abel L, Yong J, et al. 2001. SMN interacts with a novel family of hnRNP and spliceosomal proteins. EMBO J. 20:5443–5452.
92. Kozu T, Henrich B, Schafer KP. 1995. Structure and expression of the gene (HNRPA2B1) encoding the human hnRNP protein A2/B1. Genomics 25:365–371.
93. Kamma H, Satoh H, Matusi M, et al. 2001. Characterization of hnRNP A2 and B1 using monoclonal antibodies: intracellular distribution and metabolism through cell cycle. Immunol. Lett. 76:49–54.
94. Hatfield J, Rothnagel J, Smith R. 2002. Characterization of the mouse hnRNP A2/B1/B0 gene and identification of processed pseudogenes. Gene 295:33.
95. Garayoa M, Martinez A, Lee S, et al. 2000. Hypoxia-inducible factor-1 (HIF-1) up-regulates adrenomedullin expression in human tumor cell lines during oxygen deprivation: a possible promotion mechanism of carcinogenesis. Mol. Endocrinol. 14:848–862.

IV

MOLECULAR AND GENETIC TUMOR MARKERS

16

Molecular Techniques in Cancer Diagnosis and Management

Jeffrey S. Ross, Karen Gray, Rebecca Mosher, and James Stec

1. INTRODUCTION

The introduction of targeted therapeutics into clinical oncology practice has created opportunities for further development of molecular diagnostics to serve cancer patients. The approvals of Herceptin™ for the treatment of HER-2/neu overexpressing breast cancer and Gleevac™ for the treatment of chronic myelogenous leukemia featuring a *bcr/abl* translocation and gastrointestinal stromal tumors with selective *c-kit* oncogene activating mutations have brought an expanded role to the diagnostic laboratory and for the testing of patients to determine their eligibility to receive these new therapies *(1,2)*. The molecular diagnostics industry is in a state of rapid evolution, technological development, and novel clinical applications *(3–5)*. As seen in Table 1, the in vitro diagnostics industry is now believed to consist of a $33 billion market of which molecular diagnostics is currently less than 3%.

This modest market is in contrast to the worldwide pharmaceuticals industry believed to encompass more than $1 trillion. Gene-based and molecular diagnostics testing is currently listed at only one billion dollars in worldwide sales, but is growing at a 30–50% rate. It is thought that as many as 1500 genes and 5000 proteins could become test targets. From an economic viewpoint, nonmolecular types of tests average $26.34 per test charge whereas molecular diagnostics tests average $113.04. In Table 2, the oncology molecular diagnostics industry is organized by the test or biomarker target, these being DNA, RNA, and protein. From this list, it can be seen that the evolving test menu combines a strategy of new applications for well established test platforms like *in situ* hybridization (ISH) and immunohistochemistry (IHC) and the emergence of entirely new technologies. In addition, a variety of enabling technologies such as laser capture microdissection (LCM) and tissue microarrays (TMA) have accelerated the rate of biomarker discovery, validation, and introduction into clinical practice.

2. DNA TARGETS FOR ONCOLOGY MOLECULAR DIAGNOSTICS

The inherent stability of DNA and its resistance to degradation even after tissue fixation and paraffin embedding has made it the most durable target for molecular diagnostic applications. The DNA from human chromosomes has been used to demonstrate the presence of deletions, translocations, gains or losses of whole chromosomes, and a variety of other subtle defects associated with the diagnosis of cancer and disease outcome *(6,7)*. The introduction

From: *Cancer Diagnostics: Current and Future Trends*
Edited by: R. M. Nakamura, W. W. Grody, J. T. Wu, and R. B. Nagle © Humana Press Inc., Totowa, NJ

Table 1
The World-Wide In Vitro Diagnostics Industry

	Clinical pathology	Anatomic pathology	Molecular diagnostics
Market size	$26 billion	$6 billion	$1 billion
Growth rate	>5%	5–10%	30–50%
Margins	Low	Medium	High

and development of the polymerase chain reaction (PCR) has enabled more sophisticated techniques for detecting minute amounts of abnormal DNA in human tumors and relating these findings not only to patient outcome but selection of the therapy *(8)*.

2.1. Routine Metaphase Cytogenetics

Metaphase cytogenetics is arguably the first molecular diagnostic test applied to the field of cancer diagnostics. Ironically, the discovery of the Philadelphia chromosome, the small acrocentric chromosome resulting from the 9/22 (*bcr/abl*) translocation first reported in the early 1950s also became one of the first gene-based targets in the new era of directed oncology *(2)*. The approval of the tyrosine kinase inhibitor STI-471 or Gleevac™ as a direct inhibitor of the activated *bcr/abl* gene brought cytogenetics into the modern era of targeted therapeutics. In cancer patients, cytogenetics is predominately utilized for the classification of leukemia and lymphoma with significantly fewer applications for the evaluation of patients with solid tumors. Technical advancements, including trypsin banding and subsequently the introduction of fluorescence *in situ* hybridization (FISH), chromosomal bar codes, multi-color banding, spectral karyotyping, and comparative genomic hybridization (CGH) have added numerous important applications for cancer diagnostics *(6)*.

2.2. Interphase Cytogenetics: In Situ Hybridization for DNA Targets

2.2.1. Fluorescence In Situ Hybridization

2.2.1.1. ANEUSOMIES

The detection of chromosomal gains and losses or aneusomies using complementary probes for the centromeres of the human chromosomes by FISH during interphase evaluation of whole cells and tissue sections has been used in a variety of research and clinical applications *(9)*. FISH-based aneusomy detection using urinary cytology samples has outperformed conventional cytology and achieved significant clinical use for the evaluation of patients with recurrent urothelial carcinoma *(10)*.

2.2.1.2. TRANSLOCATIONS

Although not sensitive enough to detect small chromosomal changes such as point mutations, the FISH technique proved to be an excellent method for detecting specific chromosomal translocations. The FISH method for detection of the *bcr/abl* translocation can be performed on blood and bone marrow cells to detect chronic myelogenous leukemia (CML) with greater sensitivity and speed than conventional cytogenetics *(11)*. FISH has also been used as a method of subclassifying soft tissue sarcomas (Table 3), which has led to major reconsideration of the derivation of both round cell and spindle cell lesions *(12)*.

Table 2
Summary of Molecular Diagnostic Techniques in Oncology

Target	Methods	Testing samples	Current clinical examples	Future status
DNA				
	Routine cytogenetics	Blood Bone marrow Fresh tissues	Classification • Leukemia • Lymphoma • Sarcomas	Limited by low sensitivity and resolution
	ISH, FISH and CISH	Blood Bone marrow Fresh tissues Paraffin blocks	*Bcr/abl* translocation in CML HER-2/neu amplification *N-myc* amplification Sarcoma translocations HPV genotyping in gynecologic cytology	Selected growth. Limited by low resolution
	CGH CGH arrays SNPs	Blood Bone marrow Blood	Uncommon familial cancer predisposition Prediction of metabolism and toxicity of anti-cancer drugs	Continued development Major bioinformatics challenges
	PCR sequencing	Blood Bone marrow Fresh tissues	Common familial cancer predisposition • *BRCA1,2* and others Tumor suppressor gene mutations • *p53* and others Oncogene activating mutations • cKit in GIST Gene rearrangements in lymphoma Minimal residual disease after BMT High-risk HPV detection	Continued discovery of new applications Limited by low throughput
	Southern blot	Blood Bone marrow Fresh tissues	Gene rearrangements in lymphoma *N-myc* gene amplification in neuroblastoma	Little further utility due to dilutional effects and lack of automation

(*continued*)

Table 2 (*continued*)
Summary of Molecular Diagnostic Techniques in Oncology

Target	Methods	Testing samples	Current clinical examples	Future status
	Micro-satellite instability	Fresh tissues Urine	Colorectal cancer predisposition Resection margin status Urothelial carcinoma metastasis	Growth potential for selected clinical situations discovery of new applications
RNA				
	Transcriptional profiling Northern blot	Blood Bone marrow Fresh tissues	Pharmacogenomic discovery	Substantial growth
	RT-PCR	Blood Bone marrow Fresh tissues (?Paraffin blocks)	Minimal residual disease after BMT Micrometastasis detection in sentinel lymph nodes Oncogene activation CpG island hypermethylation to detect prostate cancer TS/DPD levels to predict 5-FU response Melastatin detection for melanoma prognosis	Substantial growth
	ISH, FISH and CISH	Blood (after cell capture assays) Bone marrow Fresh tissues		Limited growth
Protein				
	Western blot 2D-PAGE	Blood Blood Bone marrow Fresh tissues		Limited
	MALDI-TOF	Blood Bone marrow Body fluids		

Technique	Sample	Application	Clinical potential
SELDI	Blood	Detection of early stage ovarian cancer	Enormous potential if technique can be standardized and reproducibility improved
IHC	Bone marrow Fresh tissues	Immunophenotyping of lymphoma Solid tumor classification ER/PR status in breast cancer HER-2/neu status in breast cancer	
BioAssays			
PCR-based	Fresh tissues Urine	Telomerase TRAP assay	Limited
ligand-receptor assays	Fresh tissues	Hormone receptor (ER/PR) Others	Limited
Truncated protein assays	Blood Bone marrow	Familial polyposis (APC) detection	Limited
General enabling techniques			
Laser capture micro-dissection	Fresh tissues Paraffin blocks	Biomarker discovery	
Tissue microarrays	Fresh tissues Paraffin blocks	Biomarker discovery	
Quantitative digital image analysis	Tissue sections	Biomarker validation Quantification of ISH and IHC	
Micro-capillary electro-phoresis	Blood Body fluids Tissue-derived fluids	High throughput sequencing • Microsatellite instability High throughput proteomics	Substantial potential
Immuno-magnetic cell capture assays	Blood Bone marrow Body fluids	Detection of cancer in blood Pharmacogenomic testing Pharmacodynamic testing	Unknown potential

Table 3
Common Sarcoma Translocations (simplified)

Translocation	Tumor phenotype
11:22	Ewings sarcoma and primitive neuroectodermal tumors
2:13	Alveolar rhabdomyosarcoma
9:22	Chondrosarcoma
X:18	Synovial sarcoma
12:14	Smooth muscle tumors
12:16	Myxoid liposarcoma

2.2.1.3. GENE AMPLIFICATION DETECTION

The most significant application of the FISH technique in cancer diagnostics has been for the detection of amplification of the HER-2/neu gene for the selection of patients to receive the humanized anti-HER-2/neu monoclonal antibody, Herceptin™ *(13,14)*. The FISH test (Fig. 1) for gene amplification is performed on 5 μm thick formalin-fixed paraffin-embedded tissue sections similar to the competing immunohistochemical technique (*see* Section 4.5). Approximately, 85% of published studies have linked HER-2/neu gene amplification or protein overexpression with adverse outcome in breast cancer and the prediction of therapeutic benefit with HerceptinTM *(13,14)*. The new chromogenic *in situ* hybridization test (CISH) will be discussed in Section 2.2.2.

Other examples of FISH detection of gene amplifications in clinical practice include the prediction of disease aggressiveness and therapy selection for patients with neuroblastoma featuring amplification of the *N-myc* gene *(15)*. Additional clinically significant gene amplification tests include the topoisomerase IIα gene for the prediction of anthracycline chemotherapy response *(16)* and the *cyclin D* gene as a predictor of outcome in breast cancer *(17)*.

2.2.2. Chromogenic In Situ *Hybridization*

In situ hybridization using nonfluorescence probes has also become clinically useful for the management of patients with cancer and precancer syndromes. In contrast with other radiolabeled and fluorophore-labeled probes (Table 4), CISH has many advantages including, relative ease of use, production of permanent slides, simplicity in slide scoring, and potential for automation and high throughput

2.2.2.1. HER-2/*NEU* GENE AMPLIFICATION DETECTION

Similar to the FISH, the CISH technique has the advantages of using a sample with a built in internal control, a robust DNA target less likely to degrade after tissue processing, and the opportunity for a more objective scoring system when compared to immunohistochemistry *(18,19)*. In addition, the CISH method does not require a relatively expensive fluorescence microscope and produces slides that are easily stored and can be reviewed without loss of signal over time. With further refinement employing signal amplification strategies, there is significant potential for the CISH method to eventually become the preferred method of detection of HER-2/neu gene amplification.

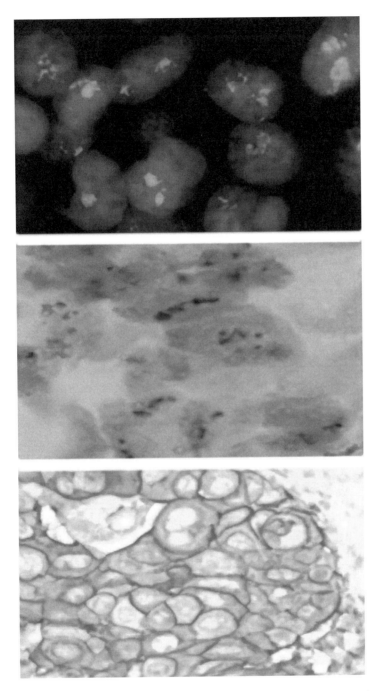

Fig. 1. HER-2/neu testing in breast cancer. *Lower:* Immunohistochemistry using Herceptest™ system (Dako, Corp.) with continuous membranous 3+ positive immunostaining for HER-2/neu protein. *Middle:* HER-2/neu gene amplification detected by FISH (Ventana Inform™ System). *Upper:* HER-2/neu gene amplification detected by CISH (Zymed System). Color figure available for viewing at **www. humanapress.com**.

Table 4
In situ **Hybridization Comparison**

	FISH Fluorescence *in situ* hybridization	CISH Chromogenic *in situ* hybridization	RISH Radiolabeled *in situ* hybridization
Sensitivity	Intermediate	Lowest	Highest
Ease of use	Intermediate	Easiest	Most cumbersome
Automation available	Yes	Yes	No
Slide Scoring	Difficult	Easiest	Most difficult
Microscope Requirements	Fluorescence	Routine	Routine with dark field condenser
Signal amplification	Limited use but complicate slide scoring	Can increase sensitivity,	Not generally required
Quantification	Excellent for gene amplification scoring	Subjective, may require digital image analysis	Autoradiographic grain counting most accurate
mRNA applications	Limited to none	Yes	Yes
Current clinical applications	Cytogenetics CGH and CGH arrays HER-2/neu gene Melastatin light-chain restriction in lymphoma /myeloma diagnosis	Viral detection (HPV, others) amplification	None

2.2.2.2. HUMAN PAPILLOMA VIRUS DETECTION

CISH has been used to identify high-risk types of human papilloma virus (HPV) in gynecologic cytology specimens *(20–22)*. Using a cocktail of probes designed to detect the HPV genotypes associated with high risk for progression of low grade to high-grade cervical lesions, CISH has compared favorably with the established hybrid capture technique for detecting HPV *(20–22)*. Large-scale studies are necessary to determine whether this method can equal or surpass the hybrid capture method for the wide scale screening of atypical gynecologic cytology specimens to determine which patients need clinical follow-up.

2.2.3. Comparative Genomic Hybridization

The FISH technology has been used to perform comparative genomic hybridization (CGH) where DNA extracted from malignant tumors can be comparatively hybridized against normal or reference DNA samples to discover chromosomal gains and losses of DNA segments in the neoplasms *(23,24)*. The CGH technology has uncovered numerous genetic defects in tumors that had previously been undetected by conventional cytogenetics *(23,24)*. Clinical applications of CGH have been limited by lack of resolution. More recently, a technique of CGH combined with analysis of arrays containing artificial human chromosomes derived from bacteria or yeast *(25–28)* has significantly enhanced the precision, sensitivity, and utility of CGH for mapping of tumor-specific genetic alterations (*see* Section 3.1.).

2.2.4. Single Nucleotide Polymorphism Detection

More than 1 million genetic markers known as single nucleotide polymorphisms (SNPs) have recently become available for genotyping and phenotyping studies *(29–32)*. SNPs are the most common type of genetic difference between individuals and provide a tool to survey the genome. With the intense competition to find disease associated genes, companies are turning to faster, more efficient means of interrogating the genome such as multiplexing using reverse transcriptase-polymerase chain reaction (RT-PCR), mass spectrometry (MS), arrays, or FACs-based fuorescent bead methods. Hundreds of thousands of gene-associated SNP candidates have been identified and uncovered numerous loci that appear to have significant potential to generate clinically useful data for patient management. Novel genotyping strategies are emerging on a regular basis using a variety of techniques, including oligonucleotide genomic arrays *(29,30)*, gel and flow cytometry, classic gene sequencing, MS *(31)*, and microarray or gene chips *(32)* all designed to increase the rate of data generation and analysis. In oncology, the SNP technology has focused on three areas of clinical applications: detecting the predisposition for cancer, the prediction of toxic responses and therapeutic benefits for anti-cancer drugs.

2.2.4.1. CANCER PREDISPOSITION TESTING

SNP genotyping and gene sequencing have uncovered a variety of familiar cancer predisposition syndromes based on single and multiple gene variances *(32–34)*. Genotyping has been introduced widely for the detection of familial cancers of the breast, ovary, colon, melanoma, and multiple endocrine neoplasia *(32–34)*.

2.2.4.2. PREDICTION OF DRUG TOXICITY

One of the earliest applications of SNP genotyping in cancer management was the discovery of variations in drug metabolism associated with genomic variations in drug metabolizing enzymes such as the cytochrome p450 and conjugating enzyme systems *(35)*. Known alternatively as pharmacogenetics and toxicogenomics, the wide potential clinical value of

Table 5
Tumor Suppressor Genes

Gene name	Designation	Location	Disease association
Adenomatous Polyposis Coli	APC	5q21	Familial polyposis coli
Breast cancer 1	BRCA1	17q21	Familial breast cancer
Breast cancer 2	BRCA2	13q12	Familial breast cancer
E-cadherin	CDH1	16q22	Familial stomach cancer Lobular breast cancer Prognosis in epithelial cancers
Cyclin-dependent kinase inhibitor 1C	CDKN1C	16q22	Beckwith-Wiedemann syndrome Wilms tumor Rhabdomyosarcoma
p16 Cyclin-dependent kinase inhibitor 2A (MTS 1; INK4A)	CDKN2A	11p15	Familial melanoma Bladder cancer Other epithelial tumors
Mitogen-activated protein kinase 4	MAP2K4	17p11	Pancreatic, breast, colorectal cancer
Multiple endocrine neoplasia type I	MEN1	11q13	Pituitary adenoma Parathyroid adenoma Islet cell carcinoma Carcinoids
Hereditary non-polyposis colorectal cancer type I	hMSH2	2p22	Colorectal cancer Ovarian cancer Endometrial cancer
Hereditary non-polyposis colorectal cancer type I	hMLH1	3p21	Colorectal cancer Ovarian cancer Endometrial cancer
Neurofibromatosis type I	NF1	17q11	Neurofibromas Gliomas Pheochromocytomas Acute myelogenous leukemia
Neurofibromatosis type II	NF2	22q12	Schwannomas Meningiomas Ependymomas
Phosphatase and tensin homolog	PTEN	10q23	Cowden's syndrome Gliomas Prostate cancer Endometrial cancer
Retinoblastoma	RB1	13q14	Retinoblastoma Osteosarcoma Small cell lung cancer Breast cancer

(continued)

Table 5 (*continued*)
Tumor Suppressor Genes

Gene name	Designation	Location	Disease association
Serine/Threonine Kinase 11	STK11	19p13	Peutz-Jehgers syndrome
TP 53	p53	17p13	Li Fraumeni syndrome Inactive in >50% of human malignancies
Tuberous sclerosis 1	TSC1 (KIAA023)	9q34	Hamartomas Renal cell carcinoma Angiomyoliopma
Tuberous sclerosis 2	TSC2	16p13	Hamartomas Renal cell carcinoma Angiomyolipoma
Von-Hippel Lindau	VHL	3p26	Hemangiomas Renal cell carcinoma Pheochromocytoma
Wilms tumor 1	WT1	11p13	Genitourinary dysplasia Familial Wilms tumor

this approach will be uncovered as more candidate polymorphisms can be associated with drug toxicities.

2.2.4.3. PREDICTION OF DRUG EFFICACY—PHARMACOGENOMICS

The application of genomic strategies to predict anticancer drug efficacy and employ the technology in drug discovery, development, and clinical trials encompasses the field of pharmacogenomics *(36–38)*. Pharmacogenomics can utilize germ line SNPs and multigenetic polymorphisms to predict drug response as well as the direct profiling of tumors for expression of genes associated with drug efficacy and resistance.

2.3. Polymerase Chain Reaction and Direct Sequencing

The PCR technique is likely the single most important technical advance in the field of cancer molecular diagnostics *(39)*. PCR approaches to DNA have yielded a variety of molecular diagnostic assays recently eclipsed by the applications of the mRNA assessment by real time PCR (*see* Section 2.3.1.).

2.3.1. Tumor Suppressor Gene Mutation Detection

PCR-based gene sequencing techniques have enhanced the ability to detect point mutations in tumor suppressor genes such as *TP53 (40)*. *TP53* mutation analysis has been used for the management of urinary bladder cancer, detection of lung and colorectal cancer, molecular assessment of resected margins, and monitoring effectiveness of anti-*p53* gene therapies *(41–44)*. A list of tumor suppressor genes sequenced by PCR for clinical use is shown in Table 5. PCR technologies are also widely used to assist in the direct sequencing of genomic DNA from family members with familial cancer syndromes; such as detection of the *BRCA1* and *BRCA2* gene mutations and predisposition for breast cancer as well as some of the other syndromes listed in Table 5 *(45)*.

2.3.2. Oncogene Activation

PCR strategies have similarly been used to detect oncogene activation associated with point mutations in a variety of malignancies. For example, the PCR technique has been used to detect *ras* oncogene point mutations for the diagnosis of pancreatic cancer in limited clinical samples, as well as predict adverse outcome in a variety of solid tumors *(46)*. Recently, PCR-based direct sequencing has been employed to detect specific therapy-responsive mutations in the *c-kit* oncogene in Gleevac™-treated gastrointestinal stromal tumors (GISTs). Although virtually all GISTs overexpress the *c-kit* protein, it has been shown that a minority of point mutations in the *c-kit* gene can produce Gleevac™ resistant tumors *(47)*. Recently, resistance or relapse in CML to Gleevac™ therapy has also shown to involve point mutations in the abl oncogene making the kinase less inhibited by the drug.

2.3.3. Gene Rearrangements

PCR methods have been developed to detect clonal gene rearrangements characteristic of malignant lymphoid neoplasms and for the detection of recurrent disease after therapy *(48,49)*. The RT-PCR method has become the preferred method for detecting successful engraftment after bone marrow transplantation and the presence of minimal residual disease in long term follow-up of lymphoma and leukemia patients in clinical remission *(48,49)*.

2.3.4. HPV Detection

In addition to the ISH and outdated Southern and dot blot methods, PCR-based testing and the hybrid capture assay have been widely used to detect high risk HPV genotypes in gynecologic cytology specimens *(50–53)*. Although the hybrid capture technique is the most widely employed, clinicians continue to express concern regarding the value of HPV detection in the management of their patients with atypical cytology reports *(53)*.

2.4. Southern Blot

The introduction of southern blot technology to clinical practice represented one of the earliest applications of the emerging field of molecular diagnostics in the 1980s. Southern blot continues to be used in many laboratories for the detection of clonal gene rearrangements in patients with malignant lymphoid neoplasms *(48,49)*. Southern blotting is also occasionally used for detection of gene amplifications and remains a major protocol test for the clinical management of children with diagnosed neuroblastoma *(15)*. The relatively cumbersome nature of the assay and potential for the target DNA to be diluted by adjacent stromal, endothelial, and inflammatory cell DNA has limited the use of southern blotting for the evaluation of solid tumors.

2.5. Microsatellite Instability

Microsatellite DNA sequences consist of 4–25 tandemly repeated nucleotide units scattered throughout the human genome *(54–57)*. The role of microsatellites in cellular homeostasis is unknown. Using PCR and sequencing strategies, abnormalities in microsatellites have been associated with a variety of cancer predisposition syndromes *(52)* and have been used as a strategy for the early detection of malignancy including assessment of patients with recurrent urothelial neoplasia *(58)*. MS including both the matrix-assisted desorption and electrospray-ionization methods has recently been introduced to measure microsatellite instability (MSI) *(59)*. MSI is also associated with promoter gene hypermethylation which will be discussed in Section 3.

3. RNA TARGETS FOR ONCOLOGY MOLECULAR DIAGNOSTICS

The measurement of gene expression by detecting absolute and relative mRNA levels has become a major approach to cancer molecular diagnostics *(3–5,32,37)*. The determination of mRNA expression for both novel and known genes by transcriptional profiling using genomic microarrays, RT-PCR, and *in situ* hybridization has found both direct clinical applications and major roles in drug discovery and development *(60,61)*.

3.1. Transcriptional Profiling and Genomic Microarrays

The development of printed and spotted genomic microarrays has allowed for the rapid screening and accumulation of new information concerning SNPs, gene mutation, and mRNA expression in human malignancies *(62–69)*. Transcriptional profiling by hybridizing labeled probes derived from disease specimens to arrayed oligo or cDNAs gives a picture of the transcriptome or mRNA levels of known and novel genes in a neoplasm often compared to the gene expression status of a reference sample. Reference samples can include cell lines, normal tissues, and cancer precursor lesions *(62–69)*. Biochip and microarray technologies have contributed to the industrialization of the genomic and proteomic discovery process and the development of personalized medicine *(32)*. Table 6 lists the major types of arrays or biochips and their associated fluorescent, radioisotope, or MS *(67)* reporter systems in current use or in development for oncology molecular diagnostics. Each of these techniques have the ability to generate hundreds of thousands of data points requiring sophisticated and complex information systems necessary for accurate and useful data analysis (*see* Section 6.6.).

3.1.1. cDNA Microarrays

cDNA microarrays were introduced in the mid-1990s *(70)* and have achieved widespread use for the expression profiling of human clinical samples and in drug and biomarker target discovery. Using sequence verified cDNA clones, robotic printing, either fluorescent or radioisotope-based signal detection, and usually either glass slide or nylon membrane hybridization surfaces (Fig. 2), this technique has generated a wealth of new information in subtyping leukemia/lymphoma, solid tumor classification, pharmacogenomics, and drug and biomarker target discovery *(62–69)*. In addition, oligonucleotide-based cDNA Microarrays produced by companies like Affymetrix, Inc. have been used extensively to map the human gene trascriptome.

3.1.2. Oligonucleotide Microarrays

Oligonucleotide arrays have been extensively used for transcriptional profiling and detection of SNPs and individual gene point mutations. This method originally employed photolithography techniques to apply the large number of oligonucleotides on the glass and nylon surfaces *(62)*. Often there is redundancy so that a single gene is represented by more than 20 oligonucleotides spanning its entire length that reduces the rate of false-negatives *(62)*. This approach has been used to profile differences in gene expression between samples from human tumors and reference test tissues when compared similar to cDNA-based microarrays. Oligonucleotide arrays are well regarded for their automated, high-throughput genome wide analysis of SNPS and other clinically relevant DNA polymorphisms *(71)*.

3.1.3. Comparative Genomic Hybridization (CGH) Microarrays

In DNA array-based CGH (array-CGH) the original CGH technique applied to metaphase chromosomes has been replaced by spots of either cloned cDNA or bacterial artificial human

Table 6
Types of Microarrays in Oncology Molecular Diagnostics

Feature	cDNA microarray (spotted arrays)	Oligonucleotide microarrays	CGH-BAC/YAC microarrays	Tissue microarrays
Target type and technology	Double-stranded cDNA made from tumor mRNA PCR products from cDNA clones Competitive hybridization	16–24 bp oligonucleotides *in situ* synthesis or printing Up to 240,000 oligos/chip Probe redundancy decreases false-positives	DNA fragment arrays Bacterial/yeast artificial chromosomes 100bp to 100kb 5000 spots 1Mb resolution	Paraffin section arrays Frozen section arrays
Types of array surfaces	Glass slides Silicon Nylon membranes	Glass slides Silicon Nylon membranes Gels Beads		Glass slides
Signal Detection Systems	Fluorophores Radioisotopes Typically dual color	Fluorophores Typically single color	Fluorophores	Fluorophores Chromagens Radioisotopes
Technical limitations	Printing inaccuracies False hybridizations	Greater density, but limited by cross-hybridization errors	Limited resolution	Tumor heterogeneity Formalin-based protein and RNA degradation
Automation capability	Robot printing Laser scanning	Robot printing Laser scanning	Fluorescence microscopy Digital imaging	Image analysis
Clinical applications	Leukemia/lymphoma classification Solid tumor classification Carcinoma of unknown primary site Drug selection	Gene re-sequencing SNP discovery Tumor classification SNP prediction of toxicity Drug selection	High-resolution cytogenetics for gains and losses Tumor classification New primary tumor vs metastasis	Currently used for research purposes only
Drug discovery and development applications	Drug target selection Pharmacogenomics discovery Biomarker discovery	Drug target selection Pharmacogenomics discovery Biomarker discovery	Drug target discovery	Drug target valida- tion Pharmacogenomic target validation Biomarker validation

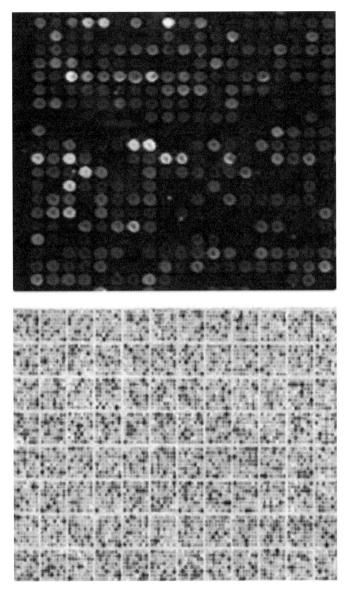

Fig. 2. cDNA microarrays. cDNA Microarrays with each circle representing a distinct cDNA. Probes are generated from isolated RNA(s) by labeling with fluorescent or radioactive nucleotides for detection of specific hybridization. *Top:* Fluorophore-based detection comparing Cy3- or Cy5-labeled probes from normal and disease specimens. After hybridization, fluorescent intensities on scanned images are quantified, corrected for background noise, and normalized. *Bottom:* Radio-isotope detection with a [^{35}S]-nucleotide labeled from a single specimen. The intensity of the densitometric signal is equivalent to the relative abundance. Color figure available for viewing at **www. humanapress.com**.

chromosomes (BAC) or yeast artificial human chromosomes (YAC) *(72)*. More recently, the CGH technique has been applied to cDNA genomic microarrays allowing for sensitive detection of single gene copy losses and gains in tumor samples compared with corresponding normal tissues *(73)*. The resolution of array-CGH is significantly greater when compared to metaphase CGH. It is possible that array-CGH will allow the original cytogenetic level of resolution to reach a molecular level *(72,73)*. The technique can be automated and will increase the throughput of comparing tumors to normal tissues for far more subtle gains and losses of genetic material on an industrial scale; opening the door to the individualization of patient therapies targeting the specific genetic alterations existing in their tumors *(72,73)*.

3.1.4. Tissue Microarrays and Target Validation

Tissue microarrays (TMA) allow a high-throughput testing of multiple characterized tumors samples often with known clinical status and follow-up on a single microscopic glass slide *(74–78)*. TMA can facilitate the discovery of biomarkers and drug targets by allowing for rapid assessment of disease association, as well as improvements in efficiency and productivity by conserving reagents and reducing hands-on time. Patient population studies as large as 600 cases can be assessed by ISH and IHC on a single microscopic slide. New digital image analysis hardware and software has been specifically designed to facilitate TMA analysis allowing for individual core slide scoring to be performed in a semi-automated manner.

3.1.5. Data Analysis and Data Display

Each DNA microarray produces tens of thousands of measurements that require significant computer-based data analysis to determine biologically relevant patterns. It is critical to have systems in place that efficiently combine association, functional, and gene expression data to assess a gene's potential as a disease marker or drug target. Four techniques have emerged as the predominant method of DNA microarray data analysis: hierarchical clustering, self-organizing maps, multidimensional scaling, and pathway associations *(79,80)*. Originally described in 1997, the arrangement of hybridization data into a cluster order based on color-coded intensities, provided clues as to which genes were signaling in groups *(81–86)*. Typically, genes whose expression was significantly greater than that of the reference sample are depicted with increasing intensity on the red scale and those with less gene expression than the reference sample displayed in increasing green signals *(81)*. In hierarchical clustering, the algorithm groups genes in the array based on similarities in their patterns of gene expression. Typically, genes featuring the most similar patterns of expression are grouped next to each other in the vertical axis and patient samples with similar clinical or disease outcome features are arranged along the horizontal axis (Fig. 3). The grouping of similar gene expression samples with similar disease outcome samples is known as a dendrogram. Cluster analysis of genes can be performed in both a supervised and unsupervised manner. In supervised analysis, the bioinformatics system uses machine learning after the computer is provided with an initial batch of categorized data known as the learning set. In unsupervised analysis, the computer attempts to perform the clustering without exposure to a set of previous training cases.

3.1.6. Transcriptional Profiling and Pharmacogenomics

Hierarchical clustering of transcriptional profiling data from clinical samples known to have responded or been resistant to a single agent or combination of anti-cancer drugs is a fundamental component of modern pharmacogenomics *(35,36,87–91)*. Using a predominantly cDNA microarray approach, several groups have now reported on their success at discovering gene expression that can be linked to resistance and responsiveness to standard

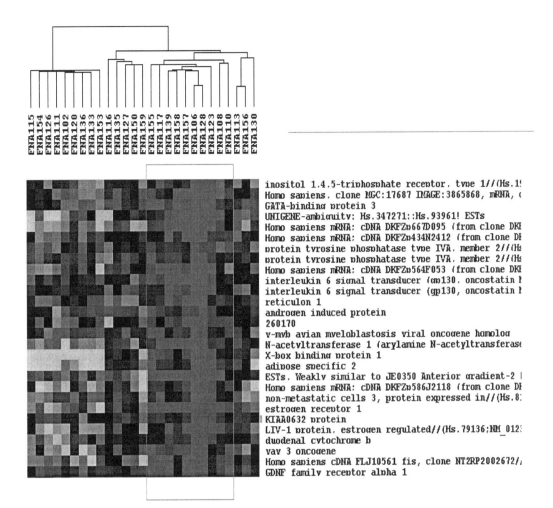

inositol 1.4.5-triphosphate receptor, type 1//(Hs.1!
Homo sapiens, clone MGC:17687 IMAGE:3865868, mRNA, c
GATA-binding protein 3
UNIGENE-ambiguity: Hs.347271::Hs.93961! ESTs
Homo sapiens mRNA: cDNA DKFZp667D095 (from clone DKI
Homo sapiens mRNA: cDNA DKFZp434N2412 (from clone DI
protein tyrosine phosphatase type IVA, member 2//(Hs
protein tyrosine phosphatase type IVA, member 2//(Hs
Homo sapiens mRNA: cDNA DKFZp564F053 (from clone DKI
interleukin 6 signal transducer (gp130, oncostatin I
interleukin 6 signal transducer (gp130, oncostatin I
reticulon 1
androgen induced protein
260170
v-myb avian myeloblastosis viral oncogene homolog
N-acetyltransferase 1 (arylamine N-acetyltransferase
X-box binding protein 1
adipose specific 2
ESTs, Weakly similar to JE0350 Anterior gradient-2 I
Homo sapiens mRNA: cDNA DKFZp586J2118 (from clone DI
non-metastatic cells 3, protein expressed in//(Hs.8:
estrogen receptor 1
KIAA0632 protein
LIV-1 protein, estrogen regulated//(Hs.79136;NM_012:
duodenal cytochrome b
vav 3 oncogene
Homo sapiens cDNA FLJ10561 fis, clone NT2RP2002672/i
GDNF family receptor alpha 1

Fig. 3. Breast cancer cDNA microarray results evaluated by hierarchical gene cluster analysis for defining specific gene expression signatures.Hierarchical clustering algorithm allows the clustering of individual tumor profiles on the basis of their similarities to their co-expression with the estrogen receptor α gene. Each row represents a tumor and each column a single gene. A group of specimens featuring a similar gene expression signature is identified by the rectangular box. Color figure available for viewing at **www.humanapress.com**.

of care chemotherapy *(85,86)*. In the next several years, the ability of this approach to personalize the treatment of newly diagnosed cancer patients with individualized selection and dosage of chemotherapeutic agents will be tested on a large scale.

3.2. Northern Analysis

Northern blotting was the first mRNA detection method used to test gene expression patterns in human cancer. Currently, Northern analysis is limited to a research role, and is not widely used for clinical assessment of human samples. The technique is cumbersome, slow, and similar to Southern blotting, at risk for the loss of sensitivity as a result of dilution of the target malignant cell mRNA levels by surrounding nonneoplastic tissues.

3.3. Differential Display

Prior to the development of high-throughput microarray technologies, the differential display of mRNA was used. Differential display is a technique in which mRNA expression levels in a cell population are reverse transcribed and then amplified by many separate PCR reactions. This robust and relatively simple procedure allows identification of genes that are differentially expressed in different cell populations and is particularly useful for the discovery of biomarkers (92). Differential display is not currently used for direct clinical testing.

3.4. Serial Analysis of Gene Expression

Serial analysis of gene expression (SAGE) is a direct and quantitative measure of gene expression based on the isolation and sequencing of unique sequence SAGE tags (93). The sequence data are then analyzed to identify the presence and level of gene expression and are combined to form a SAGE library. Similar to differential display, the SAGE method is currently applied to discovery biomarkers.

3.5. Reverse Transcriptase-Polymerase Change Reaction

The introduction of the real-time RT-PCR technique has allowed a rapid growth in gene expression studies for both hematologic malignancies and solid tumors (94). In multiplex RT-PCR, housekeeping and gene specific oligonucleotide primers and dye conjugated-probes are added to cDNA produced from RNA isolated from clinical samples and a quantitative level of mRNA expression is obtained by normalizing the amplification cycle time for the target gene against that of a housekeeping gene (94). A variety of commercial closed system RT-PCR technologies are used for clinical applications, predominantly the TaqMan™ method by ABI, Inc. and the Lightcycler™ by Roche Instruments, Inc. are the two most favored instruments. RT-PCR applications generally focus on the enhanced sensitivity associated with PCR-based strategies owing to the ability to detect RNA over a 7-log range.

3.5.1. Leukemia and Lymphoma Diagnosis and Management

RT-PCR techniques have found their first clinical applications in the field of leukemia and lymphoma management (95–98). RT-PCR can be used to detect the presence of non-Hodgkin's lymphoma in minute tissue samples (96,98), as well as the recurrence of the disease after bone marrow transplantation (97). Although the sensitivity of PCR-based methods to detect recurrent lymphoma has caused significant concern as to the specificity for clinically significant vs molecular derived disease relapse, most major cancer centers employ the technique on a regular basis to follow their patients particularly after they have received intensive treatment and bone marrow transplantation.

3.5.2. Solid Tumor Classification

The RT-PCR technique has also been extensively employed to evolve and revise the classification of solid tumors. RT-PCR has been used to detect disease-specific DNA translocations in sarcomas (99,100) and mRNA expression tumor-specific biomarkers drug target genes such as HER-2/neu (101) and PSMA (102,103).

3.5.3. Micrometastasis Detection, Sentinel Lymph Nodes, and Resection Margin Status

Recently, RT-PCR methods have been used to detect minute amounts of tumor-derived mRNA in lymph node samples and resection margin biopsies from patients suffering from a

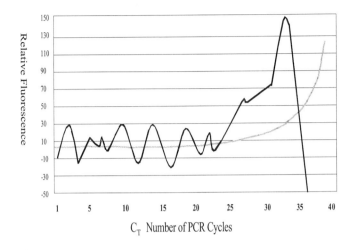

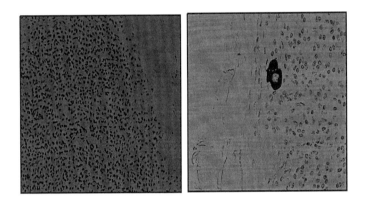

Fig. 4. Micrometastasis detection of breast cancer in a sentinel axillary lymph node biopsy. *Top panel:*Real time PCR (TaqMan™ detection of cytokeratin 19 mRNA after 25 cycles of amplification (dark curve) normalized to internal control dye (light curve). *Bottom panel left:* hematoxylin and eosin stained section of one-half of the same lymph node showing no evidence of tumor cells. *Bottom panel right:* immunohistochemical stain for cytokertain 19 demonstates a single aggregate of two malignant cells beneath the surface in the subcapsular sinusoid. Color figure available for viewing at **www.humanapress.com**.

variety of solid tumors *(104–110)*. This RT-PCR approach has been compared with serial tissue sections and immunohistochemistry *(111,112)* for the detection of micrometatsases (Fig. 4) in sentinel lymph node biopsies. The methods designed to enhance the diagnosis of micrometastasis are currently controversial. It is not certain if lymph node samples reveal malignant cells on routine microscopy, but abnormal mRNA expression detected by RT-PCR are clinically different from lymph nodes that do not contain RT-PCR derived aberrant messages *(113)*. Long-term clinical follow-up and treatment related follow-up will be needed to determine whether this ultrasensitive method of detecting tumor cells in lymph nodes or at microscopically negative surgical resection margins can guide therapy decisions and improve patient outcomes

3.5.4. Rare Event Detection in Peripheral Blood and Body Fluids

Detection of rare circulating tumor cells in peripheral blood and body fluids by RT-PCR has been used as a method for the diagnosis of early stage cancer and monitoring therapeutic response *(114–116)*. A substantial number of malignant tumors have been detected by RT-PCR in peripheral blood samples including carcinomas of the breast, lung, pancreas, colon, prostate, and melanoma *(114–116)*. Peripheral blood based RT-PCR detection of circulating prostate cancer cells has been extensively studied, and although the RT-PCR based detection of PSA mRNA in blood samples is highly sensitive, concern remains as to the specificity of this method for the diagnosis of initial or recurrent carcinoma *(117,118)*.

3.5.5. Gene Methylation Status

RT-PCR based measurement *CpG* island promoter gene hypermethylation in peripheral blood is an indicator for the existence of cancer *(119–121)*. Detection of *CpG* island hypermethylation of the glutathione-*S*-transferase-π gene appears to be a tumor specific event in prostate cancer and shows significant promise as a blood-based test to improve on the specificity of the diagnosis of prostate cancer compared with serum PSA screening *(122–124)*. Gene methylation has also been studied in a wide variety of cancers as a prognostic factor *(125–128)*. Finally, methylation enzymes have recently emerged as a target of cancer therapeutics *(129)*.

3.5.6. Pharmacogenomics

The RT-PCR technique has enabled the introduction of pharmacogenomics into clinical practice. Reflecting that the vast majority of human tumors are stored after formalin-fixation as paraffin blocks, strategies have been designed to amplify mRNA targets extracted from paraffin. Most notable is Taqman™ RT-PCR quantitation of thymidylate synthase and dihydropyrimidine dehydrogenase mRNAs extracted from paraffin-embedded tissues is a predictor of response of colorectal cancer to 5-fluorouracil-based therapy *(130)*.

3.6. ISH, FISH, and CISH for mRNA Detection

In situ hybridization techniques have been applied to detect cell-specific mRNA levels in tissue sections, aspirates, and smears of various human malignancies as well as to detect viral DNAs associated with infections and other biomarkers..

3.6.1. Melastatin

Melastatin is a calcium channel-related gene associated with the development of the nevo-melanocytic system. The expression of melastatin mRNA has been associated with normal neval cells, melanocytic proliferations, and a substantial percentage of *in situ* and invasive malignant melanomas *(131)*. Loss of expression of melastatin mRNA (Fig. 5) in either focally or diffuse patterns have been detected in malignant melanomas and linked to adverse clinical outcome, independent of all known melanoma prognostic factors including tumor thickness *(132)*. Melastatin testing has been introduced to guide follow-up diagnostic and therapeutic decisions such as sentinel lymph node biopsies based on the melastatin expression profile of the primary tumor.

3.6.2. Other Uses

In situ hybridization has also been used to detect κ and λ light-chain mRNA expression in lymphoid infiltrates. Notoriously difficult to demonstrate in paraffin-based immunohistochemistry, restriction of expression of light chain of mRNA has been demonstrated by the

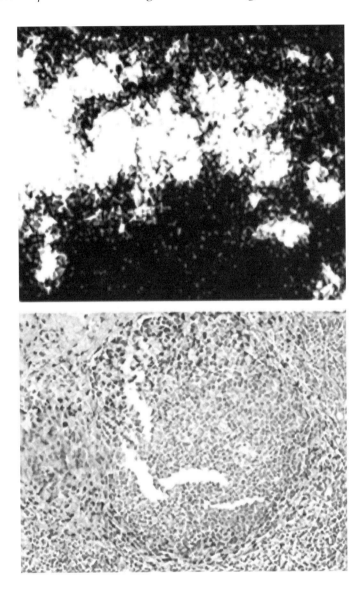

Fig. 5. Melastatin expression loss in malignant melanoma. *Top panel:* dark field view with radio-isotope-labeled probe showing melastatin expression loss in lower center of the microscopic field (arrow). *Bottom panel:* chromogenic ISH with digoxigenin-labeled probe showing melastatin loss in foci of tumor cells the center of the melanoma nodule (arrow). Color figure available for viewing at **www.humanapress.com**.

ISH method and correlated with other factors indicative of a clonal B cell malignant population *(133)*.

4. PROTEIN-BASED TARGETS FOR ONCOLOGY MOLECULAR DIAGNOSTICS

The field of proteomics has emerged as a complementary strategy to genomics for both oncology drug discovery and molecular diagnostics *(134–138)*. Proteomics is a systematic analysis and documentation of the proteins present in a biological sample. This includes measurements of post-translational modification, up-/down-regulation of proteins and absence of expression. The technique requires sophisticated instrumentation for protein separation and identification, and documentation in a standardized, easily retrievable, comparative format. Sequencing the human genome had a finite end-point; in contrast, the proteome is highly dynamic with endless possible variations. Current estimates for the human genome are between 35,000–50,000 genes, but with the fact that many genes exhibit splice variants and that most proteins are post-translationally modified, it is estimated that at least 1 million different proteins exist. With this degree of complexity, the goal of scientists is not to simply catalog protein components under static conditions but to understand how changes in the proteomes contribute to physiological function, disease, as well as to associated proteins with pathways and networks *(134–138)*. In the clinic, mass spectroscopy proteomic approaches to analyze blood and body fluids have been used to detect the existence of cancer *(139,140)*, predict responses to anti-cancer drugs *(141)*, and discover novel targets for cancer therapeutics *(142)*.

4.1. Western Analysis

Despite its major role in the development of clinical assays and validation of protein targets for therapeutics and diagnostic purposes, gel electrophoresis and immunoblotting is not commonly used as a specific diagnostic platform for oncology patients.

4.2. Two-Dimensional Gel Electrophoresis (2DGE)

Two-dimensional gel electrophoresis (2DGE) is a technique that has been available for more than two decades and used to characterize complex mixtures of proteins first by charge (isoelectric focusing) and then by molecular size (SDS-gel electrophoresis) *(135)*. The separated proteins can be imaged and quantified after detection with organic dyes (Coomassie blue) metal reduction (silver stain), fluorophores, metal chelators (Sypro Ruby—fluorescent metal chelator), or radiolabels. 2DGE has been used for identification of novel proteins in protein mixtures, as well as a method for purification of individual proteins prior to spectroscopy *(135)*. The technique is challenging, somewhat cumbersome, and requires substantial user expertise. It is predominately done in research laboratories and pharmaceutical companies as "discovery" for the search of novel proteins biomarkers, or pathway regulators that will lead to a better understanding of novel disease mechanisms. Two-dimensional gel electrophoresis also serves generally as an enabling tool to better resolve complex protein mixtures to prepare them for identification and sequencing by MS *(135)*.

4.3. Matrix-Assisted Laser Desorption/Ionization Time of Flight

Mass spectroscopy has evolved as a major method of analysis of the proteome. Matrix-assisted laser desorption/ionization time of flight (MALDI-TOF) instruments have been developed to characterize proteins and peptides obtained from 2DE samples and characterization of peptide sequences, and by inference, gene sequences *(143–145)*. MALDI-TOF is a form of comparative MS in which fragmentation patterns in peptides obtained from an electron bombardment are compared to databases of known amino acid sequences. The MALDI-TOF instruments analyze crystalline protein substrates after laser pulsation followed by energy transfer desorption and gas-phase matrix ion production *(143–145)*. Both negative and positive molecular ions are detected by the MALDI-TOF system. MALDI-TOF has been used in a variety of biologic and clinical applications including protein and peptide analysis, nucleic acid sequencing, and drug target discovery *(146,147)*. The MALDI-TOF technique is a major method of genotyping patient samples for the detection of clinically important SNPs and polymorphisms *(148)*.

4.4. Surface-Enhanced Laser Desorption and Ionization Time of Flight Mass Spectroscopy

Surface-enhanced laser desorption and ionization (SELDI) is a form of mass spectroscopy in which surface-enhanced affinity capture, desorption, and release are performed *(149,150)*. This technique separates proteins according to their mass and electrical charge generating a spectrum of mass/charge peaks or amplitudes for 15,000 or more proteins or peptides in a single analysis. The height of the peak represents the relative abundance of a protein in the sample. The speed and cost effectiveness of SELDI-time of flight (TOF) is ideal for profiling serum or bodily fluids for disease-specific patterns.

The most successful application of SELDI is a surface extraction technique in which the extraction, presentation, and structural modification or amplification of the sample is performed using a surface protein-chip array *(149,150)*. SELDI proteomic arrays allow for detection of minute amounts of proteins and peptides in complex protein mixtures such as serum and body fluids. The arrays use covalent linkage of antibodies, receptors, enzymes, ligands, and lectins, as well as DNA and RNA. After protein-chip purification on the SELDI surface, TOF-MS with laser desorption is performed to characterize the peptides present in the unknown sample. Substantial infomatics analysis is then required to evaluate the presence and amount of various peptides. The technique can be highly sensitive for the detection of low concentration peptides, that has caused concern as to possible decreases in specificity.

The SELDI technique has been applied to a wide variety of cancer in varying clinical situations *(151)*. Recently, the SELDI proteomics array method has been combined with a self-learning bioinfomatic system and successfully detected peptide patterns characteristic of early stage ovarian cancer *(152)*. Although further validation of this approach must be performed on larger groups of patients, the SELDI-TOF technique shows great promise as a potential method of developing new disease markers capable of detecting cancers at early stages.

4.5. Immunohistochemistry

Immunohistochemistry (IHC) has served as a cornerstone of paraffin-based testing of solid tumors for diagnosis, prognosis, prediction of drug response, and validation of new drug and biomarker targets *(153,154)*. The detection of HER-2/neu protein in breast cancer samples by IHC linked to use of the drug, Herceptin™ significantly increased awareness in the limitations of the technique especially when a semi-quantitative imperfect scoring system is used *(13,14,155,156)*. Pre-analytic issues, including fixation, tissue processing, and antigen retrieval can greatly impact the final results of the procedures *(157–160)*. Image analysis instruments show promise for quantifying results and reducing interobserver and intraobserver variations in slide scoring after staining *(161)* Proper standards, controls, and protocols must be adhered to whether IHC is performed manually or on automated instruments *(157–160)*. Nonetheless, owing to the wide availability of antibodies, the familiarity of the procedure in most pathology laboratories and the adaptability to fixed paraffin embedded tissues; it is likely that the role of IHC in oncology molecular diagnostics will continue for the near future.

Table 7
Protein-Based Arrays

Type of array	Utility	Current status
cDNA clone arrays	Drug development	Research
Protein microarrays	Drug development	Research
Antibody microarrays	Serum diagnostics Antibody screening	Clinical trials
Aptamer microarrays	Unknown	In development
Microfluidic arrays	Cancer screening	In development

4.6. Protein Arrays

A variety of protein arrays (Table 7) have recently been designed to facilitate biomarker discovery and clinical molecular diagnostics *(162)*.

4.7. Enzyme Immunoassays

Advances in enzyme-based serum immunodiagnostics have included increased sensitivity, expansion of automated methods, and the discovery of new shed glyocproteins allowing for closer monitoring of epithelial malignancies *(163,164)*. Furthermore, a number of inventive technologies have recently been introduced to allow multiplex ELISA based determination of up to 18 analytes in the same assay (i.e., antibody arrays or beads). Multiplexing may allow assessment of the phenotypic and physiological context that the target is expressed, by comparing with known clinical markers (e.g., PSA, CA125). Correlation with known physiological parameters will help establish the rules which a specific target gene or protein operates in normal and disease systems, what the most effective therapy may be, and what happens with therapy.

4.8. Truncated Protein Assays

Recently, assays have been designed to detect truncated proteins as indicators of both germ line and somatic genetic defects in various forms of cancer. An example of this approach is the clinically available peripheral blood-based truncated protein assay for the diagnosis of familial polyposis coli *(165)*. A fecal digital version of the truncated APC protein assay has recently shown promise as a screening test for the detection of larger high-risk colonic adenomas and cancers *(166)*.

5. BIOASSAYS

5.1. Ligand–Receptor Assays

Ligand-binding assays have largely been replaced by direct immunoassays on tissue sections and cytosols and protein extracts of tumor tissues *(167)*. The advantages of immunolocalization assays as currently used for determining estrogen receptor status in patients with breast cancer must be weighed against the risk of false positive results when compared with biochemical functional assays such as the dextran-charcoal radiolabeled estradiol binding technique *(167)*. The inherent advantages of confirming both the measurements of the presence of immunodetectable protein and of the functional status of a cancer-

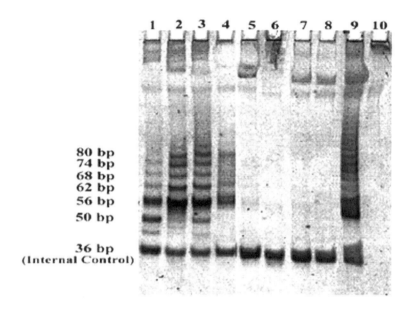

Fig. 6. Telomerase detection in urinary cytologic specimens.using the telomeric repeat amplification protocol (TRAP) method correlate to the presence of malignant cells. *Lanes 1, 2, 3* and *4* contain fluids with malignant cells from different patients that show a ladder of base-pairs indicating the presence of telomerase activity. *Lanes 5, 6, 7,* and *8* are patient fluids that were negative for malignant cells and show no base-pair ladder. *Lane 9* is the control cell line known to be positive for telomerase activity and lane 10 is the telomerase negative control fluid.

related cell receptor may achieve increasing importance in the era of targeted cancer therapeutics *(168)*.

5.2. PCR-Based Ligand–Receptor Assays

Although a variety of PCR-based bioassays have been developed, the test that has achieved the most widespread use in clinical applications is the telomere amplification protocol or TRAP procedure for determining telomerase activity *(169)*. This technique (Fig. 6) has been used in early detection strategies in several clinical settings, most notable for the surveillance of patients with recurrent urothelial carcinoma *(170–172)*. This technique appears to be more sensitive for detecting low-grade bladder tumors than conventional cytology, but has been criticized for its loss of specificity resulting from the relatively frequent finding of false-positive tests *(173)*. New slide direct measurements using both ISH and IHC have recently introduced, but have not had widespread evaluation as to their clinical utility *(170–172)*.

6. GENERAL ENABLING TECHNOLOGIES

6.1. Tissue Microarrays

Tissue microarrays (TMAs) have been described previously *(173–77)*. TMAs are facilitating drug discovery and development by industrializing the assessment of mRNA and protein target expression in large numbers of clinical defined human and animal samples *(173–174)*. TMAs are also used to validate disease specific association of novel tumor biomarkers, prognostic and predictive factors *(178)* (Fig. 7).

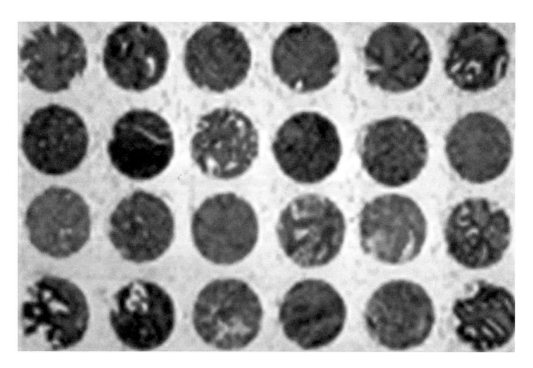

Fig. 7. Tissue microarray. A series of blocks from a set of patients with prostate cancer have been bored at 1. 2 mm and transferred to a recipient block to form the tissue microarray. Sections from the recipient block can now be used to study a variety of biomarkers using immunohistochemistry and *in situ* hybridization. Color figure available for viewing at **www.humanapress.com**.

6.2. Single Cell Analysis and Laser Capture Microdissection

The discovery of laser microdissection allowed for determining individual cell and tissue specific expression of DNA, RNA, and protein for both clinical and research samples *(179)*. Prior to this discovery, the major method of separating complex cell and tissue mixtures for individual cell or group analysis was performed using a fluorescence-based cell sorter (flow cytometry). Laser microdissection includes the techniques of laser-assisted microdissection, laser catapault microdissection, and laser capture microdissection (LCM) *(179)*. Easily applied to both frozen and paraffin sections, LCM features microscopic selection of individual cells or minute tissue areas to be detached from the surrounding sample or, alternately, the undesired components can be eliminated and the remaining cells of interest obtained for molecular analysis *(180)*. LCM has enabled the genomic profiling of small tissue biopsies by preventing the dilution of mRNA signals of the desired (i.e., tumor) cells by large numbers of benign stromal and inflammatory cells *(181,182)*. Subcomponents of individual tissues can be separately selected and the mRNA extracted from this minute material amplified by PCR-based strategies (Fig. 8). LCM has had a major impact in proteomics-based discovery where the ability to sample minute tissue areas and profile the proteins by two-dimensional gel electrophoresis and MALDI mass spectroscopy has enhanced novel peptide identification, post-translational gene modifications, and protein–protein interaction studies *(183–185)*. Similarly, LCM has been combined with cDNA microarray profiling to elucidate novel gene expression pathways in isolated populations from diseases such as prostate cancer *(186)*.

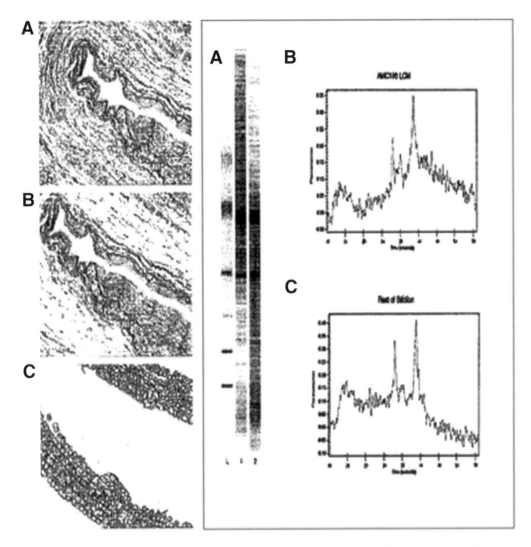

Fig. 8. Laser capture microdissection. On the left are serial pictures of artery showing intact specimen (**A**), of specimen after capture of smooth muscle (**B**), and the isolated small muscle cells (**C**). On the right are the bioanalyzer run (A) and densitometric scans (B, C) showing that high quality mRNA is obtained by extraction from 10,000 captures of artery smooth muscle as evidenced by the strong 28S and 18S ribosomal RNA bands.

6.3. Digital Image Analysis

Computer-assisted digital image analysis has been an enabling system for quantitative data accumulation for a wide variety of molecular technologies, including genomic, proteomic, and tissue microarrays. Image analysis has also continued to be applied to the scoring of slides obtained from ISH and IHC procedures *(187,188)*. Recently, image analysis has been used to improve accuracy and reproducibility of the scoring of slides stained with antibodies to HER-2/neu protein *(189–191)*. By employing cells lines of known HER-2/neu protein expression with digital image analysis, it is anticipated that more reliable assessment breast cancer specimens can be performed on archival formalin-fixed material and allow an improved selection of patients for potential Herceptin™-based therapies.

6.4. Microcapillary Electrophoresis

Microcapillary fluidic technologies including electrophoresis have enabled the development of high-throughput approaches to proteomics *(137–142,192,193)*. These methods are currently allowing for rapid miniaturized and point of care approaches to molecular diagnostics for cancer and show significant potential to create simplified, closed systems for genomic and proteomic profiling *(192)*.

6.5. Immunomagnetic Bead Peripheral Blood Cell Capture

The immunomagnetic bead cell capture system *(194,195)* has enabled the collection of small numbers of cancer cells from peripheral blood, bone marrow and body fluids *(196–198)*. Although still limited by the small numbers of cells captured in most clinical situations and the resulting minute amounts of DNA, RNA, and protein recovered for molecular analysis, this method combined with the latest, highly sensitive genomic and proteomic strategies shows promise as a method of performing drug response monitoring and pharmacogenomics to individualize therapy for cancer patients.

6.6. Bioinformatics

The wealth of data generated by the emerging high throughput genomic and proteomic biochips is totally dependent on the bioinformatics system chosen to evaluate the data *(199–201)*. Microarray technologies are having a major impact in cancer disease understanding, biomarker, and drug development, but continue to struggle with limitations created by a current lack of data comparability *(202)*. The pathway to clinical use for all new molecular diagnostics-based assays will require a sophisticated and robust bioinformatics platform that can support both the early method validation and the subsequent clinical trials required for regulatory and commercial success.

REFERENCES

1. Vogel CL, Cobleigh MA, Tripathy D, et al. 2002. Efficacy and safety of trastuzumab as a single agent in first-line treatment of HER2-overexpressing metastatic breast cancer. J. Clin. Oncol. 20:719–726.
2. O'Dwyer ME and Druker BJ. 2000. STI571: an inhibitor of the BCR-ABL tyrosine kinase for the treatment of chronic myelogenous leukaemia. Lancet Oncol. 1:207–211.
3. Keesee SK. 2002. Molecular diagnostics: impact upon cancer detection. Expert Rev. Mol. Diagn. 2:91–92.
4. Poste G. 2001. Molecular diagnostics: a powerful new component of the healthcare value chain. Expert Rev. Mol. Diagn. 1:1–5.
5. Leonard DG. 2001. The present and future of molecular diagnostics. Mol. Diagn. 6:71–72.
6. Tonnies H. 2002. Modern molecular cytogenetic techniques in genetic diagnostics. Trends Mol. Med. 8:246–249.
7. Sandberg AA and Chen Z. 1994. Cancer cytogenetics and molecular genetics: detection and therapeutic strategy. In Vivo 8:807–818.
8. Lewis F, Maughan NJ, Smith V, Hilla, K, Quirke P. 2001. Unlocking the archive gene expression in paraffin embedded tissue. J. Pathol. 195:66–71.
9. Tibiletti MG, Bernasconi B, Dionigi A, Riva C. 1999. The applications of FISH in tumor pathology. Adv. Clin. Path. 3:111–118.

10. Skacel M, Liou LS, Pettay JD, Tubbs RR. 2002. Interphase fluorescence *in- situ* hybridization in the diagnosis of bladder cancer. Front. Biosci. 7:e27–e32.

11. Pelz F, Kroning H, Franke A, Wieacker P, Stumm M. 2002. High reliability and sensitivity of the BCR/ABL1 D-FISH test for the detection of *BCR/ABL* rearrangements. Ann. Hematol. 81:147–153.

12. Fletcher JA. 1996. Cytogenetics and molecular biology of soft tissue tumors. Monogr Pathol. 38:37–64.

13. Ross JS and Fletcher JA. 1998. The HER-2/*neu* Oncogene in Breast Cancer: Prognostic Factor, Predictive Factor, and Target for Therapy. Oncologist 3:237–252.

14. Lohrisch C and Piccart M. 2001. HER2/*neu*as a predictive factor in breast cancer. Clin. Breast Cancer. 2:129–135.

15. Bown N. 2001. Neuroblastoma tumour genetics: clinical and biological aspects. J. Clin. Pathol. 54:897–910.

16. Sherr CJ. 2000. The Pezcoller lecture: cancer cell cycles revisited. Cancer Res. 60:3689–3695.

17. Tanner M, Jarvinen P, Isola J. 2001. Amplification of HER-2/*neu* and topoisomerase IIalpha in primary and Metastatic breast cancer. Cancer Res. 61:5345–5348.

18. Tanner M, Gancberg D, Di Leo A, et al. 2000. Chromogenic in situ hybridization: a practical alternative for fluorescence *in situ* hybridization to detect HER-2/*neu* oncogene amplification in archival breast cancer samples. Am. J. Pathol. 157:1467–1472.

19. Kumamoto H, Sasano H, Taniguchi T, Suzuki T, Moriya T, Ichinohasama R. 2001. Chromogenic *in situ* hybridization analysis of HER-2/*neu* status in breast carcinoma: application in screening of patients for trastuzumab (Herceptin) therapy. Pathol. Int. 51:579–584.

20. Roteli-Martins CM, Alves VA, Santos RT, Martinez EZ, Syrjanen KJ, Derchain SF. 2001. Value of morphological criteria in diagnosing cervical HPV lesions confirmed by *in situ* hybridization and hybrid capture assay. Pathol. Res. Pract. 197:677–682.

21. Unger ER. 2000. *In situ* diagnosis of human papillomaviruses. Clin. Lab. Med. 20:289–301.

22. Cheung AL, Graf AH, Hauser-Kronberger C, Dietze O, Tubbs RR, Hacker GW. 1999. Detection of human papillomavirus in cervical carcinoma: comparison of peroxidase, Nanogold, and catalyzed reporter deposition (CARD)-Nanogold in situ hybridization. Mod. Pathol. 12:689–696.

23. Houldsworth J and Chaganti RS. 1994. Comparative genomic hybridization: an overview. Am. J. Pathol. 145:1253–1260.

24. Tachdjian G, Aboura A, Lapierre JM, Viguie F. 2000. Cytogenetic analysis from DNA by comparative genomic hybridization. Ann. Genet. 43:147–154.

25. Monni O, Hyman E, Mousses S, Barlund M, Kallioniemi A, Kallioniemi OP. 2001. From chromosomal alterations to target genes for therapy: integrating cytogenetic and functional genomic views of the breast cancer genome. Semin. Cancer Biol. 11:395–401.

26. Forozan F, Karhu R, Kononen J, Kallioniemi A, Kallioniemi OP. 1997. Genome screening by comparative genomic hybridization. Trends Genet. 13:405–409.

27. Veltman JA, Schoenmakers EF, Eussen BH, et al. 2002. High-throughput analysis of subtelomeric chromosome rearrangements by use of array-based comparative genomic hybridization. Am. J. Hum. Genet. 70:1269–1276.

28. Cai WW, Mao JH, Chow CW, Damani S, Balmain A, Bradley A. 2002. Genome-wide detection of chromosomal imbalances in tumors using BAC microarrays. Nat. Biotechnol. 20:393–396.

29. Taylor JG, Choi EH, Foster CB, Chanock SJ. 2001. Using genetic variation to study human disease. Trends. Mol. Med. 7:507–512.

30. Carlson CS, Newman TL, Nickerson DA. 2001. SNPing in the human genome. Curr. Opin. Chem. Biol. 5:78–85.

31. Griffin TJ and Smith LM. 2000. Single-nucleotide polymorphism analysis by MALDI-TOF mass spectrometry. Trends Biotechnol. 2:77–84.

32. Kallioniemi OP. 2001. Biochip technologies in cancer research. Ann. Med. 33:142–147.

33. Relling MV and Dervieux T. 2001. Pharmacogenetics and cancer therapy. Nature Rev. Cancer. 1:99–108.

34. Borg A. 2001. Molecular and pathological characterization of inherited breast cancer. Semin. Cancer Biol. 11:375–385.

35. Renegar G, Rieser P, Manasco, P. 2001. Pharmacogenetics: the Rx perspective. Expert Rev. Mol. Diagn. 1:255–263.

36. Ginsburg GS and McCarthy JJ. 2001. Personalized medicine: revolutionizing drug discovery and patient care. Trends Biotechnol. 19:491–496.

37. Cordon-Cardo C. 2001. Applications of molecular diagnostics: solid tumor genetics can determine clinical treatment protocols. Mod. Pathol. 14:254–257.

38. Innocenti F and Ratain MJ. 2002. Update on pharmacogenetics in cancer chemotherapy. Eur. J. Cancer. 38:639–644.

39. Davis EG, Chao C, McMasters KM. 2002. Polymerase chain reaction in the staging of solid tumors. Cancer J. 8:135–143.

40. Weinberg RA. 1995. The molecular basis of oncogenes and tumor suppressor genes. Ann. N Y Acad. Sci. 758:331–338.

41. Sidransky D and Hollstein M. 1996. Clinical implications of the *p53* gene. Annu. Rev. Med. 47:285–301.

42. Kausch I and Bohle A. 2002. Molecular aspects of bladder cancer III. Prognostic markers of bladder cancer. Eur. Urol. 41:15–29.

43. McCormick F. 2001. Cancer gene therapy: fringe or cutting edge? Nature Rev. Cancer. 1: 130–141.

44. Soussi T and Beroud C. 2001. Assessing TP53 status in human tumours to evaluate clinical outcome. Nature Rev. Cancer. 1:233–240.

45. Borg A. 2001. Molecular and pathological characterization of inherited breast cancer. Semin. Cancer Biol. 11:375–385.

46. Apple SK, Hecht JR, Novak JM, et al. 1996. Polymerase chain reaction-based *K-ras* mutation detection of pancreatic adenocarcinoma in routine cytology smears. Am. J. Clin. Pathol. 105:321–326.

47. Heinrich MC, Blanke CD, Druker BJ, Corless CL. 2002. Inhibition of KIT tyrosine kinase activity: a novel molecular approach to the treatment of KIT-positive malignancies. J. Clin. Oncol. 20:1692–1703.

48. Rubnitz JE and Pui CH. 1999. Molecular diagnostics in the treatment of leukemia. Curr. Opin. Hematol. 229–235.

49. Gleissner B and Thiel E. 2001. Detection of immunoglobulin heavy chain gene rearrangements in hematologic malignancies. Expert Rev. Mol. Diagn. 2:191–200.

50. Unger ER and Duarte-Franco E. 2001. Human papillomaviruses: into the new millennium. Obstet. Gynecol. Clin. North. Am. 653–666.

51. Schneider A, Hoyer H, Lotz B, et al. 2000. Screening for high-grade cervical intra-epithelial neoplasia and cancer by testing for high-risk HPV, routine cytology or colposcopy. Int. J. Cancer. 89:529–534.

52. Pete I, Szirmai K, Csapo Z, et al. 2002. Detection of high-risk HPV *in situ* cancer of the cervix by PCR technique. Eur. J. Gynaecol. Oncol. 23:74–78.

53. Herbst AL, Pickett KE, Follen M, Noller KL. 2001. The management of ASCUS cervical cytologic abnormalities and HPV testing: a cautionary note. Obstet. Gynecol. 98:849–851.

54. Atkin NB. 2001. Microsatellite instability. Cytogenet. Cell. Genet. 92:177–181.

55. Peltomaki P. 2001. DNA mismatch repair and cancer. Mutat. Res. 488:77–85.

56. Saletti P, Edwin ID, Pack K, Cavalli F, Atkin WS. 2001. Microsatellite instability: application in hereditary non-polyposis colorectal cancer. Ann. Oncol. 12:151–160.

57. Frazier ML, Su LK, Amos CI, Lynch PM. 2000. Current applications of genetic technology in predisposition testing and microsatellite instability assays. J. Clin. Oncol. 18:70S–74S.

58. Steiner G, Schoenberg MP, Linn JF, Mao L, Sidransky D. 1997. Detection of bladder cancer recurrence by microsatellite analysis of urine. Nat. Med. 3:621–624.

59. van den Boom D, Jurinke C, McGinniss MJ, Berkenkamp S. 2001. Microsatellites: perspectives and potentials of mass spectrometric analysis. Expert Rev. Mol. Diagn. 1:383–393.

60. Emilien G, Ponchon M, Caldas C, Isacson O, Maloteaux JM. 2000. Impact of genomics on drug discovery and clinical medicine. QJM 93:391–423.

61. Herrmann JL, Rastelli L, Burgess CE, et al. 2001. Implications of oncogenomics for cancer research and clinical oncology. Cancer J. 7:40–51.

62. Harkin DP. 2000. Uncovering functionally relevant signaling pathways using microarray based expression profiling. Oncologist 5:501–507.

63. Snijders AM, Meijer GA, Brakenhoff RH, van den Brule AJ, van Diest PJ. 2000. Microarray techniques in pathology: tool or toy? Mol. Pathol. 53:289–294.

64. Raetz EA, Moos PJ, Szabo A, Carroll WL. 2001. Gene expression profiling. Methods and clinical applications in oncology. Hematol. Oncol. Clin. North Am. 15:911–930.

65. Polyak K and Riggins GJ. 2001. Gene discovery using the serial analysis of gene expression technique: implications for cancer research. J. Clin. Oncol. 19:2948–2958.

66. Lewis F, Maughan NJ, Smith V, Hillan K, Quirke P. 2001. Unlocking the archive-gene expression in paraffin-embedded tissue. J. Pathol. 195:66–71.

67. Maughan NJ, Lewis FA, Smith V. 2001. An introduction to arrays. J. Pathol. 195:3–6.

68. Alizadeh AA, Ross DT, Perou CM, van de Rijn M. 2001. Towards a novel classification of human malignancies based on gene expression patterns. J. Pathol. 195:41–52.

69. Ramaswamy S and Golub TR. 2002. DNA microarrays in clinical oncology. J. Clin. Oncol. 20:1932–1941.

70. Schena M., Shalon D, Davis RW, Brown PO. 1995. Quantitative monitoring of gene expression patterns with a complementary DNA microarray. Science 270:467–470.

71. Wang DG, Fan JB, Siao CJ, et al. 1998. Large-scale identification, mapping, and genotyping of singlenucleotide polymorphisms in the human genome. Science. 280:1077–1082.

72. Monni O, Hyman E, Mousses S, Barlund M, Kallioniemi A, Kallioniemi OP. 2001. From chromosomal alterations to target genes for therapy: integrating cytogenetic and functional genomic views of the breast cancer genome. Semin. Cancer Biol. 11:395–401.

73. Monni O, Barlund M, Mousses S, et al. 2001. Comprehensive copy number and gene expression profiling of the 17q23 amplicon in human breast cancer. Proc. Nat. Acad. Sci. USA 98:5711–5716.

74. Hoos A and Cordon-Cardo C. 2001. Tissue microarray profiling of cancer specimens and cell lines: opportunities and limitations. Lab. Invest. 81:1331–1138.

75. Moch H, Kononen T, Kallioniemi OP, Sauter G. 2001. Tissue microarrays: what will they bring to molecular and anatomic pathology? Adv. Anat. Pathol. 8:14–20.

76. Bubendorf L, Nocito A, Moch H, Sauter G. 2001. Tissue microarray (TMA) technology: miniaturized pathology archives for high-throughput in situ studies. J. Pathol. 195:72–79.

77. Skacel M, Skilton B, Pettay JD, Tubbs RR. 2002. Tissue microarrays: a powerful tool for high-throughput analysis of clinical specimens: a review of the method with validation data. Appl. Immunohistochem. Mol. Morphol. 10:1–6.

78. Kallioniemi OP, Wagner U, Kononen J, Sauter G. 2001. Tissue microarray technology for high-throughput molecular profiling of cancer. Hum. Mol. Genet. 10:657–662.

79. Zhang MQ. 1999. Large-scale gene expression data analysis: a new challenge to computational biologists. Genome Res. 9:681–688.

80. Werner T. 2001. Cluster analysis and promoter modeling as bioinformatics tools for the identification of target genes from expression array data. Pharmacogenomics 2:25–36.

81. Scherf U, Ross DT, Waltham M, et al. 2000. A gene expression database for the molecular pharmacology of cancer. Nat. Genet. 24:236–244.

82. Johnson KF and Lin SM. 2001. Critical assessment of microarray data analysis: the 2001 challenge. Bioinformatics 17:857–858.

83. Goryachev AB, Macgregor PF, Edwards AM. 2001. Unfolding of microarray data. J. Comput. Biol. 8:443–461.

84. Davenport J. 2001. Microarrays. Data standards on the horizon. Science 292:414–415.

85. Dougherty ER, Barrera J, Brun M, et al. 2002. Inference from clustering with application to gene-expression microarrays. J. Comput. Biol. 105–126.

86. Fryer RM, Randall J, Yoshida T, et al. 2002. Global analysis of gene expression: methods, interpretation, and pitfalls. Exp. Nephrol. 10:64–74.

87. Zanders ED. 2000. Gene expression analysis as an aid to the identification of drug targets. Pharmacogenomics 1:375–384.

88. Weinstein JN. 2000. Pharmacogenomics—teaching old drugs new tricks. N. Engl. J. Med. 343:1408–1409.

89. Diasio RB and Johnson MR. 2000. The role of pharmacogenetics and pharmacogenomics in cancer chemotherapy with 5-fluorouracil. Pharmacology 61:199–203.

90. Innocenti F and Ratain MJ. 2002. Update on pharmacogenetics in cancer chemotherapy. Eur. J. Cancer 38:639–644.

91. Los G, Yang F, Samimi G, et al. 2002. Using mRNA expression profiling to determine anticancer drug efficacy. Cytometry 47:66–71.

92. Zhang JS, Duncan EL, Chang AC, Reddel RR. 1998. Differential display of mRNA. Mol. Biotechnol. 10:155–165.

93. Yamamoto M, Wakatsuki T, Hada A, Ryo A. 2001. Use of serial analysis of gene expression (SAGE) technology. J. Immunol. Meth. 250:45–66.

94. Jung R, Soondrum K, Neumaier M. 2000. Quantitative PCR. Clin. Chem. Lab. Med. 38: 833–836.

95. Morgan GJ and Pratt G. 1998. Modern molecular diagnostics and the management of haematological malignancies. Clin. Lab. Haematol. 3:135–141.

96. Gleissner B and Thiel E. 2001. Detection of immunoglobulin heavy chain gene rearrangements in hematologic malignancies. Exp. Rev. Mol. Diagn. 1:191–200.

97. Dolken G. 2001. Detection of minimal residual disease. Adv. Cancer Res. 82:133–185.

98. Diaz-Cano SJ, Blanes A, Wolfe HJ. 2001. PCR techniques for clonality assays. Diagn. Mol. Pathol. 10:24–33.

99. Dagher R, Pham TA, Sorbara L, et al. 2001. Molecular confirmation of Ewing sarcoma. J. Pediatr. Hematol. Oncol. 23:221–4.

100. Naito N, Kawai A, Ouchida M, et al. 2000. A reverse transcriptase-polymerase chain reaction assay in the diagnosis of soft tissue sarcomas. Cancer. 89:1992–1998.

101. Bieche I, Onody P, Laurendeau I, et al. 1999. Real-time reverse transcription-PCR assay for future management of ERBB2-based clinical applications. Clin. Chem. 45:1148–1156.

102. Ghossein RA, Osman I, Bhattacharya S, et al. 1999. Detection of prostatic specific membrane antigen messenger RNA using immunobead reverse transcriptase polymerase chain reaction. Diagn. Mol. Pathol. 8:59–65.

103. Elgamal AA, Holmes EH, Su SL, et al. 2000. Prostate-specific membrane antigen (PSMA): current benefits and future value. Semin. Surg. Oncol. 18:10–16.

104. Raj GV, Moreno JG, Gomella LG. 1998. Utilization of polymerase chain reaction technology in the detection of solid tumors. Cancer 82:1419–1442.

105. Pantel K and Hosch SB. 2001. Molecular profiling of micrometastatic cancer cells. Ann. Surg. Oncol. 8:18S–21S.

106. von Knebel Doeberitz M, Weitz J, Koch M, Lacroix J, Schrodel A, Herfarth C. 2001. Molecular tools in the detection of micrometastatic cancer cells—technical aspects and clinical relevance. Recent Results Cancer Res. 158:181–186.

107. Taback B, Morton DL, O'Day SJ, Nguyen DH, Nakayama T, Hoon DS. 2001. The clinical utility of multimarker RT-PCR in the detection of occult metastasis in patients with melanoma. Recent Results Cancer Res. 158:78–92.

108. Jung R, Soondrum K, Kruger W, Neumaier M. 2001. Detection of micrometastasis through tissue-specific gene expression: its promise and problems. Recent Results Cancer Res. 158:32–39.

109. van Diest PJ, Torrenga H, Meijer S, Meijer CJ. 2001. Pathologic analysis of sentinel lymph nodes. Semin. Surg. Oncol. 20:238–245.

110. Turner RR, Giuliano AE, Hoon DS, Glass EC, Krasne DL. 2001. Pathologic examination of sentinel lymph node for breast carcinoma. World J. Surg. 25:798–805.

111. Noura S, Yamamoto H, Miyake Y, et al. 2002. Immunohistochemical assessment of localization and frequency of micrometastases in lymph nodes of colorectal cancer. Clin Cancer Res. 8:759–767.

112. Ishida M, Kitamura K, Kinoshita J, Sasaki M, Kuwahara H, Sugimachi K. 2002. Detection of micrometastasis in the sentinel lymph nodes in breast cancer. Surgery 131:S211–216.

113. Hermanek P. 1999. Disseminated tumor cells versus micrometastasis: definitions and problems. Anticancer Res. 19:2771–2774.

114. Ghossein RA, Carusone L, Bhattacharya S. 1999. Review: polymerase chain reaction detection of micrometastases and circulating tumor cells: application to melanoma, prostate, and thyroid carcinomas. Diagn. Mol. Pathol. 8:165–175.

115. Ghossein RA and Bhattacharya S. 2000. Molecular detection and characterisation of circulating tumour cells and micrometastases in solid tumours. Eur. J. Cancer 36:1681–1694.

116. Ghossein RA and Bhattacharya S. 2001. Molecular detection and characterization of circulating tumor cells and micrometastases in prostatic, urothelial, and renal cell carcinomas. Semin. Surg. Oncol. 20:304–311.

117. Nejat RJ, Katz AE, Olsson CA. 1998. The role of reverse transcriptase-polymerase chain reaction for staging patients with clinically localized prostate cancer. Semin. Urol. Oncol. 16:40–45.

118. Hamdy FC. 2001. Prognostic and predictive factors in prostate cancer. Cancer Treat. Rev. 27:143–151.

119. Herman JG and Baylin SB. 2000. Promoter-region hypermethylation and gene silencing in human cancer. Curr. Top. Microbiol. Immunol. 249:35–54.

120. Esteller M and Herman JG. 2002. Cancer as an epigenetic disease: DNA methylation and chromatin alterations in human tumours. J. Pathol. 196:1–7.

121. Wong IH. 2001. Methylation profiling of human cancers in blood: molecular monitoring and Prognostication. Int. J. Oncol. 19:1319–1324.

122. Jeronimo C, Usadel H, Henrique R, et al. 2001. Quantitation of GSTP1 methylation in non-neoplastic prostatic tissue and organ-confined prostate adenocarcinoma. J. Natl. Cancer Inst. 93:1747–1752.

123. Lin X, Tascilar M, Lee WH, et al. 2001. GSTP1 CpG island hypermethylation is responsible for the absence of GSTP1 expression in human prostate cancer cells. Am. J. Pathol. 159: 1815–1826.

124. Cairns P, Esteller M, Herman JG, et al. 2001. Molecular detection of prostate cancer in urine by GSTP1 hypermethylation. Clin Cancer Res. 7:2727–2730.

125. Jubb AM, Bell SM, and Quirke P. 2001. Methylation and colorectal cancer. J. Pathol. 195:111–134.

126. Yang X, Yan L, Davidson NE. 2001. DNA methylation in breast cancer. Endocr. Relat. Cancer 8:115–127.

127. Claij N and te Riele H. 1999. Microsatellite instability in human cancer: a prognostic marker for chemotherapy? Exp. Cell. Res. 246:1–10.

128. Paul R, Ewing CM, Jarrard DF, Isaacs WB. 1997. The cadherin cell-cell adhesion pathway in prostate cancer progression. Br. J. Urol. 79(Suppl 1):37–43.

129. Szyf M. 2001. Towards a pharmacology of DNA methylation. Trends Pharmacol. Sci. 22: 350–354.

130. Salonga D, Danenberg KD, Johnson M, et al. 2000. Colorectal tumors responding to 5-fluorouracil have low gene expression levels of dihydropyrimidine dehydrogenase, thymidylate synthase, and thymidine phosphorylase. Clin Cancer Res. 6:1322–1327.

131. Duncan LM, Deeds J, Hunter J, et al. 1998. Down-regulation of the novel gene melastatin correlates with potential for melanoma metastasis. Cancer Res. 58:1515–1520.

132. Duncan LM, Deeds J, Cronin FE, et al. 2001. Melastatin expression and prognosis in cutaneous malignant melanoma. J. Clin. Oncol. 19:568–576.

133. King G, Chambers G, Murray GI. 1999. Detection of immunoglobulin light chain mRNA by in situ hybridisation using biotinylated tyramine signal amplification. Mol. Pathol. 52:47–50.

134. Jain KK. 2000. Applications of proteomics in oncology. Pharmacogenomics 1:385–393.

135. Lee KH. 2001. Proteomics: a technology-driven and technology-limited discovery science. Trends Biotechnol. 19:217–222.

136. Simpson RJ and Dorow DS. 2001. Cancer proteomics: from signaling networks to tumor markers. Trends Biotechnol. 19:S40–S48.

137. Dua K, Williams TM, Beretta L. 2001. Translational control of the proteome: relevance to cancer. Proteomics 1:1191–1199.

138. Herrmann PC, Liotta LA, Petricoin EF III. 2001. Cancer proteomics: the state of the art. Dis. Markers 17:49–57.

139. Srinivas PR, Srivastava S, Hanash S, Wright GL Jr. 2001. Proteomics in early detection of cancer. Clin. Chem. 47:1901–1911.

140. Bichsel VE, Liotta LA, Petricoin EF III. 2001. Cancer proteomics: from biomarker discovery to signal pathway profiling. Cancer J. 7:69–78.

141. Hutter G and Sinha P. 2001. Proteomics for studying cancer cells and the development of chemoresistance. Proteomics 1:1233–1248.

142. Hanash SM, Madoz-Gurpide J, Misek DE. 2002. Identification of novel targets for cancer therapy using expression proteomics. Leukemia 16:478–485.

143. Kolchinsky A and Mirzabekov A. 2002. Analysis of SNPs and other genomic variations using gel-based chips. Hum. Mutat. 19:343–360.

144. Leushner J. 2001. MALDI TOF mass spectrometry: an emerging platform for genomics and diagnostics. Expert Rev. Mol. Diagn. 1:11–18.

145. Hamdan M, Galvani M, Righetti PG. 2001. Monitoring 2-D gel-induced modifications of proteins by MALDI-TOF mass spectrometry. Mass Spectrom Rev. 20:121–41.

146. Papac DI and Shahrokh Z. 2001. Mass spectrometry innovations in drug discovery and development. Pharm. Res. 18:131–45.

147. Andersen JS and Mann M. 2000. Functional genomics by mass spectrometry. FEBS Lett. 480:25–31.

148. Griffin TJ and Smith, LM. 2000. Single-nucleotide polymorphism analysis by MALDI-TOF mass spectrometry. Trends Biotechnol. 18:77–84.

149. Weinberger SR, Morris TS, Pawlak M. 2000. Recent trends in protein biochip technology. Pharmacogenomics 1:395–416.

150. Merchant M and Weinberger SR. 2000. Recent advancements in surface-enhanced laser desorption/ionization-time of flight-mass spectrometry. Electrophoresis 21:1164–1177.

151. Wulfkuhle JD, McLean KC, Paweletz CP, et al. 2001. New approaches to proteomic analysis of breast cancer. Proteomics 1:1205–1215.

152. Petricoin EF, Ardekani AM, Hitt BA, et al. 2002. Use of proteomic patterns in serum to identify ovarian cancer. Lancet 359:572–577.

153. Taylor CR and Cote RJ. 1997. Immunohistochemical markers of prognostic value in surgical pathology. Histol. Histopathol. 12:1039–1055.

154. Oertel J and Huhn D. 2000. Immunocytochemical methods in haematology and oncology. J. Cancer Res. Clin. Oncol. 126:425–40.

155. Hanna W. 2001. Testing for HER2 status. Oncology 2:22–30.

156. Schaller G, Evers K, Papadopoulos S, Ebert A, Buhler H. 2001. Current use of HER2 tests. Ann. Oncol. 12:S97–S100.

157. Taylor CR. 2000. The total test approach to standardization of immunohistochemistry. Arch. Pathol. Lab. Med. 124:945–951.

158. Werner M, Chott A, Fabiano A, Battifora H. 2000. Effect of formalin tissue fixation and processing on immunohistochemistry. Am. J. Surg. Pathol. 24:1016–1.

159. Miller RT, Swanson PE, Wick MR. 2000. Fixation and epitope retrieval in diagnostic immunohistochemistry: a concise review with practical considerations. Appl. Immunohist. Molec. Morph. 8:228–235.

160. Shi SR, Cote RJ, Taylor CR. 2001. Antigen retrieval techniques: current perspectives. J. Histochem. Cytochem. 4:931–937.

161. Esteva FJ, Hortobagyi GN, Sahin AA, et al. 2001. Expression of erbB/HER receptors, heregulin and P38 in primary breast cancer using quantitative immunohistochemistry. Pathol. Oncol. Res. 7:171–177.

162. Walter G, Bussow K, Lueking A, Glokler J. 2002. High-throughput protein arrays: prospects for molecular diagnosis. Trends Mol. Med. 8:250–253.

163. Johnson PJ. 2001. A framework for the molecular classification of circulating tumor markers. Ann. N Y Acad. Sci. 945:8–21.

164. Thomas CM and Sweep CG. 2001. Serum tumor markers: past, state of the art, and future. Int. J. Biol. Markers. 16:73–86.

165. Ahnen DJ. 1996. The genetic basis of colorectal cancer risk. Adv. Intern. Med. 41:531–552.

166. Traverso G, Shuber A, Levin B, et al. 2002. Detection of APC mutations in fecal DNA from patients with colorectal tumors. N. Engl. J. Med. 346:311–320.

167. Goussard J. 1998. Paraffin section immunocytochemistry and cytosol-based ligand-binding assays for ER and PR detection in breast cancer: the time has come for more objectivity. Cancer Lett. 132:61–66.

168. Thorpe R, Wadhwa M, Mire-Sluis A. 1997. The use of bioassays for the characterisation and control of biological therapeutic products produced by biotechnology. Dev. Biol. Stand. 91:79–88.

169. Kim NW and Wu F. 1997. Advances in quantification and characterization of telomerase activity by the telomeric repeat amplification protocol (TRAP). Nucleic Acids Res. 25:2595–2597.

170. Vasef MA, Ross JS, Cohen MB. 1999. Telomerase activity in human solid tumors. Diagnostic utility and clinical applications. Am. J. Clin. Pathol. 112:S68–75.

171. Mu J and Wei LX. 2002. Telomere and telomerase in oncology. Cell Res. 12:1–7.

172. Dahse R and Mey J. 2001. Telomerase in human tumors: molecular diagnosis and clinical significance. Expert Rev. Mol. Diagn. 1:201–210.

173. Ross JS and Cohen MB. 2000. Ancillary methods for the detection of recurrent urothelial neoplasia. Cancer 90:75–86.

174. Battifora H. 1986. The multitumor (sausage) tissue block: novel method for immunohistochemical antibody testing. Lab. Invest. 55:244–248.

175. Kononen J, Bubendorf L, Kallioniemi A, et al. 1998. Tissue microarrays for high-throughput molecular profiling of tumor specimens. Nat. Med. 4:844–847.

176. Zarrinkar PP, Mainquist JK, Zamora M, et al. 2001. Arrays of arrays for high-throughput gene expression profiling. Genome Res. 11:1256–1261.

177. Hoos A, Cordon-Cardo C. 2001. Tissue microarray profiling of cancer specimens and cell lines: opportunities and limitations. Lab. Invest. 81:1331–1338.

178. Torhorst J, Bucher C, Kononen J, et al. 2001. Tissue microarrays for rapid linking of molecular changes to clinical endpoints. Am. J. Pathol. 159:2249–2256.

179. Todd R and Margolin DH. 2002. Challenges of single-cell diagnostics: analysis of gene expression. Trends Mol. Med. 8:254–257.

180. Curran S, McKay JA, McLeod HL, Murray GI. 2000. Laser capture microscopy. Mol. Pathol. 53:64–68.

181. Best CJ and Emmert-Buck MR. 2001. Molecular profiling of tissue samples using laser capture microdissection. Expert Rev. Mol. Diagn. 1:53–60.

182. Maitra A, Wistuba II, Gazdar AF. 2001. Microdissection and the study of cancer pathways. Curr. Mol. Med. 1:153–162.

183. Simone NL, Paweletz CP, Charboneau L, Petricoin EF III, Liotta LA. 2000. Laser capture microdissection: beyond functional genomics to proteomics. Mol. Diagn. 5:301–307.

184. Craven RA and Banks RE. 2001. Laser capture microdissection and proteomics: possibilities and limitation. Proteomics 1:1200–1204.

185. Verma M, Wright GL Jr, Hanash SM, Gopal-Srivastava R, Srivastava S. 2001. Proteomic approaches within the NCI early detection research network for the discovery and identification of cancer biomarkers. Ann. NY Acad. Sci. 945:103–15.

186. Rubin MA. 2001. Use of laser capture microdissection, cDNA microarrays, and tissue Microarrays in advancing our understanding of prostate cancer. J. Pathol. 195:80–86.

187. Bacus SS and Ruby SG. 1993. Application of image analysis to the evaluation of cellular prognostic factors in breast carcinoma. Pathol. Annu. 28:179–204.

188. Aziz DC and Barathur RB. 1994. Quantitation and morphometric analysis of tumors by image analysis. J. Cell. Biochem. Suppl. 19:120–125.

189. Esteva FJ, Hortobagyi GN, Sahin AA, et al. 2001. Expression of erbB/HER receptors, heregulin and P38 in primary breast cancer using quantitative immunohistochemistry. Pathol. Oncol. Res. 7:171–177.

190. Wang S, Saboorian MH, Frenkel EP, et al. 2001. Assessment of HER-2/*neu* status in breast cancer. Automated Cellular Imaging System (ACIS)-assisted quantitation of immunohistochemical assay achieves high accuracy in comparison with fluorescence in situ hybridization assay as the standard. Am. J. Clin. Pathol. 116:495–503.

191. Hanna W. 2001. Testing for HER2 status. Oncology 61:22–30.

192. Bosserhoff AK, Buettner R, Hellerbrand C. 2000. Use of capillary electrophoresis for high throughput screening in biomedical applications. A minireview. Comb. Chem. High Throughput Screen. 3:455–466.

193. Celis JE, Kruhoffer M, Gromova I, et al. 2000. Gene expression profiling: monitoring transcription and translation products using DNA microarrays and proteomics. FEBS Lett. 480:2–16.

194. Haukanes BI and Kvam C. 1993. Application of magnetic beads in bioassays. Biotechnology (N Y). 11:60–63.

195. Rye PD, Hoifodt HK, Overli GE, Fodstad O. 1997. Immunobead filtration: a novel approach for the isolation and propagation of tumor cells. Am. J. Pathol. 150:99–106.

196. Park S, Lee B, Kim I, et al. 2001. Immunobead RT-PCR versus regular RT-PCR amplification of CEA mRNA in peripheral blood. J. Cancer Res. Clin. Oncol. 127:489–494.

197. Flatmark K, Bjornland K, Johannessen HO, et al. 2002. Immunomagnetic detection of micrometastatic cells in bone marrow of colorectal cancer patients. Clin. Cancer Res. 8: 444–449.

198. Barker SD, Casado E, Gomez-Navarro J, et al. 2001. An immunomagnetic-based method for the purification of ovarian cancer cells from patient-derived ascites. Gynecol. Oncol. 82:57–63.

199. Brazma A and Vilo J. 2000. Gene expression data analysis. FEBS Lett. 480:17–24.

200. Maughan NJ, Lewis FA, Smith V. 2001. An introduction to arrays. J. Pathol. 195:3–6.

201. Bayat A. 2002. Science, medicine, and the future: Bioinformatics. Br. Med. J. 324:1018–1022.

202. Bustin SA and Dorudi S. 2002. The value of microarray techniques for quantitative gene profiling in molecular diagnostics. Trends Mol. Med. 8:269–272.

17

DNA Repair Defects in Cancer

Ramune Reliene and Robert H. Schiestl

1. INTRODUCTION

Cancer is the second leading cause of death in the United States, exceeded only by heart disease. In the United States, one of every four deaths is from cancer *(1)*. It has been established that cancer is a genetic disease. Carcinogenesis can be promoted by a single dominant mutation leading to expression of an oncogene. Alternatively, according to the two-step mutation model proposed by Knudson in 1971 *(2)*, cancer may arise when a recessive mutation in a tumor suppressor gene is expressed *(3,4)*. In familial cancers, this occurs when an inherited mutation is followed by a loss of heterozygosity event removing the wildtype (Wt) allele of the gene. In sporadic cancers, a somatic mutation occurs in one allele followed by loss of heterozygosity of the second allele of a tumor suppressor gene. In a more complex model of tumorigenesis, cancer risk is enhanced by a deficiency in DNA repair. Loss of DNA repair function leads to accumulation of a high frequency of mutations, including tumor-promoting mutations. Such mutations can occur as point mutations or as result of large-scale chromosomal rearrangements, such as chromosomal deletions, duplications, and translocations. Cancer formation can be initiated by these events, if the deleted chromosomal region encodes a tumor suppressor gene or if an amplified region encodes an oncogene. In fact, the genomic instability resulting in loss and gain of whole chromosomes or large portions thereof has been observed in the majority of tumors *(5)*. Such rearrangements can lead to gene disruptions that inactivate a tumor suppressor gene or alter the function of a proto-oncogene. DNA is subject to continuous damage by noxious exogenous chemical and physical agents or oxygen radicals produced by the normal cellular metabolism. About 10,000 oxidative lesions are formed in our genome in each cell every day *(6)*. In addition, some chemical bonds in DNA undergo spontaneous hydrolysis. The cell responds to DNA damage by inducing cell-cycle arrest and DNA repair or, when damage is too severe to be repaired, undergoes cellular death by apoptosis. There are four pathways for DNA repair, such as base excision repair (BER), nucleotide excision repair (NER), mismatch repair (MMR) and double-stand-break (DSB) repair *(7,8)*. DSBs are repaired by either nonhomologous end-joining (NHEJ) or homologous recombination (HR) *(7,9–11)*. Several inherited syndromes associated with a markedly elevated incidence of cancer involve genes that are essential in DNA repair (Table 1). These include xeroderma pigmentosum (XP), hereditary nonpolyposis colorectal cancer (HNPCC), ataxia telangiectasia (AT), Nijmegen

From: *Cancer Diagnostics: Current and Future Trends*
Edited by: R. M. Nakamura, W. W. Grody, J. T. Wu, and R. B. Nagle © Humana Press Inc., Totowa, NJ

Table 1
DNA Repair Deficiency is Associated With Carcinogenesis

DNA repair deficiency	Genes affected	Syndromes	Common types of cancer	References
Nucleotide-excision	XPA-XPG, XPV	Xeroderma pigmentosum, Cockayne's, trichothiodys-trophy	Skin	17–19, 21
Mismatch	MSH, MLH	Hereditary nonpolyposis colorectal cancer	Colorectal, endometrial, gastric	28–31, 33, 34
DNA damage check point and DSB repair	ATM, Trp53, NBS, FA, BRCA1, BRCA2	Ataxia telangiectasia, Li- Fraumeni, Nijmegen breakage, Fanconi's anemia	Lymphoid, breast, ovarian, various carcinomas, squamous cell sarcoma	47, 48, 55, 56, 61, 70–72, 85–87
Other: DNA helicases	BLM, WRN	Werner's, Bloom's	WRN—primarily sarcomas, also various types of carcinomas Bloom—lymphoid, various types of carcinomas, including Wilms tumor, osteosarcoma	79–81

breakage syndrome (NBS), Li-Fraumeni syndrome, Bloom's syndrome, Werner's syndrome, and Fanconi's anemia.

1.1. Base Excision Repair

BER eliminates single damaged or inappropriate base residues by the action of specialized DNA glycosylases and AP endonucleases *(7,12)*. After removal of the damaged base by a DNA glycosylase, incision by AP endonuclease, and excision of damaged nucleotide by exonuclease, the resulting gap is filled by DNA synthesis and ligation seals the remaining single stranded break. Apparently, absence of any of the DNA glycosylases results in small or moderate changes in spontaneous mutation frequencies, that may have an effect on the long-term integrity of the genome.

1.2. Nucleotide Excision Repair

The role of nucleotide excision repair (NER) in cancer first came to light through the study of inherited disease xeroderma pigmentosum (XP) *(13)*. Patients with this autosomal recessive disease are very sensitive to ultraviolet (UV)-light that causes prominent pigmentation in the sun-exposed areas. Additionally, patients have greater than 2000-fold increased risk of developing skin cancer *(14)*. The incidence of XP varies from 1 in 250,000 in Europe and the United States to as high as 1 in 40,000 in Japan *(15,16)*. Defects in any of seven genes, designated *XPA-XPG*, give rise to this disease. XP heterozygotes are at no higher risk for neoplasia than the general population *(17)*. Deficiency in some of the XP genes may also lead to a combination of XP and Cockayne's syndromes or XP and trichothiodystrophy. Cockayne's syndrome and trichothiodystrophy alone do not show evidence of increased cancer, but are associated with congenital neurological degeneration and skeletal abnormalities *(18)*.

NER is the most flexible of all DNA repair mechanisms because of its ability to eliminate numerous structurally unrelated DNA lesions caused by many exogenous mutagens. This repair removes the major UV-induced photoproducts such as cyclobutane pyrimidine dimers, as well as other DNA adducts, including polycyclic aromatic hydrocarbons, and cisplatin lesions *(19,20)*. NER excises damage within oligomers that are 25 to 32 nucleotides long *(7,18,21)*. The NER process involves the action of about 20–30 proteins in successive steps of damage recognition, local opening of the DNA double helix around the injury, and incision of the damaged strand on both sides of the lesion. After excision of the damage-containing oligonucleotide, the resulting gap is filled by DNA repair synthesis, followed by strand ligation.

1.3. Mismatch Repair

The role of MMR in cancer came with the discovery of a group of patients with colon cancer that exhibited alterations of poly(A) or poly (AC) tracts in their genomes *(22,23)*. Such dispersed repetitive sequences consisting of 10–50 tandem repeats of 1–6 base pairs were termed microsatellites. Alterations in the length of such microsatellite sequences gave rise to the term microsatellite instability (MSI). The link between MSI and MMR deficiency has been suggested when MSI was observed in bacteria with defects in the mismatch- repair genes *mutS* or *mutL (24)* and in the yeast homologues of either *mutS* or *mutL (25)*. In humans, homologues of the *E. coli mutS*, *MSH (26)*, and homologues of the *mutL*, termed *MLH* or *PMS (27)*, were identified and their mutant forms were found in kindred with hereditary nonpolyposis colorectal cancer *(28–31)*. MSI occurs in approx 15% of sporadic (nonfamilial) colorectal cancers and in most cancer patients with hereditary nonpolyposis colorectal cancer *(22,23,32)*. About 10% of endometrial and gastric cancer cases contain defects in MMR *(33)*. Patients heterozygous for a mutation in a MMR gene are prone to cancer *(29,34)*. MMR enzymes repair mismatches of nucleotides that occur when DNA polymerase inserts the wrong base in newly synthesized DNA. Incorrectly paired nucleotides are excised from the mismatched strand and new DNA is synthesized *(7)*.

1.4. DNA Double-Strand Break Sensing and Repair

Chromosomal double-strand breaks (DSBs) can be formed by oxygen free-radicals, ionizing radiation, DNA replication or topoisomerase failure. DNA DSBs are repaired by either nonhomologous end-joining (NHEJ) or homologous recombination (HR) *(7,9–11)*. During NHEJ, the ends of broken DNA are often modified by the addition or deletion of several nucleotides prior to relegation. Impaired rejoining of DSBs may result in large-scale genomic rearrangements, including chromosomal translocations, inversions and deletions, the alterations observed in many tumor cells *(35–38)*. In HR events, the homologous sequences provide a template for the repair. The original sequence is restored when HR occurs from allelic sequences on the sister chromatid or homologous chromosome. HR is usually a precise type of DNA repair when recombination occurs between homologs. Repetitive DNA sequences comprising about 25% of mammalian genome *(39)* provide an alternative template for HR. This type of HR is not cell-cycle dependent but may lead to deletions, duplications, and translocations, events that have deleterious consequences for genome integrity and are associated with carcinogenesis. As an example, HR between Alu elements *(40)* resulting in tandem duplication in the *ALL-1* gene is associated with acute myeloid leukemia *(41)*. Therefore, HR may serve as a mechanism for both DNA repair and chromosomal instability depending on the template used.

Genes involved in signaling and repair of DNA DSBs include *ATM*, *NBS*, *Trp53*, *BRCA1* and *BRCA2*, *FANC*, *WRN* and *BLM (38,42–44)*. Mutations in these genes give rise to cancer-prone syndromes, such as AT, Nijmegen breakage (NBS), Li-Fraumeni (Trp53), Fanconi's anemia (FA), Werner's (WRN) and Bloom's (BLM) syndromes. Most of these disorders, such as AT, NBS, BRCA mutation-associated breast cancer, FA, and BLM syndrome are associated with marked sensitivity to ionizing radiation *(45)* and/or DNA cross-links, both known to strongly induce DNA strand breaks. Consequently, cells from these patients display elevated frequencies of chromosomal aberrations.

AT is an autosomal recessive disorder characterized by early onset progressive cerebellar ataxia, ocular telangiectasia (dilation of blood capillaries), immunodeficiency, sterility, and cancer predisposition *(46–48)*. This pleitropic disorder occurs in 1 of about 300,000 births *(49,50)*. Approximately 10% of the AT patients develop cancers and there is a 250-fold increased risk for lymphomas and a 70-fold excess risk for leukemias *(51)*. Other types of tumors include gastric, liver, pancreatic, ovarian, breast, and salivary gland cancers *(52)*. AT arises from a mutation of the *ATM* gene *(53,54)* that encodes a serine/threonine kinase involved in sensing of DNA damage and transcriptional activation of numerous downstream effectors resulting in cell cycle arrest followed by DNA repair.

Nijmegen breakage syndrome (NBS) patients share the phenotype of AT patients, such as immunodeficiency, radiosensitivity, and predisposition to lymphoid malignancies, but lack both ataxia and telangiectasia *(55,56)*. The NBS syndrome is caused by a recessive mutation in the *NBS1* gene *(57,58)*. NBS1 protein together with RAD50 and MRE11 form the RAD50/ MRE11/NBS1 protein complex, which has diverse functions, including recombination, telomere maintenance and S-phase checkpoint response to DSBs *(59,60)*.

Li-Fraumeni syndrome *(61,62)* is a dominantly inherited disorder (only one inherited allele is mutant) caused by a mutation in the tumor suppressor gene *Trp53*. Tumorigenesis in Li-Fraumeni patients is associated with the loss of the remaining functional allele and nearly 100% of patients develop cancer *(63)*. Some patients develop multiple primary cancers *(64)*. A variety of tumors, such as breast, brain, leukemia, lymphoma, lung carcinoma, and adeno-carcinoma usually appear in children and young adults. The p53 protein is a downstream regulator of the ATM DNA damage response pathway. This pathway plays a role in main-taining genomic integrity by suppressing excessive HR *(65–67)*. Aneuploidy often observed in tumors from p53 deficient mice suggests that the functional p53 protein prevents chromo-somal loss *(68,69)*.

Germline mutations in the tumor suppressor genes *BRCA1* and *BRCA2* show an autoso-mal dominant inheritance pattern, although tumors appear when somatic mutation occurs to alter the second allele. Individuals carrying mutations in *BRCA* genes primarily develop breast and ovarian cancers *(70,71)*. Mutations in the *BRCA1* gene are found in about 70% of families with inherited breast and ovarian cancers and 20% of the families with only breast cancer *(72)*. Mutations in one allele of *BRCA2* are associated with up to 85% risk of breast cancer and 15% risk of ovarian cancer *(72)*. *BRCA2* mutations are the most common muta-tions identified in hereditary pancreatic cancer *(73)*. Both *BRCA1* and *BRCA2* mutant cells are deficient in homologous recombination *(74,75) see* Section 2.6. The role of BRCA pro-teins in DSB repair might be implemented via its interaction with HR protein RAD51 *(70,71,76)* and cell-cycle checkpoint response to ionizing radiation *(77)*. BRCA1 appears to interact with a protein complex RAD50/MRE11/NBS1 *(78)*, the repair complex linked to both NHEJ and HR.

Several cancer prone autosomal recessive syndromes are caused by mutations in RECQ helicase genes *(79–81)*, such as Bloom's (BLM), Werner's (WRN) and Rothmund-Thomson (RecQL4) syndromes. The tumor spectrum for Bloom's syndrome patients is extremely diverse *(82)*. This includes the type of cancers that are seen in the general population, such as leukemia, various types of carcinomas and lymphomas, and cancers that are rare in the gen-eral population, such as Wilms tumor and osteosarcoma. Werner and Rothmund-Thomson patients develop primarily sarcomas. Werner's syndrome is an adult progeria syndrome that manifests into age-related traits after puberty, including osteoporosis, calcification of soft tissue, atherosclerosis, cataracts, and diabetes mellitus *(83)*. Evidence suggests that BLM protein plays a role in repairing DNA damage via interaction with RAD51 *(84)*. WRN pro-tein interacts with several proteins involved in DNA repair, including the Ku70/Ku80 heterodimer, DNA topoisomerase I, and p53 *(83)*.

Mutations in one of eight *FANC* genes give rise to Fanconi's anemia (FA), an autosomal-recessive disorder associated with aplastic anemia resulting from progressive loss of bone marrow stem cells and elevated risk of acute myeloid leukemia (15,000-fold) and squamous cell sarcoma *(85–87)*. The prevalence of the disease is about 1 in 200,000. The most charac-teristic phenotype of FA deficient cells is hypersensitivity to DNA cross-linking agents, such as mitomycin C or diepoxybutane *(88)*. The biochemical function of FANC proteins is not fully understood. The finding that the FANCD2 colocalizes with BRCA1 into irradia-tion-induced foci in the nucleus offers a hint in supporting the role of FANC in DNA repair

Table 2
Assays for DNA Repair Deficiency and Chromosomal Rearrangement

DNA repair deficiency	Assay	Ref.
NER	Host-cell reactivation	*93*
MMR	Microsatellite instability	*97*
DSB	Single-cell electrophoresis or comet	*98, 101, 104*
	DNA strand rejoining capacity	*115, 116*
	Chromosomal and extrachromosomal plasmid	*117, 118, 123, 129–131*
	Cytogenetic assays: Chromosome banding	*105*
	Multicolor FISH (M-FISH)	*108*
	Spektral karyotyping (SKY)	*109*

(89). Observation that BRCA2 restored resistance to mitomycin C in fibroblasts derived from FANCB and FANCD1 patients and that both patients have biallelic inactivation mutations of BRCA2 linked the FANC genes with BRCA1 and BRCA2 in a common pathway *(90)*. Human homologs of RAD54 harbor somatic mutation in some human cancers *(91,92)*.

2. ASSAYS FOR DNA REPAIR DEFICIENCY

Assays developed to assess the capacity of DNA repair in the different pathways or resultant chromosomal rearrangements are summarized in Table 2.

2.1. Host–Cell Reactivation Assay

Athas et al. developed a host-cell reactivation assay to measure NER capacity in response to UV irradiation and chemical-induced DNA damage *(93)*. For this assay, damaged, nonreplicating plasmid DNA harboring the chloramphenicol acetyltransferase (*cat*) reporter gene is introduced into unexposed host lymphocytes by transient transfection. Efficiency of NER of the damaged bacterial *cat* gene is monitored proportionally as a function of reactivated CAT enzyme activity following a 40 h repair/expression incubation period. The assay was validated by its ability to discriminate XP cells in severe (complementation groups A and D) and moderate (complementation group C) NER deficiencies. The host reactivation assay has been used to demonstrate reduced NER efficiency in basal cell carcinoma patients *(94,95)*. The reduced DNA repair of UV-induced DNA damage contributed to the risk of sunlight-induced skin carcinogenesis in basal cell carcinoma. This assay allows indirect measurement of the extent and efficiency of overall cellular repair of DNA but is less suitable for evaluating the repair of strand breaks, as they reduce plasmid transfer frequencies *(96)*.

2.2. Detection of Microsatellite Instability

Microsatellite instability (MSI) is a characteristic of colon cancers with underlying mutations in DNA MMR genes *(22,23,32)*. The MSI detection assay is based on PCR amplification from 5 to 10 microsatellite markers, poly(A) or poly (AC) tracks, and analysis of amplification products by denaturing polyacrylamide gel electrophoresis (PAGE) *(97)* (*see also* Chapter 19) High-frequency MSI is defined as appearance of new alleles for two or more of five microsatellite markers. MSI observed for one of five markers is reported as low-frequency MSI. If low-frequency MSI is observed, additional markers, up to a maximum of ten, are tested. Instability of between 1 and 3 out of 10 loci assayed is defined as low-frequency MSI, whereas instability at 4 or more loci is defined as high-frequencyMSI. High-frequency MSI has been found in most cases of hereditary nonpolyposis colorectal cancer *(32)*. The MSI assay is routinely used in clinical molecular diagnostic laboratories. Determination of MSI requires the presence of instability in the markers used. This method does not detect gross chromosomal alterations including large deletions, duplications, and translocations.

2.3. Comet Assay

Single-cell gel electrophoresis or comet assay is a rapid and sensitive fluorescent microscopic method to examine DNA damage and repair at the individual cell level (www.cometassay.com). It can be applied to proliferating as well as nonproliferating cells. In this assay, single cells are embedded in a thin layer of agarose on a microscope slide and lysed to remove cytoplasm and the majority of nuclear proteins. The released DNA is subjected to gel electrophoresis. If breaks are present, relaxed DNA loops and/or DNA fragments migrate into the gel, forming an image resembling a tail when viewed by fluorescence microscopy. The relative tail intensity and length is proportional to the frequency of DNA breaks. The alkaline comet assay for measuring DNA strand breaks induced by genotoxic agents was developed by Singh et al. in 1988 *(98)*. The alkaline comet assay, and further developments thereof detects various other forms of DNA damage, such as oxidative DNA base damage and DNA–DNA/DNA–protein/DNA–drug cross-linking, and DNA repair in virtually any eukaryotic cell *(99–104)*. By determining the removal (repair) of DNA damage over time, the comet assay can be used in the clinic as a diagnostic tool for monitoring DNA repair capacity, which may be used to diagnose DNA repair deficiency syndromes. The classical comet assay combined with fluorescent *in situ* hybridization facilitates identification of DNA damage at particular genes or chromosomes. Specific oligonucleotide probes labeled with the fluorescent tags are hybridized to the region of interest to evaluate gene/ chromosome specific DNA damage induction or repair. The comet assay has many important applications ranging from clinical investigations and molecular epidemiology to biomonitoring and nutritional toxicology.

2.4. Cytogenetic Assays

Chromosomal rearrangements formed because of improper DSB repair, can be detected by cytogenetic techniques (*see also* Chapter 18) Chromosome analysis is one of the most commonly performed diagnostic genetic tests in oncology, prenatal, and reproductive medicine.

The analysis typically involves identification of chromosomes based on size, morphology, and alternating light and dark band patterns *(105)*. Such a systemic examination of the karyotype allows identification of numerical chromosomal abnormalities (gain or loss of whole chromosome) and certain structural rearrangements (translocations, inversions, deletions, insertions). Classical cytogenetic methods detect primarily exchange aberrations between chromosomes in mitotic cells. Preparation of metaphase chromosomes requires successful culturing of cells, which is difficult to achieve for some types of cells. In addition, it can produce artificial chromosome abnormalities. The development of fluorescence *in situ* hybridization (FISH) techniques specific for distinct chromosomal regions has greatly advanced this methodology to allow measurement of intrachromosomal aberrations. In addition, the technique is no longer restricted to the analysis of mitotic cells. The locus-specific or whole chromosome-specific "painting" with fluorescently labeled probes allows visualization of chromosomal regions or individual chromosomes in metaphase or interphase cells and the identification of both numerical and structural chromosomal aberrations with high sensitivity and specificity *(106,107)*. Using a series of dye combinations or fluorochromes, each chromosome can be differentially labeled and detected. The multicolor chromosome painting provides the means to examine the entire genome in a single experiment. The multicolor FISH test is often referred to as either multiplex-FISH (M-FISH) *(108)* or spectral karyotyping (SKY) *(109)*. The two methods differ in the way they acquire and process the chromosome images. M-FISH is based on the use of fluorochrome-specific optical filters *(108)*, whereas SKY is based on the spectral signature of each fluorochrome in the probe cocktail *(109)*. Chromosome painting has developed into a versatile research tool for chromosomal analysis in clinical and cancer cytogenetics *(106,110)*. This technique allows identification of the structurally abnormal chromosomes (marker chromosomes), cryptic translocations, and complex rearrangements *(109,111–113)*, which cannot be identified by chromosome banding technology alone. Combination of chromosomal painting with a conventional chromosome banding technology would greatly improve the diagnostics of clinical specimen. However, the multicolor FISH tests require advanced microscopy equipment and a specialized software computer and are, therefore, limited to a few selected clinical cytogenetic laboratories. Further development and maybe automatization of this technology may increase its availability for most cytogenetic labs.

2.5. Assays for Chromosomal Double-Strand Break Rejoining Capacity

An assay with the ability to detect correct rejoining of radiation-induced DSBs would provide a useful tool to predict radiosensitivity and, hence, cancer predisposition in humans. Certain individuals cannot tolerate conventional dose of radiotherapy, thus determining radiosensitivity in cancer patients is a prerequisite prior to subjecting them to radiotherapy. The colony survival assay in which percentage of survival of irradiated cells is measured allows determination of radiosensitivity of lymphoblastoid cells from patient blood *(114)*. By using this assay, elevated radiosensitivity has been identified in cells from AT and FA patients *(45)* (*see also* Chapter 22).

There are several cellular assays available to monitor rejoining of the radiation-induced DSBs. A conventional fraction of DNA radioactivity released (FAR) assay *(115)* is designed to measure total rejoining. In this assay, cells are irradiated to induce DSB and allowed to repair. The DNA from ^{14}C-thymidine-labeled cells is then separated by pulsed-field gel electrophoresis (PFGE). The fraction of radioactivity released from the plug is measured by liquid scintillation counting of the sliced gel. An induction curve for FAR versus irradiation dose is used to obtain relative numbers of DSBs after repair.

Correct rejoining of radiation-induced DSBs can be monitored by measuring reconstitution of an original size Not I fragment on chromosome 21 *(116)*. Following cell irradiation and DNA repair, DNA is digested with a restriction enzyme NotI, separated by PFGE and hybridized with single-copy DNA probes to NotI restriction fragments (3.2, 2 and 1.2 megabase pair fragments of chromosome 21). DSB induction and joining of correct ends are estimated by comparison of the intact full size band with a smear of broken or misrejoined restriction fragments. The misrejoining frequency can be assessed by comparing results from this technique with results from a conventional FAR assay *(116)*. A limitation of the assay is its requirement of rather high radiation doses.

2.6. Plasmid Assays for Double-Strand Break Repair by NHEJ and HR

A number of plasmid-based assays allow measurement of distinct pathways of DNA DSB repair, such as NHEJ and HR. DSB repair by HR can be measured utilizing the rare-cutting I-SceI endonuclease *(117)*. The assay determines I-SceI-induced DSB repair efficiency by HR between tandem repeats of an inactivated bacterial antibiotic resistance gene or marker gene, such as *CAT, luciferase*, or *GFP* genes *(118)*. The assay is implemented by transfection of two plasmids. One plasmid contains a substrate for HR (e.g., two copies of a gene) where one copy is inactivated by introducing the 18 base pair recognition sequence for I-SceI endonuclease. The second copy is made inactive by other means. Chromosomal or extrachromosomal DSB repair can be examined. When the HR substrate is integrated into a chromosome by stable transfection, repair of chromosomal DSBs induced by I-SceI is measured. Upon transient plasmid transfection, repair of DSBs within a plasmid (e.g., extrachromosomal DNA), is monitored. A second plasmid containing the I-SceI expression cassette is transiently transfected into the cells. I-SceI endonuclease generates a DSB at an I-SceI site, which leads to HR between the tandem repeats and results in reconstitution of antibiotic resistance or a marker gene. The frequency of HR is assessed by the number of clones being able to grow on antibiotic containing media or by the expression of a fluorescent marker gene, respectively. The use of a fluorescent marker gene rather than antibiotic resistance gene is favorable, since it eliminates the need for colony formation, which might take a long time and cannot be used for primary cells. Reduced repair of I-SceI breaks has been observed in a number of cell lines deficient in recombination associated genes, such as *RAD51, RAD54, XRCC2, XRCC3, BRCA1*, and *BRCA2 (74,75,119–122)*.

Extrachromosomal HR recombination can be assessed using a transient luciferase expression assay in which HR between fragments of the luciferase gene in plasmid DNA restores a functional luciferase gene *(123)*.

Chromosomal NHEJ can be examined by estimating efficiency of colony formation on a selective media following random stable integration of a linearized plasmid bearing an intact antibiotic resistance gene *(118,124–126)*. Extrachromosomal DNA rejoining capacity can be measured by using a luciferase reporter system, in which a linearized plasmid transfected into a cell will express the luciferase gene, once NHEJ and recircularization of the plasmid occurs *(127,128)*.

Recently, several plasmid assays were developed based on reconstitution of genes encoding fluorescent proteins. Transient transfection and FACS analysis is carried out on transfected cells to estimate repair efficiency. These assays are sensitive and rapid to perform and may soon be adapted for a broad application in human cells for prognostic and diagnostic purposes. Additionally, the requirement for the cells to grow up into colonies will be eliminated. The rapid dual fluorescence (RDF) assay determines the correct rejoining of DSBs induced by a restriction enzyme *(129)*. The plasmid contains the genes for yellow fluorescent (YFP) and green fluorescent proteins (GFP), where the GFP gene is digested at a unique restriction site prior to transfection. Plasmid DNA will express YFP but not GFP unless correct repair of the DSB has taken place. A plasmid designed to measure HR capacity in human cancer cells *(130)* contains an intact, emission-shifted, blue variant of GFP (BFP) with a 300 nucleotide stretch of homology to an inactive copy of GFP. HR between two GFP sequences creates a functional GFP, whereas in the absence of HR only functional BFP is present.

A plasmid system has been developed as a rapid assay to measure the efficiency and the proficiency of both, NHEJ or HR, after transient transfection *(131)*. Two constructs allow the independent expression and simultaneous detection of the GFP protein, as a marker of transfection, expressed constitutively in the cells that have incorporated the DNA. The YFP protein, as a marker of recombination can only be expressed if the restriction enzyme introduces DSBs in the vector. The substrates are linearized by restriction digestion to create a DSB, and transiently transfected into cells. For analysis of DSB repair by NHEJ a plasmid is linearized at a multicloning site located between the promoter and *YFP* structural gene. Rejoining of the DNA termini reconstitutes the original promoter-gene sequence and the recombination marker can be expressed. For analysis of DSB repair by HR, a second plasmid is linearized at the multiple cloning site located in the intervening sequence of a duplication-deletion in the *YFP* gene. Deletion of the duplicated sequence by HR reconstitutes the intact sequence of the *YFP* gene and allows its expression. In both assays, the recombination efficiency is determined as the number of recombinants as a fraction of the number of transfectants. Finally, one can sequence through the junctions of the NHEJ events to determine the pathway of the NHEJ event, such as the occurrence and extent of microhomology. With this plasmid system it was determined that Ku86 mutation reduced NHEJ to about 30% *(131)* and a deficiency in Wrn resulted in a significantly increased length of DNA deletions during NHEJ *(132)*.

3. ASSAYS FOR GENOMICS AND PROTEOMICS

With the recent success in the sequencing of the human genome (approx 30 to 35,000 genes) and the explosion of information in the field of genetics, it seems that the importance of genetics in public health will become more important than ever. Interindividual differences in cancer predisposition occur *(133)*. Therefore, it is prudent to employ large-scale screening methods based on the sequence of the human genome to investigate such interindividual differences. Advances in automation and bioinformatics gave rise to a new discipline of biology termed genomics; a systematic approach to conduct global and comprehensive studies about genes and genomes. A full biological description of the molecular processes going on in the transition from normal to neoplastic growth is currently underway. Large-scale screening assays that can be used for cancer research include determination of the entire gene expression profile that is the entirety of the expression levels of all human genes, and the proteome that is the entirety of all proteins in a cell *(134)*.

The gene expression profile is established by using RNA isolated from normal or cancer cells, reverse transcribed into cDNA, labeled with different dyes, and hybridized to probes immobilized on glass or plastic slides in discrete spots, so that the position of each spot is assigned. The competitive hybridization of two differently labeled cDNAs hybridized to the discrete probes makes examination of differences in expression patterns possible. This analysis has been shown to have great potential for molecular diagnosis of cancer. Two types of diffuse large B-cell lymphomas in patients exhibiting vastly different survival rates after treatment that cannot be characterized by currently available micro- or macroscopical pathological examinations were classified by different gene expression patterns *(135)*. Furthermore, studies of primary breast tumors from patients with *BRCA1* mutations and patients with *BRCA2* mutations identified 176 genes differently expressed between the two different tumor genotypes *(136)*.

Cellular functions are carried out by proteins. Proteomics cannot only characterize the expression levels of all proteins but also protein modifications that may regulate their functions. Proteins are separated by two-dimensional electrophoresis and after isolation of specific protein spots from the gel, mass spectrometry is used to unequivocally identify the specific proteins. With this method, unique membrane proteins with potential roles in clinical cancer were discovered in breast cancer cells *(137)*.

In summary, both gene expression profiling and proteomics are novel evolving technologies, but by further extension, the current studies indicate that both technologies might also be useful to determine cancer predisposition in people and establishing profiles as molecular markers of predisposition.

ACKNOWLEDGMENTS

This work was supported by grants from the National Institute of Environmental Health Sciences, NIH RO1 No. ES09519 as well as National Cancer Institute, NIH RO1 No. CA82473, as well as funding from the UCLA Center for Occupational and Environmental Health (to RHS), and a post graduate research fellowship of the UC Toxic Substances Research and Teaching Program (to RR).

REFERENCES

1. American Cancer Society, 2003. Cancer Facts and Figures. American Cancer Society Inc., Atlanta, GA. Available online at http://www.cancer.org. Accessed January 10, 2004.
2. Knudson AG Jr. 1971. Mutation and cancer: statistical study of retinoblastoma. Proc. Natl. Acad. Sci. USA 68:820–823.
3. Knudson AG. 1993. Antioncogenes and human cancer. Proc. Natl. Acad. Sci. USA 90:10,914–10,921.
4. Knudson AG. 2001. Two genetic hits (more or less) to cancer. Nat. Rev. Cancer 1:157–162. Accessed January 10, 2004.
5. Mitelman F, Johansson B, Mertens F. 2003. Mitelman Database of Chromosomal Abberations in Cancer.Available at http://cgap.nci.nih.gov/Chromosomes/Mitelman.
6. Ames BN, Shigenaga MK, Hagen TM. 1993. Oxidants, antioxidants, and the degenerative diseases of aging. Proc. Natl. Acad. Sci. USA 90:7915–7922.
7. Friedberg EC, Walker GC, Siede W. 1995. DNA Repair and Mutagenesis. ASM Press:Washington DC.
8. Hansen WK and Kelley MR. 2000. Review of mammalian DNA repair and translational implications. J. Pharmacol. Exp. Ther. 295:1–9.
9. Jeggo PA. 1998. DNA breakage and repair. Adv. Genet. 38:185–218.
10. van Gent DC, Hoeijmakers JH, Kanaar R. 2001. Chromosomal stability and the DNA double-stranded break connection. Nat. Rev. Genet. 2:196–206.
11. Khanna KK and Jackson SP. 2001. DNA double-strand breaks: signaling, repair and the cancer connection. Nat. Genet. 27:247–254.
12. Krokan HE, Nilsen H, Skorpen F, Otterlei M, Slupphaug G. 2000. Base excision repair of DNA in mammalian cells. FEBS Lett. 476:73–77.
13. Cleaver JE. 1968. Defective repair replication of DNA in xeroderma pigmentosum. Nature 218:652–656.
14. Kraemer KH, Lee MM, Scotto J. 1987. Xeroderma pigmentosum. Cutaneous, ocular, and neurologic abnormalities in 830 published cases. Arch. Dermatol. 123:241–250.

15. Robbins JH, Kraemer KH, Lutzner MA, Festoff BW, Coon HG. 1974. Xeroderma pigmentosum. An inherited diseases with sun sensitivity, multiple cutaneous neoplasms, and abnormal DNA repair. Ann. Intern. Med. 80:221–248.

16. Takebe H, Miki Y, Kozuka T, Furuyama JI, Tanaka K. 1977. DNA repair characteristics and skin cancers of xeroderma pigmentosum patients in Japan. Cancer Res. 37:490–495.

17. Bootsma D, Kraemer KH, Cleaver JE, Hoeijmakers JHJ. 1998. Nucleotide excision repair syndromes: xeroderma pigmentusum, cockayne syndrome, and trichothiodystrophy, in: The Genetic Basis of Human Cancer, Kinzler KW and Vogelstein B, eds., McGraw-Hill: New York, pp. 245–274.

18. Lindahl T, Karran P, Wood RD. 1997. DNA excision repair pathways. Curr. Opin. Genet. Dev. 7:158–169.

19. Wood RD. 1996. DNA repair in eukaryotes. Annu. Rev. Biochem. 65:135–167.

20. Gunz D, Hess MT, Naegeli H. 1996. Recognition of DNA adducts by human nucleotide excision repair. Evidence for a thermodynamic probing mechanism. J. Biol. Chem. 271:25,089–25,098.

21. de Boer J and Hoeijmakers JH. 2000. Nucleotide excision repair and human syndromes. Carcinogenesis 21:453–460.

22. Ionov Y, Peinado MA, Malkhosyan S, Shibata D, Perucho M. 1993. Ubiquitous somatic mutations in simple repeated sequences reveal a new mechanism for colonic carcinogenesis. Nature 363:558–561.

23. Thibodeau SN, Bren G, Schaid D. 1993. Microsatellite instability in cancer of the proximal colon. Science 260:816–819.

24. Levinson G and Gutman GA. 1987. High frequencies of short frameshifts in poly-CA/TG tandem repeats borne by bacteriophage M13 in Escherichia coli K-12. Nucleic Acids Res. 15:5323–5338.

25. Strand M, Prolla TA, Liskay RM, Petes TD. 1993. Destabilization of tracts of simple repetitive DNA in yeast by mutations affecting DNA mismatch repair. Nature 365:274–276.

26. Fishel R and Wilson T. 1997. MutS homologs in mammalian cells. Curr. Opin. Genet. Dev. 7:105–113.

27. Peltomaki P. 1997. DNA mismatch repair gene mutations in human cancer. Environ. Health Perspect. 105(Suppl 4):775–780.

28. Fishel R, Lescoe MK, Rao MR, et al. 1993. The human mutator gene homolog MSH2 and its association with hereditary nonpolyposis colon cancer. Cell 75:1027–1038.

29. Leach FS, Nicolaides NC, Papadopoulo N, et al. 1993. Mutations of a mutS homolog in hereditary nonpolyposis colorectal cancer. Cell 75:1215–1225.

30. Bronner CE, Baker SM, Morrison PT, et al. 1994. Mutation in the DNA mismatch repair gene homologue hMLH1 is associated with hereditary non-polyposis colon cancer. Nature 368:258–261.

31. Papadopoulos N, Nicolaides NC, Wei YF, et al. 1994. Mutation of a mutL homolog in hereditary colon cancer. Science 263:1625–1629.

32. Aaltonen LA, Salovaara R, Kristo P, et al. 1998. Incidence of hereditary nonpolyposis colorectal cancer and the feasibility of molecular screening for the disease. N. Engl. J. Med. 338:1481–1487.

33. Perucho M. 1996. Cancer of the microsatellite mutator phenotype. Biol. Chem. 377:675–684.

34. Peltomaki P and de la Chapelle A. 1997. Mutations predisposing to hereditary nonpolyposis colorectal cancer. Adv. Cancer Res. 71:93–119.

35. Rabbitts TH. 1994. Chromosomal translocations in human cancer. Nature 372:143–149.

36. Sanchez-Garcia I. 1997. Consequences of chromosomal abnormalities in tumor development. Annu. Rev. Genet. 31:429–453.

37. Morgan WF, Corcoran J, Hartmann A, Kaplan MI, Limoli CL, Ponnaiya B. 1998. DNA double-strand breaks, chromosomal rearrangements, and genomic instability. Mutat. Res. 404:125–128.

38. Pierce AJ, Stark JM, Araujo FD, Moynahan ME, Berwick M, Jasin M. 2001. Double-strand breaks and tumorigenesis. Trends Cell. Biol. 11:S52–S59.

39. Schmid CW, Deka N, Matera AG. 1989. Repetitive human DNA: the shape of things to come, in: Chromosomes: Eukaryotic, Prokaryotic and Viral. Vol. I, Adolph KW A, ed., Boca Raton: CRC Press, pp. 3–29.

40. Smit AF. 1996. The origin of interspersed repeats in the human genome. Curr. Opin. Genet. Dev. 6:743–748.

41. Schichman SA, Caligiuri MA, Strout MP, et al. 1994. ALL-1 tandem duplication in acute myeloid leukemia with a normal karyotype involves homologous recombination between Alu elements. Cancer Res. 54:4277–4280.

42. Jasin M. 2000. Chromosome breaks and genomic instability. Cancer Invest. 18:78–86.

43. Thompson LH and Schild D. Recombinational DNA repair and human disease. Mutat. Res. 509:49–78.

44. Vessey CJ, Norbury CJ, Hickson ID. 1999. Genetic disorders associated with cancer predisposition and genomic instability. Prog. Nucleic Acid Res. Mol. Biol. 63:189–221.

45. Gatti RA. 2001. The inherited basis of human radiosensitivity. Acta. Oncol. 40:702–711.

46. Boder E and Sedgwick RP. 1957. Ataxia-Telangiectasia. A familiar syndrome of progressive cerrebellar ataxia, oculocutaneous telangiectasia and frequent pulmonary infection. A preliminary report on 7 children, an autopsy, and a case history. Univ. Southern Calif. Med Bull. 28:9–15.

47. Lavin MF and Shiloh Y. 1997. The genetic defect in ataxia-telangiectasia. Annu. Rev. Immunol. 15:177–202.

48. Gatti RA, Becker-Catania S, Chun HH, et al. 2001. The pathogenesis of ataxia-telangiectasia. Learning from a Rosetta Stone. Clin. Rev. Allergy Immunol. 20:87–108.

49. Woods CG, Bundey SE, Taylor AM. 1990. Unusual features in the inheritance of ataxia telangiectasia. Hum. Genet. 84:555–562.

50. Swift M, Morrell D, Cromartie E, Chamberlin AR, Skolnick MH, Bishop DT. 1986. The incidence and gene frequency of ataxia-telangiectasia in the United States. Am. J. Hum. Genet. 39:573–583.

51. Morrell D, Cromartie E, Swift M. 1986. Mortality and cancer incidence in 263 patients with ataxia- telangiectasia. J. Natl. Cancer Ins. 77:89–92.

52. Swift M, Reitnauer PJ, Morrell D, Chase CL. 1987. Breast and other cancers in families with ataxia-telangiectasia. N. Engl. J. Med. 316:1289–1294.

53. Gatti RA, Berkel I, Boder E, et al. 1988. Localization of an ataxia-telangiectasia gene to chromosome 11q22-23. Nature 336:577–580.

54. Savitsky K, Bar-Shira A, Gilad S, et al. 1995. A single ataxia telangiectasia gene with a product similar to PI-3 kinase. Science 268:1749–1753.

55. Weemaes CM, Hustinx TW, Scheres JM, van Munster PJ, Bakkeren JA, Taalman RD. 1981. A new chromosomal instability disorder: the Nijmegen breakage syndrome. Acta. Paediatr. Scand. 70:557–564.

56. Shiloh Y. 1997. Ataxia-telangiectasia and the Nijmegen breakage syndrome: related disorders but genes apart. Annu. Rev. Genet. 31:635–662.

57. Varon R, Vissinga C, Platzer M, et al. 1998. Nibrin, a novel DNA double-strand break repair protein, is mutated in Nijmegen breakage syndrome. Cell 93:467–476.

58. Matsuura S, Tauchi H, Nakamura A, et al. 1998. Positional cloning of the gene for Nijmegen breakage syndrome. Nat. Gene. 19:179–181.

59. Petrini JH. 2000. The Mre11 complex and ATM: collaborating to navigate S phase. Curr. Opin. Cell. Biol. 12:293–296.

60. Wu X, Ranganathan V, Weisman DS, et al. 2000. ATM phosphorylation of Nijmegen breakage syndrome protein is required in a DNA damage response. Nature 405:477–482.

61. Li FP, Fraumeni JF Jr. 1969. Soft-tissue sarcomas, breast cancer, and other neoplasms. A familial syndrome? Ann. Intern. Med. 71:747–752.

62. Livingstone LR, White A, Sprouse J, Livanos E, Jacks T, and Tlsty TD. 1992. Altered cell cycle arrest and gene amplification potential accompany loss of wild-type p53. Cell 70:923–935.

63. Strong LC, Williams WR, Tainsky MA. 1992. The Li-Fraumeni syndrome: from clinical epidemiology to molecular genetics. Am. J. Epidemiol. 135:190–199.

64. Hisada M, Garber JE, Fung CY, Fraumeni JF Jr, Li FP. 1998. Multiple primary cancers in families with Li-Fraumeni syndrome. J. Natl. Cancer Inst. 90:606–611.

65. Sturzbecher HW, Donzelmann B, Henning W, Knippschild U, Buchhop S. 1996. p53 is linked directly to homologous recombination processes via RAD51/RecA protein interaction. Embo. J. 15:1992–2002.

66. Willers H, McCarthy EE, Wu B, et al. 2000. Dissociation of p53-mediated suppression of homologous recombination from G1/S cell cycle checkpoint control. Oncogene 19:632–639.

67. Bishop AJ, Barlow C, Wynshaw-Boris A, Schiestl RH. 2000. Atm deficiency causes an increased frequency of intrachromosomal homologous recombination in mice. Cancer Res. 60:395–399.

68. Purdie CA, Harrison DJ, Peter A, et al. 1994. Tumour incidence, spectrum and ploidy in mice with a large deletion in the p53 gene. Oncogene 9:603–609.

69. Donehower LA, Godley LA, Aldaz CM, et al. 1995. Deficiency of p53 accelerates mammary tumorigenesis in Wnt-1 transgenic mice and promotes chromosomal instability. Genes Dev. 9:882–895.

70. Scully R and Livingston DM. 2000. In search of the tumour-suppressor functions of BRCA1 and BRCA2. Nature 408:429–432.

71. Welcsh PL, Owens KN, King MC. 2000. Insights into the functions of BRCA1 and BRCA2. Trends Genet. 16:69–74.

72. Nathanson KL, Wooster R, Weber BL, Nathanson KN. 2001. Breast cancer genetics: what we know and what we need. Nat. Med. 7:552–556.

73. Murphy KM, Brune KA, Griffin C, et al. 2002. Evaluation of candidate genes MAP2K4, MADH4, ACVR1B, and BRCA2 in familial pancreatic cancer: deleterious BRCA2 mutations in 17%. Cancer Res. 62:3789–793.

74. Moynahan ME, Chiu JW, Koller BH, Jasin M. 1999. Brca1 controls homology-directed DNA repair. Mol. Cell. 4:511–518.

75. Moynahan ME, Pierce AJ, Jasin M. 2001. BRCA2 is required for homology-directed repair of chromosomal breaks. Mol. Cell. 7:263–272.

76. Wong AK, Pero R, Ormonde PA, Tavtigian SV, Bartel PL. 1997. RAD51 interacts with the evolutionarily conserved BRC motifs in the human breast cancer susceptibility gene brca2. J. Biol. Chem. 272:31941–31944.

77. Xu B, Kim S, Kastan MB. 2001. Involvement of Brca1 in S-phase and G(2)-phase checkpoints after ionizing irradiation. Mol. Cell. Biol. 21:3445–3450.

78. Zhong Q, Chen CF, Li S, et al. 1999. Association of BRCA1 with the hRad50-hMre11-p95 complex and the DNA damage response. Science 285:747–750.

79. van Brabant AJ, Stan R, Ellis NA. 2000. DNA helicases, genomic instability, and human genetic disease. Annu. Rev. Genomics Hum. Genet. 1:409–459.

80. Karow JK, Wu L, Hickson ID. 2000. RecQ family helicases: roles in cancer and aging. Curr. Opin. Genet. Dev. 10:32–38.

81. Mohaghegh P and Hickson ID. 2001. DNA helicase deficiencies associated with cancer predisposition and premature ageing disorders. Hum. Mol. Genet. 10:741–746.

82. German J. 1993. Bloom syndrome: a mendelian prototype of somatic mutational disease. Medicine (Baltimore) 72:393–406.

83. Shen J and Loeb LA. 2001. Unwinding the molecular basis of the Werner syndrome. Mech. Ageing. Dev. 122:921–944.

84. Wu L, Davies SL, Levitt NC, Hickson ID. 2001. Potential role for the BLM helicase in recombinational repair via a conserved interaction with RAD51. J. Biol. Chem. 276:19,375–19,381.

85. Meyn MS. 1997. Chromosome instability syndromes: lessons for carcinogenesis. Curr. Top. Microbiol. Immunol. 221:71–148.

86. Grompe M and D'Andrea A. 2001. Fanconi anemia and DNA repair. Hum. Mol. Genet. 10:2253–2259.

87. Joenje H and Patel KJ. 2001. The emerging genetic and molecular basis of Fanconi anaemia. Nat. Rev. Genet. 2:446–457.

88. Sasaki MS and Tonomura A. 1973. A high susceptibility of Fanconi's anemia to chromosome breakage by DNA cross-linking agents. Cancer Res. 33:1829–1836.

89. Garcia-Higuera I, Taniguchi T, Ganesan S, et al. 2001. Interaction of the Fanconi anemia proteins and BRCA1 in a common pathway. Mol. Cell. 7:249–262.

90. Howlett NG, Taniguchi T, Olson S, et al. 2002. Biallelic inactivation of BRCA2 in Fanconi anemia. Science 297:606–609.

91. Matsuda M, Miyagawa K, Takahashi M, et al. 1999. Mutations in the RAD54 recombination gene in primary cancers. Oncogene 18:3427–3430.

92. Hiramoto T, Nakanishi T, Sumiyoshi T, et al. 1999. Mutations of a novel human RAD54 homologue, RAD54B, in primary cancer. Oncogene 18:3422–3426.

93. Athas WF, Hedayati MA, Matanoski GM, Farmer ER, Grossman L. 1991. Development and field-test validation of an assay for DNA repair in circulating human lymphocytes. Cancer Res. 51:5786–5793.

94. Grossman L and Wei Q. 1995. DNA repair and epidemiology of basal cell carcinoma. Clin. Chem. 41:1854–1863.

95. Wei Q, Matanoski GM, Farmer ER, Hedayati MA, Grossman L. 1995. DNA repair capacity for ultraviolet light-induced damage is reduced in peripheral lymphocytes from patients with basal cell carcinoma. J. Invest. Dermatol. 104:933–936.

96. Nickoloff JA and Reynolds RJ. 1992. Electroporation-mediated gene transfer efficiency is reduced by linear plasmid carrier DNAs. Anal. Biochem. 205:237–243.

97. Boland CR, Thibodeau SN, Hamilton SR, et al. 1998. A National Cancer Institute Workshop on Microsatellite Instability for cancer detection and familial predisposition: development of international criteria for the determination of microsatellite instability in colorectal cancer. Cancer Res. 58:5248–5257.

98. Singh NP, McCoy MT, Tice RR, Schneider EL. 1988. A simple technique for quantitation of low levels of DNA damage in individual cells. Exp. Cell. Res. 175:184–191.

99. Fairbairn DW, Olive PL, O'Neill KL. 1995. The comet assay: a comprehensive review. Mutat. Res. 339:37–59.

100. Anderson D, Yu TW, McGregor DB. 1998. Comet assay responses as indicators of carcinogen exposure. Mutagenesis 13:539–555.

101. Speit G and Hartmann A. 1999. The comet assay (single-cell gel test). A sensitive genotoxicity test for the detection of DNA damage and repair. Methods Mol. Biol. 113:203–212.

102. Rojas E, Lopez MC, Valverde M. 1999. Single cell gel electrophoresis assay: methodology and applications. J. Chromatogr. B. Biomed. Sci. Appl. 722:225–254.

103. Kassie F, Parzefall W, Knasmuller S. 2000. Single cell gel electrophoresis assay: a new technique for human biomonitoring studies. Mutat. Res. 463:13–31.

104. Tice RR, Agurell E, Anderson D, et al. 2000. Single cell gel/comet assay: guidelines for in vitro and in vivo genetic toxicology testing. Environ. Mol. Mutagen. 35:206–221.

105. Caspersson T, Farber S, Foley GE, et al. 1968. Chemical differentiation along metaphase chromosomes. Exp. Cell. Res. 49:219–222.

106. Ried T, Schrock E, Ning Y, Wienberg J. 1998. Chromosome painting: a useful art. Hum. Mol. Genet. 7:1619–1626.

107. Fauth C and Speicher MR. 2001. Classifying by colors: FISH-based genome analysis. Cytogenet. Cell. Genet. 93:1–10.

108. Speicher MR, Gwyn Ballard S, Ward DC. 1996. Karyotyping human chromosomes by combinatorial multi-fluor FISH. Nat. Genet. 12:368–375.

109. Schrock E, du Manoir S, Veldman T, et al. 1996. Multicolor spectral karyotyping of human chromosomes. Science 273:494–497.

110. Bayani J and Squire JA. 2001. Advances in the detection of chromosomal aberrations using spectral karyotyping. Clin. Genet. 59:65–73.

111. Henegariu O, Bray-Ward P, Artan S, Vance GH, Qumsyieh M, and Ward DC. 2001. Small marker chromosome identification in metaphase and interphase using centromeric multiplex fish (CM-FISH). Lab. Invest. 81:475–481.

112. Henegariu O, Artan S, Greally JM, et al. 2001. Cryptic translocation identification in human and mouse using several telomeric multiplex fish (TM-FISH) strategies. Lab. Invest. 81: 483–491.

113. Nietzel A, Rocchi M, Starke H, et al. 2001. A new multicolor-FISH approach for the characterization of marker chromosomes: centromere-specific multicolor-FISH (cenM-FISH). Hum. Genet. 108:199–204.

114. Huo YK, Wang Z, Hong JH, et al. 1994. Radiosensitivity of ataxia-telangiectasia, X-linked agammaglobulinemia, and related syndromes using a modified colony survival assay. Cancer Res. 54:2544–2547.

115. Rydberg B, Lobrich M, Cooper PK. 1994. DNA double-strand breaks induced by high-energy neon and iron ions in human fibroblasts. I. Pulsed-field gel electrophoresis method. Radiat. Res. 139:133–141.

116. Lobrich M, Rydberg B, Cooper PK. 1995. Repair of x-ray-induced DNA double-strand breaks in specific Not I restriction fragments in human fibroblasts: joining of correct and incorrect ends. Proc. Natl. Acad. Sci. USA 92:12,050–12,054.

117. Jasin M. 1996. Genetic manipulation of genomes with rare-cutting endonucleases. Trends Genet. 12:224–228.

118. Willers H, Xia F, Powell SN. 2002. Recombinational DNA Repair in Cancer and Normal Cells: The Challenge of Functional Analysis. J. Biomed. Biotechnol. 2:86–93.

119. Lambert S and Lopez BS. 2000. Characterization of mammalian RAD51 double strand break repair using non-lethal dominant-negative forms. Embo. J. 19:3090–3099.

120. Dronkert ML, Beverloo HB, Johnson R, Hoeijmakers JH, Jasin M, Kanaar R. 2000. Mouse RAD54 affects DNA double-strand break repair and sister chromatid exchange. Mol. Cell. Biol. 20:3147–3156.

121. Pierce AJ, Johnson RD, Thompson LH, Jasin M. 1999. XRCC3 promotes homology-directed repair of DNA damage in mammalian cells. Genes Dev. 13:2633–2638.

122. Johnson RD, Liu N, Jasin M. 1999. Mammalian XRCC2 promotes the repair of DNA double-strand breaks by homologous recombination. Nature 401:397–399.

123. Morrison C and Wagner E. 1996. Extrachromosomal recombination occurs efficiently in cells defective in various DNA repair systems. Nucleic Acids Res. 24:2053–2058.

124. Harrington J, Hsieh CL, Gerton J, Bosma G, Lieber MR. 1992. Analysis of the defect in DNA end joining in the murine scid mutation. Mol. Cell. Biol. 12:4758–4768.

125. Buhler B, Kohler G, Nielsen PJ. 1995. Efficient nonhomologous and homologous recombination in scid cells. Immunogenetics 42:181–187.

126. Manivasakam P, Aubrecht J, Sidhom S, Schiestl RH. 2001. Restriction enzymes increase efficiencies of illegitimate DNA integration but decrease homologous integration in mammalian cells. Nucleic Acids Res. 29:4826–4833.

127. Tang W, Willers H, Powell SN. 1999. p53 directly enhances rejoining of DNA double-strand breaks with cohesive ends in gamma-irradiated mouse fibroblasts. Cancer Res. 59:2562–2565.

128. Zhong Q, Chen CF, Chen PL, Lee WH. 2002. BRCA1 facilitates microhomology-mediated end joining of DNA double strand breaks. J. Biol. Chem. 277:28641–28647.

129. Collis SJ, Sangar VK, Tighe A, et al. 2002. Development of a novel rapid assay to assess the fidelity of DNA double- strand-break repair in human tumour cells. Nucleic Acids Res. 30:E1.

130. Slebos RJ and Taylor JA. 2001. A novel host cell reactivation assay to assess homologous recombination capacity in human cancer cell lines. Biochem. Biophys. Res. Commun.

131. Secretan MB, Scuric Z, Oshima J, et al. 2003. Effect of Ku86 and DNA-PKcs Deficiency on Non-Homologous End-Joining and Homologous Recombination Using a Novel Transient Screening Assay. Submitted.
132. Oshima J, Huang S, Pae C, Campisi J, Schiestl RH. 2002. Lack of WRN results in extensive deletion at nonhomologous joining ends. Cancer Res. 62:547–551.
133. Lichtenstein P, Holm NV, Verkasalo PK, et al. 2000. Environmental and heritable factors in the causation of cancer—analyses of cohorts of twins from Sweden, Denmark, and Finland. N. Engl. J. Med. 343:78–85.
134. Martin DB and Nelson PS. 2001. From genomics to proteomics: techniques and applications in cancer research. Trends Cell. Biol. 11:S60–S65.
135. Alizadeh AA, Eisen MB, Davis RE, et al. 2000. Distinct types of diffuse large B-cell lymphoma identified by gene expression profiling. Nature 403:503–511.
136. Hedenfalk I, Duggan D, Chen Y, et al. 2001. Gene-expression profiles in hereditary breast cancer. N. Engl. J. Med. 344:539–548.
137. Adam PJ, Boyd R, Tyson KL, et al. 2003. Comprehensive Proteomic Analysis of Breast Cancer Cell Membranes Reveals Unique Proteins with Potential Roles in Clinical Cancer. J. Biol. Chem. 278:6482–6489.

18

Chromosomal and Molecular Cytogenetic Assays for Evaluation of Human Tumors

Peter C. Hu, Vicki L. Hopwood, and Armand B. Glassman

1. INTRODUCTION: HISTORY OF CANCER CYTOGENETICS

1.1. Pre-Hypotonic Era and Techniques

In the *Magnificent History of Genetics,* written by Dr. Hsu *(1),* the time before 1952 was characterized as the "Dark Ages" of cytogenetics. Actually, the study of chromosomes started earlier in the 19th century. Walther Flemming discovered lampbrush chromosomes, described them in 1882, and coined the term "mitosis" *(2).* Balbiani communicated the structure of the polytene chromosomes in 1881 *(3).* Wilhelm Waldeyer-Artz coined the term "chromosome" in 1888 *(4).* Using grasshopper testes, Walter Sutton published *The Chromosome Theory of Heredity* in 1903 *(5).* Boveri, working with chromosomes of sea urchins in culture, theorized that chromosome changes were the cause of neoplasia *(6).*

Early in the 1920s, it was believed that the chromosome number of man was 48. This number was derived by Painter *(1)* by using thin slices of testes taken from executed prisoners. Subsequently, tissue culturing techniques, mitotic arrestants, and more sophisticated study of chromosomes demonstrated that this number was incorrect.

1.2. Post-Hypotonic Era and Techniques

In 1952, T.C. Hsu reported the use of low-salt-concentrate solutions, which resulted in a better spread of chromosomes *(1).* In 1956, Tjio and Levan used these techniques to identify the correct chromosome number of man as 46 *(7).* Chromosomes were still stained without the benefit of banding differentiation until 1968 when Caspersson introduced Giemsa/Trypsin/G-banding (G-banding) *(8).* Despite the fact that chromosome banding was not yet available, Nowell and Hungerford described the first consistent chromosomal abnormality associated with a human neoplasm, the Philadelphia chromosome *(9).* The Philadelphia chromosome was thought to be chromosome 22. This abnormality was a consistently demonstrated aberration associated with chronic myelogenous leukemia. At the time, chromosomes were classified by size and their centromere location. It was thought that what we now know as chromosome 22 was smaller than what we now know as chromosome 21. After Q- and G-banding, it became possible to distinguish chromosomes of similar size and shape by their distinctive banding patterns. Additional refinements of banding techniques included high-resolution banding introduced by Yunis in 1976 *(10).* GTG remains the standard for chromosome banding analysis. It is used as the initial screening technique for karyotypic

From: *Cancer Diagnostics: Current and Future Trends*
Edited by: R. M. Nakamura, W. W. Grody, J. T. Wu, and R. B. Nagle © Humana Press Inc., Totowa, NJ

abnormalities in a variety of cancers and constitutional disorders. This technique permits a general survey of the genome.

1.3. Molecular Cytogenetics Era and Techniques

The era of molecular cytogenetics has begun. The use of DNA probes is incorporated into cytogenetic practice to determine loss, gain, or rearrangement of specific genes. It has provided increased resolution and sensitivity of analysis. In 1986, Gray and Pinkel *(11)* discovered that blocking DNA could be used to suppress interspersed repetitive DNA sequences and this largely eliminated nonspecific signals and permitted better fluorescence *in situ* hybridization (FISH). From 1991 to1999, a series of advances occurred, including comparative genomic hybridization (CGH) by Kallioniemi *(12)*, spectral karyotyping (SKY) by Schrock *(13)*, MFISH by Speicher, Ballard, Ward *(14)*, Rx Fish by Muller, Rocci and Ferguson-Smith in 1997 *(15)*, and M-banding in 1999. All resulted in the expanded application of FISH technique. The techniques of CGH, RXFISH, SKY, MFISH, and M-banding are FISH techniques for screening and evaluating the entire genome. These methods complement and enhance our ability to determine chromosomal aberrations in GTG karyotyping. They have provided an increased ability to detect and describe complex chromosomal changes that are characteristic of neoplastic cells and help bridge the gap between molecular and classic cytogenetics.

2. CYTOGENETIC EVALUATION OF LEUKEMIAS

2.1. The Myeloid Leukemias

2.1.1. Acute Myelogenous Leukemia

Between 40 and 50% of patients presenting with acute myelogenous leukemias (AML) have an abnormal karyotype when examined by conventional methods. Additional information regarding cryptic translocations and subtle molecular genetic changes can be detected by using FISH, polymerase chain reaction (PCR), real-time PCR (RT-PCR), quantitative PCR, and gene sequencing. These techniques are useful for the initial diagnosis, following response to therapy, evaluation of minimal residual disease and recurrence. Conventional karyotyping is limited in its utilization to the characterization of chromosomal changes noted if the cells undergo metaphase in tissue culture. The use of molecular cytogenetic changes (i.e., locus-specific FISH and PCR), permit evaluation of cells that are in interphase and various other phases of the cell cycle.

To perform conventional karyotyping, a minimum of 20 metaphases are analyzed. Clonality requires that two of the metaphases have the same karyotypic make-up. If a patient has two out of 20 metaphases with trisomy chromosome 8 and is a male, his karyotype would be 47,XY,+8[2]/46,XY[18] to describe his 20 metaphases. On the other hand, changes that are associated with deletions of all or part of a chromosome require that three metaphases have the abnormality before clonality is declared. Exceptions to this are if the patient had a known chromosomal abnormality (i.e., translocation 9:22 [t(9;22)], was treated), and has one out of 20 metaphases with the t(9;22); that one metaphase with the translocation would be reported because of the obvious historical clinical data and clinical significance. Cells unable to undergo mitosis and having no metaphases cannot be characterized by conventional karyotyping and the techniques of FISH and or PCR must be used to evaluate chromosomal abnormalities. Tissue culture of bone marrow, peripheral blood, or lymph node specimens requires from 24 to 72 h for growth prior to harvesting to obtain metaphases. Mitogens (e.g., lipopolysaccharide [LPS] for B cells and phytohemagglutinin [PHA] for T cells) can be used to increase the yield of metaphases. There is good correlation (>90%) for conventional karyotyping and molecular techniques for assessing the known abnormalities of t(9:22), t(8:21), inv(16), t(15:17) and deletions of 11q23. Each week at the University Texas MD Anderson Cancer Center a leukemia profile meeting is held. At this meeting patient clinical information, pertinent hematopathology, flow cytometry, molecular diagnostics, and cytogenetic findings including FISH are integrated, discussed, and correlated.

Chromosomal changes seen in AML include changes in number and structure. Structural abnormalities include translocations (t); deletions (del); additions (add); and occasionally other changes such as inversions (inv); homogenously staining regions (hsr); double minutes (dm), and ring (r) alterations to the chromosomes. Unidentified chromosomes are classified as markers (mar). Because the diploid karyotypic state is either 46,XX (for females) or 46,XY (for males) any other numerical changes are considered either hyperdiploid (>46 chromosomes) or hypodiploid (<46 chromosomes). A pseudodiploid state exists where the chromosome number remains 46 but there is some structural chromosome abnormality such as a t, del, or add. An example of this would be 46,XY,t(9;22)(q34;q11.2), which is a pseudodiploid clone. Frequent chromosomal changes include the trisomy state, represented as a plus sign. For instance, a patient with a myeloproliferative disorder with a trisomy 8 would be 46,XX,+8. Various chromosomes may be added or deleted in whole or part. Loss of a chromosome is represented by a minus sign, so monosomy 7 would be represented as 45,XY, -7. Partial loss of a chromosome, for instance, a deletion of part of the q arm of chromosome 5 would be represented as 46,XX,del(5)(q31q35) *(16)*.

Cytogenetic changes that relate to the French American British (FAB) classification of AMLs include the t(8;21)(q22;q22) associated with M2; t(15;17)(q22;q11.2-12) present in M3; inv(16) seen with M4$_{EO}$ *(17)*; and t(9;11)(p22;q23) and other 11q23 deletions or translocations that are noted in M5. Alterations of 3q especially translocations or inversions of 3q have been associated with thrombocytosis, platelet abnormalities and M7.

The prognosis of AML has been clinically associated with karyotypic abnormalities. In general, t(8;21), t(15;17), and inv(16) are considered favorable cytogenetic changes and responsive to chemotherapy. Cytogenetic changes involving loss of part or all of chromosomes 5 and 7, as well as trisomies 8, are considered of poor prognostic significance. Karyotypes that are diploid or have insufficient metaphases for cytogenetic diagnosis are considered of intermediate predictive value.

Other cytogenetic abnormalities that are seen in AML include: trisomy 8, monosomy 7, deletion of 7q, monosomy 5, and deletion of 5q. Each of these occurs approx 10% of the time in patients with karyotypic abnormalities of AML. Deletion of 20q is seen in 5% or less of the patients with AML. 11q23 deletions and translocations involving 11q23 have been reported in various types of AML. Often 11q23 abnormalities are part of more complex karyotypic abnormalities. The use of karyotypes for evaluating and assisting morphology and in use for prognosis is ongoing and expanding, particularly through the use of locus specific probes applied with FISH or spectral karyotyping (SKY). Favorable vs unfavorable karyotypes may result in alteration or selection of specific chemotherapeutic protocols depending upon the institution.

2.1.2. Myelodysplastic Syndromes and Therapeutic Myelodysplastic Syndromes

Myelodysplastic syndromes (MDS) including chronic myelomonocytic leukemia (CMML) are undergoing continued evolution in terms of classification, diagnosis, and treatment. Approximately 40 to 50 ±% of MDS cases have recognizable cytogenetic abnormalities. Despite this, specific clonal karyotypic abnormalities are not as well recognized as in the AMLs. A significant percentage of MDS patients evolve into AML and many of the chromosomal changes are similar to those seen in AML. MDS abnormalities include partial chromosome deletions, additions, and losses of entire chromosomes. No specific translocations are specified. Less than 50% of the cases with refractory anemia or refractory anemia with ringed sideroblasts show clonal abnormalities. More than 50% of the cases with high-grade refractory anemia with excess blasts or refractory anemia with excess blasts in transition show clonal abnormalities *(18)*.

In a study from UTMDACC, our CMML population showed abnormal karyotypes in 34% of the patients. Reports in the literature indicate abnormalities in 30 to 40% of CMML. Karyotype abnormalities have failed to show significant independent correlation with survival in CMML.

Therapeutic myelodysplastic syndrome (tMDS) is of increasing importance and occurs primarily in patients previously treated with alkalizing chemotherapeutic agents and/or ionizing radiation and topoisomerase inhibitors. Overall, these patients may account for as many as 10 to 15% of all cases of MDS and leukemia. The number of these patients may continue to increase as patients following therapy are living longer. tMDS usually occur between 2 and 6 yr post-therapy. The karyotypic changes seen include monosomy 5 and 7 and deletion of 5q and 7q as well as 11q23 abnormalities. 11q23 abnormalities are thought to be specifically related to prior treatment with topoisomerase inhibitors.

2.1.3 Myeloproliferative Syndromes

The chronic myelogenous proliferative syndromes are represented primarily by chronic myelogenous leukemia (CML).

Nowell and Hungerford described a shortened G-group chromosome associated with CML in 1960. This was the first chromosomal abnormality to be recognized as a recurring aberration in a human cancer. Subsequently, this "Philadelphia" chromosome was identified as chromosome 22 and was the result of a reciprocal genetic exchange between chromosome 22 and chromosome 9. The genes involved include the *abl* gene in the region of chromosome 9q34 and the breakpoint cluster region *(bcr)* gene in the region of chromosome 2q11.2. Approximately 95% of the patients with CML that meet morphological and clinical criteria of the disease have the t(9;22)(q34;q11.2). Cytogenetics can aid in the initial diagnosis of CML, in the response to therapy, and in looking for minimal residual disease. Increased analytical sensitivity can come from the use of FISH techniques to identify the Philadelphia chromosome, particularly in looking for minimal residual disease or CML recurrence in the bone marrow.

CML in its early chronic phase usually presents with t(9;22) as a single chromosomal change. As the disease progresses and enters a more accelerated phase or blast crisis there may be additional chromosomal alterations. The most common alterations include an additional Philadelphia chromosome [trisomy der(22)t(9;22)], trisomy 8, isochromosome 17q [i(17)(q10)], and trisomy 19. These so-called "clonal evolutionary changes" can also occur in combinations and are associated with a poorer prognosis for patients.

It should be noted that t(9;22)(q34;q11.2) can also be seen in up to 30% of ALL in adults and about 5% of childhood ALL. Essentially, many of the ALLs are associated with a different breakpoint region and a protein of approx 185–190 kDa as a result of the fusion gene end product. In the CML, the fusion gene produces a protein of approx 210 kDa. The molecular genetic changes depend upon varying breakpoint regions and are described in other chapters. Occasionally, variant translocations are seen that involve the chromosomes 9 and 22 and an additional third or more chromosomes. It is thought that in the three-way variant translocations that the chromosome breaks occurred simultaneously and that material is translocated from the 9q region to the 22q region, the 22q region subsequently is transferred to the third chromosome, and the third chromosome then translocates back to the 9q34 breakpoint region. These derivative t(9;22) rearrangements can occur as either two or three step rearrangements. In approx 3% of the cases, a Philadelphia chromosome (der(22)t(9;22)) can not be identified by conventional cytogenetic techniques, but is identified by FISH. Even greater analytical sensitivity can be obtained by molecular diagnostic techniques such as real time quantitative PCR, especially when looking for minimal residual disease *(19)*.

2.2. The Lymphoid Leukemias

2.2.1. Acute Lymphocytic Leukemia

Acute lymphocytic leukemias (ALLs) are observed in adults and children. The majority of ALLs are of B-cell derivation. The most common leukemia subtype in children is ALL which accounts for approx 75% of the cases of childhood leukemia. Characterization of the chromosomal abnormalities in childhood leukemia is in some ways of greater significance than in adults. The number of chromosomes and type of translocation has a significant prognostic value. For instance, in childhood leukemia the modal number of chromosomes is classified into five subtypes. The first subtype is karyotypes that are hyperdiploid with greater than 50 chromosomes, including those that are near-tetraploid; a second category of hyperdiploid karyotypes that have between 47 and 50 chromosomes; a third group is the pseudodiploid karyotype with 46 chromosomes that have structural or numerical abnormalities; a fourth is the diploid karyotype with 46 apparently normal chromosomes; the fifth subtype is the hypodiploid karyotype with fewer than 46 chromosomes. The ploidy state is predictive of clinical outcome. Patients that are hyperdiploid with 51 plus chromosomes have a more favorable prognosis and a higher cure rate than other categories. The hyperdiploid 51 plus chromosome numbers represent about 25 to 30 percent of children presenting with ALL. Near triploidy (69–81 chromosomes) cases of childhood ALL are extremely rare, whereas about 3% of adult ALL cases present with this pattern. The near tetraploidy range occurs in 1 to 2% of childhood and adult cases and there appears to be a preponderance of T-cell ALLs in this group. Of those patients that present with a hyperdiploid count the median modal number of chromosomes is 55. This hyperdiploid state occurs, in 25 to 30% of children but only about ten to 20% of adult ALL. Approximately 10 to 15% of both childhood and adult ALL are diploid *(20)*.

Three categories of hypodiploid ALL are recognized. These include chromosome counts of 41–45, 30–40, and less than 30 chromosomes. Hypodiploidy with a modal number of 45 chromosomes occurs in 7–9% of both child and adult ALL. The hypodiploid state is associated with a poorer prognosis especially in childhood ALL.

Translocation t(9;22)(q34;q11.2) occurs in approx 20 to 30% of adult ALL and is associated with a poor prognosis. Childhood ALL with t(9;22) occurs in less than 5% of cases.

Translocation 9;22 ALL carries a poor prognosis both in adults and children. Translocation t(1;19)(q23;p13.3) occurs in approx 3 to 6% of childhood and adult ALL. This translocation tends to be associated with ALL of the pre-B cell type. 11q23 abnormalities involve the MLL (myeloid-lymphoid leukemia or mixed lineage leukemia) gene and are seen in approx 50 to 60% of the ALL cases in children younger than one year of age. Translocations with 11q23 have been reported with chromosome 4q21, 9p22, 10p12, and 19p13.3 among others. Translocations of t(11;19)(q23;p13.3) and t(6;11)(q27;q23) have been reported in cases of acute myelomonocytic and monocytic leukemia as well.

Other less common abnormalities include deletions of 6q, 9p additions and deletions, 12p deletions, and or translocations.

Burkitt's lymphoma, a type of B-cell ALL, is associated with three recognized translocations involving chromosome 8 and either the heavy-chain immunoglobulin gene, or the κ- or λ-light-chain genes. These. translocations are t(8;14)(q24;q32), t(2;8)(p11;q24), and t(8;22)(q24;q11) *(21)*. T-cell leukemias represent about fifteen percent of all childhood ALL and are associated with chromosomal abnormalities in T-cell receptor regions. These include the T-cell receptor for α and δ at chromosome 14q11.2, T-cell receptor β at chromosome 7q35, and T-cell receptor γ at chromosome 7p15.

2.2.2. Chronic Lymphocytic Leukemia (CLL)

CLL is the most common type of leukemia found in adults. More than 90% of the CLL patients have a proliferation of B-cell lymphocytes, and the remainder have T-cell CLL. Clonal aberrations in B-cell CLL are seen in approx 30% of cases by conventional cytogenetics. Additional chromosomal abnormalities can be observed with the use of FISH. Some of the more common chromosomal abnormalities include trisomy 12 found in approx 15 to 20% of cases, deletions of 6q, particularly in those patients progressing to prolymphocytic leukemia (PLL), and deletion of 13q, which seems to have a poor prognosis in CLL, lymphomas and multiple myeloma *(22)*.

3. CYTOGENETIC EVALUATION OF LYMPHOMAS

3.1. Non-Hodgkin's Lymphoma

Non-Hodgkins lymphoma (NHL) comprises a diverse group of lymphomas made up of B- or T-cell lymphocytes. Definitive diagnosis of B or T components requires flow cytometry and molecular diagnostic techniques (i.e., PCR). Obtaining good growth and the low proliferative index of lymphomas require consideration for the use of mitogenic stimulation (i.e., LPS or PHA) and/or molecular techniques such as FISH and PCR.

The more common translocations seen on cytogenetic evaluation include t(2;5)(p23;q35) in anaplastic large cell lymphoma (ALCL), which are often of the T-cell type, although they have also been reported in B-cell lymphomas. Translocation t(14;18)(q32;q21.3) is considered to be the cytogenetic hallmark of follicular cell lymphomas. Translocation t(11;14)(q13;q32) seen in approx 8 to 10% of adult lymphoma cases is associated with mantle cell lymphoma. In addition to these changes, there are also numerical changes, particularly trisomy 12, trisomy 7, and trisomy 3. Structural changes including the deletion of 6q and 13q abnormalities also are useful in the diagnosis and prognosis of lymphomas *(23)*. Multiple myeloma has been associated with translocation t(11;14) and carries a poorer prognosis with deletion 13q.

No specific useful conventional cytogenetic information is available for Hodgkin's lymphoma.

4. THE CYTOGENETIC EVALUATIONS OF SOLID TUMORS

4.1. Epithelial Tumors

In the field of clinical applied sciences, human cytogenetics is relatively new compared to other techniques. It was not until the mid-1950s that human chromosomes were clearly identified through the works of Hsu and others *(1,7)*. Nowell described thePhiladelphia chromosme, the first chromosomal abnormality associated with human malignancy in 1960 *(9)*. The debate of whether or not these chromosomal changes precede the development of malignancy or if they occur as secondary changes resulting from the development of malignancies, has been going on for years *(24)*.

For most of the hematopoietic cancers, initiation begins with the activation of an oncogene followed by the loss of a suppressor gene. Although little is known about the activation of solid tissue and organ tumors (STOT), the majority of these cases are the result of the loss of suppressor genes associated with the activation of an oncogene *(24)*. Part of the reason for the lack of knowledge comes from the difficulty of culturing solid tumors. However, recent culturing techniques have yielded successful analyzable karyotypes that show increasing varieties of chromosomal abnormalities for STOT compared to hematological malignancies.

Thyroid adenomas, colorectal adenomas, and salivary gland adenomas are perhaps the three most studied epithelial tumors. Over 60% of salivary gland adenomas have changes involving chromosomes 3, 8, and 12 *(25)*. However, abnormalities involving chromosomes 8 and 12 have not been reported in the same tumor. Therefore, it is expected that rearrangements involving these two chromosomes have different pathways. Rearrangements of chromosome 10q and 11q have been associated with thyroid carcinomas *(26)*.

Colorectal adenomas have been shown to have aberrations involving extra copies of chromosomes 8 and 13. Colorectal carcinomas generally have complex karyotypes. Genes located on chromosome 5 and 20 have shown to be involved with this particular cancer. Molecular studies have revealed specific genes associated with patients of familial or inherited associated polyposis and hereditary nonpolypopsis colorectal cancer (HNPCC). In addition, on the short arm of chromosome 3 lies a gene that is associated with HNPCC. The gene locus for familial adenomatous polyposis (FAP) has been mapped to the locus 5q21 and has been subsequently cloned *(24)*.

Within the malignant epithelial neoplasms, certain chromosomal changes have been reported for specific types. Deletions of the 3p region have been described in small cell and nonsmall cell undifferentiated lung epithelial carcinomas. For a hepatoblastoma, trisomy 20 has been identified in 78% of tumors. It has been known since the early 1990s that epithelial carcinomas involving the tongue, uterus corpus, ovary, breast, colorectal, and kidney have aberrations of chromosome 1, suggesting secondary changes in tumor progression *(27)*.

4.2. Connective Tissue Tumors

Two of the more studied benign mysenchymal tumors are leiomyomas and lipomas. Both show a variety of chromosomal changes. Within the group of lipomas, rearrangements involving translocations of chromosome 12 and 1, 2, 3, and 21 have been reported. Likewise for leiomyomas, chromosome rearrangements of 12 and chromosome 1, 6, and 14 have been identified *(28)*. Both types of tumors also show deletions of 13q. Other consistent changes found in uterine leiomyomas included deletion of 7q, trisomy 12, monosomy 22, and ring chromosomes *(29)*.

Sarcomas are generally difficult to classify morphologically especially when poorly differentiated or undifferentiated. In the pediatric population, the lack of differentiation often results in confusion and misdiagnosis. However, among these sarcomas, clinically significant cytogenetics findings have been reported: clear cell sarcoma +8, t(12:22)(q13;q12), alveolar rhabdomyosarcoma. t(2:13)(q35;q14), Ewing's sarcoma t(11;22)(q21;q11), synovial sarcoma t(X;18)(p12.2;q12.2), Askin's tumor t(11;22)(q21;q13), extraskeletal myxoid chondrosarcoma t(9;22)(q22;q11), and malignant mesothelioma del(3)(p13p23) *(30,31)*.

Cytogenetic findings of the specific chromosomal changes in these sarcomas have revealed potential candidate regions and location of genes, which allowed further studies into molecular cloning of these regions. Translocation breakpoints involving t(12;16)(q13;p11), t(12;22)(q13;q12), t(11;22)(q21;q13), t(2;13)(q35;q14), and others have been characterized *(32)*.

4.3. Neurological Tumors

The etiology of primary tumors of the nervous system remains unknown. The potential causes may include immunological disorders, environmental influences, viral inductions, genetic factors, hormonal factors, prior radiation therapy, and mutation. Today, two of the leading hypotheses for spontaneous neoplasms are viral and chemically induced mutagenesis. With the advance of molecular techniques, researchers have changed their focus from phenotypic characteristics to the understanding of events on the genotypic level. The discoveries of oncogenes, tumor suppressor genes, and mismatch repairs have expanded our knowledge of the pathogenesis of brain neoplasms. For benign neurogenic neoplasms, the two most studied are meningioma and neurofibroma. Monosomy 22 was the first chromosomal aberration discovered in solid tumors. This abnormality is found in meningiomas, which have their origins from the meninges. In one study this abnormality was reported in 270 out of 300 cases *(33)*.

In children, the most common primary malignant brain tumor is medulloblastoma, which often displays the cytogenetic abnormality of isochromsome 17q. Bigner et al. in 1990 demonstrated 48% of tumors with clonal changes and showed a loss of alleles for loci on chromosome 17q through molecular studies *(34)*.

The most common intraocular tumor of childhood is the retinoblastoma. This particular tumor occurs in both hereditary and spontaneous forms. A deletion of 13q is recognized by conventional cytogenetics in 5–10% of the patients. Molecular studies revealed submicroscopic deletions of the RB1 gene exist in all patients.The RB1 gene, when lost in homozygous forms, leads to the initiation of retinoblastoma formation *(35)*.

Neuroblastoma is the most commonly found extracranial tumor in children. This tumor originates from the neural crest cells and demonstrates a consistent cytogenetic abnormality of deleted 1p. Through molecular studies, it has been shown to be involved with the amplification of the NMYC oncogene. The karyotypes of these patients have also proven to be a reliable prognostic indicator. Near diploid or tetraploid karyotypes generally leads to a poor prognosis while near triploid karyotypes will have an excellent prognosis *(36)*.

4.4. Germ-Cell Tumors

Germ-cell tumors consist of a group of heterogeneous neoplasms located in different but restricted anatomical locations. There are three groups of germ cell tumors in the testis. Group I is comprised of teratomas and yolk sac tumors of infants, group II contains seminomas and nonseminomas of adolescents and adults, and group III consists of spermatocytic seminomas of the elderly. These groups are characterized epidemiologically, by chromosomal constitution and histological appearance. Proper categorization of these groups is crucial because they may require different methods of treatment. It has been established that isochromosome 12 or i(12)(p10) has been the consistent cytogenetic abnormality in testicular germ-cell tumors. Moreover, these markers often exist in multiple copies. They have also been identified in the subtypes such as seminoma, teratoma, embryonal carcinoma, combined or mixed testes germ-cell neoplasms, dysgerminoma, and immature teratoma. These findings suggest that although their histology is different, some of the origins such as seminomas and non-seminomatous tumors might be the same *(37)*.

5. TECHNIQUES

5.1. Bone Marrow Culture Set-Up

The purpose of culturing bone marrow cells is to identify chromosomal aberrations among hematopoietic cells. When a bone marrow aspirate is performed, approx 0.5–3.0 mL of early aspirate is collected in a sodium-heparinized glass tube. Sodium heparin is the anticoagulant of choice for collection purposes. Lithium heparin, EDTA, and other types of anticoagulants may be toxic to cells and have been shown to impair culture growth *(38)*. If the sample is clotted, perform a white blood cell (WBC) count immediately. If the count is sufficient, proceed with culture set up. If the cell count is insufficient, try breaking up the clot mechanically and/or warm the sample in a water bath to 37°C to dissolve the clot, which may be caused by the presence of cold auto-agglutinins.

If bone marrow samples are not available, peripheral blood containing a minimum of 30% blasts may be substituted for culture. Lower percentages of blasts have shown to yield poor to no growth when using peripheral blood. Approximately 5.0 mL of blood is needed for culture. The blood should be collected in a green-top tube containing sodium heparin. Blood may be transported at ambient room temperature, but avoid extreme temperatures. They may also be stored at 4°C but never frozen as cell viability is lost.

Lymph node biopsies should be collected in a sterile container with media. If media is not available, normal saline solution without preservatives may be substituted. The amount of specimen should be 1 cm of tissue if possible. The tissue must be minced to release individual cells for culture.

Aseptic technique must be followed when performing bone marrow culturing. This is performed under a laminar flow hood. The procedure starts by performing a cell count utilizing an automated cell counter. We are only interested in the WBCs, thus red blood cell (RBC) lysing reagents such as Zapoglobin (Coulter Beckman) may be used. Otherwise, the cell count would be falsely increased from the interference of the RBCs. For optimal growth, the WBC count should be 1–4 million per 1 mL or 10–40 million per 10-mL culture. Cultures may also be set up in different time intervals such as 24, 48, and 72 h. For example, for a bone marrow suspected of having CML, both 24 and 48 h cultures are set up.

Successful growth must provide proper media, physical, and chemical environments. Physical environmental factors such as temperatures, pH, and osmotic pressure are measured to provide proper environment. Chemicals such as vitamins, carbohydrates, and buffered salts are also added. If powdered media is used dissolve in water and sterilize before culturing. Serum is an essential part of a growth medium. Generally, 10–40% of the medium is serum. Fetal calf (bovine) serum is the most widely used. However, each batch of serum must be tested as they have been shown to exhibit different growth potentials and possibly may be toxic to specific cells.

The harvesting procedure consists of three phases: (1) arresting the cells from dividing, (2) swelling of the cells, and (3) fixing the cells so they can be dropped onto the slides.

The mitotic arresting reagent colcemid (deacetylmethyl colchicine), a synthetic form of Colchicine (naturally occurring, extracted from the autumn crocus) is the most widely used mitotic inhibitor. It prevents the formation of the spindle apparatus so that dividing cells will not enter anaphase thereby causing an accumulation of metaphases. However, the higher the concentration of colcemid in the culture, the shorter the chromosomes will become *(39)*. Generally, 0.1 mL of colcemid is added for every 10 mL of culture for 15–20 min. Certain studies, such as hypermetaphase studies require colcemid to be added for up to 24 h.

The spindle apparatus is not present because of the presence of colcemid; the chromosomes are suspended in the cytoplasmic membrane. The introduction of hypotonic solution causes the cells to swell, through a concentration gradient of fluids entering through the semi permeable cell membrane. Presently, the most widely used hypotonic solution is 0.075 M KCL. The hypotonic step usually takes 25–30 min. It is added after the colcemid step. The cells are still alive at this stage, thus during the waiting period, cultures are stored in a 37°C incubator for optimal recovery.

After the hypotonic stage, the culture is centrifuged. The revolutions per minute (RPM) and time may vary from lab to lab but generally around 1200 rpm for 7 min. After centrifugation, the supernatant (hypotonic solution) is removed and the fixative can be added. The fixative solution contains a 3:1 methanol and glacial acetic acid mixed in that order. Methanol removes excess water from the cell membrane causing shrinkage and hardening of the cell wall, while acetic acid precipitates nucleic acids and dissolves nuclear histones. The fixative is added to the culture up to the 10-mL mark for 20 min. Subsequent washes with fixative may be performed to washout debris.

When making the cell suspension for slide preparation, it is crucial not to over or under dilute. Either condition may cause poor spreading of chromosomes. Humidity and temperature can also affect the spreading. As the drop of fixative containing cells hits the microscope slide, the drying action of the fixative causes the cell membrane to pull apart, exposing, and spreading the chromosomes.

5.2. Culturing of Solid Tumors

Samples for solid tumor studies should be collected with sterile techniques, which need to be maintained throughout the entire culturing process. The sample size is generally around 1 cm³ if possible. It is transported in media but normal saline without preservatives may be substituted. This tissue can be minced or cells released by adding collagenase. Collected specimens should be kept at room temperature. There are two main categories of long-term cultures; self-terminating and continuous. The self-terminating usually contains tissues from lymph nodes, skin, and gonads. The continous is further divided into two categories: (1) malignant tumors and (2) cell types that must be transformed to create continuous cell lines.

There are many types of media used for long-term culture growth. They can be divided into three main types: growth medium (GM); maintenance medium (MM); and complete medium (CM). The main differences are CM contains all the necessary supplements and sera while GM contains the same as complete but with increased serum by 10–20%, and MM contains lower levels of serum with increased pH. New samples should be cultured in more than one type of media, and the media that requires the least amount of nutrients to sustain growth should be chosen.

Various types of factors may be added to promote growth. Fetal bovine calf serum is commonly used because of its ability to generate good results. Other media enhancements include: horse or bovine serum, epidermal growth factor, platelet derived growth factor, bovine pituitary extract, and fibroblast growth factor. These factors can be used in conjunction with fetal bovine calf serum.

Mammalian cells generally require an artificial substrate to adhere to for growth. Glass and polystyrene (type of plastic) culture vessels are suitable choices because of their negatively charged surfaces, which will attract the positively charged cells *(40)*.

The dispersion of solid tissues prior to set-up is important. They may be dispersed in the following ways: physical cutting; exposed to enzymes such as pronase, collagenase, or trypsin; and chemically by soaking in a bath containing balanced salt solution (BSS) that is free of Ca^{++} and Mg^{++}. When considering the use of enzymes it should be noted that collagenase has been shown to cause the least amount of damage to the cells *(40)*.

The incubation time for long term cultures is 5–7 d at 37°C in 5% CO_2. They should be checked for contamination after 24–48 h. Media should be changed twice per week. This is done by replacing one- to two-thirds of fresh media to the culture. If the cell line is a fast growing type, subculturing is done every 2–3 d. Sub-culturing can be done either with enzymes such as pronase or trypsin to promote cellular detachments from the flask, or by mechanical scraping. Primary cultures must be washed to remove any serum, which might interfere with the actions of the enzymes. For most cell lines, they are ready to be harvested after 6–9 d.

5.3. Giemsa Banding

There are many techniques to view chromosome banding under a microscope. The giemsa banding technique is often used in the routine cytogenetic laboratory. Banded chromosomes have helped the precision of cytogenetic diagnosis by: differentiating members of the D group chromosomes (e.g., between the G and Y group, the C and X group, and structural abnormalities). Giemsa is a complex of stains that specifically binds the phosphate group of the DNA. Giemsa or G-positive bands on a chromosome represent condensed chromatin made from the interactions of protein and DNA *(41)*. It has been suggested in the literature that these regions of the chromosome are late in replicating and gene poor.The exact mechanism of binding between Giemsa and DNA is not yet known.

There are additional steps prior to treatment with Giemsa. Aged or heated slides are recommended for achieving sharp banding patterns. A proteolytic enzyme, trypsin, must first treat chromosomes. Trypsin works by attacking specific peptide bonds in protein molecules that have carboxyl groups donated by certain amino acids (arginine and lysine). The length of trypsin exposure depends on the type of the brand being used, pH, temperature, and concentration. The time in trypsin may range from 30 s up to 5 min for old slides. The pH is between 7.2 and 7.4. After the slide is treated by trypsin, it is dipped into an antitrypsin bath such as fetal bovine serum, then quickly dipped into a Gurr's buffer bath (pH 7.2). Gurr's buffer tablets (Biomedical Specialties, Santa Monica, CA) can be used for convenience. Each tablet is mixed with 1000 mL (1 L) of water. Once the slide is in the Giemsa bath, the time may vary from 1 to 10 min. Afterwards, wash the slide with water to remove any excess dye. The slide is air-dried and ready for view under microscope.

Troubleshooting tips include: under-trypsinized chromosomes may appear to have little contrast or indistinct bands. Over-trypsinized chromosomes may have a ghost-like or grayish white appearance.

5.4. Fluorescent In Situ Hybridization Technique

Fluorescent *in situ* hybridization (FISH) is the most commonly used molecular cytogenetic technique. In conjunction with classical cytogenetic karyotypic analysis, FISH has demonstrated both specificity and reliability *(42)*. FISH can be performed on various types of specimens; bone marrow or blood smears, directly fixed cells, and formalin-fixed tissues. It is often performed on conventionally prepared cytogenetic microscopic slides. The FISHtechnique was first detailed by researchers in 1969 *(43)*. They stated that single-stranded DNA would anneal to its complementary DNA sequence, thereby tagging a specific chromosomal region with a DNA probe it would be recognized by its complementary DNA sequence within an interphase nucleus or on a metaphase chromosome. The DNA probe and its target DNA must first be denatured by heating in a solution containing formamide.

Because both of these highly repetitive nucleic acid sequences must be in single-stranded conformation. Aged cytogenetic slides are recommended for FISH. They can be aged naturally or artificially by means of incubation at 37°C in 2X standard saline citrate (SSC). They can be stored in a desiccated chamber at room temperature. The aging process is completed so that DNA can be "hardened" and survive through the harsh conditions of hybridization. Pretreatment of the slide with pepsin, proteinase K, or RNase helps reduce unwanted protein and cytoplasmic debris that might interfere with the probe from reaching its target.

For DNA to reanneal in its double-stranded form, the probe must be hybridized to the target DNA. In this cocktail of mixtures, excess repetitive sequence DNA is added to block off any nonspecific binding. Hybridization often takes 2–18 h at 37°C, and any excess repetitive sequence DNA is washed away by formamide-saline citrate solutions. To view the probe, a fluorescent tag is attached. This can be chemically modified by adding hapten molecules, such as biotin or digoxigenin, so that they can be indirectly fluorescently labeled using immunocytochemical techniques *(44)*. Using a fluorochrome of a complementary color then counterstains the target DNA. A fluorescent microscope equipped with filters specific for the fluorochrome label and the counter stain is used to detect the probe. Utilizing imaging systems, we can capture the images and enhance or increase the sensitivity of the probe via software programs. Fluorescent dyes fade under light, so proper storage must be considered when not in use.

There are three types of probes used for cytogenetics FISH studies. First, are α-satellite DNA probes. These probes are designed to specifically recognize repetitive DNA sequences such as telomeric sequences or centromers. They give out bright signals and are very useful in identification of chromosomes in interphase nuclei. The second type is the unique sequence probe, which hybridizes a single copy of DNA sequences in a specific gene region on a chromosome. Another term associated with this is the cosmid probe. They are often used to identify microdeletion syndromes. The third type of probe is the whole chromosome paint (WCP). WCP probes are comprised of a combination of unique sequence probes that recognize the entire length of genetic material of a particular chromosome. Both homologs are usually painted and fluoresce brightly. They are useful in derivative studies. WCP FISH probes can only be used on metaphase preparations. Locus specific and satellite probes may be used on interphase as well as metaphase preparations.

6. CONCLUSION

Conventional cytogenetics has been used for many years in the diagnosis, treatment, prognosis, and follow-up of myeloproliferative disorders, myelodysplastic disorders, lymphomas, and lymphocytic leukemias. Molecular techniques such as FISH, SKY, CGH, and others are complementary in evaluation of these disorders. They are useful when nonrandom patterns are identified. Because of the karyotype complexity in solid tumors, conventional cytogenetics and molecular cytogenetics are still in the developmental stages of clinical applicability. Conventional cytogenetics has demonstrated its usefulness in terms of diagnosis, treatment approaches, and as an assessment for minimal residual disease for myeloproliferative and lymphoproliferative diseases. FISH and other molecular techniques help enhance the overall sensitivity and specificity. Although we have moved towards the understanding of solid tumors through cytogenetics with their recurrent chromosomal findings, future studies on these abnormalities are crucial for better understanding of human tumorigenesis.

REFERENCES

1. Hsu TC. 1952. Mammalian chromosomes in vitro. The karyotype of man. J. Hered. 43:167–172.
2. Flemming WZ. 1882. Kern and Zelltheeilung. Leipzig, Germany: FCW Vogel.
3. Balbiani EG. 1881. [French] Sur La Structure du noyau des cellules salivaires chez les larves de Chironomus. Zool. Anz. 4:662–666.
4. Waldeyer-Hartz W. 1888. [German] Uberr Karyokinese und ihre Beziehungen zu den Befruchtungsvorgängen. Archiv für mikroskopische Anatomie und Entwicklungsmechanik. 32:1–122.
5. Sutton W. 1903. The Chromosomes in Heredity. Science 17:441–454.
6. Boveri T. 1914. Zur Frage der Enstehung maligner Tumoren. Gustov Fischer Verlag: Jena, Germany.
7. Tio JH and Levan A. 1956. The chromosome number of man. Am. J. Obstet. Gynecol. 130: 723–724.
8. Caspersson T, Farber S, Foley GE, et al. 1968. Chemical differeintiation along metaphase chromosome. Exp. Cell. Res. 49:219–222.
9. Nowell PC and Hungerford DA. 1960. A minute chromosome in human chronic myelocytic leukemia (CML). Science 132:1497–1501.
10. Yunis JJ. 1976. High resolution of human chromosomes. Science 191:1268–1270.
11. Pinkel D, Gray J, Trask B, van den Engh G, Fuscoe J, van Dekken H. 1986. Cytogenetic analysis by in situ hybridization with fluorescently labeled nucleic acid probes. Cold Spring Harbor Symp. Quant. Biol. 51:151–157.
12. Kallioniemi A, Kallioniemi OP, Suder D, et al. 1992. Comparative genome hybridization for molecular cytogenetic analysis of solid tumors. Science 258:818–821.
13. Schrock E, duManoir S, Veldman T, et al. 1996. Multicolor spectral karyotyping of human chromosomes. Science 273:494–497.

14. Speicher MR, Ballard SG, Ward DC. 1996. Karyotyping human chromosomes by combinatorial multifluor FISH. Nat. Genet. 12:368–375.

15. Muller S, Rocci M, Ferguson-Smith M, Wienberg J. 1997. Toward a multicolor chromosome bar code for the entire human karyotype by fluorescence *in situ* hybridization. Hum. Genet. 100:271–278.

16. Glassman AB. 2000. Chromosomal Abnormalities in Acute Leukemias. Clin. Lab. Med. 20:39–47.

17. Adriaansen HJ, Boekhorst PAW, Hagemeijer AM, et al. 1993. Acute myeloid leukema M4. with bone marrow eosinophlia (M4Eo) and inv(16((p13q22) exhitits a specific immunophenotype with CD2 expression. Blood 81:30–43.

18. Geddes AA, Bowen DT, Jacobs A. 1990. Clonal karyotype abnormalities and clinical progress in the Myelodysplastic syndrome. Br. J. Hematol. 76:194–202.

19. Bain BJ. 2002. Chronic Myeloproliferative Disorders: Cytogenetic and Molecular Genetic Abnormalities, vol. 108.

20. A Collaborative study of the Group Francais de Cytogenetique Hematologique. 1996. Cytogenetic abnormalities in adult acute lymphoblastic leukemia: correlations with hematologic findings outcome. Blood 8:3135–3142.

21. Bernheim A, Berger R, Lenoir G. 1981. Cytogenetic studies on African Burkitt's lymphoma cell lines: t(8;14), t(2;8) and t(8;22) translocations. Cancer Genet. Cytogenet. 4:307–315.

22. Hanson CA, Hoyer JD, Li CY, et al. 1996. Similarities between T-Cell chronic lymphocytic leukemia and the small-cell variant of T-prolymphocytic leukemia. Blood 87:3520–3521.

23. Kumari P, Mukherjee,G, Rao CR, et al. 2003. Cytogenetic study of non-hodgkin lymphoma from South India. Histologic and geographic correltations. Cancer Genet. Cytogenet. 141:14–19.

24. Glassman AB. 1997. Cytogenetics an evolving role in the diagnosis and treatment of cancer. Clin. Lab. Med. 17:21–27.

25. Sandros J, Stenman G, Mark J. 1990. Cytogenetic and molecular observations in human and experimental salivary gland tumors. Cancer Genet. Cytogenet. 44:153–167.

26. Heim S and Mitelman F. 1991. Cytogenetics of solid tumors. Recent Adv. Histopathol. 15:37–66.

27. Sandberg AA. 1990. The Chromosomes in Human Cancer and Leukemia, 2nd ed., Elsevier: New York, NY.

28. Dong SY, Morgan R, Stone J, et al. 1998. Translocation (12;14) in lipomas: a case report and review of the literature. Cancer Genet. Cytogenet. 1:59–61.

29. Pandis N, Heim S, Bardi G, et al. 1991. Chromosome analysis of 96 uterine leiomyomas. Cancer Genet. Cytogenet. 55:11–18.

30. Jelinek JS, Kransdorf MJ, Shmookler BM, Aboulafia AJ, Malawer MM. 1994. Liposarcoma of the extremities: MR and CT findings in the histologic subtypes. Radiology 2:455–459.

31. Vanni R, Dal Cin P, Marras S, et al. 1993. Endometrial polyp: Another benign tumor characterized by 12q13-q15 changes. Cancer Genet. Cytogenet. 68:32–33.

32. Barr FG, Galili N, Holick J, Biegel JA, Rovera G, Emanuel BS. 1993. Rearrangement of the PAX3 paired box gene in the pediatric solid tumor alveolar rhabdomyosarcoma. Nat. Genet. 3:113–117.

33. Sreekantaiah C, Rodriquez E, Chaganti RSK. 1994. Genetic changes in epithelial solid neoplasia. Cancer Res. 54:3398–3406.

34. Bigner SH, Mark J, Bigner DD. 1990. Cytogenetics of human brain tumors. Cancer Genet. Cytogenet. 47:141–154.

35. Laure L, Francis LM, Pascal C, Anne-Claude G, Francine T, Daniel FS. 2001. Molecular characterization of the deletion in retinoblastoma patients with 13q14 cytogenetic anomalies. Ophthalmic Genet. 1:1–10.

36. Vandesompele J. 2001. Multicentre analysis of patterns of DNA gains and losses in 204 neuroblastoma tumors: how many genetic subgroups are there? Med. Pediatr. Oncol. 36:5–10.

37. Chaganti RS and Houldsworth J. 2000. Genetics and biology of adult human male germ cell tumors. Cancer Res. 60:1475–1482.
38. Rooney DE and Czepulkowski BH. 1986. Chromosome staining and bonding technique, in: Human Cytogenetics: A Practical Approach. IRL Press: Oxford, pp. 57–84.
39. Lawce HJ and Brown MG. 1991. Harvesting, slidemaking, and chromosome elongation techniques, in: ACT Cytogenetics Laboratory Manual, 2nd ed., Raven Press: New York, NY, pp. 31–106.
40. Freshney RI. 1986. Introduction, in: Animal Cell Culture, Freshney R, ed., IRL Press: Washington.
41. Hamerton JL. 1984. Cytogenetic disorders. N. Engl. J. Med. 310:314–316.
42. Nolte M, Werner M, Ewig M, et al. 1996. Fluorescence *In Situ* Hybridization (FISH) is a reliable diagnostic tool for detection of the 9;22 translocation. Leuk. Lymph. 22:287–294.
43. Buongiorno-Nardeli M and Amaldi F. 1969. Autoradiographic detection of molecular hybrids between r RNA and DNA in tissue sections. Nature 225:946–947.
44. Trask BJ, Allen S, Massa H, Fertitta A, Sachs R, Van Den Engh G, Wu M. 1993. Studies of metaphase and interphase chromosomes using fluorescence *in situ* hybridization, in: Cold Spring Harbor Symposia on Quantitative Biology, vol. 8. Cold Spring Harbor Press: Cold Spring Harbor, NY, pp. 767–775.

19

Microsatellite Alterations as Diagnostic and Prognostic Molecular Markers in Patients With Cancer

Bret Taback and Dave S. B. Hoon

1. INTRODUCTION

Identification of specific genetic alterations associated with tumor initiation and progression offers a unique opportunity to develop nucleic acid based assays for cancer detection. Polymerase chain reaction (PCR) provides a highly sensitive and specific technique for the detection of these genetic changes in a limited amount of tissue. Recent findings of circulating nucleic acids in the plasma and serum from patients with a variety of malignancies provide a minimally invasive approach that may prove clinically useful for cancer screening, diagnosis, subclinical disease surveillance, and monitoring response to therapy.

1.2. History

Recent advances in tumor genetics have documented a variety of genetic alterations during cancer initiation and progression. These mutations, whether inherited or acquired, can result in inactivation of tumor suppressor genes and/or activation of protooncogenes. Continued accumulation of these genetic abnormalities results in cellular transformation, uncontrolled proliferation, and subsequently a phenotype with the ability for invasion and metastasis. An additional genetic mechanism associated with neoplastic transformation is aberrant hypermethylation of CpG islands in gene promoter regions, which results in transcriptional silencing of genes that regulate cell growth. However, one of the most frequent genetic changes identified in cancer is allelic imbalance manifested as loss of heterozygosity (LOH). The demonstration of LOH on multiple chromosomes across a number of different tumor types suggests the involvement of many putative tumor suppressor genes in carcinogenesis. In 1971, Knudson evaluated the presentation and distribution of retinoblastomas among inherited and noninherited cases and hypothesized that cancer could arise in as few as two mutational events (1). Many believe the first stage requires the acquisition of a minor initial mutational event (such as a base insertion, substitution or deletion) that "knocks out" one allele and is followed by a second alteration, usually LOH of the corresponding allele on the other chromosome; the combination of these two events leads to complete loss of genetic expression.

Historically, cytogenetic studies were performed on tumor tissue to characterize gross chromosomal aberrations. These karyotypic analyses provide a genome-wide assessment of changes in absolute chromosome number and in chromosome structure, including deletions, amplifications, translocations, and inversions. At best, these studies are gross assessments of

From: *Cancer Diagnostics: Current and Future Trends*
Edited by: R. M. Nakamura, W. W. Grody, J. T. Wu, and R. B. Nagle © Humana Press Inc., Totowa, NJ

regional alterations and are limited to the evaluation of tumor cells that are actively dividing. Comparative genomic hybridization (CGH) can detect changes in DNA sequence copy number across the entire genome. Minimal amount of tissue is needed, metaphase cells are not required, and results can often be obtained rapidly *(2)*. Unfortunately, the technique has limited sensitivity for detecting minimal deletions at present. Fluorescent *in situ* hybridization (FISH) technique hybridizes fluorescent genetic probes to chromosomes in nuclei of metaphase or interphase cells *(3)*. It requires a minimal amount of tissue or cells and can be performed on paraffin-embedded tumors for a rapid detection of chromosomal alterations, but is often problematic in reproducibility and sensitivity. These techniques have contributed significant insight into our understanding of cancer biology through tumor genetics *(4,5)*.

LOH analysis of microsatellite markers has provided investigators with a highly specific and focused assessment of regional chromosomal losses. LOH analysis can localize discrete regions of potential tumor suppressor genes. Simple sequence tandem repeats (STRs) of repetitive base pairs have been identified throughout the human genome *(6)*. These so called microsatellites demonstrate polymorphism characterized by high variability in length among individuals *(7)*. PCR primers that border a specific microsatellite region can be created and when amplified can be used to evaluate any loss at that particular chromosome loci. After post-PCR electrophoresis to separate fragment lengths, examination of band patterns for similarly amplified DNA primer sequences among individuals allows novel application of this technology for paternity testing as well as for forensics to establish identity. This approach has also been applied to cancer genetics. When compared to the electrophoresis band pattern of normal DNA, the pattern of tumor DNA may show a diminution of band intensity (allelic imbalance) and/or a shift in band position (microsatellite instability).

There is compelling evidence to suggest that carcinogenesis is the clonal expansion of genetically altered cells and therefore DNA polymerase chain reaction (PCR)-based assays may provide a highly sensitive method to detect early-stage cancers. The relative stability of DNA makes this assay system readily accessible and facile. Exponential amplification of a DNA target from a minimal amount of tissue or body fluids through routine PCR techniques offers a unique opportunity to assess tumor-specific genetic alterations that may serve as useful molecular surrogates of subclinical disease presence. This approach can characterize tumors and may aide in diagnosis when histopathologic assessment is inconclusive. The molecular pathogenesis for colon, melanoma, and cervical cancers has been established based on the identification of genetic events during various stages of tumor development *(8–10)*. Likewise, because genetic alterations demonstrate stability during disease progression, nucleic acid PCR affords the opportunity to identify occult lymph node and systemic metastases associated with primary tumors containing this same genetic profile *(10–13)*. Tumor-associated genetic alterations such as *k-ras* have provided unique molecular markers to look for colorectal cancer in stool specimens, lung cancer in bronchial lavage fluid, pancreatic cancer in biliary secretions, and occult metastasis in tumor-draining lymph nodes *(14–19)*. Allelic imbalance has provided a genetic basis to explain the clinical phenomenon of field cancerization in head and neck tumors by demonstrating shared nucleic acid alterations in adjacent yet histologically different tissues from hyperplasia, dyplasia, carcinoma *in situ*, and invasive lesions *(20)*. These findings suggest that molecular analysis of suspicious or high-risk lesions may be used to identify very early cancers and determine patient risk for local recurrence *(21–25)*.

Recently, specific genetic alterations in primary tumors have demonstrated promise as molecular predictors of prognosis and determinants of response to therapy for carcinomas of different organs *(26–40)*. However, examination of a primary tumor specimen may be of limited value because it is a static assessment of prior genetic events. It does not reflect the ongoing acquisition of genetic alterations throughout disease progression. Characterization of these additional aberrations may serve as supplementary predictors of patient outcome and/or more importantly treatment response *(10,12,25,41)*.

Circulating nucleic acids in the plasma and serum of cancer patients have been shown to harbor genetic alterations identical to those characterized in autologous primary tumors, which suggests their role as potential surrogate markers of disease *(42–69)*. Our group and other investigators have speculated on the potential prognostic utility of circulating microsatellite marker alterations detected in the plasma/serum from cancer patients *(70–75)*.

Examination of blood specimens for genetic markers is a minimally invasive, facile, and logistically practical approach for the detection and monitoring of cancer. There is substantial interest in circulating nucleic acids for cancer screening, diagnosis, prognosis, surveillance of occult disease progression, identifying potential therapeutic targets, and monitoring response to therapy.

1.3. Historical Aspects

The identification of circulating nucleic acids was first described by Mandel and Metais in 1948 *(76)*. Unfortunately, application in the field of cancer dod not occur until 30 yr later when circulating "free" DNA was demonstrated to be elevated in patients with cancer. During the interim, indirect tests such as antibody fixation, or hapten-inhibition, and direct measurements, including immunoprecipitation or counterimmunoelectrophoresis, had limited sensitivity for DNA and therefore resulted in debate regarding the presence, pathology, and etiology of free DNA in plasma/serum *(77–86)*. As a consequence, interest in this field was limited to illnesses where circulating DNA was assumed to have clinical importance, such as in chronic inflammatory states, particularly systemic lupus, rheumatoid arthritis, and other collagen–vascular disorders *(80,82,85,87–89)*. In 1977, Leon et al. used a highly sensitive radioimmunoassay to demonstrate markedly elevated nanogram levels of DNA in cancer patients compared to normal controls (mean concentration: 180 ng/mL vs 13 ng/mL, respectively) *(42,90)*. Serum DNA levels were twice as high in patients with metastatic disease compared to patients without metastasis, implying that circulating free DNA may be used to monitor disease progression. Patients with a decreasing absolute serum DNA concentration after radiation therapy tended to have a better tumor response and clinical outcome. This was the first study to demonstrate the potential clinical utility of circulating DNA in cancer, but the application did not gain acceptance until 1989 when Stroun, Anker, and colleagues suggested that this circulating DNA originated from tumor cells *(44,45)*. Their theory was confirmed in 1994 when two separate investigators identified *k-ras* and *N-ras* gene mutations in the plasma from patients with acute myelogenous leukemia (AML) and pancreatic cancer, respectively *(47,48)*. Currently, tumor-specific genetic alterations identified in both plasma and serum from cancer patients include oncogene mutations and amplifications, genetic rearrangements, microsatellite variations, allelic loss of tumor suppressor and metastasis inhibitor genes, tumor-associated viral DNA, and hypermethylation of gene promoter CpG islands.

This chapter will discuss microsatellite alterations, particularly LOH, as potential diagnostic and prognostic markers in epithelial cancers. Emphasis is placed on those investigations that established a precedent for tumor analysis and on subsequent studies of circulating nucleic acids in plasma and serum as molecular markers of disease. Highlights will focus on genetic markers identified in epithelial malignancies, which may demonstrate clinical utility when detected in serum and plasma.

2. TECHNIQUE

Many of the historical methods for DNA extraction, quantitation, and assessment were time-consuming, lacked specificity and sensitivity, and were associated with exposure to potentially hazardous radioactive and toxic organic solvents *(90,91)*. Utilizing current commercially available kits, quality DNA can be rapidly and efficiently extracted from plasma and serum *(92)*. Newer blood collection tubes, isolation methods and post PCR semi-automated analysis systems permit high-throughput, batch processing of samples in less time and with reduced chance for technical error, producing consistent results.

2.1. Blood Collection

Consistently reliable and reproducible results require strict adherence to standard operating procedures (SOPs) and the application of good laboratory practice (GLP). during sample collection, processing, storage, DNA isolation, PCR set-up, and analysis. When collecting blood samples for PCR analysis during venipuncture, it is important to discard the first 1–2 mL of blood in a separate vacutainer tube to avoid contamination from the skin plug. However, if blood for PCR is drawn during other blood work then these tubes can be collected last in sequence and therefore the aforementioned step is not necessary. For plasma assessment, blood is collected into sodium citrate or ethylenediamine tetraacetic acid (EDTA) tubes; tubes containing heparin should be avoided because heparin may impede PCR. For serum assessment, blood is collected in additive-free tubes kept at room temperature to permit coagulation; after centrifugation, the supernatant is collected and stored at –20°C to –80°C until utilized. Collected whole blood should not be exposed to excessive refrigeration or heat because temperature-induced cell lysis will contaminate the specimen with normal lymphocyte DNA.

There is no consensus as to whether serum or plasma is preferable for circulating nucleic acid analysis. Plasma is centrifuged unclotted blood. In one study of specimens from patients with breast cancer, the incidence of LOH was higher in serum than in plasma; however, serum and plasma were assessed from different cohorts of patients and were not matched for stage of disease *(60)*. Furthermore, a more sensitive detection method was used when evaluating serum. However, higher concentrations of genomic DNA have been shown to be present in serum vs plasma *(93)*. This finding may confound comparison of results for serum and plasma. Likewise, heating collected blood samples or storing them for prolonged periods at room temperature prior to DNA extraction may lead to increased DNA yields by lysing white blood cells and/or circulating tumor cells. We assessed DNA content in paired serum and plasma samples from ten patients with stage IV melanoma. Thirty milliliters of blood was collected from each patient; 10 mL was processed immediately for serum, 10 mL was processed immediately for plasma, and 10 mL was incubated overnight at 37°C and then processed for serum. In each instance, DNA was isolated from 800 µL of serum or

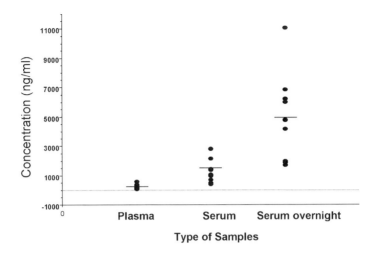

Fig. 1. DNA concentration in plasma, serum, and serum collected overnight. Blood was obtained from ten advanced stage IV melanoma patients and equivalent volumes were processed immediately for plasma and serum or after incubation for 24 h at room temperature (serum overnight) DNA was isolated from 800 μL of plasma/serum. Quantification using the Picogreen assay was as follows: plasma (median 259 ng/mL; range: 83–604 ng/mL), serum (median 1056 ng/mL; range: 411–2821 ng/mL) and serum overnight (median 4783 ng/mL; range: 1709–11054 ng/mL). Horizontal bars represent median DNA concentrations.

plasma and quantitated using the Picogreen assay (Molecular Probes). In all cases, the concentration of DNA obtained from serum was greater than for the corresponding plasma. More interestingly, serum collected from blood samples incubated overnight demonstrated the most DNA (Fig. 1). Therefore, blood samples collected for multicenter trials and during serial bleeds from patients should be obtained in a uniform fashion.

2.2. Blood Processing and Storage

To enhance preservation of serum samples and avoid potential for contamination, we use CORVAC serum separator tubes (Sherwood-Davis & Geck) for blood collection. A self-contained gel is dispersed along the sidewalls of each tube. Immediately after blood collection, the tube is centrifuged at room temperature, creating a physical gel barrier between the two compartments (clotted blood and serum). This ensures a more reliable transport by preventing ongoing contamination of the serum with any genomic DNA released by cell lysis. We then filter the serum through a 13-mm serum filter (Fisher Scientific) to remove any potential contaminating cells and/or other debris; the serum is then placed in aliquots and cryopreserved at –30°C until analysis. From a 12.5-mL draw CORVAC serum separator vacutainer tube we can reliably collect approx 4 mL of quality serum. Peripheral blood lymphocytes collected from each patient in a conventional 4.5-mL sodium citrate vacutainer tube provide genomic DNA –to serve as a control for each individual. Lymphocytes were lysed in a commercially available buffered solution and DNA isolated using DNAzol (Molecular Research Center). In addition, we spot whole-blood collected from each patient onto FTA blood cards (Fitzco, Minneapolis, MN), which can be refrigerated at 4°C for future genomic DNA extraction.

2.2.1. DNA Isolation

There are a variety of commercially available kits for DNA isolation from serum and plasma, none of which have demonstrated consistently improved yield or purity (92). The traditional organic extraction method using SDS and proteinase K digestion followed by phenol-chloroform remains the "gold standard" for DNA isolation (91,94). However, this technique is cumbersome, time-consuming, requires a larger volume of starting plasma/serum, and involves exposure to highly toxic/corrosive agents. In contrast, pre-made reagents and packaged spin columns from commercially available kits substantially reduce preparation and processing time, eliminate exposure to potentially harmful organic reagents, and facilitate collection of DNA directly suitable for PCR. We have previously demonstrated the efficiency of the QIAmp DNA Blood Mini Kit (Qiagen) for high through-put processing of a large number of blood samples for rapid LOH analysis (73). However, there are limitations with this approach when isolating small amounts of DNA.

Because of the assortment of isolation kits and methods for extraction, the quantity and quality of DNA obtained may vary between investigators and laboratories. These differences are increased by the lack of any standardized protocol for isolating circulating nucleic acids prior to PCR. Many investigators do not quantitate their starting DNA concentrations but instead choose to use a constant volume. This can be problematic when interpreting results and performing assays on multiple markers.

2.3. DNA Quantitation

Total DNA in serum from cancer patients can range from nanograms to micrograms per milliliter; the amount of DNA circulating in plasma is substantially less (42–45,84,90,95). Among normal healthy donor volunteers, free serum DNA concentrations are usually less than 200 ng/mL and most often below 50 ng/mL; free DNA in plasma is lower or not detectable (42,84,96). We have utilized the PicoGreen dsDNA Quantitation Kit (Molecular Probes, Eugene, OR) to quantify double-stranded DNA (dsDNA) in plasma and serum after extraction. This highly sensitive fluorescent nucleic acid stain can quantitate DNA down to a level of 25 pg/mL. The intensity of fluorescence is read using a standard spectrofluorometer in a multi-well plate format, without interference from contaminating RNA and single-stranded DNA. Final concentrations are extrapolated from standard curve concentrations. Using this method we found dsDNA amounts of 9–79 ng/mL in serum from 25 healthy volunteers. In a second set of normal controls, 17 of 18 plasma specimens had undetectable DNA levels. Overall, quantification of DNA levels in plasma/serum is important; however range can vary in normal individuals, cancer patients, and non-cancer patients with benign disease. Measurement of DNA levels as sole markers of malignancy can prove challenging.

2.4. Loss of Heterozygosity Analysis

For LOH assessment, post-PCR products are separated by polyacrylamide-gel electrophoresis (PAGE) and analyzed for signal intensity using densitometric software (Fig. 2). Allelic band intensity can be detected by autoradiographs of ^{32}P-labeled forward microsatellite PCR primers. Fluorescent dye-labeled primers avoid radioactivity exposure and allow effortless and more precise analysis using a laser gel scanner. Recently we have begun using capillary array electrophoresis (CAE) for post-PCR product band separation and analysis (Fig. 3). This automated high-throughput technology affords a simple user interface and permits greater resolution than conventional slab gel electrophoresis. Incorpo-

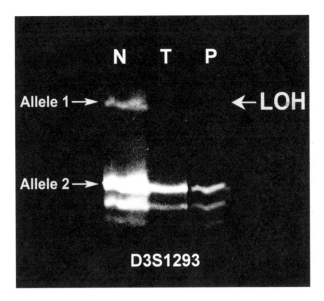

Fig. 2. Post-PCR gel electrophoresis demonstrating LOH for microsatellite marker D3S1293 in a patient's melanoma tumor (*T*) and plasma sample (*P*) compared to paired lymphocyte DNA (*N*).

ration of internal size standards for each sample can distinguish between fragment lengths that differ by a single base pair. Pool-plexing samples prior to a run allows for greater throughput and efficiency (Fig. 4). Regardless of the post-PCR separation procedure selected, allelic imbalance in the test sample must be evaluated by comparison with the individual's genomic DNA (from normal tissue or lymphocytes) run in parallel for each microsatellite marker assessed. LOH is calculated as a relative reduction in the signal intensity of one allele in tumor DNA compared to the corresponding allele in normal control DNA. The allelic ratio is calculated as (T1/T2) /(N1/N2), where T1 and T2 are the signal intensities in the two alleles in the tumor DNA, and N1 and N2 are the corresponding alleles in normal DNA. It has been suggested that LOH be defined if the allelic ratio is less than 50–80% *(97)*. However, studies in the literature have reported positive LOH for allelic loss anywhere from 25–80%. Standardization of plasma/serum analysis for LOH needs to be addressed for future validation among laboratories.

Variations in sample procurement, DNA extraction, primer design, buffers, PCR cycling conditions, and post-PCR product analysis can affect consistency among results. Attention to technique and the use of separate designated rooms for tissue processing, DNA extraction, PCR set-up, and post-PCR analysis is encouraged to prevent cross-contamination. Optimized PCR conditions must be established prior to evaluating tissue/body fluid samples to ensure accurate and reliable results. Positive and negative controls must be incorporated in each PCR run; if their respective results are not obtained, the assay should be considered invalid and repeated for verification. Highly polymorphic markers should be chosen for microsatellite analysis, to ensure a significant number of informative events. For LOH analysis, control DNA should be obtained from patients' autologous peripheral blood lymphocytes or histologically confirmed normal tissue. Control DNA should be run in parallel with the patient's test sample for every PCR experiment; this DNA serves as a reference for the comparison of test sample band patterns and intensity.

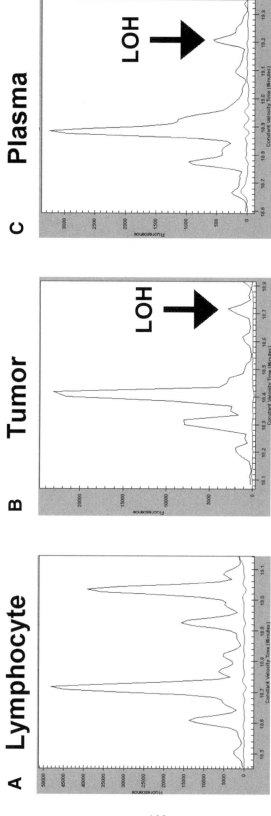

Fig. 3. Capillary array electrophoresis demonstrating LOH for microsatellite marker D12S1657 in a patient's melanoma tumor (**A**) and plasma sample (**B**) compared to paired lymphocyte DNA (**C**).

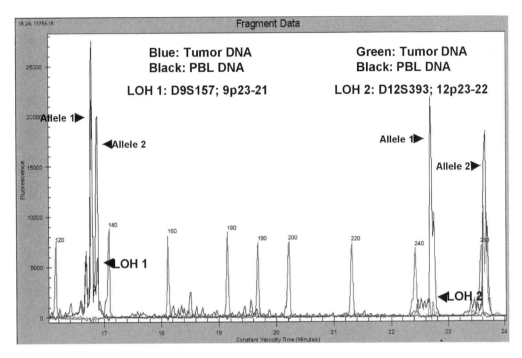

Fig. 4. Pool-multiplex microsatellite marker analysis by capillary array electrophoresis. Simultaneous demonstration of LOH for microsatellite marker D9S157 (left-side of figure) and D12S393 (right-side of figure). from a patients serum sample. Numbered peaks represent map marker.

3. CLINICAL UTILITY OF A MOLECULAR MARKER

3.1. Sensitivity and Specificity

For any diagnostic test to achieve clinical application it must have a high degree of sensitivity and specificity. Sensitivity is the ability of a test to detect a true positive result when the disease is present and is measured as: [(number of true positive cases)/(number of true positives cases + number of false negative cases)] × 100%. Specificity is the ability of a test to detect a true negative result when there is no disease present and is measured as: [(number of true negative cases)/(number of true negative cases + number of false positive cases)] × 100%. A highly sensitive assay identifies disease presence and excludes a false-negative result, whereas a highly specific assay confirms the presence of disease and rules out the possibility of other causes (i.e., a false-positive result). All diagnostic tests have a sensitivity and a specificity, however, the higher the sensitivity of a test the greater the risk of making a false-positive error and similarly, the higher the specificity of a test the greater the risk of committing a false-negative error. Thus, sensitivity and specificity are inversely related. In theory, it is better to have a false-negative result than a false-positive result because the former merely fails to identify the patient as having the disease whereas the latter misclassifies and inaccurately labels the patient with a disease (regarded as a dual error). Therefore, it is more favorable to have a test biased towards greater specificity while sacrificing some degree of sensitivity. Dilution studies that mix serially decreasing amounts of mutated DNA in normal genomic DNA can establish an assay's sensitivity. Evaluation of a

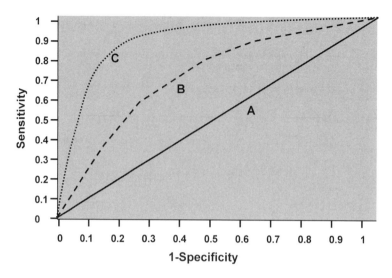

Fig. 5. Representative ROC curves demonstrating a poor (A, 0.5), good (B, 0.7), and excellent (C, 0.9) test results.

significant number of samples from healthy donor subjects (and possibly from patients with benign processes) are used to confirm specificity.

3.2. Receiver Operating Characteristic Curve

Receiver operating characteristic (ROC) curves are useful for evaluating the clinical utility of a diagnostic test based on a molecular marker *(98)*. A ROC curve is a graph that represents sensitivity vs 1-specificity, also known as the false positive rate) of a particular test. The test is assessed in two cohorts, such as patients with a disease and normal or noncancer control subjects. The area under the ROC (AUROC) curve indicates the tests' ability to discriminate between the two groups. The greater the AUROC curve the better the diagnostic test. Although there are no established guidelines, generally, an AUROC curve of less than 0.7 is associated with a poor test, an area of 0.7 to 0.8 is a marginally useful test, 0.8 to 0.9 is a good test, and those tests with an area greater than 0.9 are excellent (Fig. 5).

4. TUMOR SYSTEMS

4.1. Breast

Microsatellite analysis has demonstrated areas of common deletion in breast cancers on chromosome arms 1p, 1q, 2p, 3p, 4p, 8p, 11q, 13q, 14p, 16q, 17p, 18q, and 22q *(99–107)*. Because lymph node metastasis is the single most important prognostic factor in breast cancer, studies of primary tumors have attempted to demonstrate allelic imbalances associated with this event. This would identify putative tumor suppressor genes involved in cancer progression and could establish predictive molecular markers to evaluate primary tumors. Identifying LOH profiles that predict for metastasis would provide valuable prognostic information without the need for a diagnostic lymph node dissection. Large patient studies have reported that tumors demonstrating LOH of chromosomes 11p, 11q 13q, 17p, and 22q are associated with increased incidence of lymph node metastasis *(108,109)*. Furthermore, LOH at loci 1p34, 3p25, 8p22, 13q12, 17p13, and 22q13 has been correlated with postoperative recurrence and poorer prognosis *(30,110)*. However, in multivariate analysis only 13q LOH and 17p LOH were independently predictive of outcome.

Many of these LOH events have been identified in early (ductal and lobular carcinoma *in situ*) and preneoplastic (hyperplasia and atypia) lesions *(104,106,111)*. Additionally, LOH has been identified in morphologically normal terminal duct lobular units adjacent to cancers as well as in stromal cells distant from tumors *(106,112)*. These findings suggest that early genetic alterations in breast tumors are heterogenous and do not follow conventional progression models described in colon cancer and melanoma *(8,9,113)*. Therefore, it is doubtful that a particular marker(s) will be useful as diagnostic screening tool. Alternatively, assessing body fluids for circulating nucleic acids that are tumor associated and patient specific may serve as a valuable surrogate for disease progression. Circulating DNA with LOH has been detected in the serum and plasma from breast cancer patients *(60,62,69,114,115)*. We have correlated tumor-specific DNA microsatellites in serum with advancing AJCC stage of breast cancer *(65)*. We postulated that this method may provide a novel approach for monitoring tumor-associated genetic changes in the blood of breast cancer patients and that plasma/serum analysis for LOH may be of clinical utility in detecting subclinical disease progression. In a follow-up study we assessed microsatellite alterations in the serum of 56 patients with early-stage breast cancer *(69)*. As expected, the incidence of circulating microsatellites for LOH was higher in patients with AJCC stage II disease (27%) than in patients with stage I disease (17%). Additionally, the presence of circulating LOH was associated with primary tumors that had increased proliferation indices as characterized by an increased diploid index, elevated MIB-1 fraction, and abnormal ploidy. This study included five patients with DCIS; LOH was not detected in serum from these patients.

The literature reports a 27–66% incidence of plasma LOH in breast cancer, reflecting a very heterogeneous population of tumors, many of which were relatively large and advanced *(60,62,114,115)*. During our preliminary investigations, we evaluated paired plasma and serum from patients and found greater yields of free DNA in serum using Picogreen assay. Presently, most studies in breast cancer have not assessed or demonstrated any correlation between LOH and clinical, pathologic, or outcome parameters. However, Silva et al. found a significant correlation between plasma DNA alterations and invasive ductal histology, three or more lymph nodes positive for metastasis, and a high proliferative index *(62)*. In a follow-up study, they showed that the preoperative presence of plasma LOH was significantly associated with a worse disease-free survival rate *(75)*.

The relative paucity of reports identifying circulating DNA in the plasma/serum of breast cancer patients partially reflects difficulty with at least some aspect of this technique *(114)*. Chen et al. demonstrated that they could improve detection of circulating LOH by assessing serum instead of plasma and by the addition of laser fluorescence and an automatic sequencer in place of radioactive autoradiography (48 vs 21%, respectively) *(60)*. Although they report a higher detection rate, all of the tumors were one centimeter or greater, and more than half were associated with lymph node involvement or unknown lymph node status, indicating more advanced disease. This technique may prove more sensitive than conventional densitometric analysis of standard gels, but additional direct comparisons are required.

Recently we have identified circulating microsatellite alterations in the bone marrow of patients with early-stage breast cancer *(116)*. The incidence was greater than that found in paired serum samples from the same patients. Bone marrow may be preferable to blood because the lower flow and less turbulent environment may permit pooling of tumor DNA.

Moreover, bone is the most frequent site of breast cancer metastasis and early detection may identify those patients at increased risk for relapse. Bone marrow analysis for LOH may be an important surrogate marker for systemic metastasis. These findings may corroborate the reported association between circulating tumor cells in bone marrow and worse prognosis *(117)*. Larger studies are needed with well-defined patient populations and long-term follow-up.

4.2. Melanoma

Melanoma is characterized by significant increasing genetic instability with advancing stage *(118–120)*. The most frequent genetic alteration in melanoma is allelic imbalance *(121–128)*. This occurs commonly at certain chromosome loci in a nonrandom manner, suggesting the involvement of putative tumor suppressor and metastasis inhibitory genes. LOH at chromosomes 9p21 and 10q23.3 occurs in regions of recognized tumor suppressor genes *p16/CDKN2A* and *PTEN/MMAC1*, respectively, and is frequently identified in tumors of all thickness, implicating an early potential role in the development and progression of primary melanomas *(124,129)*. In contrast, LOH on chromosome 6q and the distal arm of 1p occurs more frequently in thicker primary tumors and metastases *(13,124,130,131)*.

The demonstration of additional LOH events in systemic metastases suggests that genetic alterations continue to occur throughout disease progression and might serve as supplemental predictors of patient outcome. In an allelotypic analysis of 47 melanomas, Healy and colleagues found frequent 3p and 10q LOH in thin lesions; by comparison, 6q, 11q, and 17p LOH were predominant in thicker tumors *(123)*. LOH at 9p was most frequent and appeared in all tumor sizes. Melanoma appears to follow a tumor genetic progression model in which early LOH at 9p is followed by LOH at 10q, 3p, 6q, and later by LOH at 11q, 17p, and 1p *(9,118)*. To date, no molecular marker identified in primary melanomas has consistently shown independent prognostic utility. There is more convincing evidence to suggest that the frequency of LOH may be more predictive of patient outcome in melanoma and other cancers *(41,96,124,132)*. Careful scrutiny is warranted when reviewing frequency of allelic loss and patient outcome data because LOH increases with tumor size and other more aggressive histopathologic features; this must be considered in any statistical analysis.

We initially demonstrated the presence of circulating microsatellite markers in the plasma of melanoma patients and showed a significant concordance with genetic alterations in paired melanoma tumor tissues *(58)*. This early study evaluated ten microsatellite markers corresponding to six chromosome arms (1p, 3p, 6q, 9p, 10q, and 11q) that were associated with frequent LOH in melanoma tumors. Increased LOH frequency was significantly associated with advanced AJCC stage, but follow-up was too short for outcome correlations. In a second study, we evaluated preoperative plasma from 57 patients undergoing surgical resection of all clinically apparent disease. Again, LOH presence correlated significantly with stage of disease *(74)*. At a median follow-up of 21 mo, the presence of LOH was associated with a statistically significant reduction in overall survival of patients with stage III and IV melanoma. This correlation was particularly significant for the expression of microsatellite marker D1S228 alone or in combination with D9S157. Similarly, poorer prognosis has been ascribed to ovarian, gastrointestinal stromal tumors, adenocarcinomas of the colon, hematologic malignancies, and neuroblastomas that show LOH at these sites *(35,38,40,133,134)*. These two markers correspond to recognized tumor suppressor gene regions retinoblastoma (RB) and p16[INK4a], which play an integral role in cell cycle and differentiation *(135,136)*. In addition,

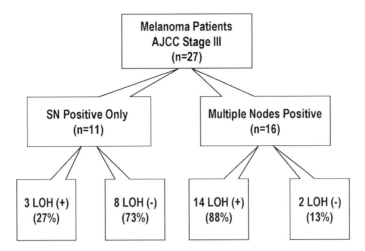

Fig. 6. Plasma LOH analysis relative to nodal tumor burden in same stage (III) melanoma patients undergoing sentinel lymph node (SLN) dissection followed by completion lymphadenectomy. First tier segregates patients according to lymph node involvement by H&E and IHC (for SLN) and second tier according to pre-operative plasma LOH status. +, plasma sample positive for LOH; –, plasma sample negative for LOH

when we evaluated the presence of lymph node involvement in stage III melanoma patients we found a correlation with plasma LOH and the number of lymph node metastases (Fig. 6). These results provide evidence that circulating nucleic acids demonstrating LOH not only correspond to subclinical tumor burden but also may have prognostic significance.

Recently, we have assessed the role of LOH as a molecular determinant of response to therapy. In this pilot study we retrospectively assessed serum collected from advanced melanoma patients at the time of enrollment onto a biochemotherapy protocol *(137)*. Because treatment with this regimen can be toxic and its outcome uncertain, we examined whether molecular analysis of serum could differentiate between responders and nonresponders to biochemotherapy *(138)*. At a median follow-up of 13 mo, we found an overall response rate of 56% (23 of 41 patients) LOH was present in serum from 12 of 41 (29%) patients and there was a significant association between biochemotherapy response rate and the absence of LOH. Only 2 of 23 (9%). responders demonstrated LOH, vs 10 of 18 (56%) nonresponders (multivariate analysis, $p = 0.003$). Furthermore, serum LOH was a statistically significant independent predictor of disease progression ($p = 0.003$). Current AJCC staging criteria do not consider treatment outcome *(139)*. Assessment of serum for molecular determinants provides a novel approach for evaluating prognosis and treatment response. Molecular diagnostics may improve risk stratification and identification of those patients most likely to benefit from a particular therapy.

4.3. Gastrointestinal

The presence of microsatellite alterations, including LOH and instability, has been well described for esophageal, gastric, colorectal, pancreatic, and hepatic tumors. Some of the earliest investigations of a molecular pathogenesis for cancer were described in colorectal cancers *(140–145)*. Vogelstein et al. established a genetic tumor progression model for colorectal cancer by characterizing the frequency of allelic deletions on chromosome 5q

(APC region), 17 and 18q, as well as the presence of *k-ras* mutation in advancing histologic stages of polyps and a set of invasive cancers *(8)*. Their findings identified the following temporal relationship: *k-ras* mutations occurred early during colorectal cancer development, with most presenting in adenomas larger than 1 cm, whereas 5q alterations became more prominent in larger adenomas often with some degree of dysplasia. This was followed by LOH of 18q in larger adenomas and finally by 17p LOH in invasive colorectal cancers. In a follow-up study, the same group showed that stage II and III colorectal cancer patients with 18q LOH in their primary tumors had a much worse 5 yr overall survival than same stage patients whose tumors did not contain this loss *(32)*.

The frequency of these tumor-specific genetic alterations led to their assessment in blood (plasma/serum) as unique molecular markers of disease. Hibi et al. performed a comprehensive assessment of 44 colorectal cancers and paired serum samples for LOH and microsatellite instability (MSI) using a panel of microsatellite markers mapped to chromosomes 18q, 17p, and 8p as well as mutational analysis for *p53* and *k-ras (70)*. Although 31 (70%) and 15 (34%) of 44 tumors had LOH and microsatellite instability, respectively, neither could be identified in the paired serum samples. In contrast, *k-ras* mutations were detected in the serum from 3 (19%) of 16 patients with positive tumors, and *p53* mutations were detected in 7 (70%) of 10 patients with this alteration in their primary tumor. Kolble et al. successfully demonstrated LOH and MSI in 7 (26%) and 13 (48%) of 27 serum samples, respectively, from patients with colorectal cancer *(59)*. LOH was most frequently demonstrated in serum from patients with extensive lymph node involvement or systemic metastasis, but no associations could be shown between tumor stage and patient outcome. These discouraging findings in plasma/serum have led many investigators to examine other sources, such as stool specimens, for the presence of tumor associated genetic markers that could be used for colorectal cancer diagnosis *(14,146,147)*.

k-ras mutation is under intense investigation because of its high frequency in gastrointestinal cancers *(148)*. Approximately 50% of colorectal and 90% of pancreatic tumors have *k-ras* mutations. Unlike other gene mutations, *k-ras* occurs most often at a single codon(12) which allows for a highly simplified and thus practical approach for developing a gene-based detection assay. Published series have identified circulating *k-ras* mutations in 19–86% of plasma/serum from colorectal cancer patients *(52,53,70)*. However, further refinements in specificity and sensitivity of the various assays are needed before this approach is uniformly accepted.

k-ras mutations may be more valuable for the diagnosis of pancreatic cancer. Although this disease represents only 2% of all new cancer cases in the United States each year, 80% of patients will die within 1 yr. Pancreatic cancer frequently develops and spreads without symptoms, making it difficult to diagnose and assess. Mutated *k-ras* has been detected in pancreatic secretions, biliary fluid, and duodenal juices from patients with pancreatic cancer *(16,149,150)*. Unfortunately, similar genetic aberrations in patients with chronic pancreatitis have limited the clinical application of this assay as a diagnostic marker for cancer *(151–154)*. Assessing plasma/serum has been proposed as an alternative because DNA levels are lower in blood than in pancreatic secretions; circulating levels of this DNA mutation are higher in patients with cancer vs those with chronic pancreatitis *(43,155)*. A review of the literature by Sorenson found a 53% overall incidence of *k-ras* mutation in plasma/serum from 144 patients *(156)*. He also noted an overall false-positive rate of only 2.5% in plasma/serum from normal healthy individuals, patients with nonmalignant pancreatic lesions, those with acute and chronic pancreatitis, and patients with non-*k-ras* mutant colorectal and pancreatic cancers. However, the sensitivity of detection was lower for blood than enteric secretions; thus, most patients whose serum contained *k-ras* mutation already had metastatic disease. Theodor et al., identified *k-ras* mutations in the serum from 14 (70%) of 20 patients diagnosed with pancreatic cancer and was able to improve the assay sensitivity to 95% by combining it with an elevated CA19-9 level *(155)*. Further studies are needed to evaluate the combination of markers, but the rarity of pancreatic cancer and the lack of disease-specific risk factors make any prospective marker investigation study unlikely. A more practical application would be as an aide in the diagnostic work-up of patients with a pancreatic mass or as a surrogate marker for monitoring subclinical disease progression.

4.4. Urologic

There are no proven tumor markers for urologic malignancies, except PSA for prostate cancer. Because symptom presentation is often subtle, molecular diagnostics would not only provide insight into the tumor's origin but might facilitate early detection. Urologic tumor types have been differentiated by unique alterations of chromosomal profile patterns. Initial studies were based on differences in cytogenetics *(3,157,158)*. Microsatellite markers that map chromosome regions with greater detail provide a precise tool for accurately assessing allelic imbalances. These markers can potentially distinguish between tumor types that are morphologically similar but have different biologic behaviors and treatments, such as lesions in the aerodigestive tract or in the collecting ducts of the kidney *(20,21,159–161)*.

Among renal cell carcinomas, of which clear cell histology accounts for the majority, LOH is a frequent event. In particular, 3p LOH occurs with a frequency of over 95%; most genetic aberrations present at the von Hippel-Lindau tumor suppressor gene site locus 3p25-26 *(162–164)*. In contrast to renal clear cell carcinomas, which arise in the proximal collecting tubules of the kidney, those tumors arising from the distal collecting ducts display a different pattern of LOH with frequent allelic loss on chromosome arms 1q, 6p, 8p, 13q, and 21q *(36,165)*. These results imply that proximal and distal renal cancers arise from distinct tumor genetic pathways and microsatellite analysis may facilitate their diagnosis as well as provide unique tumor-specific markers for plasma/serum/urine surveillance.

Based on 3p LOH frequency in renal cancers, Goessl et al. evaluated four microsatellite markers on this chromosome for LOH and MSI in the plasma of 40 patients with clear cell carcinoma *(54)*. LOH for at least one microsatellite marker was detected in plasma DNA from 25 (63%) patients, and 14 (35%) demonstrated LOH at more than one locus. MSI occurred in only one patient's tumor and another patient's plasma sample. No correlation with plasma LOH and tumor stage was found and outcome data was not evaluated. Although LOH specificity may be low for cancer screening, it may be useful for patient follow-up when combined with other microsatellite markers such as those found on chromosome 9 and 17 *(166,167)*. von Knobloch and colleagues used multiple fluorescent microsatellite markers and an automated laser sequencer to identify LOH in the serum of 20 (87%). of 23 patients with renal cell carcinoma, with 85% specificity *(168)*. Most frequent serum LOH detected was for 3p and 5q chromosomal regions. Although no association was found with tumor grade, this is the first study to correlate serum LOH with disease stage in kidney cancer patients. This same group evaluated serum and urine specimens from 39 patients with transitional cell carcinoma of the bladder cancer *(169)*. Serum LOH was present in 33 (85%) patients, and the most frequent alteration occurred on chromosome 8p. LOH on 8p was also the most frequent alteration in urine, but the incidence of LOH in urine was only 36%. There were no clinical correlations. The disparity may reflect differences in the stability and/or clearance of free DNA in blood vs urine.

Cairns et al. found frequent LOH on chromosome 9p in bladder tumors and Mao et al. demonstrated that identical microsatellite aberrations could be detected in the urine from patients with bladder cancer *(170,171)*. In a study of 20 patients with suspicious bladder lesions 19 demonstrated microsatellite alterations in their urine as compared to 50% of patients with abnormal cytologies suggesting the potential role of microsatellite analysis for bladder cancer screening *(51,172)*. Utting et al. analyzed tumors, plasma, serum, and urine from 44 patients with bladder cancer for six microsatellite markers on three chromosomes: 4, 9, and 17 *(173)*. The incidence of microsatellite alterations detected was as follows: tumor (27%), plasma (50%), serum (44%), and urine (54%). However, assay specificity for correctly identifying LOH for any of the body fluids evaluated was only 24–28%. The inconsistent results suggest that the presence of tumor DNA from these sources is highly variable. Clinically relevant microsatellite analysis of various body fluids to detect urologic malignancies or follow tumor progression will require specific tumor markers that are stable and obtained from a reliable source *(174)*.

4.5. Gynecologic

Ovarian cancer may go relatively unnoticed until considerable clinical symptoms become evident, at which time the disease is already advanced, and patient prognosis is poor. In addition, the pathogenesis for many of these tumors remains unknown *(175,176)*. A number of investigators have attempted to delineate the molecular events associated with ovarian carcinoma to:

1. Elucidate a tumor genetic cancer progression model.
2. Identify potential precursor lesions of invasive cancer.
3. Better characterize biologic behavior of morphologically similar tumor types.
4. Identify molecular markers of disease progression and potential targets for therapy.

It is becoming evident that diverse tumorigenic pathways for various ovarian cancers can be demonstrated by molecular genetics and that these findings may provide early detection markers *(177–181)*. Cliby and colleagues performed a comprehensive allelotypic analysis of 37 epithelial ovarian cancers using 70 polymorphic microsatellite markers and showed a high frequency of LOH for the following chromosome arms: 5q (43%); 6p (62%); 6q (57%); 7p (36%); 8p (40%); 9q (54%); 13q (56%); 14q (47%); 15q (36%); 17p (81%); 17q (76%); 18q (43%); 21q (36%); and 22q (71%) *(180)*. Moreover, they showed a significantly increased frequency of LOH for chromosome arms 6p, 13q, 17p, and 17q in high-grade as compared to low-grade tumors. Dodson et al. employed LOH analysis to explore whether genetic differences could be used to discriminate between low-grade, high-grade, and borderline epithelial ovarian cancers *(179)*. They found that LOH on chromosome arms 13q and 15q was significantly more frequent in high-grade tumors, LOH on 3p was more frequent in low-grade tumors, and LOH on 6p, 17p, and 17q was lost with equal frequency regardless of grade. The findings suggest that LOH during tumorigenesis occurs initially on chromosomes 6 and 17 and then on 13q and 15q. However, in this study, allelic loss was infrequent for low-grade and borderline tumors, and no common genetic events could be identified between borderline and invasive tumors. These findings are in agreement with other investigators

Table 1
ROC Curve Analysis of DNA Concentration in Patients With Cancer, Nonneoplastic Disease, and Healthy Donors

| Patient characteristics | No. of patients | DNA Concentration (ng/mL) | | ROC curve results |
		Median plasma	Range (10–90 percentile)	
Healthy	44	7	0–20	> 0.9
Nonneoplastic disease	164	16	7–71	
Cancer	122	59	10–844	> 0.74

Adapted from ref. *96*.

who reported an increased frequency of LOH from more mitotically active tumors *(69,111,178)*. To date no study has successfully divided different histologic tumor types based on characteristic LOH profile expression panels.

Iwabuchi et al. used CGH, LOH, and MSI analysis to evaluate various ovarian cancers for genetic changes *(181)*. They found a high rate of DNA-sequence copy number abnormalities in high-grade ovarian cancers as compared to low-grade tumors. Increased copy number abnormalities at 3q25-26 and 20q13 were most frequent in low-grade tumors whereas increased copy number abnormalities at 8q24 were more likely to occur in high-grade tumors. Tumors demonstrating many copy number abnormalities were associated with decreased patient survival. One of the first studies to demonstrate the presence of tumor-specific genetic alterations in body fluids of ovarian cancer patients was by Hickey and colleagues *(61)*. In their preliminary series, they found LOH in 17 (85%) of 20 patients' serum samples and 12 (63%) of 19 peritoneal fluid samples. Interestingly, they observed these findings in few early-stage patients using a select panel of six microsatel-lite markers on four chromosome arms. This provided an incentive for future investigations to evaluate circulating DNA markers as a diagnostic test for ovarian cancer.

The largest study of circulating DNA microsatellites for LOH as a diagnostic test for ovarian cancer was recently reported by Chang et al. *(96)*. Plasma was analyzed from 330 patients as follows: 54 with ovarian cancer, 68 with other non-ovarian cancers, 164 with nonneoplastic diseases and 44 healthy normal control donors. DNA was isolated using the QIAamp DNA Blood Kit; in most cases, 200 µL of plasma was quantitated with Picogreen. Results are summarized in Table 1. Digital single nucleotide polymorphism (SNP) PCR was performed to assess allelic imbalance in the plasma samples from 54 patients with ovarian cancer and 31 patients with nonneoplastic disease. All plasma samples had DNA concentrations greater than 50 ng/mL. The median number of informative markers per patient was four. When a cut-off level of 0.6 for allelic proportion was used to define imbalance, the results demonstrated a sensitivity of 87% for stage I/II and 95% for stage III/IV ovarian cancer patients. The AUROC curve was 0.95 when utilizing allelic imbalance to differentiate between 54 patients with ovarian cancer and 31 control patients with nonneoplastic disease. In contrast, the AUROC curve was 0.76 when plasma DNA concentration was used as a discriminant. Interestingly, the AUROC curve was 0.78 for CA 125. The AUROC curve increased to 0.84 when CA 125 was combined with plasma DNA concentration and used to evaluate serum from 45 patients with ovarian cancer and 18 patients with nonneoplastic diseases. The authors concluded that the sensitivity and specificity were too low for plasma DNA concentration alone to serve as a useful screening tool for ovarian cancer, but assessment of allelic imbalance using digital SNP analysis might show promise. Digital SNP technology is costly and rigorous to perform. Certain technical issues need to be resolved and validated prior to widespread acceptance of this approach.

Cervical cancer is one of the most frequent gynecologic malignancies worldwide *(182)*. Detailed molecular analysis has identified human papilloma virus (HPV) types 16 and 18 as most commonly associated with cervical cancer. After HPV DNA integration into the host genome, the specific expression of viral oncogenes E6 and E7, most often from HPV types 16 and 18, leads to genomic instability and subsequent neoplastic transformation of the cervical epithelial cell. Although HPV infection is causally related to the development of cervical cancer, most women with HPV infection will not develop a malignancy *(183–186)*. To further elucidate specific genetic events associated with cervical cancer, Kersemaekers and colleagues assessed 67 stage IB and IIA cervical cancers with 81 microsatellite markers *(37)*. Although LOH occurred frequently on chromosomes 3p, 4p, 6p, 6q, 11q, 17p, and 18q, only 18q LOH correlated significantly with decreased overall survival. Correlations with other known clinical and pathologic prognostic parameters were not significant. The same group evaluated ten patients with cervical intraepithelial neoplasia (CIN) and synchronous invasive carcinomas and lymph node metastasis to chronicle the genetic events associated with cancer progression *(10)*. They found frequent LOH on chromosome arms 3p, 6p, and 11q for CIN lesions, with additional LOH at 6q, 17p, and 18q for the corresponding invasive component. Lymph node metastasis was associated with additional LOH on chromosome X. Mitra et al. found LOH on chromosomes 1q, 3q, 5q, 10q, 11p, and 18p in 26–42% of cervical cancers *(187)*. LOH was most frequent on chromosomes 4q (46%) and 5p (53%). These authors identified a potential tumor suppressor gene site at locus 5p15 and suggested its role as a potential marker for progression of precancerous cervical lesions *(188)*. Interestingly, HPV status did not correlate with any of the sites showing frequent LOH. In a comprehensive allelotypic analysis of cervix tumors, Mullokandov et al. reported a 39–43% incidence of LOH for 3p, 6p, and 18q *(189)*. No pattern of LOH could be identified and no correlation with HPV status could be demonstrated. It appears that 3p LOH is an early event in cervical carcinoma, most often preceded by HPV infection, whereas 1p LOH occurs later during tumor progression and is most often noted in metastatic lesions *(190–192)*. The genetic alterations that develop between these two anchoring events remain far from resolved.

The Pap smear remains the standard for diagnosis of cervical cancer, but its analysis is subjective. In an attempt to improve the diagnostic efficacy of cervical cytology, Rha et al. used nine microsatellite markers to evaluate Pap smears from 21 patients *(193)*. Microsatellite alterations were detected in smears from 16 (76%) patients. However, only 11 (85%) of 13 invasive squamous cell cancers and 5 (63%) of 8 earlier CIN lesions were identified, suggesting inferior sensitivity. In contrast, genetic alterations were detected in two cytologically normal Pap smears. Outcomes were not available but one may speculate a role for microsatellite analysis when the Pap smear is suspicious but not diagnostic. Recently this group assessed plasma HPV-16 and HPV-18 E7 DNA levels in patients with cervical cancer *(194)*. HPV DNA was identified in only 11 (6.9%) of 175 cases of invasive cancer and 1 (1.8%) of 57 patients with pre-invasive disease. A similarly low incidence of HPV DNA has been found in the pretreatment serum of cervical cancer patients *(195)*. These findings demonstrate the limited diagnostic utility of this blood assay. Its role as a potential marker for recurrent disease will require further evaluation.

4.6. Lung

The identification of circulating DNA in plasma/serum for LOH was first reported in lung cancer in 1996, in the same journal issue as that for head and neck cancers *(49,50)*. Because lung cancer is one of the most frequent cancer diagnoses and remains the leading cause of cancer death worldwide, numerous reports have focused on the potential clinical utility of prominent genetic changes in this disease. Lung cancer is associated with a significant degree of genomic instability of which the most frequently reported events include LOH and MSI; both have been identified in patients' plasma samples *(196,197)*.

In their original report Chen et al. used three markers corresponding to chromosomes 6, 21, and X to detect microsatellite alterations (LOH or MSI) in 16 (76%) tumor specimens and 15 (71%) plasma samples from 21 patients with small cell lung cancer (SCLC), with excellent concordance *(49)*. Using those same markers in 43 patients with SCLC, Bruhn et al. found that the incidence of microsatellite alterations was 19% in tumors and 25% in plasma samples, but concordance between tumor and plasma was only 40% *(196)*. Differences between the two studies are attributed to different techniques and degrees of clinical tumor burden.

Sanchez-Cespedes et al. used four microsatellite markers that map to chromosome 3p to evaluate serum from 22 patients with non-SCLC. Serum specimens from 6 patients (28%) contained alterations, and in four patients these were identical to those in the primary tumor for at least one of the markers assessed *(57)*. No clinical correlations were made in this study.

Gonzalez et al. utilized the same three microsatellite markers as Chen and others in conjunction with an assessment for TP53 mutations in the plasma of 35 SCLC patients *(66)*. They found concordance for at least one molecular marker in 71% of cases. Although no difference in survival was demonstrated with respect to the presence or absence of plasma alterations, those patients with plasma TP53 mutation and microsatellite alterations demonstrated a significantly reduced overall survival rate as compared to other patients. In less than one-half of all of the cases, a correlation was found between regression or progression of the tumor and the loss or persistence of the plasma DNA abnormality, respectively. Chromosomal alterations including allelic imbalance and mutations such as *k-ras* and TP53 occur more frequently in lung cancers from smokers than non-smokers, and therefore may represent a potential screening tool in this high-risk population *(198–200)*. LOH on chromosomes 3p, 6q, 9p, 16p 17p, 19p, and *k-ras* mutations were demonstrated more often in adenocarcinomas from smokers than nonsmokers, however clinical correlations with patient outcome are inconsistent and lacking *(31,201)*.

Others have assessed sputum and bronchoalveolar lavage fluid for genetic changes associated with lung cancers but in general assay sensitivities were low and sample sizes were small *(15,170)*. Radiographic imaging, fiberoptic bronchoscopic examination, and cytologic sputum analysis have shown limited effectiveness for early cancer diagnosis and their routine use has yet to demonstrate a survival advantage. The field of molecular diagnostics offers promise, but highly specific markers with improved sensitivity must be demonstrated in large-scale clinical trials.

4.7. Head and Neck

The first report to document circulating microsatellite alterations in serum was assessed in patients with head and neck cancer *(50)*. This group had previously demonstrated microsatellite alterations in lung and bladder tumors and found similar alterations in corresponding sputum and urine samples, respectively, leading to speculation that shed tumor-associated free DNA may serve as "clonal markers for cancer detection" *(170)*. This theory was tested by screening serum samples from 21 head and neck squamous cell cancer patients with a panel of 12 microsatellite markers. These markers mapped to chromosome sites 3p, 9p, and 17p which were likely to harbor tumor suppressor genes and to two chromosomes regions on 14 and 21 which demonstrated a high propensity for MSI in primary tumors *(50)*. Microsatellite alterations were found in 18 (86%) primary tumors and 6 (29%) serum samples. All alterations in serum were also identified in the corresponding primary tumor. More relevant was the statistically significant association between the presence of serum tumor DNA and poor outcome. It must be noted that many patients had advanced disease, which may have contributed to the favorable clinical correlations. Additionally, almost one-half of the patients with no detectable serum alterations had advanced disease. Thus, the assay's sensitivity was limited.

Microsatellite markers have been used in the field of head and neck cancer to characterize site of origin for unknown primary aerodigestive tract tumors *(21)*, to establish a genetic basis for field cancerization *(22,202,203)*, to assess occult primary and recurrent oral malignancies *(202)*, and to differentiate between various salivary gland tumors *(159)*. These reports demonstrate the vast potential clinical applicability for microsatellite analyses. However, although primary head and neck squamous cell carcinoma (HNSCC) is associated with a number of genetic alterations (with greater than 70% of LOH noted on chromosome 9p; 50% LOH on chromosomes 3, 11q, 13q, and 17p; and greater than 35% LOH on chromosomes 4, 6p, 8, 14q, and 19q), few evaluations have shown prognostic significance *(204,205)*. A study that used 20 microsatellite markers to assess LOH at 14q in 73 primary HNSCC demonstrated an incidence of LOH of 40% for at least one loci *(39)*. Among 53 patients with known clinical outcome, those with primary tumors showing LOH for any one marker, had a three-fold higher risk of death than patients whose primary tumors retained heterozygosity at 14q. Again, most patients (79%) had stage III/IV disease; the fact that no specific marker had particular prognostic significance may merely reflect the overall genomic instability associated with more progressive disease.

Molecular markers may serve as indicators of more advanced disease and/or aggressive tumors that are not appreciated by current staging criteria. The detection of increasing amounts of circulating DNA alterations may serve as a surrogate marker of subclinical tumor burden and/or as a minimally invasive procedure for monitoring the increasing tumor instability that is associated with progression. The identification of those genetic aberrations that occur in premalignant head and neck lesions and have greater predictive value as a stratification factor for those morphologically similar lesions at increased risk for progression may be more informative. This has been demonstrated in leukoplakic lesions that express deletions at 3p14 and 9p21 *(24,25,206,207)*.

4.8. Nasopharyngeal

Nasopharyngeal carcinoma (NPC), relatively uncommon in the Western world, is one of the most frequent malignancies in Southeast Asia; it is endemic in China and Hong Kong.

The detection of markedly elevated circulating levels of Epstein-Barr virus (EBV) antibody titers in almost all patients with NPC led to the presumption of a viral etiology *(208,209)*. The identification of EBV DNA in NPC tumors confirmed the association; however, the demonstration of identical EBV DNA terminal repeat sequences among common primary tumors, carcinomas *in situ* and dyplastic lesions suggests clonal progression from an infected progenitor cell *(210)*. Although EBV infection is an early event in NPC development, the fact that most viral transforming genes are not expressed in these tumors suggests that other genetic changes, such as loss of tumor suppressor genes, are required for tumorgenesis *(211)*. Genetic aberrations demonstrated in NPC include LOH on chromosomes 3, 5, 6, 9, 11, 14, 16, and 17; the most frequent sites of LOH (i.e., greater than 30%) are on chromosomes 3p, 9p, 11q, 13q, and 14q *(212,213)*. These losses identified by CGH have been further delineated by microsatellite analysis.

LOH of 3p is one of the most frequent genetic events in NPC and in one investigation it was reported in 100% of informative cases, most frequently at loci 3p14 and 3p25 (RAF-1 locus) *(214)*. However, only half of the tumors were informative for any one marker. In contrast, EBV DNA was identified in all 36 tumors. The findings demonstrate limitations of LOH analysis compared to analysis based on gene amplification. LOH assesses for allelic loss, which is more difficult to evaluate among a background of normal wild-type DNA than a chromosomal gain, particularly when the gain is a heterotopic fragment. Allelic analysis can be confounded by contamination from normal DNA as well as its relative "uninformativity" for any given marker in any particular patient.

LOH has also been described distally on the short arm of chromosome 3 in the VHL region, but mutations of this gene in NPC appear infrequent *(215,216)*. Likewise, frequent LOH has been described on chromosome 9. In one study, up to 61% (11 of 18 cases) of tumors demonstrated an allelic deletion when assessed with a panel of 21 microsatellite markers *(217)*. Many of these deletions included the p15 and p16 tumor suppressor gene regions and were bi-allelic. Failure to find significant point mutations suggests that homozygous genetic deletions may be the dominant mechanism for NPC development *(218)*. Additionally, LOH on chromosome 11 occurs frequently in NPC; one study reported a 54% incidence among 52 primary tumors *(219)*. Two separate sites of frequent major chromosome deletions were identified: 11q13.2-22 and 11q22-24. Genes *PYGM, cyclin D1, FOLR1* and the proto-oncogene *INT-2* reside in the 11q13 region, whereas the *ATM* gene is found in the 11q22-23 region. Recently, 14q LOH has been shown to occur quite frequently (74%) *(220)*. These findings were confirmed by another group that evaluated a series of 60 patients and found 78% LOH on 13q and 80% LOH on 14q. LOH at 3q31-q32 correlated with a lower level of EBV infection, whereas LOH at 14q was associated with more poorly differentiated tumors *(221)*.

A recent study performed a comprehensive allelotyping of 27 microdissected NPC primary tumors. Allelic losses were greater than 80% on 3p, 9p, 9q, 11q, and 14q, greater than 70% on 11q and 12q, greater than 50% on 13q and 16q, but only 35–50% on 1p, 5q and 12p. Similar findings have been reported by Miturangura et al. with the additional demonstration of LOH at 3q, 6p, 19q,and 22q between 35 and 50% *(222)*. Despite these findings, the unique association of EBV DNA in almost all tumors makes this a highly desirable molecular marker for this disease. Miturangura et al. successfully identified circulating EBV DNA in the serum from 13 (31%) of 42 NPC patients *(56)*. In this pilot trial, no prominent correlations could be demonstrated with clinical data or tumor pathology. Lo et al. used a highly sensitive quantitative PCR technique to detect EBV DNA in the plasma from 55 (96%) of 57 patients *(72)*. The median copy number of EBV DNA was 47,047/mL in patients with stage III/IV disease and only 5918/mL in patients with stage I/II disease. Seven of the 15 patients who received radiotherapy had complete remission of their disease and plasma EBV DNA levels became undetectable; six of the remaining eight patients with persistently elevated EBV DNA copy levels (75%) demonstrated residual or progressive disease. In a follow-up study, the same investigators showed that a rise in circulating EBV DNA predicted disease recurrence whereas a persistently undetectable level correlated with clinical remissions.

Lo et al. speculated that an initial rise in free EBV DNA after the initiation of radiotherapy most likely reflected tumor lysis *(223)*. The "decay rate" of this circulating EBV DNA was assessed in serial bleeds from patients undergoing treatment. The median half-life was determined to be 3.8 d. In a larger study, evaluating 170 NPC patients undergoing radiotherapy alone, this group found that elevated post-treatment EBV plasma DNA levels were more significantly associated with recurrence than elevated pretreatment levels: relative risk ratio 11.9 (95% confidence interval [CI] = 5.53 to 25.43) vs 2.5 (95% CI = 1.14 to 5.70), respectively *(224)*. Because of the uniqueness of this disease, its associated highly specific DNA marker, the homogenous treatment regimen, and the logistics of performing serial blood assessments, these studies remain pivotal in the assessment of plasma kinetics of tumor-associated circulating nucleic acid markers *(225–232)*.

5. PITFALLS AND CONSIDERATIONS

Current advances in molecular oncology have transformed microsatellite marker evaluations into a powerful tool for the identification of genes associated with malignancy. Microsatellite analysis has been used to diagnose cancer, evaluate recurrence, assess response to therapy, and predict outcome. Many early studies evaluated primary tumor tissue. However, the usefulness of this specimen is limited by genotypic heterogeneity among tumor cells and by infiltration with normal cells including lymphocytes and macrophages. More importantly, assessment of primary tumors cannot reflect the ongoing tumor alterations that characterize progression and metastasis. By contrast, assessment of plasma/serum for circulating tumor DNA is a minimally invasive approach that is logistically practical for serial genetic analysis and may prove clinically relevant because it is dynamic rather than static in nature.

Microsatellite analysis can detect chromosomal alterations, but marker selection has been too inconsistent to allow clinically relevant application across various patient populations. Moreover, LOH results are affected by the primer sequences selected, the labeling technique used, and the purity and quality of the commercially prepared marker product. PCR must be optimized on test samples prior to a definitive analysis. Care must be taken to avoid DNA contamination and to follow strictly established standard operating techniques that include separate designated areas for tissue/body fluid sample processing, DNA extraction, pre-PCR set-up, and PCR thermocycling. Methodologies for post PCR product analysis include standard gel electrophoresis followed by autoradiography of radioisotope or nonradioisotope products with densitometric analysis or laser scanning of fluorescently labeled products. Recently, CAE using an automated sequencer has been employed for fluorescent microsatellite analysis. This is extremely accurate for high-throughput evaluation of multiple samples. Results are shown as peaks instead of bands, and the area under the peak represents post-PCR product amount. LOH is calculated from the ratios of peak heights.

However, a multicenter trial found no superiority in sensitivity with this technique as compared to conventional gel analysis *(233)*. Other approachs for screening LOH now include single nucleotide polymorphism analysis (SNPs).

Currently, no standard exists for defining LOH. A positive LOH result has been described for allelic ratios of 25–80%; this wide range reflects contamination of tumor DNA with normal DNA. A variety of methods have been proposed for extracting DNA from body fluids and tissues *(92,234–237)*. Laser capture microdissection (LCM), which permits selective extraction of single cells from a tumor specimen, can avoid contamination of tissue specimens, but cannot be used for serum and plasma *(238)*. LOH assessment of DNA from blood depends on the method of blood processing. Some laboratories allow the plasma/serum to sit at room temperature while others heat the sample before processing; both techniques appear to enrich circulating DNA levels and may affect the purity of results.

Microsatellite analysis requires the comparison of tumor DNA to each patient's normal genomic DNA. For tissue and body fluid analyses, we recommend peripheral blood lymphocytes, which can be readily collected and processed for DNA. Retrospective tissue analysis often uses morphologically normal tissue from the tumor specimen, but adjacent normal-appearing tissue may contain genetic alterations identical to those in the tumor *(112)*. We therefore suggest utilizing normal-appearing tissue furthest from the tumor, preferably with a mixed cell type to enhance the chance of having a predominance of normal DNA.

Ideally, a tumor marker should be highly selective for occult tumor, highly specific for cancer, closely correlated with extent of disease, stable in plasma/serum, and easy to assess. Because tumor initiation and progression is associated with a variety of different genetic alterations that are not consistent for most tumor types, assessing multiple markers may improve results. The multimarker approach also accommodates the heterogeneity that exists within a tumor and among tumor lesions from the same patient. Protein markers are stable, easy to detect, and can be readily quantitated, but their limited sensitivity and specificity are suboptimal for screening and early diagnosis. mRNA markers are more sensitive and specific, but mRNA is relatively unstable and often require fresh/frozen tissue. Assay efficiencies can vary with specific primer sets, and false positives may result from the presence of pseudogenes, illegitimate expression, and/or contaminating RNA and DNA sequences *(239)*. More importantly, specificity is affected by any change in the expression or the abundance of gene transcription. Sources of these changes include tumor heterogeneity, cytokines, growth factors, hormones, and the tumor microenvironment. DNA-based methods are highly specific for tumor cell detection, however DNA PCR amplification is less sensitive than RT-PCR because of a lower copy number per cell *(73)*. Variations in clonal selection and deletion may affect results in a similar fashion as for mRNA assays.

6. CONCLUSION

Assessment of circulating genetic markers provides an appealing approach for monitoring subclinical disease progression and response to treatment in cancer patients. These molecular surrogates may eventually be used to screen high-risk populations for cancer and to develop novel therapeutics more patient specific. Serial assessment of blood and/or body fluids for tumor-specific molecular genetic alterations may provide valuable prognostic information that is less static and more practical than standard tumor analyses. We do not understand the mechanisms that elevate levels of circulating nucleic acids in cancer patients—is DNA released from tumor cells undergoing apoptosis, necrosis or is there a means for active release? *(45,71,240–242)*. Additionally, we do not know whether certain chromosome loci DNA may be more efficient in "surviving" in blood and for how long. Nor do we know whether free tumor DNA is from circulating tumor cells, the primary tumor site, occult subclinical lesions, or metastasis. Further translational studies will help answer these questions and should firmly establish the role of these circulating DNA markers in cancer detection.

ACKNOWLEDGMENTS

From the Gonda (Goldschmied) Research Laboratories of the John Wayne Cancer Institute. Supported in part by the California Breast Cancer Research Program Grant 7WB-0021, NCI P01CA29605 and P01CA12582, Department of Defense DAMD-17-03-1-0261, the Ben B. and Joyce E. Eisenberg Foundation (Los Angeles), Rachel Goodman Cancer Research Grant and the Fashion Footwear Association of New York. We wish to thank Ms. Gwen Berry for outstanding editorial assistance. We apologize to studies not cited in this review due to space.

REFERENCES

1. Knudson AG Jr. 1971. Mutation and cancer: statistical study of retinoblastoma. Proc. Natl. Acad. Sci. USA 68:820–823.
2. Kallioniemi A, Kallioniemi OP, Sudar D, et al. 1992. Comparative genomic hybridization for molecular cytogenetic analysis of solid tumors. Science 258:818–821.
3. Gray JW, Kallioniemi A, Kallioniemi O, Pallavicini M, Waldman F, Pinkel, D. 1992. Molecular cytogenetics: diagnosis and prognostic assessment. Curr. Opin. Biotechnol. 3:623–631.
4. Mertens F, Johansson B, Hoglund M, Mitelman F. 1997. Chromosomal imbalance maps of malignant solid tumors: a cytogenetic survey of 3185 neoplasms. Cancer Res. 57:2765–2780.
5. Mitelman F, Johansson B, Mandahl N, Mertens F. 1997. Clinical significance of cytogenetic findings in solid tumors. Cancer Genet. Cytogenet. 95:1–8.
6. Beckman JS and Weber JL. 1992. Survey of human and rat microsatellites. Genomics 12: 627–631.
7. Weber JL and May PE. 1989. Abundant class of human DNA polymorphisms which can be typed using the polymerase chain reaction. Am. J. Hum. Genet. 44:388–396.
8. Vogelstein B, Fearon ER, Hamilton SR, et al. 1988. Genetic alterations during colorectal-tumor development. N. Engl. J. Med. 319:525–532.
9. Walker GJ, Palmer JM, Walters MK, Hayward NK. 1995. A genetic model of melanoma tumorigenesis based on allelic losses. Genes Chromosomes Cancer 12:134–141.
10. Kersemaekers AM, van de Vijver MJ, Kenter GG, Fleuren GJ. 1999. Genetic alterations during the progression of squamous cell carcinomas of the uterine cervix. Genes Chromosomes Cancer 26:346–354.
11. Losi L, Benhattar J, Costa J. 1992. Stability of K–*ras* mutations throughout the natural history of human colorectal cancer. Eur. J. Cancer 28:1115–1120.
12. Nakayama T, Taback B, Turner R, Morton DL, Hoon DS. 2001. Molecular clonality of in-transit melanoma metastasis. Am. J. Pathol. 158:1371–1378.
13. Morita R, Fujimoto A, Hatta N, Takehara K, Takata M. 1998. Comparison of genetic profiles between primary melanomas and their metastases reveals genetic alterations and clonal evolution during progression. J. Invest. Dermatol. 111:919–924.
14. Dong SM, Traverso G, Johnson C, et al. 2001. Detecting colorectal cancer in stool with the use of multiple genetic targets. J. Natl. Cancer Inst. 93:858–865.
15. Ahrendt SA, Chow JT, Xu LH, et al. 1999. Molecular detection of tumor cells in bronchoalveolar lavage fluid from patients with early stage lung cancer. J. Natl. Cancer. Inst. 91:332–339.

16. Tada M, Omata M, Kawai S, et al. 1993. Detection of *ras* gene mutations in pancreatic juice and peripheral blood of patients with pancreatic adenocarcinoma. Cancer Res. 53:2472–2474.

17. Hayashi N, Arakawa H, Nagase H, et al. 1994. Genetic diagnosis identifies occult lymph node metastases undetectable by the histopathological method. Cancer Res. 54:3853–3856.

18. Hashimoto T, Kobayashi Y, Ishikawa Y, et al. 2000. Prognostic value of genetically diagnosed lymph node micrometastasis in non-small cell lung carcinoma cases. Cancer Res. 60: 6472–6478.

19. Yamada T, Nakamori S, Ohzato H, et al. 2000. Outcome of pancreatic cancer patients based on genetic lymph node staging. Int. J. Oncol. 16:1165–1171.

20. Califano J, van der Riet P, Westra W, et al. 1996. Genetic progression model for head and neck cancer: implications for field cancerization. Cancer Res. 56:2488–2492.

21. Califano J, Westra WH, Koch W, et al. 1999. Unknown primary head and neck squamous cell carcinoma: molecular identification of the site of origin. J. Natl. Cancer Inst. 91:599–604.

22. Califano J, Westra WH, Meininger G, Corio R, Koch WM, Sidransky D. 2000. Genetic progression and clonal relationship of recurrent premalignant head and neck lesions. Clin. Cancer Res. 6:347–352.

23. Brennan JA, Mao L, Hruban RH, et al. 1995. Molecular assessment of histopathological staging in squamous-cell carcinoma of the head and neck. N. Engl. J. Med. 332:429–435.

24. Zhang L, Cheung KJ Jr, Lam WL, et al. 2001. Increased genetic damage in oral leukoplakia from high risk sites: potential impact on staging and clinical management. Cancer 91: 2148–2155.

25. Rosin MP, Cheng X, Poh C, et al. 2000. Use of allelic loss to predict malignant risk for low-grade oral epithelial dysplasia. Clin. Cancer Res. 6:357–362.

26. Harima Y, Sawada S, Nagata K, Sougawa M, Ohnishi,T. 2001. Chromosome 6p21.2, 18q21.2 and human papilloma virus (HPV) DNA can predict prognosis of cervical cancer after radiotherapy. Int. J. Cancer 96:286–296.

27. Tsuneizumi M, Emi M, Hirano A, et al. 2002. Association of allelic loss at 8p22 with poor prognosis among breast cancer cases treated with high-dose adjuvant chemotherapy. Cancer Lett. 180:75–82.

28. Utada Y, Emi M, Yoshimoto M, et al. 2000. Allelic loss at 1p34–36 predicts poor prognosis in node-negative breast cancer. Clin. Cancer Res. 6:3193–3198.

29. Utada Y, Haga S, Kajiwara T, et al. 2000. Allelic loss at the 8p22 region as a prognostic factor in large and estrogen receptor negative breast carcinomas. Cancer 88:1410–1416.

30. Emi M, Yoshimoto M, Sato T, et al. 1999. Allelic loss at 1p34, 13q12, 17p13.3, and 17q21.1 correlates with poor postoperative prognosis in breast cancer. Genes Chromosomes Cancer 26:134–141.

31. Zhou X, Kemp BL, Khuri FR, et al. 2000. Prognostic implication of microsatellite alteration profiles in early-stage non-small cell lung cancer. Clin. Cancer Res. 6:559–565.

32. Jen J, Kim H, Piantadosi S, et al. 1994. Allelic loss of chromosome 18q and prognosis in colorectal cancer. N. Engl. J. Med. 331:213–221.

33. Gryfe R, Kim H, Hsieh ET, et al. 2000. Tumor microsatellite instability and clinical outcome in young patients with colorectal cancer. N. Engl. J. Med. 342:69–77.

34. Watanabe T, Wu TT, Catalano PJ, et al. 2001. Molecular predictors of survival after adjuvant chemotherapy for colon cancer. N. Engl. J. Med. 344:1196–1206.

35. Ogunbiyi OA, Goodfellow PJ, Gagliardi G, et al. 1997. Prognostic value of chromosome 1p allelic loss in colon cancer. Gastroenterology 113:761–766.

36. Schoenberg M, Cairns P, Brooks JD, et al. 1995. Frequent loss of chromosome arms 8p and 13q in collecting duct carcinoma (CDC) of the kidney. Genes Chromosomes Cancer 12:76–80.

37. Kersemaekers AM, Kenter GG, Hermans J, Fleuren GJ, van de Vijver MJ. 1998. Allelic loss and prognosis in carcinoma of the uterine cervix. Int. J. Cancer 79:411–417.

38. Alvarez AA, Lambers AR, Lancaster JM, et al. 2001. Allele loss on chromosome 1p36 in epithelial ovarian cancers. Gynecol. Oncol. 82:94–98.

39. Lee DJ, Koch WM, Yoo G, et al. 1997. Impact of chromosome 14q loss on survival in primary head and neck squamous cell carcinoma. Clin. Cancer Res. 3:501–505.

40. O'Leary T, Ernst S, Przygodzki R, Emory T, Sobin L. 1999. Loss of heterozygosity at 1p36 predicts poor prognosis in gastrointestinal stromal/smooth muscle tumors. Lab. Invest. 79: 1461–1467.

41. Hampl M, Hampl JA, Reiss G, Schackert G, Saeger HD, Schackert HK. 1999. Loss of heterozygosity accumulation in primary breast carcinomas and additionally in corresponding distant metastases is associated with poor outcome. Clin. Cancer Res. 5:1417–1425.

42. Leon SA, Shapiro B, Sklaroff DM, Yaros MJ. 1977. Free DNA in the serum of cancer patients and the effect of therapy. Cancer Res. 37:646–650.

43. Shapiro B, Chakrabarty M, Cohn EM, Leon SA. 1983. Determination of circulating DNA levels in patients with benign or malignant gastrointestinal disease. Cancer 51:2116–2120.

44. Stroun M, Anker P, Lyautey J, Lederrey C, Maurice PA. 1987. Isolation and characterization of DNA from the plasma of cancer patients. Eur. J. Cancer. Clin. Oncol. 23:707–712.

45. Stroun M, Anker P, Maurice P, Lyautey J, Lederrey C, Beljanski M. 1989. Neoplastic characteristics of the DNA found in the plasma of cancer patients. Oncology 46:318–322.

46. Maebo A. 1990. Plasma DNA level as a tumor marker in primary lung cancer. Nihon Kyobu Shikkan Gakkai Zasshi. 28:1085–1091.

47. Sorenson GD, Pribish,DM, Valone FH, Memoli VA, Bzik DJ, Yao SL. 1994. Soluble normal and mutated DNA sequences from single-copy genes in human blood. Cancer Epidemiol. Biomarkers Prev. 3:67–71.

48. Vasioukhin V, Anker P, Maurice P, Lyautey J, Lederrey C, Stroun M. 1994. Point mutations of the *N-ras* gene in the blood plasma DNA of patients with myelodysplastic syndrome or acute myelogenous leukaemia. Br. J. Hematol. 86:774–779.

49. Chen XQ, Stroun M, Magnenat JL, et al. 1996. Microsatellite alterations in plasma DNA of small cell lung cancer patients. Nat. Med. 2:1033–1035.

50. Nawroz H, Koch W, Anker P, Stroun M, Sidransky D. 1996. Microsatellite alterations in serum DNA of head and neck cancer patients. Nat. Med. 2:1035–1037.

51. Mao L, Schoenberg MP, Scicchitano,M, et al. 1996. Molecular detection of primary bladder cancer by microsatellite analysis. Science 271:659–662.

52. Anker P, Lefort F, Vasioukhin V, et al. 1997. K-*ras* mutations are found in DNA extracted from the plasma of patients with colorectal cancer. Gastroenterology 112:1114–1120.

53. Kopreski MS, Benko FA, Kwee C, et al. 1997. Detection of mutant K-*ras* DNA in plasma or serum of patients with colorectal cancer. Br. J. Cancer 76:1293–1299.

54. Goessl C, Heicappell R, Munker R, et al. 1998. Microsatellite analysis of plasma DNA from patients with clear cell renal carcinoma. Cancer Res. 58:4728–4732.

55. Mulcahy HE, Lyautey J, Lederrey C, et al. 1998. A prospective study of K-*ras* mutations in the plasma of pancreatic cancer patients. Clin. Cancer Res. 4:271–275.

56. Mutirangura A, Pornthanakasem W, Theamboonlers A, et al. Epstein-Barr viral DNA in serum of patients with nasopharyngeal carcinoma. Clin. Cancer Res. 1998. 4:665–669.

57. Sanchez-Cespedes M, Monzo M, Rosell R, et al. 1998. Detection of chromosome 3p alterations in serum DNA of non-small-cell lung cancer patients. Ann. Oncol. 9:113–116.

58. Fujiwara Y, Chi DDJ, Wang H, et al. 1999. Plasma DNA microsatellites as tumor-specific markers and indicators of tumor progression in melanoma patients. Cancer Res. 59:1567–1571.

59. Kolble K, Ullrich OM, Pidde H, et al. 1999. Microsatellite alterations in serum DNA of patients with colorectal cancer. Lab. Invest. 79:1145–1150.

60. Chen X, Bonnefoi H, Diebold-Berger S, et al. 1999. Detecting tumor-related alterations in plasma or serum DNA of patients diagnosed with breast cancer. Clin. Cancer Res. 5: 2297–2303.

61. Hickey KP, Boyle KP, Jepps HM, Andrew AC, Buxton EJ, Burns PA. 1999. Molecular detection of tumour DNA in serum and peritoneal fluid from ovarian cancer patients. Br. J. Cancer 80:1803–1808.

62. Silva JM, Dominguez G, Garcia JM, et al. 1999. Presence of tumor DNA in plasma of breast cancer patients: clinicopathological correlations. Cancer Res. 59:3251–3256.

63. Silva JM, Dominguez G, Villanueva MJ, et al. 1999. Aberrant DNA methylation of the p16INK4a gene in plasma DNA of breast cancer patients. Br. J. Cancer 80:1262–1264.

64. Silva JM, Gonzalez R, Dominguez G, Garcia JM, Espana P, Bonilla F. 1999. TP53 gene mutations in plasma DNA of cancer patients. Genes Chromosomes Cancer 24:160–161.

65. Taback B, Giuliano AE, Nguyen DH, et al. 2000. Tumor-related free DNA microsatellites detected in breast cancer patients serum correlates with disease progression. Proc. Am. Soc. Clin. Oncol. 19:606a.

66. Gonzalez R, Silva JM, Sanchez A, et al. 2000. Microsatellite alterations and TP53 mutations in plasma DNA of small-cell lung cancer patients: follow-up study and prognostic significance. Ann. Oncol. 11:1097–1104.

67. Mulcahy HE, Lyautey J, Lederrey C, et al. 2000. Plasma DNA K-*ras* mutations in patients with gastrointestinal malignancies. Ann. NY Acad. Sci. 906:25–28.

68. Mutirangura A. 2001. Serum/plasma viral DNA: mechanisms and diagnostic applications to nasopharyngeal and cervical carcinoma. Ann. NY Acad. Sci. 945:59–67.

69. Taback B, Giuliano AE, Hansen NM, Hoon DS. 2001. Microsatellite alterations detected in the serum of early stage breast cancer patients. Ann. NY Acad. Sci. 945:22–30.

70. Hibi K, Robinson CR, Booker S, et al. 1998. Molecular detection of genetic alterations in the serum of colorectal cancer patients. Cancer Res. 58:1405–1407.

71. Anker P, Mulcahy H, Chen XQ, Stroun M. 1999. Detection of circulating tumour DNA in the blood (plasma/serum) of cancer patients. Cancer Metastasis Rev. 18:65–73.

72. Lo YM, Chan LY, Lo KW, et al. 1999. Quantitative analysis of cell-free Epstein-Barr virus DNA in plasma of patients with nasopharyngeal carcinoma. Cancer Res. 59:1188–1191.

73. Nakayama T, Taback B, Nguyen DH, et al. 2000. Clinical significance of circulating DNA microsatellite markers in plasma of melanoma patients. Ann. NY Acad. Sci. 906:87–98.

74. Taback B, Fujiwara Y, Wang H, Foshag L, Morton D, Hoon D. 2001. Prognostic significance of circulating microsatellite markers in the plasma of melanoma patients. Cancer Res. 61: 5723–5726.

75. Silva JM, Silva J, Sanchez A, et al. 2002. Tumor DNA in plasma at diagnosis of breast cancer patients is a valuable predictor of disease-free survival. Clin. Cancer Res. 8:3761–3766.

76. Mandel P and Metais P. 1948. Les acides nucleiques du plasma sanguin chez l'homme. CR. Acad. Sci. Paris. 142:241–243.

77. Barnett EV. 1968. Detection of nuclear antigens (DNA) in normal and pathologic human fluids by quantitative complement fixation. Arthritis Rheum. 11:407–417.

78. Stollar BD. 1970. Immunochemical measurement of DNA in nucleoprotein with the use of anti-DNA antibodies from patients with systemic lupus erythematosus. Biochim. Biophys. Acta. 209:541–549.

79. Rosenberg BJ, Erlanger BF, Beiser SM. 1972. Radioimmunochemical studies on nucleoside-specific antibodies using iodinated DNA. J. Immunol. 108:271–274.

80. Tan EM, Schur PH, Carr RI, Kunkel HG. 1966. Deoxybonucleic acid (DNA) and antibodies to DNA in the serum of patients with systemic lupus erythematosus. J. Clin. Invest. 45: 1732–1740.

81. Davis GL Jr, and Davis JS. 1973. Detection of circulating DNA by counterimmuno-electrophoresis (CIE) Arthritis Rheum. 16:52–58.

82. Barnett EV. 1968. Role of nuclear antigens and antinuclear antibodies in inflammation. Biochem. Pharmacol. (Suppl.):77–86.

83. Perlin E and Moquin RB. 1972. Serum DNA levels in patients with malignant disease. Am. J. Clin. Pathol. 58:601–602.

84. Steinman CR. 1975. Use of nucleic acid hybridization for specific detection of submicrogram quantities of DNA, and its application to human plasma. Clin. Chem. 21:407–411.

85. Steinman CR. 1975. Free DNA in serum and plasma from normal adults. J. Clin. Invest. 56:512–515.

86. Cox RA and Gokcen M. 1977. A rapid sensitive radioassay for serum native and denatured DNA. Res. Commun. Chem. Pathol. Pharmacol. 17:309–318.

87. Hughes GR, Cohen SA, Lightfoot RW Jr, Meltzer JI, Christian CL. 1971. The release of DNA into serum and synovial fluid. Arthritis Rheum. 14:259–266.

88. Koffler D, Agnello V, Winchester R, Kunkel HG. 1973. The occurrence of single-stranded DNA in the serum of patients with systemic lupus erythematosus and other diseases. J. Clin. Invest. 52:198–204.

89. Li JZ and Steinman CR. 1989. Plasma DNA in systemic lupus erythematosus. Characterization of cloned base sequences. Arthritis Rheum. 32:726–733.

90. Leon SA, Green A, Yaros MJ, Shapiro B. 1975. Radioimmunoassay for nanogram quantities of DNA. J. Immunol. Methods 9:157–164.

91. Sambrook J and Russell DW. 2001. Molecular cloning: a laboratory manual. Cold spring harbor: Cold Spring Harbor Laboratory.

92. Dixon SC, Horti J, Guo Y, Reed E, Figg WD. 1998. Methods for extracting and amplifying genomic DNA isolated from frozen serum. Nat. Biotechnol. 16:91–94.

93. Lee TH, Montalvo L, Chrebtow V, Busch MP. 2001. Quantitation of genomic DNA in plasma and serum samples: higher concentrations of genomic DNA found in serum than in plasma. Transfusion 41:276–282.

94. Goelz SE, Hamilton SR, Vogelstein B. 1985. Purification of DNA from formaldehyde fixed and paraffin embedded human tissue. Biochem. Biophys. Res. Commun. 130:118–126.

95. Kamm RC and Smith AG. 1972. Nucleic acid concentrations in normal human plasma. Clin. Chem. 18:519–522.

96. Chang HW, Lee SM, Goodman SN, et al. 2002. Assessment of plasma DNA levels, allelic imbalance, and CA 125 as diagnostic tests for cancer. J. Natl. Cancer Inst. 94:1697–1703.

97. Goessl C, Krause H, Muller M, et al. 2000. Fluorescent methylation-specific polymerase chain reaction for DNA-based detection of prostate cancer in bodily fluids. Cancer Res. 60: 5941–5945.

98. Metz CE. 1978. Basic principles of ROC analysis. Semin. Nucl. Med. 8:283–298.

99. Chen LC, Kurisu W, Ljung BM, Goldman ES, Moore D, Smith HS. 1992. Heterogeneity for allelic loss in human breast cancer. J. Natl. Cancer. Inst. 84:506–510.

100. Deng G, Chen LC, Schott DR, et al. 1994. Loss of heterozygosity and p53 gene mutations in breast cancer. Cancer Res. 54:499–505.

101. Chen LC, Matsumura K, Deng G, et al. 1994. Deletion of two separate regions on chromosome 3p in breast cancers. Cancer Res. 54:3021–3024.

102. Patel U, Grundfest-Broniatowski S, Gupta M, Banerjee S. 1994. Microsatellite instabilities at five chromosomes in primary breast tumors. Oncogene 9:3695–3700.

103. Driouch K, Dorion-Bonnet F, Briffod M, Champeme MH, Longy M, Lidereau R. 1997. Loss of heterozygosity on chromosome arm 16q in breast cancer metastases. Genes Chromosomes Cancer 19:185–191.

104. O'Connell P, Pekkel V, Fuqua SA, Osborne CK, Clark GM, Allred DC. 1998. Analysis of loss of heterozygosity in 399 premalignant breast lesions at 15 genetic loci. J. Natl. Cancer. Inst. 90:697–703.

105. Aubele M, Mattis A, Zitzelsberger H, et al. 1999. Intratumoral heterogeneity in breast carcinoma revealed by laser-microdissection and comparative genomic hybridization. Cancer Genet. Cytogenet. 110:94–102.

106. Moinfar F, Man YG, Arnould L, Bratthauer GL, Ratschek M, Tavassoli FA. 2000. Concurrent and independent genetic alterations in the stromal and epithelial cells of mammary carcinoma: implications for tumorigenesis. Cancer Res. 60:2562–2566.

107. Regitnig P, Moser R, Thalhammer M, et al. 2002. Microsatellite analysis of breast carcinoma and corresponding local recurrences. J. Pathol. 198:190–197.

108. Takita K, Sato T, Miyagi M, et al. 1992. Correlation of loss of alleles on the short arms of chromosomes 11 and 17 with metastasis of primary breast cancer to lymph nodes. Cancer Res. 52:3914–3917.

109. Nagahata T, Hirano A, Utada Y, et al. 2002. Correlation of allelic losses and clinicopathological factors in 504 primary breast cancers. Breast Cancer. 9:208–215.

110. Ragnarsson G, Eiriksdottir G, Johannsdottir JT, Jonasson JG, Egilsson V, Ingvarsson S. 1999. Loss of heterozygosity at chromosome 1p in different solid human tumours: association with survival. Br. J. Cancer 79:1468–1474.

111. Radford DM, Fair KL, Phillips NJ, et al. 1995. Allelotyping of ductal carcinoma in situ of the breast: deletion of loci on 8p, 13q, 16q, 17p and 17q. Cancer Res. 55:3399–3405.

112. Deng G, Lu Y, Zlotnikov G, Thor AD, Smith HS. 1996. Loss of heterozygosity in normal tissue adjacent to breast carcinomas. Science 274:2057–2059.

113. Driouch K, Briffod M, Bieche I, Champeme MH, Lidereau R. 1998. Location of several putative genes possibly involved in human breast cancer progression. Cancer Res. 58:2081–2086.

114. Mayall F, Fairweather S, Wilkins R, Chang B, Nicholls R. 1999. Microsatellite abnormalities in plasma of patients with breast carcinoma: concordance with the primary tumour. J. Clin. Pathol. 52:363–366.

115. Shaw JA, Smith BM, Walsh T, et al. 2000. Microsatellite alterations in plasma DNA of primary breast cancer patients. Clin. Cancer Res. 6:1119–1124.

116. Taback B, Giuliano AE, Hansen NM, Singer FR, Shu S, Hoon DS. 2003. Detection of tumor-specific genetic alterations in bone marrow from early-stage breast cancer patients. Cancer Res. 63:1884–1887.

117. Braun S, Pantel K, Muller P, et al. 2000. Cytokeratin-positive cells in the bone marrow and survival of patients with stage I, II, or III breast cancer. N. Engl. J. Med. 342:525–533.

118. Healy E, Belgaid CE, Takata M, et al. 1996. Allelotypes of primary cutaneous melanoma and benign melanocytic nevi. Cancer Res. 56:589–593.

119. Parmiter A, Balaban G, Clark W, Nowell P. 1988. Possible involvement of the chromosome region 10q24–q26 in early stages of melanocytic neoplasia. Cancer Genet. Cytogenet. 30: 313–317.

120. Fountain J, Bale S, Housman D, Dracopoli N. 1990. Genetics of melanoma. Cancer Surv. 9: 645–671.

121. Goldberg EK, Glendening JM, Karanjawala Z, et al. 2000. Localization of multiple melanoma tumor-suppressor genes on chromosome 11 by use of homozygosity mapping-of-deletions analysis. Am. J. Hum. Genet. 67:417–531.

122. Gonzalgo ML, Bender CM, You EH, et al. 1997. Low frequency of p16/CDKN2A methylation in sporadic melanoma: comparative approaches for methylation analysis of primary tumors. Cancer Res. 57:5336–5347.

123. Healy E, Rehman I, Angus B, Rees JL. 1995. Loss of heterozygosity in sporadic primary cutaneous melanoma. Genes Chromosomes Cancer 12:152–156.

124. Healy E, Belgaid C, Takata M, et al. 1998. Prognostic significance of allelic losses in primary melanoma. Oncogene 16:2213–2218.

125. Haluska F and Housman D. 1995. Recent advances in the molecular genetics of malignant melanoma. Cancer Surv. 25:277–292.

126. Flores JF, Walker GJ, Glendening JM, et al. 1996. Loss of the p16INK4a and p15INK4b genes, as well as neighboring 9p21 markers, in sporadic melanoma. Cancer Res. 56:5023–5032.

127. Jimenez P, Canton J, Concha A, et al. 2000. Microsatellite instability analysis in tumors with different mechanisms for total loss of HLA expression. Cancer Immunol. Immunother. 48:684–690.

128. Palmieri G, Cossu A, Ascierto PA, et al. 2000. Definition of the role of chromosome 9p21 in sporadic melanoma through genetic analysis of primary tumours and their metastases. Br. J. Cancer 83:1707–1714.

129. Herbst RA, Weiss J, Ehnis A, Cavenee WK, Arden KC. 1994. Loss of heterozygosity for 10q22–10qter in malignant melanoma progression. Cancer Res. 54:3111–3114.

130. Dracopoli N, Harnett P, Bale S, et al. 1989. Loss of alleles from the distal short arm of chromo-some 1 occurs late in melanoma tumor progression. Proc. Natl. Acad. Sci. 86:4614–4618.

131. Millikin D, Meese E, Vogelstein B, Witkowski C, Trent J. 1991. Loss of heterozygosity for loci on the long arm of chromosome 6 in human malignant melanoma. Cancer Res. 51:5449–5453.

132. Zhou W, Goodman SN, Galizia G, et al. 2002. Counting alleles to predict recurrence of early-stage colorectal cancers. Lancet 359:219–225.

133. Carter TL, Watt PM, Kumar R, et al. 2001. Hemizygous p16(INK4A). deletion in pediatric acute lymphoblastic leukemia predicts independent risk of relapse. Blood 97:572–574.

134. Caron H, van Sluis P, de Kraker J, et al. 1996. Allelic loss of chromosome 1p as a predictor of unfavorable outcome in patients with neuroblastoma. N. Engl. J. Med. 334:225–230.

135. Classon M and Harlow E. 2002. The retinoblastoma tumour suppressor in development and cancer. Nat. Rev. Cancer 2:910–917.

136. Sherr CJ. 1996. Cancer cell cycles. Science 274:1672–1677.

137. O'Day SJ, Gammon G, Boasberg PD, et al. 1999. Advantages of concurrent biochemotherapy modified by decrescendo interleukin-2, granulocyte colony-stimulating factor, and tamoxifen for patients with metastatic melanoma. J. Clin. Oncol. 17:2752–2761.

138. Taback B, O'day S, Fournier PJ, Hoon DS. 2002. Serum genetic markers as surrogates of response to biochemotherapy in patients with melanoma. Proc. Amer. Soc. Clin. Oncol. 21:339a.

139. Eton O, Legha SS, Moon TE, et al. 1998. Prognostic factors for survival of patients treated systemically for disseminated melanoma. J. Clin. Oncol. 16:1103–1111.

140. Bos JL, Fearon ER Hamilton SR, et al. 1987. Prevalence of *ras* gene mutations in human colorectal cancers. Nature 327:293–297.

141. Forrester K, Almoguera C, Han K, Grizzle WE, Perucho M. 1987. Detection of high incidence of K-*ras* oncogenes during human colon tumorigenesis. Nature 327:298–303.

142. Solomon E, Voss R, Hall V, et al. 1987. Chromosome 5 allele loss in human colorectal carcino-mas. Nature 328:616–619.

143. Bodmer WF, Bailey CJ, Bodmer J, et al. 1987. Localization of the gene for familial adenomatous polyposis on chromosome 5. Nature 328:614–616.

144. Leppert M, Dobbs M, Scambler P, et al. 1987. The gene for familial polyposis coli maps to the long arm of chromosome 5. Science 238:1411–1413.

145. Fearon ER, Hamilton SR, Vogelstein B. 1987. Clonal analysis of human colorectal tumors. Science 238:193–197.

146. Sidransky D, Tokino T, Hamilton SR, et al. 1992. Identification of *ras* oncogene mutations in the stool of patients with curable colorectal tumors. Science 256:102–105.

147. Prix L, Uciechowski P, Bockmann B, Giesing M, Schuetz AJ. 2002. Diagnostic biochip array for fast and sensitive detection of K-*ras* mutations in stool. Clin. Chem. 48:428–435.

148. Sorenson GD. 2000. Detection of mutated KRAS2 sequences as tumor markers in plasma/serum of patients with gastrointestinal cancer. Clin. Cancer Res. 6:2129–2137.

149. Kondo H, Sugano K, Fukayama N, et al. 1994. Detection of point mutations in the K-*ras* oncogene at codon 12 in pure pancreatic juice for diagnosis of pancreatic carcinoma. Cancer. 73:1589–1594.

150. Iguchi H, Sugano K, Fukayama N, et al. 1996. Analysis of Ki-*ras* codon 12 mutations in the duodenal juice of patients with pancreatic cancer. Gastroenterology 110:221–226.

151. Tada M, Ohashi M, Shiratori Y, et al. 1996. Analysis of k-*ras* gene mutation in hyperplastic duct cells of the pancreas without pancreatic disease. Gastroenterology 110:227–231.

152. Yanagisawa A, Ohtake K, Ohashi K, et al. 1993. Frequent c-Ki-*ras* oncogene activation in mucous cell hyperplasias of pancreas suffering from chronic inflammation. Cancer Res. 53:953–956.

153. Kondo H, Sugano K, Fukayama N, et al. 1997. Detection of k-*ras* gene mutations at codon 12 in the pancreatic juice of patients with intraductal papillary mucinous tumors of the pancreas. Cancer 79:900–905.

154. Furuya N, Kawa S, Akamatsu T, Furihata K. 1997. Long-term follow-up of patients with chronic pancreatitis and k-*ras* gene mutation detected in pancreatic juice. Gastroenterology 113:593–598.

155. Theodor L, Melzer E, Sologov M, Bar-Meir S. 2000. Diagnostic value of K-*ras* mutations in serum of pancreatic cancer patients. Ann. NY Acad. Sci. 906:19–24.

156. Sorenson GD. 2000. A review of studies on the detection of mutated KRAS2 sequences as tumor markers in plasma/serum of patients with gastrointestinal cancer. Ann. NY Acad. Sci. 906:13–16.

157. LaForgia S, Lasota J, Latif F, et al. 1993. Detailed genetic and physical map of the 3p chromosome region surrounding the familial renal cell carcinoma chromosome translocation, t(3.8).(p14.2.q24.1). Cancer Res. 53:3118–3124.

158. Fadl-Elmula I, Gorunova L, Mandahl N, et al. 1999. Cytogenetic analysis of upper urinary tract transitional cell carcinomas. Cancer Genet. Cytogenet. 115:123–127.

159. Johns MM III, Westra WH, Califano JA, Eisele D, Koch WM, Sidransky D. 1996. Allelotype of salivary gland tumors. Cancer Res. 56:1151–1154.

160. Steiner G and Sidransky D. 1996. Molecular differential diagnosis of renal carcinoma: from microscopes to microsatellites. Am. J. Pathol. 149:1791–1795.

161. Kenck C, Wilhelm M, Bugert P, Staehler G, Kovacs G. 1996. Mutation of the VHL gene is associated exclusively with the development of non-papillary renal cell carcinomas. J. Pathol. 179:157–161.

162. Gnarra JR, Tory K, Weng Y, et al. 1994. Mutations of the VHL tumour suppressor gene in renal carcinoma. Nat. Genet. 7:85–90.

163. Chudek J, Wilhelm M, Bugert P, Herbers J, Kovacs G. 1997. Detailed microsatellite analysis of chromosome 3p region in non-papillary renal cell carcinomas. Int. J. Cancer 73:225–229.

164. Wilhelm M, Bugert P, Kenck C, Staehler G, Kovacs G. 1995. Terminal deletion of chromosome 3p sequences in nonpapillary renal cell carcinomas: a breakpoint cluster between loci D3S1285 and D3S1603. Cancer Res. 55:5383–5385.

165. Polascik TJ, Cairns P, Epstein JI, et al. 1996. Distal nephron renal tumors: microsatellite allelotype. Cancer Res. 56:1892–1895.

166. Cairns P, Tokino K, Eby Y, Sidransky D. 1995. Localization of tumor suppressor loci on chromosome 9 in primary human renal cell carcinomas. Cancer Res. 55:224–227.

167. Reiter RE, Anglard P, Liu S, Gnarra JR, Linehan WM. 1993. Chromosome 17p deletions and p53 mutations in renal cell carcinoma. Cancer Res. 53:3092–3097.

168. von Knobloch R, Hegele A, Brandt H, et al. 2002. High frequency of serum DNA alterations in renal cell carcinoma detected by fluorescent microsatellite analysis. Int. J. Cancer. 98:889–894.

169. von Knobloch R, Hegele A, Brandt H, Olbert P, Heidenreich A, Hofmann R. 2001. Serum DNA and urine DNA alterations of urinary transitional cell bladder carcinoma detected by fluorescent microsatellite analysis. Int. J. Cancer. 94:67–72.

170. Mao L, Lee DJ, Tockman MS, Erozan YS, Askin F, Sidransky D. 1994. Microsatellite alterations as clonal markers for the detection of human cancer. Proc. Natl. Acad. Sci. USA 91:9871–9875.

171. Cairns P, Tokino K, Eby Y, Sidransky D. 1994. Homozygous deletions of 9p21 in primary human bladder tumors detected by comparative multiplex polyme*rase* chain reaction. Cancer Res. 54:1422–1424.

172. Wang Y, Hung SC, Linn JF, et al. 1997. Microsatellite-based cancer detection using capillary array electrophoresis and energy-transfer fluorescent primers. Electrophoresis 18:1742–1749.

173. Utting M, Werner W, Muller G, Schubert J, Junker K. 2001. A possible noninvasive method for the detection of bladder cancer in patients: microsatellite analysis of free DNA in urine and blood. Ann. NY Acad. Sci. 945:31–35.

174. Gazdar AF and Czerniak B. 2001. Filling the void: urinary markers for bladder cancer risk and diagnosis. J. Natl. Cancer. Inst. 93:413–415.

175. Seidman JD and Kurman RJ. 1996. Subclassification of serous borderline tumors of the ovary into benign and malignant types. A clinicopathologic study of 65 advanced stage cases. Am. J. Surg. Pathol. 20:1331–1345.

176. Seidman JD and Kurman RJ. 2000. Ovarian serous borderline tumors: a critical review of the literature with emphasis on prognostic indicators. Hum. Pathol. 31:539–557.

177. Singer G, Kurman RJ, Chang HW, Cho S, Shih IM. 2002. Diverse tumorigenic pathways in ovarian serous carcinoma. Am. J. Pathol. 160:1223–1228.
178. Zborovskaya I, Gasparian A, Karseladze A, et al. 1999. Somatic genetic alterations (LOH) in benign, borderline and invasive ovarian tumours: intratumoral molecular heterogeneity. Int. J. Cancer 82:822–826.
179. Dodson MK, Hartmann LC, Cliby WA, et al. 1993. Comparison of loss of heterozygosity patterns in invasive low-grade and high-grade epithelial ovarian carcinomas. Cancer Res. 53:4456–4460.
180. Cliby W, Ritland S, Hartmann L, et al. 1993. Human epithelial ovarian cancer allelotype. Cancer Res. 53:2393–2398.
181. Iwabuchi H, Sakamoto M, Sakunaga H, et al. 1995. Genetic analysis of benign, low-grade, and high-grade ovarian tumors. Cancer Res. 55:6172–6180.
182. Pisani P, Bray F, Parkin DM. 2002. Estimates of the world-wide prevalence of cancer for 25 sites in the adult population. Int. J. Cancer 97:72–81.
183. Gissmann L, Pfister H, Zur Hausen H. 1977. Human papilloma viruses (HPV): characterization of four different isolates. Virology 76:569–580.
184. zur Hausen H. 1977. Human papillomaviruses and their possible role in squamous cell carcinomas. Cur. Top. Microbiol. Immunol. 78:1–30.
185. zur Hausen H. 1976. Condylomata acuminata and human genital cancer. Cancer Res. 36:794.
186. zur Hausen H, Meinhof W, Scheiber W, Bornkamm GW. 1974. Attempts to detect virus-secific DNA in human tumors. I. Nucleic acid hybridizations with complementary RNA of human wart virus. Int. J. Cancer. 13:650–656.
187. Mitra AB, Murty VV, Li RG, Pratap M, Luthra UK, Chaganti RS. 1994. Allelotype analysis of cervical carcinoma. Cancer Res. 54:4481–4487.
188. Mitra AB, Murty VV, Singh V, et al. 1995. Genetic alterations at 5p15: a potential marker for progression of precancerous lesions of the uterine cervix. J. Natl. Cancer. Inst. 87:742–745.
189. Mullokandov MR, Kholodilov NG, Atkin NB, Burk RD, Johnson AB, Klinger HP. 1996. Genomic alterations in cervical carcinoma: losses of chromosome heterozygosity and human papilloma virus tumor status. Cancer Res. 56:197–205.
190. Wistuba II Montellano FD, Milchgrub S, et al. 1997. Deletions of chromosome 3p are frequent and early events in the pathogenesis of uterine cervical carcinoma. Cancer Res. 57:3154–3158.
191. Larson AA, Kern S, Curtiss S, Gordon R, Cavenee WK, Hampton GM. 1997. High resolution analysis of chromosome 3p alterations in cervical carcinoma. Cancer Res. 57:4082–4090.
192. Cheung TH, Chung TK, Poon CS, Hampton GM, Wang VW, Wong YF. 1999. Allelic loss on chromosome 1 is associated with tumor progression of cervical carcinoma. Cancer 86: 1294–1298.
193. Rha SH, Dong SM, Jen J, Nicol T, Sidransky D. 2001. Molecular detection of cervical intraepithelial neoplasia and cervical carcinoma by microsatellite analysis of Papanicolaou smears. Int. J. Cancer. 93:424–429.
194. Dong SM, Pai SI, Rha SH, et al. 2002. Detection and quantitation of human papillomavirus DNA in the plasma of patients with cervical carcinoma. Cancer Epidemiol. Biomarkers Prev. 11:3–6.
195. Liu VW, Tsang P, Yip A, Ng TY, Wong LC, Ngan HY. 2001. Low incidence of HPV DNA in sera of pretreatment cervical cancer patients. Gynecol. Oncol. 82:269–272.
196. Bruhn N, Beinert T, Oehm C, et al. 2000. Detection of microsatellite alterations in the DNA isolated from tumor cells and from plasma DNA of patients with lung cancer. Ann. NY Acad. Sci. 906:72–82.
197. Sanchez-Cespedes M. 2003. Dissecting the genetic alterations involved in lung carcinogenesis. Lung Cancer 40:111–121.
198. Sanchez-Cespedes M, Ahrendt SA, Piantadosi S, et al. 2001. Chromosomal alterations in lung adenocarcinoma from smokers and nonsmokers. Cancer Res. 61:1309–1313.

199. Ahrendt SA, Decker PA, Alawi EA, et al. 2001. Cigarette smoking is strongly associated with mutation of the *k-ras* gene in patients with primary adenocarcinoma of the lung. Cancer 92:1525–1530.
200. Mao L, Lee JS, Kurie JM, et al. 1997. Clonal genetic alterations in the lungs of current and former smokers. J. Natl. Cancer. Inst. 89:857–862.
201. Sanchez-Cespedes M, Rosell R, Pifarre A, et al. 1997. Microsatellite alterations at 5q21, 11p13, and 11p15.5 do not predict survival in non-small cell lung cancer. Clin. Cancer Res. 3: 1229–1235.
202. Guo Z, Yamaguchi K, Sanchez-Cespedes M, Westra WH, Koch WM, Sidransky, D. 2001. Allelic losses in OraTest-directed biopsies of patients with prior upper aerodigestive tract malignancy. Clin. Cancer Res. 7:1963–1968.
203. Califano J, Leong PL, Koch WM, Eisenberger CF, Sidransky D, Westra WH. 1999. Second esophageal tumors in patients with head and neck squamous cell carcinoma: an assessment of clonal relationships. Clin. Cancer Res. 5:1862–1867.
204. van der Riet P, Nawroz H, Hruban RH, et al. 1994. Frequent loss of chromosome 9p21–22 early in head and neck cancer progression. Cancer Res. 54:1156–1158.
205. Nawroz H, van der Riet P, Hruban RH, Koch W, Ruppert JM, Sidransky D. 1994. Allelotype of head and neck squamous cell carcinoma. Cancer Res. 54:1152–1155.
206. Mao L, Lee JS, Fan YH, et al. 1996. Frequent microsatellite alterations at chromosomes 9p21 and 3p14 in oral premalignant lesions and their value in cancer risk assessment. Nat. Med. 2:682–685.
207. Mao L, El-Naggar AK, Papadimitrakopoulou V, et al. 1998. Phenotype and genotype of advanced premalignant head and neck lesions after chemopreventive therapy. J. Natl. Cancer. Inst. 90:1545–1551.
208. Henle G and Henle W. Serum IgA antibodies of Epstein-Barr virus (EBV).-related antigens. A new feature of nasopharyngeal carcinoma. Bibl. Haematol. 1975:322–325.
209. Henle W, Henle G, Ho JH. Epstein-Barr virus-related serology in nasopharyngeal carcinoma and controls. IARC. Sci. Publ. 1978:427–437.
210. Raab-Traub N and Flynn K. 1986. The structure of the termini of the Epstein-Barr virus as a marker of clonal cellular proliferation. Cell 47:883–889.
211. Farrell PJ, Cludts I, Stuhler A. 1997. Epstein-Barr virus genes and cancer cells. Biomed. Pharmacother. 51:258–267.
212. Chen YJ, Ko JY, Chen PJ, et al. 1999. Chromosomal aberrations in nasopharyngeal carcinoma analyzed by comparative genomic hybridization. Genes Chromosomes Cancer 25:169–175.
213. Fan CS, Wong N, Leung SF, et al. 2000. Frequent c-myc and Int-2 overrepresentations in nasopharyngeal carcinoma. Hum. Pathol. 31:169–178.
214. Choi PH, Suen MW, Huang DP, Lo KW, Lee JC. 1993. Nasopharyngeal carcinoma: genetic changes, Epstein-Barr virus infection, or both. A clinical and molecular study of 36 patients. Cancer 72:2873–2878.
215. Sun Y, Hildesheim A, Li H, et al. 1995. The von Hippel-Lindau (VHL). disease tumor-suppressor gene is not mutated in nasopharyngeal carcinomas. Int. J. Cancer 61:437–438.
216. Hu LF, Eiriksdottir G, Lebedeva T, et al. 1996. Loss of heterozygosity on chromosome arm 3p in nasopharyngeal carcinoma. Genes Chromosomes Cancer. 17:118–126.
217. Huang DP, Lo KW, van Hasselt CA, et al. 1994. A region of homozygous deletion on chromosome 9p21–22 in primary nasopharyngeal carcinoma. Cancer Res. 54:4003–4006.
218. Lo KW, Huang DP, Lau KM. 1995. p16 gene alterations in nasopharyngeal carcinoma. Cancer Res. 55:2039–2043.
219. Hui AB, Lo KW, Leung SF, et al. 1996. Loss of heterozygosity on the long arm of chromosome 11 in nasopharyngeal carcinoma. Cancer Res. 56:3225–3229.
220. Mutirangura A, Pornthanakasem W, Sriuranpong V, Supiyaphun P, Voravud N. 1998. Loss of heterozygosity on chromosome 14 in nasopharyngeal carcinoma. Int. J. Cancer 78:153–156.

221. Shao J, Li Y, Wu Q, et al. 2002. High frequency loss of heterozygosity on the long arms of chromosomes 13 and 14 in nasopharyngeal carcinoma in Southern China. Chin Med. J. (Engl.) 115:571–575.

222. Mutirangura A, Tanunyutthawongese C, Pornthanakasem W, et al. 1997. Genomic alterations in nasopharyngeal carcinoma: loss of heterozygosity and Epstein-Barr virus infection. Br. J. Cancer 76:770–776.

223. Lo YM, Leung SF, Chan LY, et al. 2000. Kinetics of plasma Epstein-Barr virus DNA during radiation therapy for nasopharyngeal carcinoma. Cancer Res. 60:2351–2355.

224. Chan AT, Lo YM, Zee B, et al. 2002. Plasma Epstein-Barr virus DNA and residual disease after radiotherapy for undifferentiated nasopharyngeal carcinoma. J. Natl. Cancer Inst. 94: 1614–1619.

225. Lo KW, Lo YM, Leung SF, et al. 1999. Analysis of cell-free Epstein-Barr virus associated RNA in the plasma of patients with nasopharyngeal carcinoma. Clin. Chem. 45:1292–1294.

226. Lo KW, Teo PM, Hui AB, et al. 2000. High resolution allelotype of microdissected primary nasopharyngeal carcinoma. Cancer Res. 60:3348–3353.

227. Lo YM. 2001. Prognostic implication of pretreatment plasma/serum concentration of Epstein-Barr virus DNA in nasopharyngeal carcinoma. Biomed. Pharmacother. 55:362–365.

228. Lo YM. 2001. Quantitative analysis of Epstein-Barr virus DNA in plasma and serum: applications to tumor detection and monitoring. Ann. NY Acad. Sci. 945:68–72.

229. Lo YM, Chan AT, Chan LY, et al. 2000. Molecular prognostication of nasopharyngeal carcinoma by quantitative analysis of circulating Epstein-Barr virus DNA. Cancer Res. 60: 6878–6881.

230. Lo YM, Chan LY, Chan AT, et al. 1999. Quantitative and temporal correlation between circulating cell-free Epstein-Barr virus DNA and tumor recurrence in nasopharyngeal carcinoma. Cancer Res. 59:5452–5455.

231. Lo YM, Leung SF, Chan LY, et al. 2000. Plasma cell-free Epstein-Barr virus DNA quantitation in patients with nasopharyngeal carcinoma. Correlation with clinical staging. Ann. NY Acad. Sci. 906:99–101.

232. Johnson PJ and Lo YM. 2002. Plasma nucleic acids in the diagnosis and management of malignant disease. Clin. Chem. 48:1186–1193.

233. Bocker T, Diermann J, Friedl W, et al. 1997. Microsatellite instability analysis: a multicenter study for reliability and quality control. Cancer Res. 57:4739–4743.

234. Emanuel SL and Pestka S. 1993. Amplification of specific gene products from human serum. Genet. Anal. Tech. Appl. 10:144–146.

235. Lin Z and Floros J. 1998. Genomic DNA extraction from small amounts of sera to be used for genotype analysis. Biotechniques 24:937–940.

236. Sandford AJ and Pare PD. 1997. Direct PCR of small genomic DNA fragments from serum. Biotechniques 23:890–892.

237. Blomeke B, Bennett WP, Harris CC, Shields PG. 1997. Serum, plasma and paraffin-embedded tissues as sources of DNA for studying cancer susceptibility genes. Carcinogenesis 18:1271–1275.

238. Hoon DS, Fujimoto A, Shu S, Taback B. 2002. Assessment of genetic heterogeneity in tumors using laser capture microdissection. Methods Enzymol. 356:302–309.

239. Bostick PJ, Chatterjee S, Chi DD, et al. 1998. Limitations of specific reverse-transcriptase polymerase chain reaction markers in the detection of metastases in the lymph nodes and blood of breast cancer patients. J. Clin. Oncol. 16:2632–2640.

240. Jahr S, Hentze H, Englisch S, et al. 2001. DNA fragments in the blood plasma of cancer patients: quantitations and evidence for their origin from apoptotic and necrotic cells. Cancer Res. 61:1659–1665.

241. Stroun M, Lyautey J, Lederrey C, Olson-Sand A, Anker P. 2001. About the possible origin and mechanism of circulating DNA apoptosis and active DNA release. Clin. Chim. Acta. 313: 139–142.

242. Stroun M, Maurice P, Vasioukhin V, et al. 2000. The origin and mechanism of circulating DNA. Ann. NY Acad. Sci. 906:161–168.

20

Recent Advances in Molecular Classification and Prognosis of Colorectal Cancer

Tsung-Teh Wu and Asif Rashid

1. INTRODUCTION

Colorectal cancer is the fourth most common cancer and the second most common cause of cancer death in the United States, with approx 130,000 new cases and 55,000 deaths per year *(1)*. It is currently believed that most colorectal cancers arise from pre-existing precursor lesions (adenoma and dysplasia), but a small percentage of colorectal cancers can arise *de novo* without identifiable precursor lesions *(2–8)*. A majority of the colorectal cancers are sporadic and only 5 to 10% of colorectal cancers are associated with inherited syndromes. The molecular pathogenesis of colorectal cancer, including genetic and epigenetic alterations has been extensively studied in the past two decades and is among one of the best-understood human neoplasms. Although inherited forms of colorectal cancer constitute a minority of all colorectal cancers, the identification of underlying genetic defects responsible for the inherited syndrome has been instrumental for our understanding of the pathogenesis of colorectal neoplasia.

Three major molecular pathways have been characterized in colorectal cancers (Fig. 1). The conventional pathway involves accumulation of alterations of multiple tumor suppressor genes including adenomatous polyposis coli (*APC*), deleted in colorectal cancer (*DCC*), deleted in pancreatic cancer 4 (*DPC4*), and *p53* and oncogenes including *k-ras*, and *β-catenin* in the adenoma-carcinoma sequence accounts for a majority of colorectal cancer *(9,10)*. Approximately 15% of sporadic colorectal cancers arise through a second distinct pathway involving "DNA mismatch repair genes" that is also responsible for the hereditary nonpolyposis colorectal cancer (HNPCC) syndrome. Mutations of the DNA repair genes (*hMLH-1*, *hMSH-2*, and *hMSH-6*) cause insertions or deletions of nucleotides in the unstable repeated sequences such as microsatellites *(11–14)*. This subset of colorectal cancers has unusual pathologic features such as poor differentiation, medullary or mucinous histologic type, and prominent lymphoid inflammatory response *(15–17)*. In addition to the genetic alterations described above, inactivation of tumor suppressor genes by promoter hypermethylation is a frequent epigenetic alteration in human cancer *(18)*. In colorectal cancer, it has been shown that methylation of CpG islands is a common molecular defect in colorectal cancer *(19,20)*. "DNA methylator pathway" is the third novel pathway characterized by methylation of multiple CpG islands in a subset of colorectal carcinomas, including genes known to be important in tumorigenesis such as the *p16* tumor suppressor gene and *hMLH1* mismatch repair gene.

From: *Cancer Diagnostics: Current and Future Trends*
Edited by: R. M. Nakamura, W. W. Grody, J. T. Wu, and R. B. Nagle © Humana Press Inc., Totowa, NJ

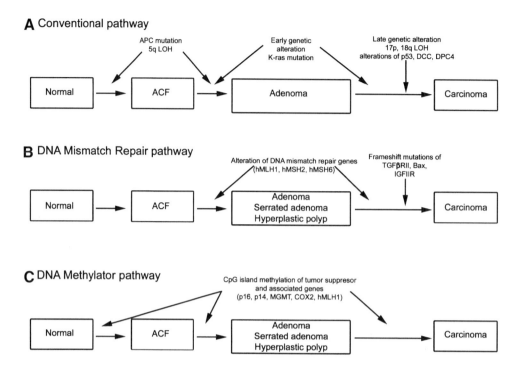

Fig. 1. Schematic summary of genetic alterations involved in the three major pathways of colorectal tumorigenesis. Aberrant crypt foci (ACF) are the earliest precursors lesion. Sequential accumulation of alterations in multiple tumor suppressor genes and oncogenes occur in conventional pathway (**A**). A total of 15 to 20% of sporadic colorectal cancer have MSI-H genotype owing to inactivation of DNA mismatch repair genes. These tumors frequently have mutations in the tumor suppressor genes with short nucleotide repeats (**B**). Inactivation of gene function by DNA hypermethylation in tumor-specific (type C) genes including methylation of *hMLH1* gene plays an important role in DNA methylator pathway (**C**). In addition to adenomas, serrated adenomas and hyperplastic polyps are also precursor lesions in DNA mismatch repair and DNA methylator pathways following the hyperplastic polyp-serrated adenoma-carcinoma sequence.

1.1. Conventional Pathway

The standard pathogenic pathway is the adenoma-carcinoma sequence, first described by Morson, and Hill and colleagues plays an important role in the majority of colorectal carcinoma *(21,22)*. Fearon and Vogelstein described sequential stepwise involvement of multiple tumor suppressor genes and oncogenes in the adenoma-carcinoma sequence *(9)*. In this model, a combination of multiple genetic alterations is required for the ultimate development of colorectal cancer and the presence of a single genetic alteration is not sufficient for malignant transformation.

1.1.1. Tumor Suppressor Genes in Conventional Pathway

Multiple tumor suppressor genes are involved in the development of colorectal cancers as evidenced by frequent chromosomal allelic losses of 1p, 5q (*APC*), 8p, 17p (*p53*), 18q (*DCC*), and 22q *(9,23–25)*. The earliest genetic change occurs in the *APC* gene. *APC* is a tumor suppressor gene located on chromosome 5q21 and was first identified through its involvement in familial adenomatous polyposis (FAP) syndrome *(26–29)*. *APC* gene has been regarded as a "gatekeeper" gene and plays a critical role in colorectal carcinogenesis. The inactivation of *APC* gene in colorectal neoplasm follows the Knudson's two-hit hypothesis. Allelic loss of chromosome 5q is present in 40–50% of sporadic colorectal adenomas and carcinomas, and somatic mutation of *APC* gene can be identified in up to 70% of sporadic colorectal cancer by sensitive in vitro synthesizing protein assay *(30,31)*. The identification of *APC* mutation in dysplastic aberrant crypt foci, the earliest morphologic colorectal precursor lesion, further supports the critical function of *APC* gene in the colorectal pathogenesis *(32)*. The function of *APC* gene has been recently characterized. *APC* gene product interacts with GSK-3β and β-catenin, and is an essential component in the Wnt pathway. *APC* gene also play an important role in cell adhesion through interaction with Cadherins *(37)*.

In contrast to *APC* gene, alterations of other tumor suppressor genes occur in the later stages of colorectal carcinogenesis. Mutations of *p53* gene and allelic loss of chromosome 17p occur in up to 75% of colorectal cancers, but rarely in adenomas *(38–41)*. The p53 protein can function as a transcription factor and is involved in the cell cycle regulation and programmed cell death. The presence of frequent *p53* alterations in carcinoma but not in adenomas suggests that *p53* may play an important role in progression of adenoma into carcinoma *(39,40)*.

Allelic loss of chromosomal 18q occurs in 70% of sporadic colorectal cancers and is less frequent in adenomas *(10)*. DCC, DPC4 (SMAD4) and JV-18(SMAD2) genes are present on chromosome 18q. A candidate tumor suppressor gene designated *DCC* that belongs to the neural cell adhesion molecule (N-CAM) family has been identified *(42)*. Only a minority of colorectal cancers demonstrated somatic mutations of *DCC* in limited mutation analysis of the whole gene, but the protein expression is frequently reduced or absent in colorectal cancers. The presence of allelic loss and loss of protein expression supports the role of *DCC* in colorectal carcinogenesis. Another tumor suppressor gene, *DPC4 (SMAD4)*, first identified in pancreatic adenocarcinoma is also located in chromosome 18q. *SMAD4* is a downstream mediator of the TGFβ signal pathway. Mutation of *DPC4* gene has been identified in 16% of colorectal cancer *(43)* and DPC4 protein expression is absent in 8% of colorectal cancer *(44)*. Although the tumor suppressor gene in chromosome 18q involved in colorectal cancer remains unclear, the presence of chromosomal 18q allelic loss appears to predict a worse outcome especially in stage II colorectal cancer *(45,46)*.

1.1.2. Oncogenes in Conventional Pathway

Among the oncogenes, *k-ras* is the most frequently mutated in colorectal adenomas and cancer. Activation mutation of *k-ras* oncogene has been detected in 50% of colorectal cancers and large (> 1 cm) adenomas, but is less frequent (approx 10%) in smaller (< 1 cm) adenomas *(9,10)*. The majority of *k-ras* mutations are present at codons 12 and 13, and less frequently at codon 61. The role of aberrant crypt and hyperplastic polyps in the development of colorectal cancer is controversial but *k-ras* mutations have been frequently detected in aberrant crypt foci and hyperplastic polyps supporting the clonal nature of these lesions *(32,47)*. The presence of *k-ras* mutations in colorectal adenomas and cancers are associated with a polypoid growth pattern rather than a flat growth pattern, but the significance of these findings is unclear *(48)*.

In addition to *k-ras*, other oncogenes such as *Her-2/neu, myc, myb,* and *trk* are infrequently involved in the colorectal carcinogenesis. β-catenin is also an oncogene and interacts with *APC* gene in the *APC/β-catenin* pathway. Mutations of *β-catenin* gene have been reported in up to 50% of colorectal cancers lacking *APC* gene mutations, and in small colorectal adenomas *(49,50)*.

1.2. DNA Mismatch Repair Pathway

Microsatellites are tandem repeat mono, di, tri, or tetranucleotides that are present throughout the human genome. The functions of microsatellites are not known but have been postulated to act as promoter sites for recombination or DNA topoisomerase binding sites *(51–53)*. Microsatellite instability (MSI) is characterized by alterations of microsatellites owing to defective mismatch repair mechanisms and has been observed in a subset (15%) of sporadic colorectal cancer. Colorectal carcinoma can be classified into microsatellite stable (MSS), microsatellite instability-low (MSI-L), and microsatellite instability-high (MSI-H). The criterion for MSI-H varies with each study, but colorectal cancers with instability in more than 40% of microsatellite markers are generally regarded as MSI-H. The National Cancer Institute (NCI) standardized the criteria for classification of MSS, MSI-L, and MSI-H in a consensus conference. The conference proposed a panel comprising of five microsatellite makers including two mononucleotide markers (BAT 25 and BAT26) and three dinucleotide markers (D2S123, D5S346, and D17S250). Colorectal cancers with instability in two or more of these five markers are classified as MSI-H *(54)*.

In contrast to the conventional pathway, colorectal cancer with MSI-H tends to have less frequent 18q allelic loss or alterations of *p53* and *k-ras* genes compared to colorectal cancer with MSS *(55,56)*. Mutations of *β-catenin* are more common in MSI-H colorectal cancer *(49,57,58)*. In addition, a distinct set of tumor suppressor genes containing short mononucleotide repeats in the encoding region such as transforming growth factor β receptor type II (*TGFβRII*), insulin growth factor 2 receptor (*IGFIIR*) and *BAX* genes are frequently mutated in MSI-H colorectal cancer *(59–61)*. Most mutations in these genes are small deletions or insertions that result in frameshifts and result from mismatch repair gene defects during the DNA synthetic phase of the cell cycle. Interesting, not all mononucleotide repeats are subjected to the same rate of mutation in MSI-H colorectal cancer, a mononucleotide repeat with poly(G) tract is more prone to mutation than poly(A) tract *(62)*.

1.2.1. Mismatch Repair Genes and Microsatellite Instability

The human mismatch repair (*MMR*) gene family consists of several genes homologues to *Escherichia coli MMR* genes: *hMLH1, hMSH2, hMSH3, hMSH6, hPMS1,* and *hPMS2* *(63–68)*. In contrast, to HNPCC patients that have similar frequency of alterations of *hMLH1* and *hMLH2*, more than 95% of the sporadic MSI-H colorectal cancers are owing to the inactivation of *hMLH1* in the majority (80 to 95%) of patients, and inactivation of *hMSH2* in a smaller subset (5 to 20%) of patients *(69,70)*. The inactivation of *hMLH1, hMSH2* and *hMSH6* in MSI-H colorectal cancer can be evaluated by the absence of protein expression in tumor cells by immunohistochemical stains (Fig. 2). The majority (95%) of the MSI-H colorectal cancer demonstrate absence of either *hMLH1* or *hMSH2* expression in the tumor cells *(63,69)*.

In the majority of patients with sporadic colorectal carcinoma the loss of hMLH1 protein expression results from promoter methylation of the *hMLH1* gene rather than mutations *(70–73)*. No methylation of *hMSH2* gene promoter has been reported, but allelic loss or somatic mutation have been reported in colorectal cancer with absent hMSH2 protein expression *(70)*. Two other *MMR* genes, *hMSH3* and *hMSH6* are not directly responsible for

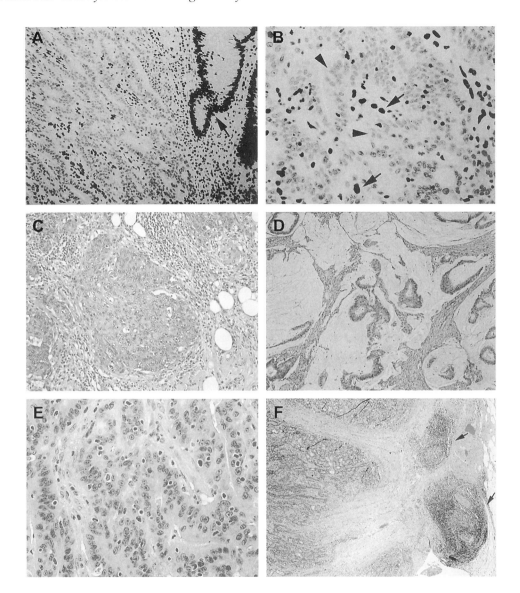

Fig. 2. Immunohistochemical stain of *hMLH1* and histological features of sporadic MSI-H colorectal cancer. The tumor cells show absence of *hMLH1* nuclear expression in contrast to normal colonic crypt epithelium (arrow) with positive staining **(A)**. In a high power view from panel A, the tumor cells (arrowheads) are negative for *hMLH1* staining, but the infiltrating lymphocytes (arrowheads) demonstrate nuclear *hMLH1* expression **(B)**. Histological characteristics of MSI-H colorectal cancer include poor differentiation with solid growth pattern **(C)**, mucinous differentiation with abundant extracellular mucin pool formation **(D)** prominent intratumor lymphocytic infiltrates **(E)**, and Crohn's-like lymphoid response (arrows) at the tumor invading front **(F)**.

MSI-H phenotype but are associated with somatic slippage-related frameshift mutations in MSI-H tumors, and probably secondary to inactivation of *hMLH1* or *hMSH2* genes *(74,75)*.

The involvement of *MMR* genes in the MSI-L colorectal cancer is not clear. Germ-line mutation of *hMSH6* gene has been reported in small subset of HNPCC families, and some of tumors in these families have MSI-L phenotype *(14,76,77)*. However, *hMSH6* mutations appear to play a minor if any role in the pathogenesis of sporadic MSI-L colorectal cancer *(78)*.

1.2.2. Histological Characteristics of Sporadic Colorectal Cancer With Microsatellite Instability

There are several distinct clinicopathological features of sporadic MSI-H colorectal cancers as compared with MSS colorectal cancers. Clinically, MSI-H cancers are more likely to present at a more advanced local stage, be proximally located, and have a better stage-specific survival after surgical and adjuvant therapies *(11,12,79–84)*. Histologically, characteristics of MSI-H cancers include exophytic growth pattern, large tumor size, poor differentiation, mucinous differentiation, Crohn's-like lymphoid response, and intratumoral lymphocytic infiltrate *(15–17)* (Fig. 2). Sporadic colorectal cancers with these features should warrant genetic testing to confirm the MSI-H genotype. A frequent association with contiguous serrated adenomas in sporadic MSI-H colorectal cancer, in contrast to the traditional adenomas seen in HNPCC colorectal cancer has also been reported *(85)*. However, no single clinicopathological feature mentioned above can sensitively predict MSI-H genotype or be used to select colorectal cancer for microsatellite instability testing *(17)*. Immunohistochemical stains for the MMR proteins (*hMLH1*, *hMSH2*, and *hMSH6*) expression can be used as an adjunct for the microsatellite instability testing. The absence of MMR protein expression typically correlated well with MSI-H, and presence of protein expression with MSS or MSI-L as predicted by microsatellite instability testing using the five NCI markers.

1.3. DNA Methylator Pathway

Epigenetic alterations have been extensively studied in colorectal cancers in the last two decades. The emphasis of epigenetic changes has switched from global hypomethylation to hypermethylation of tumor specific genes in neoplasm. Inactivation of gene function by methylation of promoter region in the DNA methylator pathway overlaps closely with the genetic alterations observed in both the conventional and DNA mismatch repair pathways. Methylation of CpG islands present in the promoter region can silence tumor suppressor genes in the absence of mutations or chromosomal loss that are typically seen in the conventional pathway.

1.3.1. DNA Methylation and CpG Islands

CpG islands are 0.5- to 2-kb regions rich in cytosine-guanine dinucleotides and are present in the 5' region of approximately half of all human genes *(86)*. DNA methylation in CpG islands is essential for mammalian development *(87)*. In neoplasia, CpG island methylation (CIM) is also an important mechanism for suppression of transcription of genes *(87,88)*. Methylation of CpG islands is a molecular defect common in colorectal cancer *(19)*. Genes with methylation can be classified as type A (age-related methylation) or type C (tumor-specific methylation) *(89)*. The methylation of type A genes in colonic mucosa increases with increasing age and include *ER, IGF2, MYOD1, N33, PAX6,* and *CSPG2 (89–92)*. The methylation of type C genes including *p16, p14, MGMT, COX-2,* and *hMLH1* is tumor specific and responsible for the carcinogenesis of sporadic colorectal cancer. Inactivation of tumor suppressor genes such as *APC* (18% of colorectal cancer) and *p16* (28–55% of colorectal cancer) by DNA methylation is a new model of inactivation in addition to the mutations of the gene and chromosomal allelic loss that accounts for the "two hit hypothesis" proposed by Kundson *(93)*. There is also a close association between the methylation of *MGMT*, a ubiquitous DNA repair enzyme, and mutation of *k-ras* gene in colorectal cancer *(94)*. Inac-

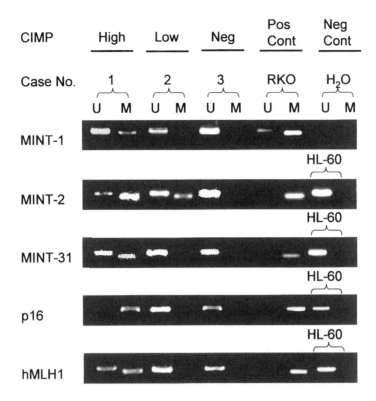

Fig. 3. CpG island methylator phenotype (CIMP) in colorectal cancer. Colorectal cancers are classified as CIMP+ if multiple loci are methylated (CIMP-high), or CIMP- if none (CIMP-negative) or only one locus was methylated (CIMP-low). Methylation status of tumor is determined by methylation-specific PCR (MSP) at *MINT1, MINT2, MINT31, p16* and *hMLH1* using primers for methylated (M) and unmethylated (U) alleles of bisulfite-treated DNA. RKO, a colon cancer cell line used as a positive control; dH$_2$O, samples without DNA used as negative control for *MINT1; HL-60*, a promyelocytic cell line used as negative control for *MINT2, MINT31, p16,* and *hMLH1.*

tivation of *MGMT* by methylation also appears to precede *k-ras* mutation in small adenomas and underscores the role of DNA methylation in the early colorectal carcinogenesis *(94)*. As discussed in the previous section, inactivation of MMR gene, *hMLH1*, by DNA methylation is responsible for the majority of the sporadic MSI-H colorectal cancer. An association between methylation of *MGMT* and MSI-L colorectal cancer has been recently described in addition to the association to *K-ras* mutation *(95)*.

1.3.2. Methylator Phenotype in Colorectal Cancer

A major subset (approx 50%) of colorectal cancer, including sporadic MSI-H colorectal cancers have methylation of multiple CpG islands termed CpG island methylator phenotype (CIMP) (Fig. 3). CIMP positive (CIMP+) colorectal cancers have methylation of genes known to be important in tumorigenesis, such as the *p16* tumor suppressor gene, *hMLH1* mismatch repair gene, and *THBS1 (19)*. Approximately 75% of he MSI-H colorectal cancer also have CIMP+ phenotype owing to the presence of methylation of *hMLH1* gene *(19)*. This CIMP phenotype can be observed in colorectal adenomas and aberrant crypt foci, the

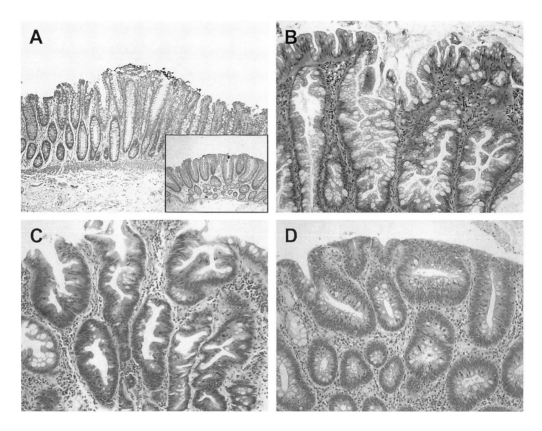

Fig. 4. Precursor lesions of colorectal cancer. Aberrant crypt foci are the earliest morphologic precursor lesion and can be subclassified into dysplastic (insert) or heteroplastic with hyperplastic features **(A)**. Hyperplastic polyp with classic saw-tooth pattern **(B)** a large hyperplastic polyp or hyperplastic polyps from patients with hyperplastic polyposis can be a precursor lesion for colorectal cancer. Serrated adenoma is distinct from hyperplastic polyp by the presence of epithelial dysplasia with saw-tooth architecture **(C)**. The classic precursor lesion, adenoma is characterized by the presence of dysplastic epithelium with tubular architecture **(D)**.

putative earliest lesion for colorectal cancers indicating the importance of DNA methylation pathway in early colorectal carcinogenesis *(19,96,97)*. In addition, CIMP+ adenomas and carcinomas have a distinct genetic profile with frequent mutation of the *k-ras* gene, but uncommon *p53* mutation *(20)*.

2. PRECURSOR LESIONS

The molecular alterations present in the precursor lesion in the adenoma-carcinoma sequence of colorectal cancer have been extensively analyzed, especially for the conventional pathway. In addition to the classic adenoma, other colorectal precursor lesions including aberrant crypt foci, hyperplastic polyp, and serrated adenoma (polyp with mixed hyperplastic and adenomatous features) have also been extensively studied (Fig. 4). An alternative pathway of colorectal carcinogenesis with a hyperplastic polyp-serrated adenoma-adenocarcinoma sequence has been proposed *(98–105)*.

2.1. Aberrant Crypt Foci: The Earliest Precursors Lesion

Aberrant crypt foci (ACFs) are the earliest morphological precursor lesions for colorectal cancer defined by the distinct macroscopic appearance in colonic mucosa stained with dyes, such as methylene blue. ACFs are phenotypically diverse lesions and can be subclassified into dysplastic and heteroplastic (hyperplastic) *(106)*. Dysplastic ACFs have histological features of adenoma and are more common in familial adenomatous polyposis (FAP) patients than in sporadic colorectal cancer patients. ACFs, especially dysplastic ones are considered precursors of colorectal cancer *(106–111)*.

Molecular alterations involving colorectal cancers have been evaluated in ACFs. Mutations of *APC* gene have been identified in up to 100% of dysplastic ACFs from FAP patients but not from sporadic colorectal cancers *(110,111)*. In contrast, heteroplastic ACFs have frequent *k-ras* (up to 82%) mutations but no *APC* or *β-catenin* mutations *(106,110,111)*. Microsatellite instability is present in 100% of ACFs from HNPCC patients *(112)*, but less frequently (3–23%) in ACFs from sporadic colorectal cancers *(97,113,114)*. An increased *p16* protein expression has been reported in ACFs *(115)*. DNA methylation of p16, *hMLH1* and *MGMT* genes and other CpG islands (MINT31, MINT1 and MINT3) is present in 34% of ACFs and is more frequent in sporadic ACFs (53%) than ACFs from FAP patients (11%) *(96)*. Furthermore, methylation is more common in dysplastic ACFs from sporadic patients (75%) than in FAP patients (8%), but no difference is present in heteroplastic ACFs between these two groups of patients *(96)*.

2.2. Hyperplastic Polyps

Hyperplastic polyps (HPs) are morphologically regarded as non-neoplastic lesions, and their roles as precursor lesions remain controversial. However, recent genetic analyses of HPs have shown that at least a subset of HPs, especially in patients with hyperplastic polyposis, are precursors of colorectal cancer *(98,116–119)*.

Genetic alterations typically seen in colorectal cancers such as *k-ras* mutation, chromosomal allelic loss of 1p, and microsatellite instability can occur in HPs *(32,98,120–123)*. The genotype appears to be different among HPs in hyperplastic polyposis (more than 20 HPs), multiple HPs (5–20 HPs) and large HPs (HPs more than 1 cm in size), with frequent chromosomal allelic loss 1p in HPs from hyperplastic polyposis *(98)*. Patients with a large HP in the right colon or hyperplastic polyposis have increased risk of colorectal cancer *(98,116–119)*. No DNA methylation of the CpG islands that are commonly methylated in colorectal carcinomas is present in sporadic HPs, but frequent concordant methylation of multiple loci is present in 43% of large HPs and HPs from hyperplastic polyposis *(124)*. A putative anti-adhesion gene *HPP1/TPEF* on chromosome 2q32–q33 identified from hyperplastic polyps can be inactivated by methylation in 63% of the HPs *(125)*.

2.3. Serrated Adenomas

Serrated adenoma (SA) is an uncommon variant of colorectal adenoma, characterized by the saw-toothed architectural features of hyperplastic polyp, but with the presence of unequivocal epithelial dysplasia *(126,127)*. The role of serrated adenomas in colorectal carcinogenesis is not established, but it has been reported that intramucosal carcinoma occurs in 11% of serrated adenomas and that colorectal cancer is common in patients with serrated adenomatosis *(127,128)*. The close morphological resemblance between HP and SA, frequent occurrence of SA in hyperplastic polyposis, and adenocarcinoma arising in the setting of colorectal hyperplastic polyps or serrated adenomas, especially in patients with hyperplastic polyposis, or serrated adenomatous polyposis has propelled a hyperplastic polyp-serrated adenoma-adenocarcinoma sequence as an alternative pathway of colorectal carcinogenesis *(98–105,116–118,126,129,130)*.

SA has been reported to have a lower frequency of *APC* gene mutation than in sporadic tubular adenomas *(131)*. Other studies have shown heterogeneity of genetic alterations in serrated adenomas, including *k-ras* mutations, *p53* gene mutations and MSI *(98,100,130, 132,133)*. The frequency of *k-ras* gene mutations has been reported to be as high as 58%, i.e., higher than in tubular adenomas *(133)*. Overexpression of p53 protein of the type associated with *p53* gene mutation (100%, 11 of 11) and mutation of *p53* (47%, 9 of 19) have been demonstrated in serrated adenomas in one study by Hiyoma et al *(133)*. However, other studies have shown low rate of *k-ras* mutation and p53 overexpression *(134,135)*. The development of microsatellite instability in serrated adenoma may have a role in the pathogenesis of colorectal carcinomas *(98,100,124,130)*. Jass and colleagues, have proposed that SA can be implicated in MSI-H and MSI-L colorectal cancers *(129,130,136)*.

Concordant CpG island methylation has been described in SAs in patients with multiple hyperplastic polyps and/or right-sided hyperplastic polyposis *(124)*. Recent data has shown that concordant methylation (CIMP+) is also more frequent in sporadic serrated adenomas (68%) than in tubular adenomas (18%) indicating that CpG island methylation is common in sporadic serrated adenomas and may play an important role in their pathogenesis *(137)*.

2.4. Adenomas

The majority of the colorectal cancers follow the adenoma-adenocarcinoma sequence. Adenomas are well-recognized precursor lesions for colorectal cancers irrespective of their underlying molecular pathway or genetic defects *(21,22)*. Mutations of the gatekeeper gene, *APC*, allelic loss of chromosome 5q, and *k-ras* oncogenes mutations (20–70%) are frequently present in adenomas *(138–146)*. Alterations frequently seen in the later stage of colorectal cancer development such as *p53* mutation (5–26%), 18q allelic loss (2–7%) are less frequently seen in adenomas *(145,146,149,150)*. MSI-H is frequently seen in adenomas from HNPCC patients (60–95%), but only occasionally in sporadic adenomas (3–7%) *(151–155)*. Methylation at multiple loci (CIMP+) is present in 25–50% of sporadic colorectal adenomas *(19,20,97)*. CIMP+ phenotype is more common in adenomas with villous histology, a characteristic associated with frequent predisposition to invasive colorectal cancer *(97)*.

3. FAMILIAL COLORECTAL CANCER

Colorectal cancer can arise in inherited syndromes including familial adenomatous polyposis (FAP), hereditary nonpolyposis colorectal cancer syndrome (HNPCC), juvenile polyposis (JPS), Peutz-Jegher syndrome (PJS), and hyperplastic polyposis and account for 5–10% of colorectal cancers.

3.1. Familial Adenomatous Polyposis Syndrome

Familial adenomatous polyposis syndrome (FAP) affecting approx 1 in 10,000 individuals, is an autosomal dominantly inherited disease with hundreds of colorectal polyps and germline mutation of the *APC* gene on the long arm of chromosome 5 *(26–29)*. If left untreated, more than 85% of the FAP patients will have colorectal cancer by the age of 45 yr. Gardner syndrome is categorized by colonic polyps and with various extracolonic manifestations such as osteoma, epidermoid cysts, and desmoid tumors.

In FAP patients, two-thirds of the *APC* mutations are small insertions or deletions that cause frameshifts in the coding region, and the remaining one-third are single base substitutions that result in stop codons. The location of the mutations can affect the clinical phenotype. Patients with attenuated FAP have *APC* mutations at the extreme 5' and 3' end of the gene *(156–158)*. The location of the germline *APC* mutation also appear to have influence on the second *APC* hit in colorectal polyps in FAP patients: germline *APC* mutations within a small region (codons 1194–1392) have predominantly allelic loss in colorectal adenomas as compared to other FAP patients that frequently have truncating mutations *(159)*.

APC gene polymorphism in I1307K allele is associated with increased risk of colorectal cancer in Ashkenazi Jews *(160,161)*. This allele is found in 6% of Ashkenazi Jews lacking a family history and 28% with a family history of colorectal cancer *(160)*. The I1307K allele contains an adenosine rich sequence A_3TA_4 at nucleotide 3920 that changes to A_8, and creates a small hypermutable region in *APC* gene *(160)* with frequent insertion mutation at this A_8 sequence *(162)*.

3.2. Hereditary Nonpolyposis Colorectal Cancer (HNPCC)

HNPCC is an autosomal dominant disorder caused by a germline mutation in MMR genes and accounts for 3–6% of colorectal cancers *(163,164)*. The inactivation of MMR genes results in high frequency of microsatellite instability (MSI-H) similar to the sporadic MSI-H colorectal cancer. More than 90% of the HNPCC patients have mutations in *hMLH1* and *hMSH2* genes *(165)*. Somatic frameshift mutation in *hMSH3* and *hMSH6* have been shown to occur in 53 and 33% of colorectal cancer in HNPCC patients secondary to germline inactivation of *hMLH1* or *hMSH2* genes *(61)*. DNA hypermethylation in *hMLH1* promoter frequently seen in sporadic MSI-H colorectal cancers is infrequently detected in 46% of colorectal cancers in HNPCC patients *(70)*. Similar to sporadic MSI-H colorectal cancers, mutations of *TGFβRII* are frequent in colorectal cancers from HNPCC patients, but mutations of *BAX* gene are more frequent in colorectal cancers of HNPCC patients (55%) than in sporadic MSI-H colorectal cancers (13%) *(55)*.

3.3. Juvenile Polyposis Syndrome

Juvenile polyposis syndrome (JPS) is an autosomal dominantly inherited syndrome characterized by multiple gastrointestinal hamartomatous polyps with increased risk of colorectal cancers *(166–168)*. The underlying genetic alterations are heterogeneous for JPS with approximately half of the JPS families having disease-specific germline mutations. Mutations of the *SMAD4 (DPC4)* gene on chromosome 18q21.1 have been identified in a subset (up to 50%) of the JPS *(169–173)*. In addition, a small subset of JPS has been linked to chromosome 10q22-23 with germline mutations of bone morphogenetic protein receptor 1A *(BMPR1A)* or *PTEN* genes *(174–179)*.

JPS can be a component of Cowden syndrome (CD) and Bannayan-Riley-Ruvalcaba syndrome (BRRS) *(175,176)*. Germline mutations of *PTEN* gene have identified in some families of CD and BRRS *(180,181)*. Somatic mutation of *PTEN* gene are present in up to 19% sporadic colorectal cancer, and more frequently (60%) in MSI-H colorectal cancer *(182,183)*.

3.4. Peutz-Jegher Syndrome

Peutz-Jegher syndrome (PJS) is an autosomal dominant disease characterized by gastrointestinal hamartomatous polyps with an arborizing smooth muscle in the lamina propria, mucocutaneous pigmentation, and increased risk of colon, pancreas, stomach, and breast cancers *(184)*. The *PJS* gene, *STK11 (LKB1)* gene, is located on chromosome 19p *(185–187)*. Germline mutations of *STK11* can be identified in half of the PJS families. No somatic mutation of *STK11* has been identified in sporadic colorectal cancer *(188,189)*.

3.5. Hyperplastic Polyposis

Hyperplastic polyposis is characterized by patients with numerous hyperplastic polyps (HPs) and increased risk of colorectal cancer *(98,117–119)*. Patients with hyperplastic polyposis can be familial and are characterized by multiple large HPs or with serrated polyposis with multiple serrated adenomas *(98,116,119)*. The genetic basis of hyperplastic polyposis remains unclear. Somatic genetic alterations in HPs in patients with hyperplastic polyposis have been discussed previously (*see* Section 2.2.).

4. PROGNOSTIC IMPLICATION OF MOLECULAR MARKERS IN COLORECTAL CANCER

Molecular alterations involving the pathogenesis of colorectal cancer, such as chromosomal allelic loss of 18q, 17p, 1p and 8p; altered level of expression of *DCC* (deleted in colorectal cancer), *p53* and *p27^{Kip1}* and high level of microsatellite instability have been reported as prognostic markers in colorectal cancers *(11,45,79–84,190–195)*. Postoperative adjuvant chemotherapy can improve the outcome in stage III (Dukes' stage C) colon cancer *(196,197)*. The benefit of postoperative chemotherapy for stage II (Duckes' stage IIB) is uncertain and molecular markers such as chromosomal allelic loss in the conventional pathway and microsatellite instability in the DNA mutator pathway may help in stratifying stage II colon-cancer patients with or without further treatment.

4.1. 18q Chromosomal Allelic Loss as a Prognostic Marker

Chromosomal allelic loss of 18q is frequently detected in up to 70% of colorectal cancers, and indicates a poor prognosis in colorectal cancers *(10,11,45,190–195)*. In the initial study series of Jen et al., the 5-yr survival rate is 93% in patients with stage II colorectal cancer with no 18q loss and 54% in those with 18q loss, indicating the prognostic value of chromosome 18q loss in patients with stage II colorectal cancers *(45)*. Several subsequent studies further confirm that 18q loss is a prognostic maker in colorectal cancers *(11,45,190–195)*, except for the study by Carethers and colleagues *(198)*. The loss of expression of *DCC* (a tumor suppressor gene on chromosome 18q21.1), similar to loss of 18q can predict a worse survival in patients with stage II or stage III colorectal cancers *(46)*. The second tumor suppressor gene on chromosome 18q21, *DPC4*, is altered in up to 33% of colorectal cancers, and loss of *DPC4* expression can correlate with presence of metastatic disease at presentation *(43,44)*.

The prognostic value of 18q loss appears to be applicable to post-operative adjuvant chemotherapy. In a large retrospective study analyzing 319 patients by Watababe and colleagues have shown that retention of chromosome 18q in microsatellite-stable cancers can predict a better outcome after post-operative adjuvant chemotherapy with fluorouracil-based regimens for stage III colon cancer *(199)*.

4.2. Microsatellite Instability Phenotype With Favorable Outcome

Colorectal cancers with high levels of microsatellite instability (MSI-H) tend to have a better prognosis and metastasize less often than compared to microsatellite stable colorectal cancers *(79–84,200,201)*. In a large series of population based studies of 607 patients by Gryfe and colleagues, 17% of the colorectal cancers were MSI-H and were associated with a significant survival advantage as compared to microsatellite stable colorectal cancers *(84)*. A similar result was shown by Samowitz and colleagues in another population based study *(200)*. In addition, patients with MSI-H colorectal cancers tend to have better prognosis after postoperative adjuvant chemotherapy *(202–204)*.

The reason MSI-H colorectal cancers have a better prognosis is unknown. Transforming growth factor β (TGFβ) is a potent inhibitor of epithelial cell growth. MSI-H colorectal cancers have a high rate (up to 90%) of mutations in the *TGFβ RII* gene *(205)*. The presence of mutation of *TGFβ RII* gene in colorectal cancers with MSI-H appears to predict a better outcome after postoperative adjuvant chemotherapy in stage III colorectal cancers *(199)*. MSI-H colorectal cancers tend to carry a higher number of activated cytotoxic intraepithelial lymphocytes as compared to MSI-L or microsatellite stable colorectal cancers *(206)*, suggesting a local cytotoxic immune response may be responsible for the better outcome for MSI-H cancers *(207)*. In addition, tumor infiltrating lymphocytes against frameshift-mutation-derived peptides resulting from the common frame shift mutation *TGFβ RII* gene have been identified in peripheral blood from patients with MSI-H colorectal cancers *(208–210)*.

5. CONCLUSIONS

The molecular genetics of familial colorectal cancers, including juvenile polyposis and Peutz-Jeghler's syndrome have been identified in the past decade. The molecular pathogenesis of sporadic colorectal cancers has three major pathways: the conventional pathway involving accumulation of alterations of tumor suppressor genes and oncogenes, DNA mismatch repair pathway, and DNA methylator pathway. Through the advance of molecular analysis, the precursor lesions for colorectal cancer have expanded from classic adenomas and currently include hyperplastic polyps and aberrant crypt foci; the earliest morphological precursor lesion. Although, prognostic molecular makers are still limited for colorectal cancers, with the recent advances in gene expression profiling more prognostic molecular markers can be identified for both therapeutic and early detection purpose.

REFERENCES

1. American Cancer Society (ACS). 1997. Cancer Facts and Figures. ACS: Atlanta, GA, pp. 10–11.
2. Bedenne L, Faivre J, Boutron MC, Piard F, Cauvin JM, Hillon P. 1992. Adenoma-carcinoma sequence or "de novo" carcinogenesis?: a study of adenomatous remnants in a population-based series of large bowel Cancer. Cancer 69:883–888.
3. Kuramoto S and Oohara T. 1989. Flat early Cancer of the large intestine. Cancer 64:950–955.
4. Shimoda T, Ikegami M, Fujisaki J, Matsui T, Aizawa S, Ishikawa E. 1989. Early colorectal carcinoma with special reference to its development de novo. Cancer 64:1138–1146.
5. Iishi H, Kitamura S, Nakaizumi A, et al. 1993. Clinicopatholgical features and endoscopic diagnosis of superficial early adenocarcinomas of the large intestine. Dig. Dis. Sci. 38:1333–1337.
6. Tada S, Yao T, Iida M, Koga H, Hizawa K, Fujishima M. 1994. A clincopathologic study of small flat colorectal carcinoma. Cancer 74:2430–2435.
7. Matsumoto T, Iida,M, Yao T, and Fujishima M. 1994. Role of nonpolypoid neoplastic lesions in the pathogenesis of colorectal cancer. Dis. Colon Rectum. 37:450–455.

8. Wada R, Matsukuma S, Abe H, et al. 1996. Histopathological studies of superficial-type early colorectal carcinoma. Cancer 77:44–50.

9. Fearon ER and Vogelstein B. 1990. A genetic model for colorectal tumorigenesis. Cell 61: 759–767.

10. Vogelstein B, Fearon ER, Hamilton SR, et al. 1988. Genetic alterations during colorectal-tumor development. N. Engl. J. Med. 319:525–532.

11. Ionov Y, Peinado MA, Malkhosyan S, Shibata D, Perucho M. 1993. Ubiquitous somatic mutations in simple repeated sequences reveal a new mechanism for colonic carcinogenesis. Nature 363:558–561.

12. Thibodeau SN, Bren G, Schaid D. 1993. Microsatellite instability in cancer of the proximal colon. Science 260:816–819.

13. Thibodeau SN, French AJ, Cunningham JM, et al. 1998. Microsatellite instability in colorectal cancer: different mutator phenotypes and the principal involvement of hMLH1. Cancer Res. 58:1713–1718.

14. Akiyama Y, Sato H, Yamada T, et al. 1997. Germ-line mutation of the hMSH6/GTBP gene in an atypical hereditary nonpolyposis colorectal cancer kindred. Cancer Res. 57:3920–3923.

15. Ruschoff J, Dietmaier W, Luttges J, et al. 1997. Poorly differentiated colonic adenocarcinoma, medullary type: clinical, phenotypic, and molecular characteristics. Am. J. Pathol. 150: 1815–1825.

16. Kim H, Jen J, Vogelstein B, Hamilton SR. 1994. Clinical and pathological characteristics of sporadic colorectal carcinomas with DNA replication errors in microsatellite sequences. Am. J. Pathol. 145:148–156.

17. Alexander J, Watanabe T, Wu T-T, Rashid A, Li S, Hamilton SR. 2001. Histopathological identification of colon cancer with microsatellite instability. Am. J. Pathol. 158:527–535.

18. Baylin SB, Herman JG, Graff JR, Vertino PM, Issa, JP. 1998. Alterations in DNA methylation: a fundamental aspect of neoplasia. Adv. Cancer Res. 72:141–196.

19. Toyota M, Ahuja N, Ohe-Toyota M, Herman JG, Baylin,SB, Issa J-PJ. 1999. CpG island methylator phenotype in colorectal cancer. Proc. Natl. Acad. Sci. USA 96:8681–8686.

20. Toyota M, Ohe-Toyota M, Ahuja N, Issa J-PJ. 2000. Distinct genetic profiles in colorectal tumors with or without the CpG island methylator phenotype. Proc. Natl. Acad. Sci. USA 97:710–715.

21. Morson BC. 1974. The polyp-cancer sequence in the large bowel. Proc. R. Soc. Med. 67: 451–457.

22. Hill MJ, Morson BC, Bussey HJ. 1978. Aetiology of adenoma-carcinoma sequence in large bowel. Lancet 1:245–247.

23. Leister I, Weith A, Bruderlein S, Cziepluch C, Kanwanpong D, Schlag P. 1990. Human colorectal Cancer: high frequency of deletions at chromosome 1p35. Cancer Res. 50: 7232–7235.

24. Vogelstein B, Fearon ER, Kern,SE, et al. 1989. Allelotype of colorectal carcinomas. Science 244:207–211.

25. Delattre O, Olschwang S, Law DJ, et al. 1989. Multiple genetic alterations distinguish distal from proximal colorectal cancer. Lancet 2:353–356.

26. Groden J, Thliveris A, Samowitz W, et al. 1991. Identification and characterization of the familial adenomatous polyposis coli gene. Cell 66:589–600.

27. Joslyn G, Carlson M, Thliveris A, et al. 1991. Identification of deletion mutations in three new genes at the familial polyposis locus. Cell 66:601–613.

28. Kinzler KW, Nilbert MC, Su L-K, et al. 1991. Identification of FAP locus genes from chromosome 5q21. Science 253:661–665.

29. Nishisho I, Nakamura Y, Miyoshi Y, et al. 1991. Mutations of chromosome 5q21 genes in FAP and colorectal cancer patients. Science 253:665–669.

30. Miyaki M, Konishi M, Kikuchi-Yanoshita R, et al. 1994. Characteristics of somatic mutation of the adenomatous polyposis of coli gene in colorectal tumors. Cancer Res. 54:3011–3020.

31. Powell SM, Zilz N, Beazer-Barclay Y, et al. 1992. APC mutations occur early during colorectal tumorigenesis. Nature 359:235–237.
32. Jen J, Powell SM, Papadopoulos N, et al. 1994. Molecular determinants of dysplasia in colorectal lesions. Cancer Res. 54:5523–5526.
33. Morin PJ, Sparks AB, Korinek V, et al. 1997. Activation of β-Catenin-Tcf signaling in colon cancer by mutations in β-Catenin or APC. Science 275:1787–1790.
34. Korinek V, Barker N, Morin PJ, et al. 1997. Constitutive transcriptional activation by a β-Catenin-Tcf complex in APC–/– colon carcinoma. Science 275:1784–1787.
35. Su L-K, Vogelstein B, Kinzler KW. 1993. Association of the APC tumor suppressor protein with catenins. Science 262:1734–1737.
36. Rubinfeld B, Souza B, Albert I, et al. 1993. Association of the APC gene product with β-Catenin. Science 262:1731–1734.
37. Hulsken J, Birchmeier W, Behrens J. 1997. E-cadherin and APC compete for the interaction with beta-catenin and the cytoskeleton. J. Cell. Biol. 127:2061–2069.
38. Baker SJ, Fearon ER, Nigro JM, et al. 1989. Chromosome 17 deletions and p53 gene mutations in colorectal carcinomas. Science 244:217–221.
39. Kikuchi-Yanoshita R, Konishi M, Ito S, et al. 1992. Genetic changes of both p53 alleles associated with the conversion from colorectal adenoma to early carcinoma in familial adenomatous polyposis and non-familial adenomatous polyposis patients. Cancer Res. 52:3965–3971.
40. Ohue M, Tomita N, Monden T, et al. 1994. A frequent alteration of p53 gene in carcinoma in adenoma of colon. Cancer Res. 54:4798–4804.
41. Baker SJ, Preisinger AC, Jessup JM, et al. 1990. p53 gene mutations occur in combination with 17p allelic deletions as late events in colorectal tumorigenesis. Cancer Res. 50:7717–7722.
42. Fearon ER, Cho KR, Nigro JM, et al. 1990. Identification of a chromosome 18q gene that is altered in colorectal cancer. Science 247:49–56.
43. Takagi Y, Kohmura H, Futamura M, et al. 1996. Somatic alterations of the DPC4 gene in human colorectal Cancer in vivo. Gastroenterology 111:1369–1372.
44. Maitra A, Molberg K, Albores-Saavedra J, Lindberg G. 2000. Loss of Dpc4 expression in colonic adenocarcinomas correlates with the presence of metastatic disease. Am. J. Pathol. 157:1105–1111.
45. Jen J, Kim H, Piantadosi S, et al. 1994. Allelic loss of chromosome 18q and prognosis in colorectal cancer. N. Engl. J. Med. 331:213–221.
46. Shibata D, Reale MA, Lavin P, et al. 1996. The DCC protein and prognosis in colorectal cancer. N. Engl. J. Med. 335:1727–1732.
47. Smith AJ, Stern HS, Penner M, et al. 1994. Somatic APC and K-ras codon 12 mutations in aberrant crypt foci from human colons. Cancer Res. 54:5527–5530.
48. Yashiro M, Carethers JM, Laghi L, et al. 2001. Genetic pathways in the evolution of morphologically distinct colorectal neoplasms. Cancer Res. 61:2676–2683.
49. Sparks AB, Morin PJ, Vogelstein B, Kinzler KW. 1998. Mutational analysis of the APC/beta-catenin/Tcf pathway in colorectal Cancer. Cancer Res. 58:1130–1134.
50. Samowitz WS, Powers MD, Spirio LN, Nollet F, van Roy F, Slattery ML. 1999. β-Catenin Mutations are more frequent in small colorectal adenomas than in larger adenomas and invasive carcinomas. Cancer Res. 59:1442–1444.
51. Hamada H, Seidman M, Howard BH, Gorman CM. 1984. Enhanced gene expression by the poly(dT-dG)Poly(dC-dA) sequence. Mol. Cell. Biol. 4:2622–2639.
52. Slightom JL, Blechl AE, and Smithies O. 1980. Human fetal $^{G}\gamma$ and $^{A}\gamma$-globin genes: complete nucleotide sequences suggest that DNA can be exchanged between these duplicated genes. Cell 21:627–638.
53. Spitzner JR, Chung IK, Muller MT. 1990. Eukaryotic topoisomerase II preferentially cleaves alternating purine-pyrimidine repeats. Nucleic Acids Res. 18:1–11.
54. Boland CR, Thibodeau SN, Hamilton SR, et al. 1998. A national cancer institute workshop on microsatellite instability for cancer detection and familial predisposition: development of inter-

national criteria for the determination of microsatellite instability in colorectal cancer. Cancer Res. 58:5248–5257.

55. Fujiwara T, Stolker JM, Watanabe T, et al. 1998. Accumulated clonal genetic alterations in familial and sporadic colorectal carcinomas with widespread instability in microsatellite sequences. Am. J. Pathol. 153:1063–1078.

56. Samowitz WS, Holden JA, Curtin K, et al. 2001. Inverse relationship between microsatellite instability and K-ras and p53 gene alterations in colon cancer. Am. J. Pathol. 158:1517–1524.

57. Kitaeva MN, Grogan L, Williams JP, et al. 1997. Mutations in β-catenin are uncommon in colorectal cancer occurring in occasional replication error-positive tumors. Cancer Res. 57:4478–4481.

58. Mirabelli-Primdahl L, Gryfe R, Kim H, et al. 1999. Beta-catenin mutations are specific for colorectal carcinomas with microsatellite instability but occur in endometrial carcinomas irrespective of mutator pathway. Cancer Res. 59:3346–3351.

59. Markowitz S, Wang J, Myeroff L, et al. 1995. Inactivation of the type II TGF-b receptor in colon cancer cells with microsatellite instability. Science 268:13336–13338.

60. Souza RF, Appel R, Yin J, et al. 1996. Microsatellite instability in the insulin-like growth factor II receptor gene in gastrointestinal tumours. Nat. Genet. 14:255–257.

61. Yamamoto H, Sawai H, Weber TK, Rodriguez-Bigas MA, Perucho M. 1998. Somatic frameshift mutations in DNA mismatch repair and proapoptosis genes in hereditary nonpolyposis colorectal cancer. Cancer Res. 58:997–1003.

62. Zhang L, Yu J, Willson JKV, Markowitz SD, Kinzler KW, Vogelstein B. 2001. Short mononucleotide repeat sequence variability in mismatch repair-deficient cancers. Cancer Res. 61:3801–3805.

63. Peltomaki P, Aaltonen LA, Sistonen P, et al. 1993. Genetic mapping of a locus predisposing to human colorectal cancer. Science 260:810–812.

64. Lindblom A, Tannergard P, Werelius B, Nordenskjold M. 1993. Genetic mapping of a second locus predisposing to hereditary non-polyposis colon cancer. Cell 5:279–282.

65. Fujii H and Shimada T. 1989. Isolation and characterization of cDNA clones derived from the divergently transcribed gene in the region upstream from the human dihydrofolate reductase gene. J. Biol. Chem. 264:10,057–10,064.

66. Palombo F, Gallinari P, Iaccarino I, et al. 1995. GTBP, a 160-kilodalton protein essential for mismatch-binding activity in human cells. Science 268:1912–1914.

67. Papadopoulos N, Nicolaides NC, Liu B, et al. 1995. Mutations of GTBP in genetically unstable cells. Science 268:1915–1917.

68. Kolodner RD. 1996. Biochemistry and genetics of eukaryotic mismatch repair. Genes. Dev. 10:1433–1442.

69. Kuismanen S., Holmberg MT, Salovaara R, de la Chapelle A, Peltomaki P. 2000. Genetic and epigenetic modification of MLH1 accounts for a major share of microsatellite unstable colorectal cancers. Am. J. Pathol. 156:1773–1779.

70. Deng G, Chen A, Hong J, Chae HS, Kim YS. 1999. Methylation of CpG in a small region of the hMLH1 promoter invariably correlates with the absence of gene expression. Cancer Res. 59:2029–2033.

71. Kane MF, Loda M, Gaida GM, et al. 1997. Methylation of the hMLH1 promoter correlates with lack of expression of hMLH1 in sporadic colon tumors and mismatch repair-defective human tumor cell lines. Cancer Res. 57:808–811.

72. Cunningham JM, Christensen ER, Tester DJ, et al. 1998. Hypermethylation of the hMLH1 promoter in colon cancer with microsatellite instability. Cancer Res. 58:3455–3460.

73. Veigl ML, Kasturi L, Olechnowicz J, et al. 1998. Biallelic inactivation of hMLH1 by epigenetic gene silencing, a novel mechanism causing human MSI cancers. Proc. Natl. Acad. Sci. 95: 8698–8702.

74. Malkhosyan S, Rampino N, Yamamoto H, Perucho M. 1996. Frameshift mutator mutations. Nature 382:499–500.

75. Yamamoto H, Sawai H, Perucho M. 1997. Frameshift somatic mutations in gastrointestinal cancer of the microsatellite mutator phenotype. Cancer Res. 57:4420–4426.

76. Wu Y, Berend MJ, Mensink RG, et al. 1999. Association of hereditary nonpolyposis colorectal cancer-related tumors displaying low microsatel-lite instability with MSH6 germline mutations. Am. J. Hum. Genet. 65:1291–1298.

77. Wijnen JT, de Leeuw W, Vasen H, et al. 1999. Familial endometrial cancer in female carriers of MSH6 mutations. Nat. Genet. 23:142–144.

78. Parc YR, Halling KC, Wang L, et al. 2000. HMSH6 alterations in patients with microsatellite instability-low colorectal cancer. Cancer Res. 60:2225–2231.

79. Lothe RA, Peltomaki P, Meling GI, et al. 1993. Genomic instability in colorectal cancer: relationship to clinicopathological variables and family history. Cancer Res. 53:5849–5852.

80. Halling KC, French AJ, McDonnell SK, et al. 1999. Microsatellite instability and 8p allelic imbalance in stage B2 and C colorectal cancers. J. Natl. Cancer Inst. 91:1295–1303.

81. Johannsdottir JT, Bergthorsson JT, Gretarsdottir S, et al. 1999. Replication error in colorectal carcinoma: association with loss of heterozygosity at mismatch repair loci and clinicopathological variables. Anticancer Res. 19:1821–1826.

82. Jernvall P, Makinen MJ, Karttunen TJ, Makela J, Vihko P. 1999. Microsatellite instability: impact on cancer progression in proximal and distal colorectal cancers. Eur. J. Cancer 35:197–201.

83. Lukish JR, Muro K, DeNobile J, et al. 1998. Prognostic significance of DNA replication errors in young patients with colorectal cancer. Ann. Surg. 227:51–56.

84. Gryfe R, Kim H, Hsieh ET, et al. 2000. Tumor microsatellite instability and clinical outcome in young patients with colorectal cancer. N. Engl. J. Med. 342:69–77.

85. Young J, Simms LA, Biden KG, et al. 2001. Features of colorectal cancers with high-level microsatellite instability occurring in familial and sporadic settings: parallel pathways of tumorigenesis. Am. J. Pathol. 159:2107–2116.

86. Bird AP. 1986. CpG-rich islands and the function of DNA methylation. Nature 321: 209–213.

87. Li E, Bestor TH, Jaenisch R. 1992. Targeted mutation of the DNA methyltransferase gene results in embryonic lethality. Cell 69:915–926.

88. Baylin SB, Herman JG, Graff JR, Vertino PM, Issa JP. 1998. Alterations in DNA methylations: a fundamental aspect of neoplasia. Adv. Cancer Res. 72:141–196.

89. Issa J-P, Ottaviano YL, Celano P, Hamilton SR, Davidson NE, Baylin SB. 1994. Methylation of the oestrogen receptor CpG island links aging and neoplasia in the human colon. Nat. Genet. 7:536–540.

90. Issa JP. 2000. CpG island methylation in aging and cancer. Curr. Top. Microbiol. Immunol. 249:101–118.

91. Issa J-P, Vertino PM, Boehm CD, Newsham IF, Baylin SB. 1996. Switch from monoallelic to biallelic human IGF2 promoter methylation during ageing and carcinogenesis. Proc. Natl. Acad. Sci. USA 93:11757–11762.

92. Ahuja N, Li Q, Mohan AL, Baylin SB, Issa J-P. 1998. Ageing and DNA methylation in colorectal mucosa and cancer. Cancer Res. 58:5489–5494.

93. Jones PA and Laird PW. 1999. Cancer epigenetics comes of age. Nat. Genet. 21:163–167.

94. Esteller M, Toyota M, Sanchez-Cespedes M, et al. 2000. Inactivation of the DNA repair gene O6-methylguanine-DNA methyltransferase by promoter hypermethylation is associated with G to A mutations in K-ras in colorectal tumorigenesis. Cancer Res. 60:2368–2371.

95. Whitehall VLJ, Walsh MD, Young J, Leggett BA, Jass JR. 2001. Methylation of O-6-methylguanine DNA methyltransferase characterizes a subset of colorectal cancer with low-level DNA microsatellite instability. Cancer Res. 61:827–830.

96. Chan AO-O, Broaddus RR, Houlihan PS, Issa J-PJ, Hamilton SR, Rashid A. 2002. CpG island methylation in aberrant crypt foci of the colorectum. Am. J. Pathol. 160:1823–1830.

97. Rashid A, Shen L, Morris JS, Issa JPJ, Hamilton SR. 2001. CpG island methylation in colorectal adenomas. Am. J. Pathol. 159:1129–1135.

98. Rashid A, Houlihan PS, Booker S, Petersen GM, Giardiello FM, Hamilton SR. 2000. Phenotypic and Molecular Characteristics of Hyperplastic Polyposis. Gastroenterology 119:323–332.

99. Jass JR, Cottier DS, Pokos V, ParryS, Winship IM. 1997. Mixed epithelial polyps in association with hereditary non-polyposis colorectal cancer providing an alternative pathway of cancer histogenesis. Pathology 29:28–33.

100. Iino H, Jass JR, Simms LA, et al. 1999. DNA microsatellite instability in hyperplastic polyps, serrated adenomas, and mixed polyps: a mild mutator pathway for colorectal cancer? J. Clin. Pathol. 52:5–9.

101. Jass JR, Iino H, Ruszkiewicz A, et al. 2000. Neoplastic progression occurs through mutator pathways in hyperplastic polyposis of the colorectum. Gut 47:43–49.

102. Jass JR. 2001. Serrated route to colorectal cancer: back street or super highway? J. Pathol. 193:283–285.

103. Hawkins NJ and Ward RL. 2001. Sporadic colorectal cancers with microsatellite instability and their possible origin in hyperplastic polyps and serrated adenomas. J. Natl. Cancer Inst. 93: 1307–1313.

104. Jass JR, Young J, Leggett BA. 2000. Hyperplastic polyps and DNA microsatellite unstable cancers of the colorectum. Histopathology 37:295–301.

105. Jass JR, Biden KG, Cummings MC, et al. 1999. Characterization of a subtype of colorectal cancer combining features of suppressor and mild mutator pathways. J. Clin. Pathol. 52: 455–460.

106. Nucci MR, Robinson CR, Longo P, Campbell P, Hamilton SR. 1997. Phenotypic and genotypic characteristics of aberrant crypt foci in human colorectal mucosa. Hum. Pathol. 28:1396–1407.

107. Pretlow TP, Brasitus TA, Fulton NC, Cheyer C, Kaplan EL. 1993. K-ras mutations in putative preneoplastic lesions in human colon. J. Natl. Cancer Inst. 85:2004–2007.

108. Heinen CD, Shivapurkar N, Tang Z, Groden J, Alabaster O. 1996. Microsatellite instability in aberrant crypt foci from human colons. Cancer Res. 56:5339–5341.

109. Yamashita N, Minamoto T, Ochiai A, Onda M, Esumi H. 1995. Frequent and characteristic K-ras activation and absence of p53 protein accumulation in aberrant crypt foci of the colon. Gastroenterology 108:434–440.

110. Otori K, Konishi M, Sugiyama K, et al. 1998. Infrequent somatic mutation of the adenomatous polyposis coli gene in aberrant crypt foci of human colon tissue. Cancer 83:896–900.

111. Takayama T, Ohi M, Hayashi T, et al. 2001. Analysis of K-ras, APC, and β-catenin in aberrant crypt foci in sporadic adenoma, cancer, and familial adenomatous polyposis. Gastroenterology 121:599–611.

112. Pedroni M, Sala E, Scarselli A, et al. 2001. Microsatellite instability and mismatch-repair protein expression in hereditary and sporadic colorectal carcinogenesis. Cancer Res. 61:896–899.

113. Augenlicht LH, Richards C, Corner G, Pretlow TP. 1996. Evidence for genomic instability in human colonic aberrant crypt foci. Oncogene 12:1767–1772.

114. Heinen CD, Shivapurkar N, Tang, Groden J, Alabaster O. 1996. Microsatellite instability in aberrant crypt foci from human colons. Cancer Res. 56:5339–5341.

115. Dai CY, Furth EE, Mick R, et al. 2000. p16(INK4a) expression begins early in human colon neoplasia and correlates inversely with markers of cell proliferation. Gastroenterology 119: 929–942.

116. Lieverse RJ, Kibbelaar RE, Griffioen G, Lamers, CBHW. 1995. Colonic adenocarcinoma in a patient with multiple hyperplastic polyps. Neth. J. Med. 46:185–188.

117. Orii S, Nakamura S, Sugai T, et al. 1997. Hyperplastic (metaplastic) polyposis of the colorectum associated with adenomas and an adenocarcinoma. J. Clin. Gastroenterol. 25:369–372.

118. Bengoechea O, Martinez-Penuela JM, Larrinaga B, Valerdi J, Borda F. 1987. Hyperplastic polyposis of the colorectum and adenocarcinoma in a 24-year-old man. Am. J. Surg. Pathol. 11:323–327.

119. Jeevaratnam P, Cottier DS, Browett PJ, van de Water, NS, Pokos V, Jass JR. 1996. Familial giant hyperplastic polyposis predisposing to colorectal cancer: a new hereditary bowel Cancer syndrome. J. Pathol. 179:20–25.

120. Lothe RA, Andersen SN, Hofstad B, et al. 1995. Deletion of 1p loci and microsatellite instability in colorectal polyps. Genes Chromosomes Cancer 14:182–188.

121. Bardi G, Pandis N, Fenger C, Kronborg O, Bomme L, Heim S. 1993. Deletion of 1p36 as a primary chromosomal aberration in intestinal tumorigenesis. Cancer Res. 53:1895–1898.

122. Otori K, Oda Y, Sugiyama K, et al. 1997. High frequency of K-ras mutations in human colorectal hyperplastic polyps. Gut 40:660–663.

123. Leggett BA, Devereaux B, Biden K, Searle J, Young, J, Jass J. 2001. Hyperplastic polyposis: association with colorectal cancer. Am. J. Surg. Pathol. 25:177–184.

124. Chan AO-O, Issa J-PJ, Morris JS, Hamilton SR, Rashid A. 2002. Concordant CpG island methylation in hyperplastic polyposis. Am. J. Pathol. 160:529–536.

125. Young J, Biden KG, Simms LA, et al. HPP1: 2001. A transmembrane protein-encoding gene commonly methylated in colorectal polyps and Cancer. PNAS 98:265–270.

126. Urbanski SJ, Kossakowska AE, Marcon N, Bruce WR. 1984. Mixed hyperplastic adenomatous polyps-an underdiagnosed entity. Am. J. Surg. Pathol. 8:551–556.

127. Longacre TA and Fenoglio-Preiser CM. 1990. Mixed hyperplastic adenomatous polyps/serrated adenomas. A distinct form of colorectal neoplasia. Am. J. Surg. Pathol. 14: 524–537.

128. Torlakovic E and Snover DC. 1996. Serrated adenomatous polyposis in humans. Gastroenterology 110:748–755.

129. Makinen MJ, George SM, Jernvall P, Makela J, Vihko P, Karttunen TJ. 2001. Colorectal carcinoma associated with serrated adenoma-prevalence, histological features and prognosis. J. Pathol. 193:286–294.

130. Leggett BA, Devereaux B, Biden K, Searle J, Young J, Jass J. 2001. Hyperplastic polyposis: association with colorectal cancer. Am. J. Surg. Pathol. 25:177–184.

131. Dehari R. 2001. Infrequent APC mutations in serrated adenoma. Tohoku J. Exp. Med. 193: 181–186.

132. Fogt F, Brien T, Brown CA, Hartmann CJ, Zimmerman RL, Odze RD. 2002. Genetic alterations in serrated adenomas: Comparison to conventional adenomas and hyperplastic polyps. Hum. Pathol. 33:87–91.

133. Hiyama T, Yokozaki H, Shimamoto F, et al. 1998. Frequent *p53* gene mutations in serrated adenomas of the colorectum. J. Pathol. 186:131–139.

134. Ajioka Y, Watanabe H, Jass JR, Yokota Y, Kobayashi M, Nishikura K. 1998. Infrequent K-ras codon 12 mutation in serrated adenomas of human colorectum. Gut 42:680–684.

135. Kang M, Mitomi H, Sada M, et al. 1999. Ki-67, p53, and Bcl-2 expression of serrated adenomas of the colon. Am. J. Surg. Pathol. 23:1158–1160.

136. Jass JR, Whitehall VLJ, Young J, Leggett BA. 2002. Emerging concepts in colorectal neoplasia. Gastroenterology 123:862–876.

137. Park S-J, Rashid A, Lee J-H, Kim SG, Hamilton SR, Wu T-T. 2003. Frequent CpG Island Methylation in Serrated Adenomas of the Colorectum. Am. J. Pathol. 3:815–822.

138. De Benedetti L, Varesco L, Pellegata NS, et al. 1993. Genetic events in sporadic colorectal adenomas: K-ras and p53 heterozygous mutations are not sufficient for malignant progression. Anticancer Res. 13:667–670.

139. Scott,N, Bell SM, Sagar P, Blair GE, Dixon MF, Quirke P. 1993. p53 expression and K-ras mutation in colorectal adenomas. Gut 34:621–624.

140. McLellan EA, Owen RA, Stepniewska KA, Sheffield JP, Lemoine NR. 1993. High frequency of K-ras mutations in sporadic colorectal adenomas. Gut 34:392–396.

141. Yamagata S, Muto T, Uchida Y, et al. 1994. Lower incidence of K-ras codon 12 mutations in flat colorectal adenomas than in polypoid adenomas. Jpn. J. Cancer Res. 85:147–151.

142. Ajiki T, Fujimori T, Ikehara H, Saitoh, Maeda S. 1995. K-ras gene mutation related to histological atypias in human colorectal adenomas. Biotech. Histochem. 70:90–94.
143. Giaretti W, Pujic N, Rapallo A, et al. 1995. K-ras-2 G-C and G-T transversions correlate with DNA aneuploidy in colorectal adenomas. Gastroenterology 108:1040–1047.
144. Morris RG, Curtis LJ, Romanowski P, et al. 1996. Ki-ras mutations in adenomas: a characteristic of cancer-bearing colorectal mucosa. J. Pathol. 180:357–363.
145. Nusko G, Sachse R, Mansmann U, Wittekind C, Hahn EG. 1997. K-ras-2 gene mutations as predictors of metachronous colorectal adenomas. Scand. J. Gastroenterol. 32:1035–1041.
146. Saraga E, Bautista D, Dorta G, et al. 1997. Genetic heterogeneity in sporadic colorectal adenomas. J. Pathol. 181:281–286.
147. Darmon E, Cleary KR, Wargovich MJ. 1994. Immunohistochemical analysis of p53 overexpression in human colonic tumors. Cancer Detect. Prev. 18:187–195.
148. Kaklamanis L, Gatter KC, Mortensen N, et al. 1993. p53 expression in colorectal adenomas. Am. J. Pathol. 142:87–93.
149. Ohue M, Tomita N, Monden T, et al. 1994. A frequent alteration of p53 gene in carcinoma in adenoma of colon. Cancer Res. 54:4798–4804.
150. Yamaguchi A, Makimoto K, Goi T, et al. 1994. Overexpression of p53 protein and proliferative activity in colorectal adenoma. Oncology 51:224–227.
151. Akiyama Y, Iwanaga R, Saitoh K, et al. Transforming growth factor (type II receptor gene mutations in adenomas from hereditary nonpolyposis colorectal cancer. Gastroenterology 112:33–39.
152. Aaltonen LA, Peltomaki P, Mecklin J-P, et al. 1994. Replication errors in benign and malignant tumors from hereditary nonpolyposis colorectal cancer patients. Cancer Res 54:1645–1648.
153. Jocoby RF, Marshall DJ, Kailas S, Schlack S, Harms B, Love R. 1995. Genetic instability associated with adenoma to carcinoma progression in hereditary nonpolyposis colon cancer. Gastroenterology 109:73–82.
154. Konishi M, Kikuchi-Yanoshita R, Tanaka K, et al. 1996. Molecular nature of colon tumors in hereditary nonpolyposis colon cancer, familial polyposis, and sporadic colon cancer. Gastroenterology 111:307–317.
155. Samowitz WS and Slattery ML. 1997. Microsatellite instability in colorectal adenomas. Gastroenterology 112:1515–1519.
156. Spirio L, Olschwang S, Groden J, et al. 1993. Alleles of the APC gene: an attenuated form of familial polyposis. Cell 75:951–957.
157. Friedl W, Meuschel S, Caspari R, et al. 1996. Attenuated familial adenomatous polyposis due to a mutation in the 3' part of the APC gene. A clue for understanding the function of the APC protein. Hum. Genet. 97:579–584.
158. Hodgson,SV, Coonar AS, Hanson PJ, et al. 1993. Two cases of 5q deletions in patients with familial adenomatous polyposis: possible link with Caroli's disease. J. Med. Genet. 30: 369–375.
159. Lamlum H, Ilyas M, Rowan A, et al. 1999. The type of somatic mutation at APC in familial adenomatous polyposis is determined by the site of the germline mutation: a new facet to Knudson's 'two-hit' hypothesis. Nat. Med. 5:1071–1075.
160. Laken SJ, Petersen GM, Gruber SB, et al. 1997. Familial colorectal cancer in Ashkenazim due to a hypermutable tract in APC. Nat. Genet. 17:79–83.
161. Stern HS, Viertelhausen S, Hunter AGW, et al. 2001. APC I1307K increases risk of transition from polyp to colorectal carcinoma in Ashkenazi Jews. Gastroenterology 120:392–400.
162. Gryfe R, Di Nicola N, Gallinger S, Redston M. 1998. Somatic instability of the APC I1307K allele in colorectal neoplasia. Cancer Res. 58:4040–4043.
163. Aaltonen LA, Salovaara R, Kristo P, et al. 1998. Incidence of hereditary nonpolyposis colorectal cancer and the feasibility of molecular screening for the disease. N. Engl. J. Med. 338: 1481–1487.

164. Evans DG, Walsh S, Jeacock J, et al. 1997. Incidence of hereditary non-polyposis colorectal cancer in a population-based study of 1137 consecutive cases of colorectal cancer. Br. J. Surg. 84:1281–1285.

165. Peltomaki P and Vasen,HF. 1997. Mutations predisposing to hereditary nonpolyposis colorectal cancer: database and results of a collaborative study. The International Collaborative Group on Hereditary Nonpolyposis Colorectal Cancer. Gastroenterology. 113:1146–1158.

166. Giardiello FM, Hamilton SR, Kern SE, et al. 1991. Colorectal neoplasia in juvenile polyposis or juvenile polyps. Arch. Dis. Child. 66:971–975.

167. Grotsky HW, Rickert RR, Smith WD, Newsome JF. 1982. Familial juvenile polyposis coli: a clinical and pathologic study of a large kindred. Gastroenterology 82:494–501.

168. Rozen P and Baratz M. 1982. Familial juvenile colonic polyposis with associated colon cancer. Cancer 49:1500–1503.

169. Howe JR, Shellnut J, Wagner B, et al. 2002. Common deletion of SMAD4 in juvenile polyposis is a mutational hotspot. Am. J. Hum. Genet. 70:1357–1362.

170. Houlston R, Bevan S, Williams A, et al. 1998. Mutations in DPC4 (SMAD4) cause juvenile polyposis syndrome, but only account for a minority of cases. Hum. Mol. Genet. 7:1907–1912.

171. Friedl W, Kruse R, Uhlhaas S, et al. 1999. Frequent 4-bp deletion in exon 9 of the SMAD4/MADH4 gene in familial juvenile polyposis patients. Genes Chromosomes Cancer 25:403–406.

172. Howe JR, Roth S, Ringold JC, et al. 1998. Mutations in the SMAD4/DPC4 gene in juvenile polyposis. Science 1086–1088.

173. Woodford-Richens K, Williamson J, Bevan S, et al. 2000. Allelic loss at SMAD4 in polyps from juvenile polyposis patients and use of fluorescence in situ hybridization to demonstrate clonal origin of the epithelium. Cancer Res. 60:2477–2482.

174. Huang SC, Chen CR, Lavine JE, et al. 2000. Genetic heterogeneity in familial juvenile polyposis. Cancer Res. 60:6882–6885.

175. Liaw D, Marsh DJ, Li J, et al. 1997. Germline mutation of the PTEN gene in Cowden disease, an inherited breast and thyroid cancer syndrome. Nat. Genet. 16:64–67.

176. Marsh DJ, Dahia PLM, Zheng Z, et al. 1997. Germline mutations in PTEN are present in Bannayan-Zonana syndrome. Nat. Genet. 16:333–334.

177. Howe JR, Bair JL, Sayed MG, et al. 2001. Germline mutations of the gene encoding bone morphogenetic protein receptor 1A in juvenile polyposis. Nat. Genet. 28:184–187.

178. Friedl W, Uhlhaas S, Schulmann K, et al. 2002. Juvenile polyposis: massive gastric polyposis is more common in MADH4 mutation carriers than in BMPR1A mutation carriers. Hum. Genet. 111:108–111.

179. Zhou XP, Woodford-Richens K, Lehtonen R, et al. 2001. Germline mutations in BMPR1A/ALK3 cause a subset of cases of juvenile polyposis syndrome and of Cowden and Bannayan-Riley-Ruvalcaba syndromes. Am. J. Hum. Genet. 69:704–711.

180. Jones KL. 1997. Bannayan-Riley-Ruvalcaba syndrome, in: Smith's Recognizable Patterns of Human Malformation, Jones KL, ed., WB Saunders: Philadelphia, pp. 522–523.

181. Longy M and Lacomb D. 1996. Cowden disease. Report of a family and review. Ann. Genet. 39:35–42.

182. Guanti G, Resta N, Simone C, et al. 2000. Involvement of PTEN mutations in the genetic pathways of colorectal cancerogenesis. Hum. Mol. Genet. 9:283–287.

183. Dicuonzo G, Angeletti S, Garcia-Foncillas J, et al. 2001. Colorectal carcinomas and PTEN/MMAC1 gene mutations. Clin. Cancer Res. 7:4049–4053.

184. Giardiello FM, Brensinger JD, Tersmette AC, et al. 2000. Very high risk of Cancer in familial Peutz-Jeghers Syndrome. Gastroenterology 119:1447–1453.

185. Hemminki A, Markie D, Tomlinson I, et al. 1998. A serine/threonine kinase gene defect in Peutz-Jeghers syndrome. Nature 391:184–187.

186. Jenne DE, Reimann H, Nezu J, et al. 1998. Peutz-Jeghers syndrome is caused by mutations in a novel serine threonine kinase. Nat. Genet. 18:38–43.

187. Hemminki A, Tomlinson I, Markie D, et al. 1997. Localization of a susceptibility locus for Peutz-Jeghers syndrome to 19p using comparative genomic hybridization and targeted linkage analysis. Nat. Genet. 15:87–90.

188. Launonen V, Avizienyte E, Loukola A, et al. 2000. No evidence of Peutz-Jeghers syndrome gene LKB1 involvement in left-sided colorectal carcinomas. Cancer Res. 60:546–548.

189. Resta N, Simone C, Mareni C, et al. 1998. STK11 mutations in Peutz-Jeghers syndrome and sporadic colon cancer. Cancer Res. 58:4799–4801.

190. McLeod HL and Murray GI. 1999. Tumour markers of prognosis in colorectal cancer. Br. J. Cancer. 79191–203.

191. Ookawa K, Sakamoto M, Hirohashi S, et al. 1993. Concordant p53 and DCC alterations and allelic losses on chromosomes 13q and 14q associated with liver metastases of colorectal carcinoma. Int. J. Cancer 53:382–387.

192. Ogunbiyi OA, Goodfellow PJ, Herfarth K, et al. 1998. Confirmation that chromosome 18q allelic loss in colon cancer is a prognostic indicator. J. Clin. Oncol. 16:427–433.

193. Lanza G, Matteuzzi M, Gafa R, et al. 1998. Chromosome 18q allelic loss and prognosis in stage II and III colon cancer. Int. J. Cancer. 79:390–395.

194. Martinez-Lopez E, Abad A, Font A, et al. 1998. Allelic loss on chromosome 18q as a prognosis in stage II and III colon cancer. Gastroenterology 114:1180–1187.

195. Jernvall P, Makinen MJ, Karttunen TJ, Makela J, Vihko P. 1999. Loss of heterozygosity at 18q21 is indicative of recurrence and therefore poor prognosis in a subset of colorectal cancers. Br. J. Cancer 79:903–908.

196. Galanis E, Alberts SR, O'Connell MJ. 2000. New adjuvant therapy for colon cancer: justified hope or commercial hype. Surg. Oncol. Clin. North Am. 9:813–823.

197. Macdonald JS. 1999. Adjuvant therapy of colon cancer. CA Cancer J. Clin. 49:202–219.

198. Carethers JM, Hawn MT, Greenson JK, Hitchcock CL, Boland CR. 1998. Prognostic significance of allelic loss at chromosome 18q21 for stage II colorectal cancer. Gastroenterology 114:1188–1195.

199. Watanabe T, Wu T-T, Catalano PJ, et al. 2001. Molecular predictors of survival after adjuvant chemotherapy for colon cancer. N. Engl. J. Med. 344:1196–1206.

200. Samowitz WS, Curtin K, Ma KN, et al. 2001. Microsatellite instability in sporadic colon cancer is associated with an improved prognosis at the population level. Cancer Epidemiol. Biomar. Prev. 10:917–923.

201. Choi SW, Lee KJ, Bae YA, et al. 2002. Genetic classification of colorectal cancer based on chromosomal loss and microsatellite instability predicts survival. Clin. Cancer Res. 8:2311–2322.

202. Elsaleh H, Powell B, Soontrapornchai P, et al. 2000. p53 Gene mutation, microsatellite instability and adjuvant chemotherapy: impact on survival of 388 patients with Dukes' C colon carcinoma. Oncology 58:52–59.

203. Elsaleh H, Powell B, McCaul K, et al. 2001. P53 alteration and microsatellite instability have predictive value for survival benefit from chemotherapy in stage III colorectal carcinoma. Clin. Cancer Res. 7:1343–1349.

204. Hemminki A, Mecklin J-P, Jarvinen H, Aaltonen LA, Joensuu H. 2000. Microsatellite instability is a favorable prognostic indicator in patients with colorectal cancer receiving chemotherapy. Gastroenterology 119:921–928.

205. Grady WM, Rajput A, Myeroff L, et al. 1998. Mutation of the type II transforming growth factor-beta receptor is coincident with the transformation of human colon adenomas to malignant carcinomas. Cancer Res. 58:3101–3104.

206. Dolcetti R, Viel A, Doglioni C, et al. 1999. High prevalence of activated intraepithelial cytotoxic T lymphocytes and increased neoplastic cell apoptosis in colorectal carcinomas with microsatellite instability. Am. J. Pathol. 154:1805–1813.

207. Guidoboni M, Gafa R, Viel A, et al. 2001. Microsatellite instability and high content of activated cytotoxic lymphocytes identify colon cancer patients with a favorable prognosis. Am. J. Pathol. 159:297–304.
208. Saeterdal I, Bjorheim J, Lislerud K, et al. 2001. Frameshift-mutation-derived peptides as tumor-specific antigens in inherited and spontaneous colorectal cancer. Proc. Natl. Acad. Sci. USA 98:13255–260.
209. Saeterdal I, Gjertsen MK, Straten P, Eriksen JA, Gaudernack G. 2001. A TGF betaRII frameshift-mutation-derived CTL epitope recognized by HLA-A2-restricted CD8+ T cells. Cancer Immunol. Immun. 50:469–476.
210. Linnebacher M, Gebert J, Rudy W, et al. 2001. Frameshift peptide-derived T-cell epitopes: a source of novel tumor-specific antigens. Int. J. Cancer 93:6–11.

21

Genetic Counseling for Hereditary Cancer Predisposition Testing

Joyce L. Seldon and Patricia A. Ganz

1. INTRODUCTION

All cancer is "genetic" in that the uncontrolled proliferation of cells is the result of numerous genetic mutations, however, we currently estimate that only 5–10% of all cancer arises in individuals with an inherited susceptibility to cancer. The malignant transformation of a cell is not the result of one mutation, but rather a complex process resulting from numerous molecular mutations associated with gene–environment interactions. The rapid advancement of molecular biology has recognized that these molecular mutations fall into at least three distinct categories: oncogenes, tumor suppressor genes, and DNA mismatch repair genes. Lifetime cancer risks for individuals with an inherited predisposition can be high for certain hereditary syndromes. It is critical to identify high-risk individuals and families to provide targeted cancer screening and prevention counseling. Effective cancer screening and surveillance may aid in the diagnosis of cancer at its earliest stages when prognosis and treatment options are more favorable. Chemoprevention, prophylactic surgery, lifestyle modifications, and other therapies may reduce the risk of developing cancer for those with a hereditary predisposition.

As new discoveries are made, the field of cancer genetics will grow to encompass new findings in gene–gene interactions and gene–environment interactions. New discoveries will also aid in our understanding of cellular processes, such as genes that affect the metabolism of hormones and other environmental agents, or how an individual may respond to specific therapies. This chapter will review genetic counseling issues involved with hereditary cancer predisposition testing. Because cancer genetic counseling is frequently requested for families with the most common hereditary neoplasms of breast, ovary, and colon, we will discuss these associated syndromes in detail.

2. FEATURES OF HEREDITARY CANCER SYNDROMES

Over 200 hereditary syndromes with cancer as a component have been described (Table 1) *(1)*. Most hereditary cancer syndromes follow an autosomal dominant pattern of inheritance with incomplete penetrance and variable expressivity. Penetrance refers to the proportion of individuals with a mutant allele (heterozygotes) who will express the associated trait or phenotype. A condition (most commonly inherited in an autosomal dominant manner) is said to have reduced or incomplete penetrance if clinical symptoms are not always present in indi-

From: *Cancer Diagnostics: Current and Future Trends*
Edited by: R. M. Nakamura, W. W. Grody, J. T. Wu, and R. B. Nagle © Humana Press Inc., Totowa, NJ

Table 1
Selected Inherited Cancer Syndromes

Syndrome	Features and associated cancers	Inheritance	Gene
Hereditary breast and ovarian cancer syndrome	Early onset breast cancer, ovarian cancer, and male breast cancer.	Autosomal dominant	*BRCA1, BRCA2*
Hereditary nonpolyposis colon cancer	Early onset colon cancer, uterine, ovarian, stomach, breast, and other GI/GU cancers.	Autosomal dominant	*hMLH1, hMSH2, hPMS1, hPMS2, MSH6*
Ataxia telangectasia	Neurologic degeneration, cerebellar ataxia, telangiectasia, immuno-deficiency, sensitivity to ionizing radiation, leukemia, and lymphomas; breast cancer in heterozygotes.	Autosomal recessive	*ATM*
Li Fraumeni syndrome	Sarcoma, breast cancer, brain, adrenocortical tumors, and leukemia	Autosomal dominant	*p53*
Cowden syndrome	Breast cancer, thyroid cancer, hamartomas, cerebellar gangliocytomas, macrocephaly, and mucocutaneous lesions	Autosomal dominant	*MMAC1, PTEN*
Peutz-Jeghers syndrome	Melanin spots of lips, buccal mucosa, and digits, GI hamartomatous polyps (especially in the jejunum) colon, breast, cervical, ovarian, testicular, and pancreatic cancer	Autosomal dominant	*STK11*
Basal cell nevus Syndrome (Gorlin syndrome)	Multiple basal cell cancers, medulloblastoma, ovarian carcinomas, fibrosarcomas, jaw cysts, palmar/plantar pits, congenital skeletal anomalies, odontogenic keratocysts, or polyostocitc bone cyst.	Autosomal dominant	*PTC*
Familial adenomatous polyposis	Colon cancer, bile duct, thyroid, small intestine. Also associated with Gardner and Turcot syndrome.	Autosomal dominant	*APC*
Multiple endocrine neoplasia, type 1	Tumors of the parathyroid glands, pancreatic islets, and pituitary glands. Increased risk for parathyroid carcinomas, pancreatic islet cell tumors, and carcinoid tumors.	Autosomal dominant	*MEN1*
Multiple endocrine neoplasia, type 2	Medullary thyroid carcinomas (MTC), pheochromocytomas, and benign parathyroid tumors.	Autosomal dominant	*RET*

Table 2
Cardinal Features of Hereditary Cancer Syndromes

1. Multiple affected family members (usually two or more) with the same type of cancer or cancers that are known to be related in certain syndromes (i.e., colon, ovarian, and uterine cancer are related types of cancers in HNPCC families)
2. Multiple generations of related affected individuals (i.e., mother, daughter, and maternal aunt)
3. Younger age of onset than is typical for type of cancer (i.e., <50 yr for breast and colon cancer)
4. Presence of rare cancers (i.e., breast cancer in males)
5. Excess of multifocal or bilateral cancers (i.e., synchronous and metasynchronous colon cancer is found in HNPCC)
6. Multiple primary cancers in the same individual (i.e., breast and ovarian cancer primaries in the same woman)
7. Physical findings that may suggest a hereditary syndrome (i.e., gastrointestinal hamartomatous polyps and excessive melanin deposits on the skin are possible characteristics of Peutz-Jeghers' syndrome)

viduals who have the disease-causing mutation. In hereditary cancer syndromes, the penetrance is usually not 100% because the phenotype is not always present in individuals who have the disease causing mutation(s). Variable expressivity refers to the extent that the phenotype is expressed. Variations in the clinical features of a hereditary cancer syndrome (e.g., type of cancer, pathologic features of a tumor, or age of onset) are observed between family members with the same deleterious mutation (intrafamilial variable expressivity) and between families with the same deleterious mutation (interfamilial variable expressivity).

The interpretation of family history is important in determining whether to suspect a possible hereditary cancer syndrome. Features of a family history, such as early age at diagnosis and multiple affected individuals demonstrating autosomal dominant inheritance are some of the "red flags" for a possible hereditary syndrome (Table 2). These concepts are important when providing cancer genetic counseling because an individual does not inherit cancer, but rather an increased risk for cancer or an inherited predisposition to cancer.

3. GENETIC COUNSELING

Genetic counseling is the process of communicating genetic, medical, and scientific knowledge into understandable and practical information for the patient so an educated and fully informed choice about testing can be made. Health care providers should also be prepared to discuss all possible consequences of testing and options for the medical and psychological management of the patient post-testing. The American Society of Clinical Oncology, the National Society of Genetic Counselors, the American Society of Human Genetics, and the National Action Plan on Breast Cancer have all issued position papers on cancer genetic susceptibility testing *(2–5)*. Cancer susceptibility testing should only be performed after comprehensive genetic counseling and informed consent. Genetic counseling should be provided before, during, and after susceptibility testing.

3.1. Family History

Because hereditary cancer syndromes only occur in a small proportion of the population, the key to identifying a family at risk for a hereditary cancer syndrome is taking an adequate family history. The gathering of family history should be represented in a pedigree structure using standard nomenclature *(6)*. At a minimum, the initial family history should include the current age or age at death, medical history, cause of death (if applicable), and cancer history of all first- and second-degree relatives of the patient, not just affected relatives. The pedigree should be extended, as appropriate, to more distant relatives. Important features to identify are the number of cancer cases in the family, type of primary cancer, multiple primary cancers, age of onset/diagnosis, degree of relationship, location/laterality of cancer, bilateral disease in paired organs, rare cancers, possible environmental exposures, and possible cancer risk reducing procedures or interventions (e.g., oophorectomy, hysterectomy). Ethnicity and the presence of consanguinity are also important to document in the pedigree. Family histories can often be inaccurately reported by patients *(7)*, therefore, confirmation of cancer history by medical records, pathology reports, death certificates, and autopsy reports should be obtained whenever possible. It is important to note that a family history of cancer is dynamic and can change over time; therefore, it must be updated periodically. Unaffected relatives can develop cancer in the interim between visits to a healthcare provider and change the risk assessment of the pedigree.

3.2. Risk Assessment

The following aspects of the family history can identify average-risk, moderate-risk, and high-risk individuals:

1. Number of affected relatives.Most inherited cancer syndromes will have multiple affected individuals (on the same side of the family) with the same type of cancer or cancers that are known to be related. The more family members with cancer, the more likely there is an inherited susceptibility. Small families might be difficult to assess.
2. Ratio of affected to unaffected relatives. It is important not to neglect unaffected relatives. A 65-yr-old patient with a history of breast cancer at 39 might seem significant until you learn that she has five older sisters with no cancer history. In assessing autosomal dominant patterns of inheritance, it is important to recognize the ratio of affected relatives to unaffected relatives. Again, small families will be difficult to assess.
3. Closeness of biological relationship of affected relatives. Family history should include affected individuals who are at least first or second degree relatives. Keep in mind that most hereditary cancer syndromes are not fully penetrant, so unaffected obligate carriers are always a possibility. Additionally, some syndromes predominantly affect females (i.e., BRCA1/2), so males are sometimes unaffected obligate carriers.
4. Ages at cancer diagnoses. Most hereditary cancer syndromes typically have earlier ages of onset for specific tumors than their sporadic counterparts.
5. Presence of bilateral/multifocal or multiple primary cancers. Affected individuals with an inherited susceptibility frequently present with bilateral or multifocal cancers. These same individuals are also at risk for second primary cancers associated with the hereditary syndrome.
6. Case(s) of rare cancer. The familial clustering of cancers that rarely occur in the general population are difficult to explain by chance alone. Rare cancers such as male breast cancer and childhood adrenal gland tumors are "flags" for certain hereditary cancer syndromes and a careful family history should be obtained and assessed.

3.3. *Informed Consent: Risks, Benefits, and Limitations of Testing*

The complexities and special nature of hereditary cancer susceptibility testing requires adequate informed consent and genetic counseling. In the process of offering cancer predisposition testing to a patient or family, both the healthcare provider and the individual being tested must be prepared to not only deal with the medical aspects of testing, but also with the psychological, legal, and social consequences of testing. Proper informed consent should include discussion of basic principles of cancer biology; basic genetic concepts such as inheritance, genes, mutations, patterns of inheritance, variable expression of genes, heterogeneity, polymorphisms, and penetrance of genes. Additionally, implications of a positive, negative, or ambiguous result and informative testing; limitations; possible benefits of testing; genetic risk to relatives and transmission of mutation to offspring should be discussed. Accuracy of testing, costs, risk of psychological distress and strain on family relationships, risk of employment/insurance discrimination and stigmatization, confidentiality and sharing of results should be discussed along with the limitations of medical surveillance, screening, prophylactic surgery, chemoprevention, and alternatives to testing.

3.4. *Interpretation of Results*

Whenever possible, informative genetic cancer susceptibility testing should begin with an affected relative at high risk to carry a hereditary mutation (Fig. 1). A positive test result means that the patient has an increased likelihood of developing cancer associated with deleterious mutations in a particular gene. It allows for informative testing of other affected and unaffected relatives who may be at risk for carrying the familial mutation based on the inheritance of the syndrome.

Negative test results can be difficult to interpret and to convey to patients. A negative test result in an affected individual from a high risk family has the following interpretations: false negative (individual is really positive for a mutation in tested gene, but the mutation was either not tested for or undetectable using particular lab method); a different (untested) gene(s) is responsible; the familial clustering is actually sporadic and the result of a chance event; or this is a family with a hereditary cancer syndrome, but the patient initially tested is a sporadic case (phenocopy). Therefore, testing of an unaffected individual is most informative in the context of a known mutation; however, this is not always possible. A negative test result in an unaffected individual is only a "true negative" if a mutation is known in the family. A negative test result in an unaffected individual from a family with no known hereditary mutation is considered "uninformative." What this means is that a negative result does not allow the health care professional to reassure the patient that his/her chances of developing cancer are the same as the general population because a mutation has not been previously identified. The patient may still have an inherited susceptibility because of an alteration in the gene tested or because of an alteration in a different gene that was not tested. Of course, it is also possible that the patient does not have an inherited susceptibility at all. The patient has learned little about his/her cancer after the test is performed and a negative result does not mean that the patient should stop close cancer screening procedures or give up actions and behaviors that reduce cancer risk.

Ambiguous test results are a challenge associated with cancer predisposition testing. The most common example is a DNA sequence variant of undetermined clinical significance

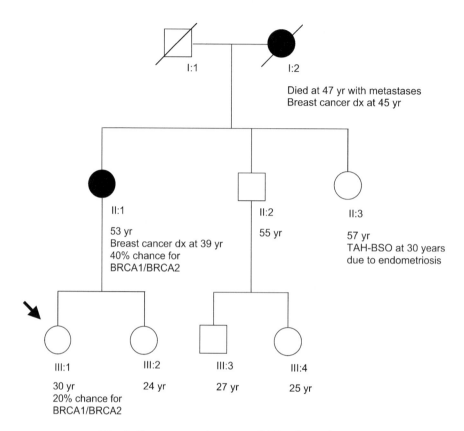

Ashkenazi Jewish Ancestry

I:1

I:2

Died at 47 yr with metastases
Breast cancer dx at 45 yr

II:1

53 yr
Breast cancer dx at 39 yr
40% chance for
BRCA1/BRCA2

II:2

55 yr

II:3

57 yr
TAH-BSO at 30 years
due to endometriosis

III:1

30 yr
20% chance for
BRCA1/BRCA2

III:2

24 yr

III:3

27 yr

III:4

25 yr

Fig. 1. Cancer genetic susceptibility flow diagram

(VUS). For some VUS, there will be published scientific reports of an increased risk for cancer associated with this particular alteration, although for others there are no published scientific reports. Therefore, it is difficult to interpret whether there is an increased risk for cancer. In the future, as more is discovered about these genes, new information may clarify the risk for cancer associated with these particular alterations. Follow-up studies such as linkage analysis or testing the parents of a patient or other affected relatives may provide some useful data in interpreting the VUS *(8)*. Individualized management options should be discussed with the patient as well as encouragement to continue high-risk cancer screening procedures and actions and behaviors to reduce cancer risk.

4. BREAST AND OVARIAN CANCER: BRCA1 AND BRCA2

4.1. Background

An estimated 5–10% of breast and ovarian cancers have an inherited component *(9–12)*. Familial breast and ovarian cancer is characterized by breast cancer diagnosis at less than 50 yr of age, bilateral breast and ovarian tumors, multiple affected related individuals within a family, multiple affected generations, and a strong association with male breast cancer. In 1994 and 1995, the BRCA1 and BRCA2 genes, respectively, were isolated by positional cloning methods *(13–15)*. BRCA1 and BRCA2 have autosomal dominant inheritance with incomplete penetrance and variable expressivity. The BRCA1 and BRCA2 genes account for an estimated 84% of hereditary breast and ovarian cancers *(16,17)*. Over 400 different deleterious BRCA1 and BRCA2 mutations have been identified *(18)*. However, the existence of other breast and ovarian cancer susceptibility genes (BRCA3, BRCA4) is suspected by the identification of a high incidence of breast/ovarian cancer within families that do not show linkage to either BRCA1 or BRCA2 *(17,19–25)*. Additionally, other low-penetrance genes are being studied and may have clinical significance *(26,27)*.

4.2. Ashkenazi Jewish Population

After the finding of a BRCA1 (185delAG frameshift) mutation in several Ashkenazi Jewish breast/ovarian families, a study was conducted in 858 Ashkenazim (unselected for cancer history) and 815 control subjects (unselected for ethnic origin). The investigators found that almost 1% of the Ashkenazi Jewish population carried this mutation as compared to none of the controls, suggesting that in 100 women of Ashkenazi descent may be at an increased risk of developing breast/ovarian cancer *(28)*. Further studies confirmed a recurrent BRCA2 mutation (6174delT) at an increased carrier frequency among the Ashkenazi Jewish population *(29,30)*. Subsequent large-scale population studies found that over 2% of Ashkenazi Jews carry BRCA1 or BRCA2 mutations (185delAG, 5382insC, and 6174delT) that confer increased risks for breast, ovarian, and prostate cancer *(31,32)*. Many studies have confirmed the higher prevalence of these founder mutations among early onset breast and ovarian cancer patients *(33–39)*. Therefore, Ashkenazi Jewish ancestry is a risk factor when evaluating a family history of breast and ovarian cancer.

4.3. Risk of Cancer in Mutation Carriers

There is little doubt that women who carry a mutation for either BRCA1 or BRCA2 are at significantly increased risk of developing breast and ovarian cancer. However, estimates regarding the degree of risk for these women are still being refined. It is important for the healthcare provider and the patient to remember that hereditary cancer susceptibility testing cannot determine, with absolute certainty, whether or not an individual will develop cancer. It cannot predict what kind of cancer a patient may or may not develop or when a patient might develop cancer. Cancer risk may vary depending on the specific mutation identified and other modifying factors. According to several different studies, the lifetime risk of breast cancer for a BRCA1 or BRCA2 carrier ranges from approx 56 to 87% *(16,17,32,40–42)*. The risk for ovarian cancer ranges from approx 16–63% for BRCA1 carriers and as high as 27% for BRCA2 carriers *(16,17,32,40–42)*.

Additionally, there are other associated risks for mutation carriers. BRCA1/2 carriers with diagnosis of a first primary breast cancer are at an approx 40–65% lifetime risk for a second primary contralateral or ipsilateral breast cancer *(41,43,44)*. Male breast cancer has also been associated with BRCA1/2 mutations *(17,18,45,46)*. Studies have reported that BRCA1/2 mutation carriers are at statistically increased risks for the following cancers: pancreatic, uterine body, cervix, prostate, colon, liver, stomach, fallopian tube, melanoma, gallbladder, and bile duct *(43,44,47)*.

4.4. Probability of Detecting a BRCA1/2 Mutation

Several models exist for predicting the likelihood of detecting BRCA1/2 mutations given a certain family history and ethnic background *(48–52)*. These models may be useful in identifying families who are likely to carry a predisposing mutation in BRCA1 or BRCA2.

Table 3
Modeled Probabilities of BRCA1/2 Mutation in Women
With Early Onset Breast Cancer (<50 yr)

First- or Second-degree relative with breast cancer <50	First- or Second-degree relative with ovarian cancer (any age)	Patient with ovarian or bilateral breast cancer	Patient with breast cancer <40	Probability of BRCA1/2 or BRCA2 mutation
•				25%
•			•	40%
		•		51%
•		•	•	76%
	•			35%
	•		•	35%
	•	•		71%
	•	•	•	71%
•	•			35%
•	•		•	59%
•	•	•		71%
•	•	•	•	89%

Note: Based on analysis of women with at least 1 first- or second-degree relative with ovarian cancer or breast cancer before 50 yr of age. Adapted from ref. *48*.

Table 3 presents the modeled probability of carrying a BRCA1 or BRCA2 mutation in women with breast cancer before age 50 or ovarian cancer at any age and at least one first- or second-degree relative with either diagnosis *(48)*.

Figure 2 illustrates an example of a clinical risk assessment for a patient. This example illustrates a three-generation pedigree with two affected women with breast cancer. Individual III:1 is a 30-yr-old female who presented for genetic counseling because she was concerned about her risk for breast/ovarian cancer and was considering prophylactic surgeries. We calculate her risk of being positive for a BRCA1/BRCA2 mutation by first calculating her mother's risk (because the data apply to affected women, not unaffected women). We find that her mother, individual II:1, is alive at 53 yr of age with a previous diagnosis of breast cancer at 39 yr of age. Our patient's maternal grandmother died at 47 yr of age from breast cancer diagnosed at 45 years of age. The family is of Ashkenazi Jewish ancestry. Looking at Table 3 we see that individual II:1 fits two risk factors ("first- or second-degree relative with breast cancer <50" and "Patient with breast cancer <40") from this modeled probability, which gives her a 40% chance of carrying a gene for BRCA1 or BRCA2. Therefore, given Mendelian autosomal dominant inheritance for BRCA1/BRCA2, individual III:1 has an approx 20% risk of carrying a gene for BRCA1/BRCA2 (one-half of her mother's risk of 40%). Risk calculations, however, are not the only factors to discuss with this patient. The patient seeking genetic counseling should also have a complete discussion of the risks, benefits, and limitations of cancer genetic susceptibility testing as well as informed consent and a discussion of who in her family should have testing first (informative testing).

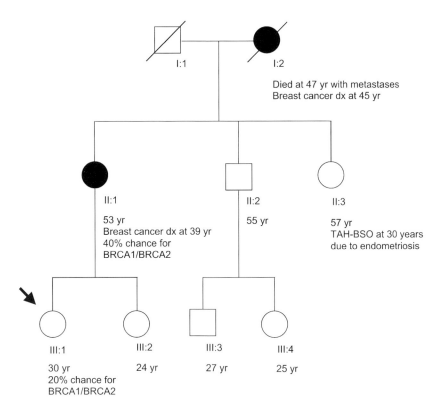

Ashkenazi Jewish Ancestry

I:1

I:2

Died at 47 yr with metastases
Breast cancer dx at 45 yr

II:1

53 yr
Breast cancer dx at 39 yr
40% chance for
BRCA1/BRCA2

II:2

55 yr

II:3

57 yr
TAH-BSO at 30 years
due to endometriosis

III:1

30 yr
20% chance for
BRCA1/BRCA2

III:2

24 yr

III:3

27 yr

III:4

25 yr

Fig. 2. A three-generation pedigree with breast cancer. Individual III:1 is the initial patient seeking genetic testing because she is concerned about her risk for breast and ovarian cancer and is considering prophylactic surgery. Note that testing should be done on an affected individual first, if possible, to establish informative testing for unaffected family members. The ideal individual to test first in this pedigree would be II:1 because she is still alive and a first degree relative to the initial patient. Also note that the modeled probability of detecting a BRCA1 or BRCA2 mutation (using Table 3) in individual II:1 is 40%. Therefore, the *a priori* chance of detecting a BRCA1 or BRCA2 mutation in her daughter is 20% (1/2 of her mother's risk given autosomal dominant inheritance). If individual II:1 tests positive for a mutation in either BRCA1 or BRCA2, then the chance that either III:1 or her sister, III:2, are positive for the same mutation is 50% each. Additionally, a positive test result in II:1 would mean that the chances for II:2, II:3, III:3, and III:4 to test positive for the same mutation would be 50%, 50%, 25%, and 25%, respectively.

4.5. Medical Management Options

The medical management of a woman with BRCA1/2 mutation is challenging and often requires a multi-disciplinary approach. The need for shared decision-making between health care providers and the patient is critical. Patients should weigh the risks, benefits, and limitations of all management options carefully. In 1997, a task force reported on the recommendations for follow-up care in BRCA1/2 carriers *(53)*. Breast cancer surveillance options include: monthly self-breast examinations (starting at 18 yr of age), annual or semiannual clinical breast exams starting at age 25, and annual mammography beginning at age 25–35 yr (or 10 yr younger than the youngest diagnosis in the family). Ovarian cancer screening options include: annual or semiannual transvaginal ultrasound with color Doppler and CA-125 blood levels *(53)*.

Prophylactic mastectomy and oophorectomy are options that should be addressed with BRCA1/2 mutation carriers. Prophylactic mastectomy has been associated with a 90% or greater reduction in the incidence of breast cancer among women with a family history of breast cancer and women who carry BRCA1/2 mutations *(54,55)*. Data regarding prophylactic oophorectomy has been shown to reduce the risk for ovarian cancer by as much as 95% and the risk of breast cancer by as much as 50% in BRCA1/2 carriers *(56–58)*. It should be emphasized to patients considering a surgical option that although prophylactic mastectomy and oophorectomy may reduce the risk of breast and ovarian cancer, the risk is never zero. Chemoprevention using tamoxifen or oral contraceptives is another option for patients to consider. In a matched case-control study, BRCA1/2 mutation carriers who used tamoxifen for 2 to 4 yr reduced their risk of developing a contralateral breast cancer by 75% *(59)*. The Breast Cancer Prevention Trial (BCPT) reported a 49% reduction in risk for invasive breast cancer and a 50% reduction in risk for noninvasive breast cancer in women at increased risk for breast cancer who took tamoxifen, a nonsteroidal anti-estrogen *(60)*. BRCA1/2 analysis from the BCPT trial has reported a 62% reduction in breast cancer incidence resulting from tamoxifen among women with BRCA2 mutations, which is consistent with the reduction in incidence as a result of tamoxifen of ER positive tumors. In contrast, the data suggested that there is no risk reduction in breast cancer incidence in BRCA1 carriers, which is consistent with the lack of effect of tamoxifen on ER negative tumors *(61)*.

The salutary effects of oral contraceptives in reducing ovarian cancer risk in the general population appear to extend to BRCA1/2 mutation carriers. A multicenter case-control study reported that the use of oral contraceptives was associated with a significant reduction in the risk of ovarian cancer among female carriers of BRCA1/2 mutations. The risk reduction was approx 20% for up to 3 yr of use and 60% for more than 6 yr of use *(62)*. In contrast, a population-based case-control in Israel did not find clear evidence of a protective effect of oral-contraceptive use among women who had a founder mutation in BRCA1/2 *(63)*.

5. HEREDITARY NONPOLYPOSIS COLORECTAL CANCER (HNPCC)

5.1. Background

Colorectal cancer is the third most common cancer in men and women. It is estimated that it will affect approx 135,400 individuals per year in the United States and is responsible for 10% of cancer mortality *(64)*. An estimated 5% of colon cancer can be attributed to highly penetrant autosomal dominant susceptibility syndromes *(65,66)*. The most common syndrome is hereditary nonpolyposis colon cancer syndrome (HNPCC), which is also known as Lynch syndrome. The rare familial adenomatous polyposis (FAP) syndrome also constitutes a small percent of inherited colon cancers. Studies of these syndromes have provided unique insights into both inherited and sporadic forms of human tumors. The HNPCC syndrome is characterized by early onset colon cancer (average onset is approx 44 yr of age) with a proximal predominance (approx 70% are proximal to the splenic flexure), multiple synchronous and metachronous colorectal cancers, and other associated cancers such as breast, ovarian carcinoma, stomach, small bowel, urinary tract (ureter and renal pelvis carcinoma),

Table 4
Clinical Criteria for HNPCC and MSI

Amsterdam criteria for HNPCC *(70)*

1. Three or more family members with colorectal cancer. One family member should be a first degree relative of the other two family members.
2. Families with familial adenomatous polyposis excluded.
3. At least two successive generations represented.
4. At least one individual younger than 50 yr at diagnosis.

Bethesda Criteria for MSI Testing *(81)*

1. Individuals with cancer in families that meet the Amsterdam criteria.
2. Individuals with two HNPCC-related cancers, including synchronous and metachronous colorectal cancers or extracolonic cancers.
3. Individuals with colorectal cancer and a first-degree relative with colorectal cancer and/or HNPCC-related extracolonic cancer and/or a colorectal adenoma; one of the cancers diagnosed at less than 45 yr, and the adenoma diagnosed at less than 40 yr.
4. Individuals with:
   a. colorectal or endometrial cancer diagnosed <45
   b. right-sided colorectal cancer with an undifferentiated pattern (solid/ cribriform) on histopathology or signet-ring-cell-type diagnosed <45 yr
   c. adenomas diagnosed <40 yr

endometrial, and pancreatic carcinoma *(67–69)*. In 1991, the International Collaborative Group on HNPCC met in Amsterdam and put forth a list of clinical criteria (Table 4) for the diagnosis of HNPCC *(70)*. Limitations of the Amsterdam criteria are that they are too restrictive in that certain features of HNPCC such as proximal colon cancer, multiple synchronous and metachronous colon cancers, and other malignancies besides colon cancer are not considered. Additionally, small pedigrees are not likely to meet the criteria.

HNPCC shows genetic heterogeneity and the syndrome is associated with mutations in the *MSH2* gene on chromosome 2p22-21 *(71,72)*, the *MLH1* gene on chromosome 3p21 *(73,74)*, the hpms1 gene on chromosome 2q31-33 *(75)*, and the *PMS2* gene on chromosome 7p22 *(75)*, and *MSH6* on chromosome 2p16 *(76)*. Thus far, all genes linked with HNPCC have been DNA mismatch repair (MMR) genes. The majority of germline mutations have been found in the *MSH2* and *MLH1* genes *(77,78)*. For many HNPCC families, a locus has yet to be discovered. The heterozygous phenotype is apparently normal. However, when the normal MMR allele is inactivated by a somatic mutation, the tissue develops a hypermutable phenotype (*see* Subheading 5.2.), which then accelerates the carcinogenic multi-step process.

5.2. Microsatellite Instability (MSI)

Microsatellites are repetitive DNA sequences that naturally occur and are highly variable from one individual to another. Microsatellite instability (MSI) refers to the hypermutable phenotype of an expanded or contracted pattern of microsatellites found in tumor tissues. MSI is infrequently found in sporadic colon cancers (10–15%) *(79)*, but is common in HNPCC kindreds (92%) *(77)* and in young patients less that 35 yr of age (58%) *(80)*. Testing for MSI can be used to identify families at high risk for HNPCC. In 1997, the Bethesda criteria (Table 4) were established for testing colorectal tumors for MSI *(81)*. MSI testing can serve as a surrogate functional marker for defective MMR function, however, it is not a direct indicator of HNPCC (because MSI does occur in sporadic tumor tissue), nor is it indicative of specific mutations in a particular mismatch repair gene.

5.3. Risks of Cancer in Mutation Carriers

The lifetime risks of cancer in HNPCC mutation carriers are approximated as follows: colorectal (78%), endometrial (43%), stomach (19%), biliary tract (18%), urinary tract (10%), and ovarian (9%) *(82)*. There is an increased risk for cancer at several other extracolonic sites such as small bowel, pancreas, and renal pelvis, and possibly breast *(68,83)*. These risks are based on gene positive HNPCC families and may be subject to ascertainment bias. Estimates regarding the degree of risk for these HNPCC families are still being refined.

Figure 3 illustrates a three-generation pedigree affected with HNPCC related cancers and some of the complexity involved in hereditary cancer testing. Individual III:1 is the initial patient seeking genetic counseling because of his concern about his family history of colon cancer. His father died when the patient was a young boy and the patient is concerned because he is getting close to the age his father was when diagnosed with colon cancer. The family does not meet the Amsterdam Criteria, but it does meet the Bethesda criteria. In doing the risk assessment, the healthcare provider should note the following: there are few family members in the first and third generation; the individuals in the third generation are some-what young; the history does include HNPCC related cancers in multiple affected individuals in multiple generations; and the affected aunt (II:3) has had uterine cancer and her treatment included an oophorectomy (reduced the risk for an ovarian cancer primary) and she has not had any colon cancer screening. One could test the patient (III:1) directly for a germline mutation. This is likely to be uninformative. One could test the patient's deceased father's (II:1) tumor tissue for MSI, but insurance is not likely to cover the cost of testing in a family member and it is not certain whether or not tumor tissue will be available and reliable. One could recommend testing commence with the patient's aunt (II:3) with either MSI testing on the uterine tumor or direct DNA analysis for the possible germline mutation. For this patient, this involves contacting a family member he barely knows and he is not sure how she will react to hearing the information and request for testing. Additionally, the test-ing has a potential impact on many family members including the patient's siblings, uncle, aunt, and numerous cousins (including a sister and female cousins possible at risk for HNPCC related cancers such as uterine and ovarian cancer). Regardless of the testing that may or may not be done, the patient and his siblings are at increased risk for colorectal cancer and should be adhering to high-risk screening recommendations.

5.4. Medical Management Options

For HNPCC carriers, an expert task force recommends colonoscopy every 1–3 yr begin-ning at age 20–25 yr *(84)*. It should be noted that colonoscopy as opposed to flexible sigmoi-doscopy is recommended owing to the characteristic right-sided colon cancers in HNPCC that the sigmoidoscopy would not detect. For women specifically, the task force recom-mended annual endometrial cancer screening with transvaginal ultrasound and/or endome-

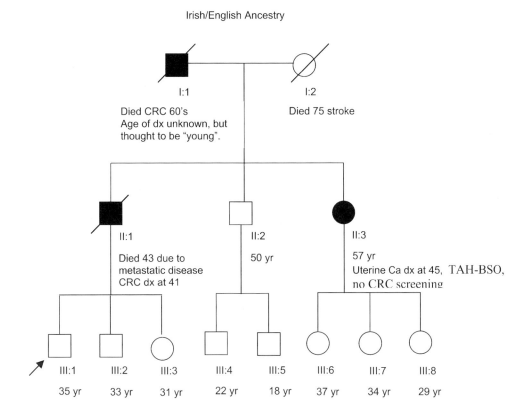

Fig. 3. A three-generation pedigree with colon and uterine cancer. Individual III:1 is the initial patient seeking genetic counseling because of his concern about his family history of colon cancer. The family does not meet the Amsterdam Criteria, but it does meet the Bethesda criteria. Note that the family history is small; the individuals in the third generation are somewhat young; the history does include HNPCC related cancers in multiple affected individuals in multiple generations; and that the affected aunt (II:3) has had uterine cancer and that her treatment included an oophorectomy (reduced the risk for an ovarian cancer primary) and that she has not had any colon cancer screening. There are different ways to approach testing this family for HNPCC, which illustrates some of the complexity of hereditary susceptibility testing. One could test the patient (III:1) directly for a germline mutation. One could test the patient's deceased father's (II:1) tumor tissue for MSI. One could recommend testing commence with the patient's aunt (II:3) with either MSI testing on the uterine tumor or DNA analysis for the possible germline mutation.

trial biopsy beginning at 25–35 yr of age. Additionally, even though there is no recommendation at this time for or against these surgeries for HNPCC mutation carriers, prophylactic subtotal colectomy, hysterectomy, and oophorectomy should be discussed as options for the patient *(84).*

6. FAMILIAL ADENOMATOUS POLYPOSIS (FAP)

6.1. Background

Familial adenomatous polyposis (FAP), also known as Gardner syndrome, is a rare colon cancer syndrome that accounts for less than 1% of colon cancer cases. FAP is an autosomal dominant condition with clinical heterogeneity expected to demonstrate complete penetrance. Classically, it is characterized by the progressive development of greater than 100 adenomatous colorectal polyps, some of which will inevitably progress to cancer. Most of these polyps are usually less than five millimeters in diameter and so thickly grown that they carpet the entire surface of the colon. The clinical diagnosis of FAP is based on the finding of 100 or more colorectal adenomas (85). Up to one-third of FAP cases result from *de novo* germline mutations in the *APC* gene. Other features of FAP and its variants include jaw and sebaceous cysts, osteomata, a retinal lesion known as congenital hypertrophy of the retinal pigment (CHRPE), desmoid tumors, and cancers of the ampulla of Vater, bile duct, thyroid, and small intestine (1). There is also an attenuated form of FAP that is characterized by a fewer number of colorectal adenomas and a later age of onset of colorectal cancer (86).

The gene responsible for FAP, known as the adenomatous polyposis coli gene (*APC* on chromosome 5q, has been identified and characterized (87–90). A study of 79 unrelated patients with FAP searched for germline mutations in the APC gene. A total of 67% carried germline mutations and of the mutations found, 92% resulted in the truncation of the APC protein (91). All affected individuals should be tested for mutations in the APC gene and appropriate relatives should consider testing given the high risk of colon cancer and the early age of onset.

6.2. Medical Management Options

For FAP carriers, annual flexible sigmoidoscopy beginning at age 10–11 is recommended. Once polyps are detected by endoscopy, counseling regarding prophylactic colectomy should commence. Surveillance for extracolonic neoplasms, specifically gastrointestinal tract adenomatous polyps is also recommended. For APC negative individuals, flexible sigmoidoscopy at age 18, 25, and 35 is recommended. If no polyps are detected, then conventional colon cancer screening with colonoscopy every 3–5 yr starting at age 50 is recommended (92).

Nonsteroidal anti-inflammatory drugs (NSAIDs) have been experimentally shown to promote apoptosis and to inhibit angiogenesis, two mechanisms that facilitate the suppression of malignant tumor growth (93). A number of epidemiologic (nonrandomized) studies have found that long-term users of aspirin or other NSAIDs have a lower risk of colorectal adenomatous polyps and colorectal cancer than nonusers (93). More specifically, randomized clinical trials have established that two nonsteroidal anti-inflammatory drugs, sulindac (94–96) and celecoxib (a selective cyclooxygenase-2 inhibitor) (97,98), suppress adenomatous polyps and cause regression of existing polyps in patients with FAP. With regard to FDA approval, celecoxib was evaluated in a randomized, double-blind, placebo-controlled trial in 83 FAP patients (97). Analysis showed a significant reduction in a surrogate endpoint—colorectal polyp counts—observed after 6 mo of therapy with celecoxib. The tolerability of celecoxib treatment in FAP patients was consistent with labeled adverse events for the drug. In December 1999, celecoxib (Celebrex) was granted accelerated FDA approval for the reduction in the number of colorectal polyps in FAP patients, as an adjunct to usual care (e.g., endoscopic surveillance or surgery).

7. SUMMARY

It is critical that healthcare providers appreciate the complexities and special nature of genetic testing in order to accurately and responsibly interpret results for patients and their families. Further research is essential to fully understand the function of these genes and to develop effective prevention strategies and therapies. Although preventive surgical treatments may be effective in reducing the risk of some organ confined cancers, these interventions are extreme and may have both physical and psychological sequelae. As individuals with hereditary predisposition genes are detected earlier in the cancer process, it is important to include them in chemoprevention trials that may prevent the progression/development of disease. This becomes extremely important given the variable penetrance of these mutations. The Division of Cancer Prevention at the NCI currently supports a number of studies in high-risk and genetically susceptible populations, and when possible, health care providers should refer suitable participants to these studies. The NCI also maintains a website for information about hereditary cancer predisposition testing and a directory of healthcare professionals who provide cancer genetic counseling.

REFERENCES

1. Schneider K. 2002. Hereditary Cancer Syndromes, Counseling About Cancer. 2nd ed. Wiley-Liss: New York, pp. 73–118.
2. American Society of Clinical Oncology. 1996. Statement of the American Society of Clinical Oncology on genetic testing for cancer susceptibility. Adopted on February 20, 1996. J. Clin. Oncol. 14(5):1730–1736.
3. American Society of Clinical Oncoloy. 1994. Statement of the American Society of Human Genetics on genetic testing for breast and ovarian cancer predisposition. Am. J. Hum. Genet. 55(5):i–iv.
4. National Society of Genetic Counselors. 1997. Predisposition genetic testing for late-onset disorders in adults. JAMA 278(15):1217–1220.
5. National Action Plan on Breast Cancer. 1996. National Action Plan on Breast Cancer position paper: Herediatry susceptibility testing for breast cancer. J. Clin. Oncol. 14(5):1737–1740.
6. Bennett RL, Steinhaus KA, Uhrich SB, et al. 1995. Recommendations for standardized human pedigree nomenclature. Pedigree Standardization Task Force of the National Society of Genetic Counselors. Am. J. Hum. Genet. 56(3):745–752.
7. Love RR, Evans AM, Josten DM. 1985. The accuracy of patient reports of a family history of cancer. J. Chronic Dis. 38(4):289–293.
8. ACMG Laboratory Practice Committee Working Group. 2000. ACMG recommendations for standards for interpretation of sequence variations. Genet. Med. 2(5):302–303.
9. Whittemore AS, Gong G, Itnyre J. 1997. Prevalence and contribution of BRCA1 mutations in breast cancer and ovarian cancer: results from three U.S. population-based case-control studies of ovarian cancer. Am. J. Hum. Genet. 60(3):496–504.
10. Ford D, Easton DF, Peto, J. 1995. Estimates of the gene frequency of BRCA1 and its contribution to breast and ovarian cancer incidence. Am. J. Hum. Genet. 57(6):1457–1462.
11. Anton-Culver H, Cohen PF, Gildea ME, Ziogas A. 2000. Characteristics of BRCA1 mutations in a population-based case series of breast and ovarian cancer. Eur. J. Cancer 36(10):1200–1208.
12. Claus EB, Schildkraut JM, Thompson WD, Risch NJ. 1996. The genetic attributable risk of breast and ovarian cancer. Cancer 77(11):2318–2324.
13. Miki Y, Swensen J, Shattuck-Eidens D, et al. 1994. A strong candidate for the breast and ovarian cancer susceptibility gene BRCA1. Science 266(5182):66–71.
14. Wooster R, Bignell G, Lancaster J, et al. 1995 Identification of the breast cancer susceptibility gene BRCA2. Nature 378(6559):789–792.

15. Tavtigian SV, Simard J, Rommens J, et al. 1996. The complete BRCA2 gene and mutations in chromosome 13q-linked kindreds. Nat. Genet. 12(3):333–337.

16. Easton DF, Bishop DT, Ford D, Crockford GP. 1993. Genetic linkage analysis in familial breast and ovarian cancer: results from 214 families. The Breast Cancer Linkage Consortium. Am. J. Hum. Genet. 52(4):678–701.

17. Ford D, Easton DF, Stratton M, et al. 1998. Genetic heterogeneity and penetrance analysis of the BRCA1 and BRCA2 genes in breast cancer families. The Breast Cancer Linkage Consortium. Am. J. Hum. Genet. 62(3):676–689.

18. Frank TS, Deffenbaugh AM, Reid JE, Hulick M, Ward BE, Lingenfelter B, et al. 2002. Clinical characteristics of individuals with germline mutations in BRCA1 and BRCA2: analysis of 10,000 individuals. J. Clin. Oncol. 20(6):1480–1490.

19. Serova OM, Mazoyer S, Puget N, Dubois V, Tonin P, Shugart YY, et al. 1997. Mutations in BRCA1 and BRCA2 in breast cancer families: are there more breast cancer-susceptibility genes? Am. J. Hum. Genet. 60(3):486–495.

20. Rebbeck TR, Couch FJ, Kant J, Calzone K, DeShano M, Peng Y, et al. 1996 Genetic heterogeneity in hereditary breast cancer: role of BRCA1 and BRCA2. Am. J. Hum. Genet. 59(3):547–553.

21. Antoniou AC, Pharoah PD, McMullan G, Day NE, Stratton MR, Peto J, et al. 2002. A comprehensive model for familial breast cancer incorporating BRCA1, BRCA2 and other genes. Br. J. Cancer 86(1):76–83.

22. Antoniou AC, Pharoah PD, McMullan G, Day NE, Ponder BA, Easton D. 2001. Evidence for further breast cancer susceptibility genes in addition to BRCA1 and BRCA2 in a population-based study. Genet. Epidemiol. 21(1):1–18.

23. Seitz S, Rohde K, Bender E, Nothnagel A, Kolble K, Schlag PM, et al. 1997 Strong indication for a breast cancer susceptibility gene on chromosome 8p12-p22: linkage analysis in German breast cancer families. Oncogene 14(6):741–743.

24. Kainu T, Juo SH, Desper R, Schaffer AA, Gillanders E, Rozenblum E, et al. 2000. Somatic deletions in hereditary breast cancers implicate 13q21 as a putative novel breast cancer susceptibility locus. Proc. Natl. Acad. Sci. USA 97(17):9603–9608.

25. Vehmanen P, Friedman LS, Eerola H, McClure M, Ward B, Sarantaus L, et al. 1997. Low proportion of BRCA1 and BRCA2 mutations in Finnish breast cancer families: evidence for additional susceptibility genes. Hum. Mol. Genet. 6(13):2309–2315.

26. Vahteristo P, Bartkova J, Eerola H, Syrjakoski K, Ojala S, Kilpivaara O, et al. 2002. A CHEK2 genetic variant contributing to a substantial fraction of familial breast cancer. Am. J. Hum. Genet. 71(2):432–438.

27. Meijers-Heijboer H, van den OA, Klijn J, Wasielewski M, de Snoo A, Oldenburg R, et al. 2002. Low-penetrance susceptibility to breast cancer due to CHEK2(*)1100delC in noncarriers of BRCA1 or BRCA2 mutations. Nat. Genet. 31(1):55–59.

28. Struewing JP, Abeliovich D, Peretz T, Avishai N, Kaback MM, Collins FS, et al. 1995. The carrier frequency of the BRCA1 185delAG mutation is approximately 1 percent in Ashkenazi Jewish individuals. Nat. Genet. 11(2):198–200.

29. Neuhausen S, Gilewski T, Norton L, Tran T, McGuire P, Swensen J, et al. 1996. Recurrent BRCA2 6174delT mutations in Ashkenazi Jewish women affected by breast cancer. Nat. Genet. 13(1):126–128.

30. Oddoux C, Struewing JP, Clayton CM, Neuhausen S, Brody LC, Kaback M, et al. 1996. The carrier frequency of the BRCA2 6174delT mutation among Ashkenazi Jewish individuals is approximately 1%. Nat. Genet. 14(2):188–190.

31. Roa BB, Boyd AA, Volcik K, Richards CS. 1996. Ashkenazi Jewish population frequencies for common mutations in BRCA1 and BRCA2. Nat. Genet. 14(2):185–187.

32. Struewing JP, Hartge P, Wacholder S, Baker SM, Berlin M, McAdams M, et al. 1997. The risk of cancer associated with specific mutations of BRCA1 and BRCA2 among Ashkenazi Jews. N. Engl. J. Med. 336(20):1401–1408.

33. Fodor FH, Weston A, Bleiweiss IJ, et al 1998. Frequency and carrier risk associated with common BRCA1 and BRCA2 mutations in Ashkenazi Jewish breast cancer patients. Am. J. Hum. Genet. 63(1):45–51.

34. Warner E, Foulkes W, Goodwin P, et al. 1999. Prevalence and penetrance of BRCA1 and BRCA2 gene mutations in unselected Ashkenazi Jewish women with breast cancer. J. Natl. Cancer Inst. 91(14):1241–1247.

35. Moslehi R, Chu W, Karlan B, et al. 2000. BRCA1 and BRCA2 mutation analysis of 208 Ashkenazi Jewish women with ovarian cancer. Am. J. Hum. Genet. 66(4):1259–1272.

36. Levy-Lahad E, Catane R, Eisenberg S, et al. 1997. Founder BRCA1 and BRCA2 mutations in Ashkenazi Jews in Israel: frequency and differential penetrance in ovarian cancer and in breast-ovarian cancer families. Am. J. Hum. Genet. 60(5):1059–1067.

37. Abeliovich D, Kaduri L, Lerer I, et al. 1997. The founder mutations 185delAG and 5382insC in BRCA1 and 6174delT in BRCA2 appear in 60% of ovarian cancer and 30% of early-onset breast cancer patients among Ashkenazi women. Am. J. Hum. Genet. 60(3):505–514.

38. Beller U, Halle D, Catane R, Kaufman B, Hornreich G, Levy-Lahad E, 1997. High frequency of BRCA1 and BRCA2 germline mutations in Ashkenazi Jewish ovarian cancer patients, regardless of family history. Gynecol. Oncol. 67(2):123–126.

39. Muto MG, Cramer DW, Tangir J, Berkowitz R, Mok S. 1996. Frequency of the BRCA1 185delAG mutation among Jewish women with ovarian cancer and matched population controls. Cancer Res. 56(6):1250–1252.

40. Ford D, Easton, DF, Bishop DT, Narod SA, Goldgar DE. 1994. Risks of cancer in BRCA1-mutation carriers. Breast Cancer Linkage Consortium. Lancet 343(8899):692–695.

41. Easton DF, Ford D, Bishop DT. 1995. Breast and ovarian cancer incidence in BRCA1-mutation carriers. Breast Cancer Linkage Consortium. Am. J. Hum. Genet. 56(1):265–271.

42. Wooster R, Neuhausen SL, Mangion J, et al. 1994. Localization of a breast cancer susceptibility gene, BRCA2, to chromosome 13q12-13. Science 265(5181):2088–2090.

43. Brose MS, Rebbeck TR, Calzone KA, Stopfer JE, Nathanson KL, Weber BL. 2002. Cancer Risk Estimates for BRCA1 Mutation Carriers Identified in a Risk Evaluation Program. J. Natl. Cancer Inst. 94(18):1365–1372.

44. Breast Cancer Linkage Consortium. 1999. Cancer Risks in BRCA2 Mutation Carriers. JNCI Cancer Spectrum 91(15):1310–1316.

45. Friedman LS, Gayther SA, Kurosaki T, et al. 1997. Mutation analysis of BRCA1 and BRCA2 in a male breast cancer population. Am. J. Hum. Genet. 60(2):313–319.

46. Couch FJ, Farid LM, DeShano ML, et al. 1996. BRCA2 germline mutations in male breast cancer cases and breast cancer families. Nat. Genet. 13(1):123–125.

47. Thompson D, Easton DF. 2002. Cancer Incidence in BRCA1 Mutation Carriers. J Natl. Cancer Inst. 94(18):1358–1365.

48. Frank TS, Manley SA, Olopade OI, et al. 1998. Sequence analysis of BRCA1 and BRCA2: correlation of mutations with family history and ovarian cancer risk. J. Clin. Oncol. 16(7):2417–2425.

49. Shattuck-Eidens D, Oliphant A, McClure M, et al. 1997. BRCA1 sequence analysis in women at high risk for susceptibility mutations. Risk factor analysis and implications for genetic testing. JAMA 278(15):1242–1250.

50. Couch FJ, DeShano ML, Blackwood MA, et al. 1997. BRCA1 mutations in women attending clinics that evaluate the risk of breast cancer. N. Engl. J. Med. 336(20):1409–1415.

51. Berry DA, Iversen ES Jr, Gudbjartsson DF, et al. 2002. BRCAPRO validation, sensitivity of genetic testing of BRCA1/BRCA2, and prevalence of other breast cancer susceptibility genes. J. Clin. Oncol. 20(11):2701–2712.

52. Parmigiani G, Berry D, Aguilar O. 1998. Determining carrier probabilities for breast cancer-susceptibility genes BRCA1 and BRCA2. Am. J. Hum. Genet. 62(1):145–158.

53. Burke W, Daly M, Garber J, et al. 1997. Recommendations for follow-up care of individuals with an inherited predisposition to cancer. II. BRCA1 and BRCA2. Cancer Genetics Studies Consortium. JAMA 277(12):997–1003.

54. Hartmann LC, Schaid DJ, Woods JE, et al. 1999. Efficacy of bilateral prophylactic mastectomy in women with a family history of breast cancer. N. Engl. J. Med. 340(2):77–84.

55. Hartmann LC, Sellers TA, Schaid DJ, et al. 2001. Efficacy of Bilateral Prophylactic Mastectomy in BRCA1 and BRCA2 Gene Mutation Carriers. JNCI Cancer Spectrum 93(21):1633–1637.

56. Rebbeck TR, Levin AM, Eisen A, et al. 1999. Breast cancer risk after bilateral prophylactic oophorectomy in BRCA1 mutation carriers. J. Natl. Cancer Inst. 91(17):1475–1479.

57. Kauff ND, Satagopan JM, Robson ME, et al. 2002. Risk-reducing salpingo-oophorectomy in women with a BRCA1 or BRCA2 mutation. N. Engl. J. Med. 346(21):1609–1615.

58. Rebbeck TR, Lynch HT, Neuhausen SL, et al. 2002. Prophylactic oophorectomy in carriers of BRCA1 or BRCA2 mutations. N. Engl. J. Med. 346(21):1616–1622.

59. Narod SA, Brunet JS, Ghadirian P, et al. 2000. Tamoxifen and risk of contralateral breast cancer in BRCA1 and BRCA2 mutation carriers: a case-control study. Hereditary Breast Cancer Clinical Study Group. Lancet 356(9245):1876–1881.

60. Fisher B, Costantino JP, Wickerham DL, et al. 1998. Tamoxifen for prevention of breast cancer: report of the National Surgical Adjuvant Breast and Bowel Project P-1 Study. J. Natl. Cancer Inst. 90(18):1371–1388.

61. King MC, Wieand S, Hale K, et al. 2001. Tamoxifen and breast cancer incidence among women with inherited mutations in BRCA1 and BRCA2: National Surgical Adjuvant Breast and Bowel Project (NSABP-P1) Breast Cancer Prevention Trial. JAMA 286(18):2251–2256.

62. Narod SA, Risch H, Moslehi R, et al. 1998. Oral contraceptives and the risk of hereditary ovarian cancer. Hereditary Ovarian Cancer Clinical Study Group. N. Engl. J. Med. 339(7):424–428.

63. Modan B, Hartge P, Hirsh-Yechezkel G, et al. 2001. Parity, oral contraceptives, and the risk of ovarian cancer among carriers and noncarriers of a BRCA1 or BRCA2 mutation. N. Engl. J. Med. 345(4):235–240.

64. The American Cancer Society. 2001. The American Cancer Society: Cancer Facts and Figures 2001. Atlanta, GA.

65. Mecklin JP, Jarvinen HJ, Hakkiluoto N, et al. 1995. Frequency of hereditary nonpolyposis colorectal cancer. A prospective multicenter study in Finland. Dis. Colon Rectum 38(6): 588–593.

66. Ponz dL, Sassatelli R, Benatti P, Roncucci L. 1993. Identification of hereditary nonpolyposis colorectal cancer in the general population. The 6-year experience of a population-based registry. Cancer 71(11):3493–3501.

67. Lynch HT and Smyrk T. 1996. Hereditary nonpolyposis colorectal cancer (Lynch syndrome). An updated review. Cancer 78(6):1149–1167.

68. Risinger JI, Barrett JC, Watson P, Lynch HT, Boyd J. 1996. Molecular genetic evidence of the occurrence of breast cancer as an integral tumor in patients with the hereditary nonpolyposis colorectal carcinoma syndrome. Cancer 77(9):1836–1843.

69. Pal T, Flanders T, Mitchell-Lehman M, et al. 1998. Genetic implications of double primary cancers of the colorectum and endometrium. J. Med. Genet. 35(12):978–984.

70. Vasen HF, Mecklin JP, Khan PM, Lynch HT. 1991. The International Collaborative Group on Hereditary Non-Polyposis Colorectal Cancer (ICG-HNPCC). Dis. Colon Rectum 34(5):424–425.

71. Fishel R, Lescoe MK, Rao MR, et al. 1993. The human mutator gene homolog MSH2 and its association with hereditary nonpolyposis colon cancer. Cell 75(5):1027–1038.

72. Leach FS, Nicolaides NC, Papadopoulos N, et al. 1993. Mutations of a mutS homolog in hereditary nonpolyposis colorectal cancer. Cell 75(6):1215–1225.

73. Papadopoulos N, Nicolaides NC, Wei YF, et al. 1994. Mutation of a mutL homolog in hereditary colon cancer. Science 263(5153):1625–1629.

74. Bronner CE, Baker SM, Morrison PT, et al. 1994. Mutation in the DNA mismatch repair gene homologue hMLH1 is associated with hereditary non-polyposis colon cancer. Nature 368(6468):258–261.

75. Nicolaides NC, Papadopoulos N, Liu B, et al. 1994. Mutations of two PMS homologues in hereditary nonpolyposis colon cancer. Nature 371(6492):75–80.

76. Akiyama Y, Sato H, Yamada T, et al. 1997. Germ-line mutation of the hMSH6/GTBP gene in an atypical hereditary nonpolyposis colorectal cancer kindred. Cancer Res 57(18):3920–3923.
77. Liu B, Parsons R, Papadopoulos N, et al. 1996. Analysis of mismatch repair genes in hereditary non-polyposis colorectal cancer patients. Nat. Med. 2(2):169–174.
78. Muller A and Fishel R. 2002. Mismatch repair and the hereditary non-polyposis colorectal cancer syndrome (HNPCC). Cancer Invest. 20(1):102–109.
79. Aaltonen LA, Peltomaki P, Leach FS, et al. 1993. Clues to the pathogenesis of familial colorectal cancer. Science 260(5109):812–816.
80. Liu B, Farrington SM, Petersen GM, et al. 1995. Genetic instability occurs in the majority of young patients with colorectal cancer. Nat. Med. 1(4):348–352.
81. Rodriguez-Bigas MA, Boland CR, Hamilton SR, et al. 1997. A National Cancer Institute Workshop on Hereditary Nonpolyposis Colorectal Cancer Syndrome: meeting highlights and Bethesda guidelines. J. Natl. Cancer Inst. 89(23):1758–1762.
82. Aarnio M, Sankila R, Pukkala E, et al. 1999. Cancer risk in mutation carriers of DNA-mismatch-repair genes. Int. J. Cancer 81(2):214–218.
83. Lynch HT, and de la CA. 1999. Genetic susceptibility to non-polyposis colorectal cancer. J. Med. Genet. 36(11):801–818.
84. Burke W, Petersen G, Lynch P, et al. 1997. Recommendations for follow-up care of individuals with an inherited predisposition to cancer. I. Hereditary nonpolyposis colon cancer. Cancer Genetics Studies Consortium. JAMA 277(11):915–919.
85. Bussey HJ. 1979. Familial polyposis coli. Pathol. Annu. 14(1):61–81.
86. Spirio L, Olschwang S, Groden J, et al. 1993. Alleles of the APC gene: an attenuated form of familial polyposis. Cell 75(5):951–957.
87. Kinzler KW, Nilbert MC, Su L, et al. 1991. Identification of FAP locus genes from chromosome 5q21. Science 253(5020):661–665.
88. Groden J, Thliveris A, Samowitz W, et al. 1991. Identification and characterization of the familial adenomatous polyposis coli gene. Cell 66(3):589–600.
89. Joslyn G, Carlson M, Thliveris A, et al. 1991. Identification of deletion mutations and three new genes at the familial polyposis locus. Cell 66(3):601–613.
90. Nishisho I, Nakamura Y, Miyoshi Y, et al. 1991. Mutations of chromosome 5q21 genes in FAP and colorectal cancer patients. Science; 253(5020):665–669.
91. Miyoshi Y, Ando H, Nagase H, et al. 1992. Germ-line mutations of the APC gene in 53 familial adenomatous polyposis patients. Proc. Natl. Acad. Sci. USA 89(10):4452–4456.
92. Petersen GM. 1996. Genetic testing and counseling in familial adenomatous polyposis. Oncology 10(1):89–94.
93. Thun MJ, Henley SJ, Patrono C. 2002. Nonsteroidal anti-inflammatory drugs as anticancer agents: mechanistic, pharmacologic, and clinical issues. J. Natl. Cancer Inst. 94(4):252–266.
94. Giardiello FM, Yang VW, Hylind LM, et al. 2002. Primary chemoprevention of familial adenomatous polyposis with sulindac. N. Engl. J. Med. 346(14):1054–1059.
95. Giardiello FM, Offerhaus JA, Tersmette AC, et al. 1996. Sulindac induced regression of colorectal adenomas in familial adenomatous polyposis: evaluation of predictive factors. Gut 38(4):578–581.
96. Giardiello FM, Hamilton SR, Krush AJ, et al. 1993 Treatment of colonic and rectal adenomas with sulindac in familial adenomatous polyposis. N. Engl. J. Med. 328(18):1313–1316.
97. Phillips RK, Wallace MH, Lynch PM, et al. 2002. A randomised, double blind, placebo controlled study of celecoxib, a selective cyclooxygenase 2 inhibitor, on duodenal polyposis in familial adenomatous polyposis. Gut 50(6):857–860.
98. Steinbach G, Lynch PM, Phillips RK, et al. 2000. The effect of celecoxib, a cyclooxygenase-2 inhibitor, in familial adenomatous polyposis. N. Engl. J. Med. 342(26):1946–1952.

22

Diagnosis of Ataxia-Telangiectasia

ATM Mutations Associated With Cancer

Midori Mitsui, Shareef A. Nahas, Helen H. Chun, and Richard A. Gatti

1. INTRODUCTION

Prior to cancer therapy, it should be determined whether an underlying hereditary disorder might exist. A diagnosis of Ataxia-telangiectasia (A-T) should be considered in every child that develops a malignancy before 5 yr of age because A-T patients are unusually sensitive to radiation and conventional doses of radiotherapy can lead to devastating clinical consequences.

1.2. Early Diagnosis of A-T

Once A-T is suspected, confirming the diagnosis clinically can be difficult in young children because most of the signs and symptoms do not manifest fully until much later: (1) the onset of ataxia can be subtle in a child just learning to walk, (2) dysarthria is difficult to assess until speech patterns are well established, (3) detecting ocular apraxia requires the cooperation of the patient, (4) telangiectasias usually do not appear until several years after the onset of ataxia, (5) cerebellar atrophy may not be obvious on magnetic resonance imaging (MRI) studies until 7 or 8 yr of age, and (6) hereditary patterns may not yet be appreciated in a young family. Additionally, although the serum α-fetoprotein (AFP) is elevated in most A-T patients, 5–10% of A-T patients have normal levels. AFP can also remain above the normal laboratory range in normal infants until about 18 mo of age, further limiting the diagnostic value of this test. Karyotyping, with special attention to translocations involving chromosomes 7 and 14, can be useful; however, harvesting metaphases from A-T cells is technically difficult because these lymphocytes do not respond well to most mitogens. Nevertheless, an astute parent will often notice even mild neurological symptoms, if present, and, when asked, will volunteer enough information to allow the oncologist to either rule out A-T or prompt a neurological consultation.

Despite the need for a rapid solution to this problem, a laboratory confirmation of A-T currently take 2–3 mo because both immunoblotting and radiosensitivity testing depend upon first establishing a lymphoblastoid cell line (LCL) (Table 1). Faster methods are under development.

From: *Cancer Diagnostics: Current and Future Trends*
Edited by: R. M. Nakamura, W. W. Grody, J. T. Wu, and R. B. Nagle © Humana Press Inc., Totowa, NJ

Table 1
Laboratory Confirmation of Clinical A-T

Laboratory procedure	False negative (%)
1. α-fetoprotein[a] (after 2 yr of age)	5
2. Immunological status[a] (immunoglobulins; T and B cells)	approx 30
3. Karyotyping[a] (technically difficult with A-T cells)	approx 10
4. Radiosensitivity testing	
Radioresistant DNA synthesis (RDS)	<1?
Colony Survival Assay[a] (CSA)	approx 10
Chromatid breaks	approx 15
5. Western blots (for ATM protein in nuclear lysates of LCLs)[a]	<1
6. Deficient phosphorylation of ATM substrates	approx 1
7. Mutation detection	
If known from a prior affected*[a]	<1
If unknown—Haplotyping (compare to database of affected haplotypes)[a,b]	
Protein truncation test (uses mRNA)	approx 20
SSCP, CSGE, DOVAM, or REF	approx 20
Automated sequencing (including interpretation of data)	approx 15
dHPLC (heteroduplex detection; misses homozygotes)	approx 10
8. Haplotyping, to establish linkage to 11q23.1 (requires a prior affected)[a]	25

[a]Available in clinical laboratories.
[b]Depends upon genetic homogeneity/inbreeding of ethnic population.

1.3. A-T Syndrome

A-T is primarily an early onset, and relentlessly progressive cerebellar ataxia transmitted as an autosomal recessive disorder *(1–5)*. It occurs in approx 1 per 40,000 live births in the United States. This frequency varies considerably from country to country depending upon the frequency of cousin-to-cousin matings.

Infants appear normal and walk at a normal age (1 yr), begin to stagger by age 3, and generally require a wheelchair by age 10. Oculocutaneous telangiectasias appear several years after onset of neurological symptoms. Ocular apraxia and dysarthria become apparent early and are hallmarks of the disease. Frequent sinopulmonary infections are common. Cancer, usually lymphoid, occurs in one-third of A-T patients.

There is presently no treatment for A-T, although some of the secondary symptoms, such as drooling, are amenable to supportive therapy. Patients that do not die of early incurable cancers or overwhelming infections, sometimes survive into their 40s and even 50s.

When infections are seen, they are usually sinopulmonary and are usually the result of, not opportunistic infections, but conventional ones—unlike that of other immunodeficiency disorders. Almost half of A-T patients die with pulmonary failure and an associated pneumonia. In this regard, ATM protein is quite prominent in the bronchial epithelial cells of normal tissue; perhaps the absence of this protein in the lungs of A-T patients plays an important role in the development of the chronic cough and poor oxygenation that precede the irreversible pulmonary failure of many A-T patients. Poor swallowing coordination and excessive drooling in some patients can also lead to frequent aspiration pneumonia. This late-stage syndrome is initially responsive to steroids although eventually even these become ineffective. The T-cell system is abnormal, usually in subtle ways. T-cell responses to viral antigens and to histocompatibility antigens are often impaired to various degrees *(6,7)*.

T-cell responses to various mitogens are often subnormal, although this is not a consistent finding and should not influence the diagnosis of new patients *(8,9)*. CD45-RA+ (naïve) memory cells are below normal levels in the peripheral blood of most A-T patients *(10)*. High natural killer (NK) cell levels have been observed in many A-T patients, although some studies report normal levels *(7)*. Patients are often allergic when skin tested. Because these findings are not common to all A-T patients, they are assumed secondary effects, perhaps of inappropriate cell signaling.

The most consistent immune defects of A-T patients are those of IgA, IgE, IgG2, or IgG4 deficiencies *(3,7)*. In general, approximately one-third of A-T patients do not manifest any obvious immunodeficiency, nor do they have increased infections. Antigenic challenge of patients with polyvalent pneumococcal polysaccharide vaccine reveals a generally poor IgG response *(11)*. A consistent finding is the inappropriate rejoining of V(D)J regions in A-T cells *(12,13)*. The thymus is dystrophic, with poor corticomedullary differentiation, and no Hassall's corpuscles *(14,15)*. This probably reflects a perturbation in the maturation of T cells, as they try to rearrange the T-cell receptor (TCR) genes—a form of nonhomologous recombination. A similar situation probably arises during the differentiation of B cells. Interestingly, the severe humoral deficiencies observed in A-T patients (IgA, IgE and IgG2 are deficient in over 80% of patients) correlate loosely with the physical distance between the heavy chain variable genes in the V(D)J region and those in the heavy chain constant regions *(16)*. Conversely, other mechanisms might also influence the immune development and function of A-T cells. ATM protein phosphorylates many important substrates. ATM protein appears, in general, in the nucleus of replicating cells but in the cytoplasm of differentiating cells. ATM protein plays a role in apoptosis, which could be pivotal to negative selection in the thymus (and in the central nervous system). Lim et al. *(17)* suggested that β-adaptins and movement of vesicles may be abnormal in A-T cells and may play a role in the secretion of immunoglobulin molecules. Studies by Rivero-Carmena et al. *(18)* suggest that membrane function of T cells from A-T patients is intact. Regueiro et al. *(7)* exhaustively reviewed the immunological literature of A-T.

2. CANCER RISK

2.1. ATM Homozygotes

The *ATM* gene plays a major role in oncogenesis *(19–22)*. These patients develop new cases of cancer at approx 100 times the age-specific population rate *(23)*. Most cancers (85% for patients under 20 yr) involve the lymphoid system, either as lymphomas or leukemias; lymphomas are more common. A characteristic T-cell leukemia (T-proliferative lympho-cytic leukemia) occurs in older A-T patients in which TCL-1 is upregulated *(24)*. Younger A-T patients typically develop a T-acute lymphocytic leukemia. In patients over 20 yr, approximately half of the cancers are nonlymphoid, occurring in the following order of decreasing frequency: stomach, breast, medulloblastoma, basal cell carcinoma, ovarian dysgerminoma, hepatoma, and uterine leiomyoma *(23)*. Homogyous $Atm^{-/-}$ knockout mice develop thymic lymphomas; by 5 mo of age, virtually all of these mice have such tumors *(25)*.

2.2. ATM Heterozygote

ATM mutations and loss of heterozygosity across the 11q22–23 region have been reported in association with breast, prostate and ovarian cancer, head and neck cancer, lymphoma, and leukemia *(26–29)*. However, on closer inspection several caveats become apparent. First, ATM mutations for some human cancers are somatic, not inherited. Thus, such individuals would not be at an increased risk for cancer, at least with regard to the *ATM* gene *(30)*. Although it is clear that the ATM gene and protein are involved in the pathogenesis, only about one-third of T-PLL and chronic lymphocytic leukemia (CLL) patients were genomic ATM heterozygotes *(31–33)*. Two mechanisms are implicated in such patients: a 'second hit' to disable the remaining normal allele, or a dominant negative mutation, whereby the abnormal allele interferes with the functions of the normal allele, such as by blocking its access to a substrate (*see* below).

When members of A-T families were studied for breast cancer incidence, a three to eight fold increase was found in almost every study *(34–38)*. Paradoxically, when large breast cancer cohorts were screened for ATM mutations, the incidence of ATM mutations has seldom been higher than that in the control populations *(39–46)*. Rare allelic variants are seen in certain populations and make such studies difficult to interpret. For example, Vorechovsky et al. *(47)* screened 81 breast cancer patients and found 3 mutations and 5 rare variants. When FitzGerald et al. *(43)* used the protein truncation test (PTT) to screen 401 late onset breast cancer patients and 200 controls, only 2 ATM mutations were found in each group, with no significant difference between them. However, because PTT did not detect missense mutations, attention subsequently focused on the relevance of rare variants and missense mutations, rather than truncating mutations.

Only about 10% of mutations in A-T patients are of the missense type, whereas >85% of ATM mutations associated with breast cancer (and not A-T) have been of the missense type. This prompted the hypothesis that perhaps the phenotypes are different for nonsense and missense ATM mutations *(48)* (i.e., perhaps certain missense changes have dominant negative effects that cause cancer but not the A-T syndrome). Most enzymes have two complementary functions: they *bind* specifically and then they *catalyze* generically. If a mutation interferes with one function but not the other, the defective molecule can actually create additional harm by keeping its natural substrates 'in complex' indefinitely. In this way, a single defective copy of a gene that normally functions in a recessive way for null alleles (those not producing any protein), would now function in a dominant way. This would further suggest that defective proteins should be immediately targeted for destruction. Table 2 summarizes the expected phenotypes that might be present from having two types of A-T carriers in the general population, $ATM^{nonsense/wt}$ and $ATM^{missense/wt}$. This concept would also necessitate a reanalysis of cancer risks based on epidemiological studies, using different frequencies for each type of heterozygote. Current evidence suggests that the frequency of ATM missense mutations in the general population may be as high as 5–8%, and these do not generally appear to cause A-T. Accumulating data suggests that ATM missense mutations may play a more significant role in some A-T cancers, such as breast cancer, than in others, such as childhood leukemia, in which the mutation spectrum seems to resemble that of A-T patients *(49)*.

Two large ongoing NIH-funded epidemiological studies are addressing the above issue. The IMECAT (International Molecular Epidemiology Consortium for Ataxia Telangiectasia) study is evaluating the cancer risk of A-T relatives in eight countries, encompassing 600 A-T families; the cancer epidemiology is being collected in parallel. The ATM mutation carriers in each family are being distinguished from noncarriers by haplotyping. The types of ATM mutations in each family are also being determined to later assess cancer-causing ATM mutations. A second independent study, WECARE (Women's Environment, Cancer, and Radiation Epidemiology), is using denaturing high performance liquid chromatography

Table 2
Phenotype/genotype Relationships for ATM Mutations

Genotype	Phenotype
ATM$^{wt/wt}$	Normal
ATM$^{trunc/trunc}$	Ataxia-telangiectasia/cancer susceptibility
ATM$^{mis/mis}$	Ataxia-telangiectasia/cancer susceptibility?
ATM$^{mis/trunc}$	Ataxia-telangiectasia/cancer susceptibility
ATM$^{trunc/wt}$	Cancer susceptibility?
ATM$^{mis/wt}$	Cancer susceptibility/neurological symptoms?

(dHPLC) to identify the frequency and types of ATM mutations in over 2500 breast cancer patients from Europe, Australia, and the US *(50)*.

In addition, studies are underway to test the functional status of DNA changes (rare variants) in the ATM gene to distinguish mutations from polymorphisms, such as: 2546delSRI, S707P, P1054R, IVS10-6T>G, and 7271T>G. Scott et al. *(51)* have recently demonstrated that 2546delSRI and S2592C have dominant interfering effects on ATM function. In follow-up studies, Spring et al. *(52)* have further tested the dominant negative model of cancer risk by creating knock-in mice carrying the delSRI mutation. The delSRI$^{-/-}$ (i.e., homozygous) mice manifested a high frequency of tumors, as do ATM$^{-/-}$ knockout mice *(25)*. Most interestingly, the delSRI$^{+/-}$ (i.e., heterozygous) mice also manifested an increased incidence of tumors, as compared to controls. This was different than the cancer risk of the heterozygous ATM knockout mice, in which the incidence of tumors did not differ from that of normal mice of the same genetic background *(25)*. Thus, some ATM mutations increase the risk of cancer even when in a heterozygous state *(53)*.

2.3. Radiosensitivity testing

Cells from patients with A-T are typically sensitive to gamma ray radiation. The colony survival assay (CSA) was established as a diagnostic test, taking advantage of this characteristic radiosensitivity *(54,55)*. From a 5 mL heparinized whole blood sample, peripheral blood lymphocytes are immortalized by Epstein-Barr virus transformation and maintained in 15% fetal bovine serum (FBS) and incubated in 5% CO_2 at 37°C. This provides enough cells in the laboratory for testing both radiosensitivity, immunoblotting, kinase function, and mutation detection—an important issue when multiple assays must be performed on very small patients.

CSA begins by plating 200 and 100 cells/well in duplicate 96-well plates. The plates are then exposed to ionizing radiation (IR) at a dose of 1 Gy (Fig. 1). After incubation for 10–13 d at 37°C, the surviving cells are stained with vital dye (tetrazolium-based colorimetric assay), followed by another 2–4 h incubation.

The wells of each plate are then scored under a microscope for the formation of viable cell colonies (stained dark blue): "positive" (survival) is defined as >32 cells/well (indicating at least five cell divisions); "negative" signifies no colony formation in that well. Colony-forming efficiency (CFE) is calculated by comparing the ratio of negative wells to positive wells. The survival fraction (SF) is calculated by dividing the CFE of irradiated plates by the CFE of unirradiated control plates. An LCL with a SF of <21% is considered radi-

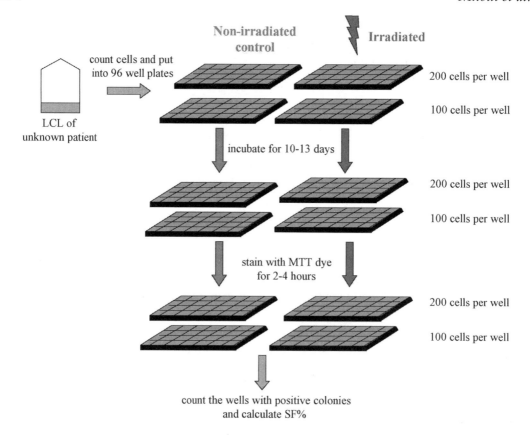

Fig. 1. Colony survival assay (CSA). For each test, a normal LCL and known A-T LCL are included as controls. The number of positive wells per plate is scored (>32 cells/well = a positive well).Colony forming efficiency, CFE, is calculated for irradiated plates (CFEi) and non-irradiated plates (CFEc). Survival fraction percentage (SF%) = CFEi/CFEc *(54)*. Color image available for viewing at **www.humanapress.com**.

osensitive, while LCLs with a SF of >37% is considered radionormal. A SF between 21 and 36% is considered as intermediate radiosensitivity. A-T LCLs typically fall in the radiosensitive range. An LCL with intermediate radiosensitivity is non-diagnostic and requires further testing. Roughly, 7% of A-T LCLs fall within this range; when such cells are retested across a range of radiation exposure rates (0.5 to 2 Gy), they are almost always radiosensitive at higher exposures (Fig. 2) *(55)*. A-T patients with intermediate radiosensitivity typically have mutations that fall within the functional domains of the ATM gene; the reason for this remains unclear *(55)*. There is also suggestive evidence that such patients may have a slower progression of neurological symptoms *(56)*.

The CSA is a useful test for confirming an early clinical diagnosis of A-T. However, this assay is also abnormal in other chromosomal instability and immunodeficiency disorders *(5)*. CSA sensitivity is >99%; specificity is approx 90%. Therefore, it is important to combine CSA data with other diagnostic testing *(57)*.

2.3.1. Immunoblotting

Recently, immunoblotting or western blot analysis has been adapted as a diagnostic test for A-T to detect ATM protein levels from nuclear lysates of LCLs *(57–60)* (Fig. 3). The

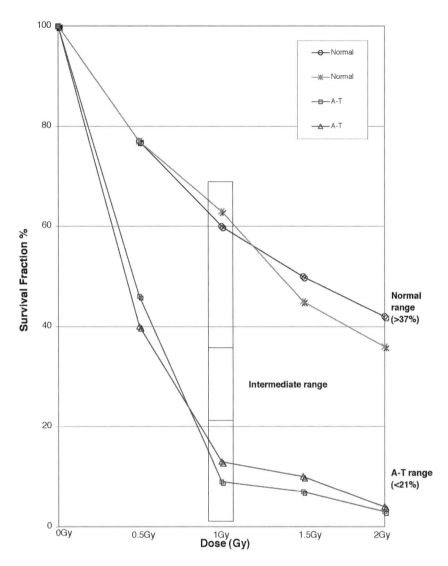

Fig. 2. Dose-response followup CSA testing for intermediate radiosensitivity. Four doses of irradiation are used: 0.5, 1.0, 1.5, and 2.0 Gy. Curves shown are for two normal and two A-T LCLs. Bar depicts CSA ranges when only one gray is used. Color image available for viewing at **www.humanapress.com**.

protein is 370 kDa in size and contains 3056 amino acids (aa). At least 5 million lymphoblastoid cells are necessary for immunoblotting. Anti-ATM antisera are used to detect ATM protein, which is visualized by enhanced chemiluminescence, and is semi-quantitated by densitometry. ATM protein levels are compared to normal protein from a non-A-T patient, and are semi-quantitatively scored over a range of 0–100%: <5%, undetectable; 5–15%, low; 16–75%, intermediate; and >75%, normal protein levels. Patients with A-T typically have <5% protein levels. Heterozygotes typically have intermediate levels *(57)*. An LCL with intermediate protein levels is not diagnostically conclusive; however, this is rarely encountered. The sensitivity and specificity of immunoblotting for A-T diagnosis are >99%.

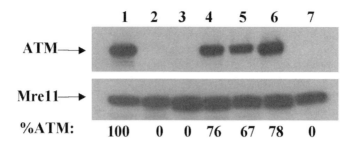

Fig. 3. Immunoblot analysis of nuclear lysates from 5 million LCLs, for evaluating ATM protein levels. Percentages below indicate densitometry readings for upper blot. Antibody to Mre 11 is used as a loading control (lower blot). *Lane 1,* normal control; *lane 2,* A-T control; *lanes 3* and *7,* newly-diagnosed A-T samples; *lanes 4–6,* not A-T patients.

Occasionally, we encounter a sample with normal ATM protein levels and radiosensitivity. The recommended followup testing would be: functional assessment of ATM protein (i.e., kinase activity on a p53 substrate), ATM mutation screening, and immunoblotting for deficiency of other proteins. The Ligase IV deficiency syndrome was discovered in this way *(61).* Because Mre11 deficiency manifests an early onset ataxia similar to A-T, our laboratory uses an antibody to Mre11 protein as a loading control in ATM testing. However, to date, only three families with Mre11 deficiency (also known as A-T Like Deficiency, ATLD) have been described *(62,63).*

2.3.2. ATM Protein Kinase Activity: A Functional Assay

Examining the protein kinase activity of ATM often helps the interpretation of an intermediate ATM protein level or CSA. Generally, cells from A-T patients do not have kinase function. However, rare patients have been described with near normal levels of ATM protein and greatly reduced kinase activity *(64–66).*

ATM phosphorylates many substrates involved in cell cycle control, DNA damage repair, and oxidative stress responses, for example, p53, MDM2, NBS1, BRCA1, CHEK1, SMC1, H2AX, and FANC D2 (67). ATM is activated by autophosphorylation after DNA double-strand breakage events and chromatin changes, such as those produced by IR and radiomimetic agents *(68).*

An ATM kinase test can be performed as an ex vivo assay on LCLs, examining p53 serine 15 (Ser15) as the phosphorylation target of ATM protein, or as an in vitro assay, by adding p53 and ^{32}P-ATP. In the former assay, cells are exposed to 2 Gy of irradiation and lysed 15 to 60 min after IR *(57).* Phosphorylation of p53 by the ATM homologue, ATR, occurs after 1 hr, so ATM-specific phosphorylation of Ser15 is controlled by time of harvest after IR. Whole cell lysates for irradiated and unirradiated control and A-T LCLs are prepared and analyzed by immunoblot analysis, using a p53 phosphoserine 15 antibody to identify ATM-specific phosphorylated p53. Typically, A-T cells have no inducible kinase activity following IR (Fig. 4). Normal cells phosphorylate p53 Ser15 immediately after exposure.

Similar assays using different ATM substrates may be used to further evaluate ATM protein kinase activity. Many phosphoserine-specific antibodies to ATM phosphorylation QS sites are commercially available, allowing considerable flexibility in choosing a phosphorylation target.

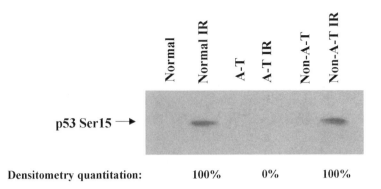

Densitometry quantitation: 100%   0%   100%

Fig. 4. ATM protein kinase assay, using p53 as substrate. LCLs were exposed to 2 Gy ionizing radiation (IR) to induce ATM kinase activity. Whole cell lysates were prepared, blotted, and immunoblots developed with antibody to phosphorylated Serine 15 of p53. Positive bands are seen in *lanes 2* and *6*. Induced ATM kinase activity is semi-quantitated by densitometry. *Lanes 1* and *2*, normal control; *lanes 3* and *4*, A-T cells; *lanes 5* and *6*, newly-diagnosed non-A-T sample.

2.4. ATM Mutations

Identifying mutations in the ATM gene has been difficult owing to its large size *(69–74)*. The gene extends over 150,000 nucleotides of genomic DNA, includes 66 exons, and has an open reading frame (ORF) of 9168 nucleotides. Most A-T patients are compound heterozygotes; they inherit a different mutation from each parent. Mutations in A-T patients are present throughout the ATM gene. Approximately 85% are nonsense mutations (many resulting from aberrant splicing), 10% are missense, and 3% are large genomic deletions or pseudoexon insertions. The latter are not detected by PCR-based methods, especially when present in heterozygous form. A compilation of almost 400 unique mutations is contained in the ATM Mutation Database (www.benaroyaresearch.org/bri_investigators/atm.htm). Although mRNA is present in virtually all A-T patients, mature truncated proteins are not detected. This is probably because of instablility; however, the role of nonsense-mediated mRNA decay (NMD) in A-T cells is being evaluated. Missense mutations have been associated with an increased risk for malignancy, particularly breast cancer (as discussed above).

The first method used to screen the large ATM gene for mutations is the Protein Truncation Test (PTT) *(71)*. PTT detects about 70% of ATM mutations *(72–74)*. If PTT does not identify both mutations, Single Strand Conformation Polymorphism (SSCP) *(75,76)* is performed, using RNA/cDNA as the starting template. This detects almost all types of mutations but involves screening of more fragments. Large genomic deletions are analyzed by loss of heterozygosity (LOH) on the gDNA, using several microsatellite and single nucleotide polymorphism (SNP) markers *(77,78)*.

Other methods have been developed for mutation screening. These include: Conformation sensitive gel electrophoresis (CSGE), restriction endonuclease fingerprinting (REF), detection of virtually all mutations (DOVAM) *(79)*, denaturing high performance liquid chromatography (dHPLC) *(50,80)*, high-density oligonucleotide arrays, and direct sequencing. None of these methods is 100% efficient owing to several limitations. The large size of the gene makes direct sequencing difficult. Certain regions of the gene are usually not included in the screening, such as deep introns, promoter, and untranslated regions, because they

	SPAT 3.2		SPAT 4.3		SPAT 5.3		SPAT 6.1		SPAT 7.3	
S1819	133	133	131	141	133	131	133	133	131	131
NS22	161	161	165	163	171	159	161	161	163	163
S2179	141	141	139	139	143	143	141	141	139	139
S1818	154	154	160	156	144	160	154	154	158	158
	[A]	[A]	[6]	[B]	[C]	[2]	[A]	[A]	[D]	[D]

	SPAT 8.3		SPAT 9.4		SPAT 10.3		SPAT 11.4		SPAT 12	
S1819	137	141	137	141	133	139	131	131	131	131
NS22	163	151	163	163	165	173	169	161	161	161
S2179	139	139	137	141	137	143	143	147	147	147
S1818	152	152	158	160	160	152	164	158	158	158
	[5]	[E]	[F]	[G]	[H]	[I]	[J]	[K]	[K]	[K]

	SPAT 13		SPAT 14		SPAT 16		SPAT 18		SPAT 19.3	
S1819	133	135	137	131	147	147	137	133	135	141
NS22	167	173	163	161	163	163	163	163	159	163
S2179	143	141	143	139	137	137	141	141	143	141
S1818	160	160	160	154	154	154	160	162	160	158
	[L]	[M]	[S]	[T]	[N]	[N]	[U]	[V]	[3]	[O]

	SPAT 20.3		SPAT 22.3		SPAT 23		SPAT 24.3		SPAT 27.3	
S1819	131	127	135	135	133	139	133	133	131	131
NS22	165	163	175	175	165	173	161	161	165	165
S2179	139	139	143	143	137	141	141	141	139	139
S1818	160	154	164	164	160	158	154	154	160	160
	[6]	[P]	[Q]	[Q]	[H]	[R]	[A]	[A]	[6]	[6]

Fig. 5. Haplotypes of probands from 20 Spanish A-T families. Recurring haplotypes are color shaded. Note that 65% of families show recurring haplotypes. Haplotypes are assigned numbers instead of letters whenever the haplotype has also been observed in other countries. Mutations have been defined for each haplotype. Color image available for viewing at **www.humanapress.com**.

yield very few mutations and DNA changes are difficult to interpret. Finally, heterozygous large genomic deletions are "masked" by the second allele when DNA fragments are amplified by PCR.

In ethnically homogeneous populations, standardized haplotyping is especially efficient for identifying founder mutations (Fig. 5) *(78)*. Four highly polymorphic microsatellite markers are used to construct the haplotypes. This finding simplifies mutation screening in these populations because in almost all cases identical mutations are carried by identical haplotypes. For example, in Costa Rica, four founder haplotypes accounted for 85% of the affected chromosomes (Table 3) *(81)*; in Brazil and Spain, 65% of the A-T patients carried at least one founder haplotype with a mutation already identified *(78,82)* (Fig. 5). Our laboratory has established a haplotype-mutation database for many ethnic populations, and we use this approach as the first step in mutation screening.

Many founder effect mutations have been identified in international studies (Table 3). Only about a dozen mutations have been observed with >1% global frequency. These recurring mutations appear to be ancestrally related *(77)* rather than independent mutational events (hot spots) *(78)*; some ATM mutations appear to be thousands of years old *(77)*. Taken together these dozen recurring mutations account for about one-third of all ATM mutations in A-T patients, the other mutations being of very low frequency.

Table 3
ATM Mutations in Ethnic Populations

Population (haplotype)	Mutation	Frequency (% alleles)
Costa Rican		
A	5908C>T	56
C	7449G>A	13
D	4507C>T	9
B	IVS63del17kb	7
Polish		
B	6095G>A	11
A	IVS53-2A>C	9
E	5546delT	5
C	7010delGT	3
D	5932G>T	3
Italian		
A	7517del4	20
B	3576G>A	7
S1	3894insT	Sardinia (>95)
United Kingdom		
FM7	5762ins137	7
FM10	7636del9	6
N African Jews	103C>T	>99
Amish	1563delAG	>99
Japanese		
A	7883del5	28
B	IVS33+2T>A	22
Norwegian	3245ATC>TGAT	55
Spanish		
6	8977C>T	18
A	9010del28	15
H	2413C>T	5
Brazilian		
2	IVS28+1711del3450	15
I	7913G>A	9
1	3802delG	9
5	8264delATAAG	7
T	IVS11-2A>G	4
Hispanic American		
H	103C>T	6
M	1348delG	6
J	IVS20-579delAAGT	6
Turkish		
A	3576G>A	17
G	6188G>A	7
H	IVS44-1G>T	7
B	5554insC	4
D	1563delAG	4
E	9170G>C	4
F	IVS21+1G>A	4

3. SUMMARY

Much has been learned about A-T within the past two decades. Perhaps the most progress has been made in the areas of early diagnosis and prenatal testing, as well as in understanding the role of ATM protein in cell signaling, DNA repair, and oxidative stress. ATM mutations have been identified in over 600 families, as well as in non-A-T patients with various types of cancers. Surprisingly, the spectra of mutations for breast cancer and for A-T patients are quite different. Radiosensitivity (RS) studies of A-T have led to the discovery of other hereditary RS disorders, such as NBS, Mre11 deficiency, Ligase IV deficiency, Fanconi anemia, and X-linked agammaglobulinemia. Mostly, the RS disorders also manifest immunodeficiency and cancer susceptibility *(5)*. Despite these advances, major questions remain unanswered:

1. How does ATM deficiency lead to cerebellar degeneration and ataxia?
2. What is the mechanism by which ATM deficiency results in RS?
3. How can the relentlessly progressive neurological degeneration be treated?

REFERENCES

1. Boder E and Sedgwick RP. 1958. Ataxia-telangiectasia: a familial syndrome of progressive cerebellar ataxia, oculocutaneous telangiectasia and frequent pulmonary infection. Pediatrics 21:526–554.
2. Gatti RA, Boder E, Vinters, HV, Sparkes S, Norman A, Lange K. 1991. Ataxia-telangiectasia: an interdisciplinary approach to pathogenesis. Medicine 70:99–117.
3. Gatti RA. 2002. Ataxia-telangiectasia, in: The Genetic Basis of Human Cancer, Vogelstein B and Kinzler KW, eds., McGraw-Hill: New York, pp. 239–266.
4. Perlman S, Becker-Catania S, Galti RA. 2003. Ataxia-Telangiectasia Diagnosis and Treatment. Sem. Pediat. Neurol. 10:173–182.
5. Gatti RA. 2001.The inherited basis of human radiosensitivity. Acta Oncologica 40:702–711.
6. Yarchoan R, Kurman CC, Nelson DL. Defective specific antiinfluenza virus antibody production in vitro by lymphocytes from patients with ataxia-telangiectasia, in: Ataxia-Telangiectasia: Genetics, Neuropathology, and Immunology of a Degenerative Disease of Childhood, Gatti RA and Swift M, eds., Alan R. Liss, Inc: New York, pp. 315–329.
7. Regueiro JR, Porras O, Lavin M, and Gatti RA. 2000. Ataxia-Telangiectasia; a primary immunodeficiency revisited. Immunol. Allergy Clin. N. Amer. 20:177–206.
8. Gatti RA, Bick M, Tam CF, et al. 1982. Ataxia-telangiectasia: a multiparameter analysis of eight families. Clin. Immunol. Immunopath. 23:501–516.
9. Woods CG and Taylor AMR. 1992. Ataxia telangiectasia in the British Isles: the clinical and laboratory features of 70 affected individuals. Quart. J. Med. New. 298:169–179.
10. Paganelli R, Scala E, Scarselli E, et al. 1992. Selective deficiency of CD4+/CD45RA+ lymphocytes in patients with ataxia-telangiectasia. J. Clin. Immunol. 12:84–91.
11. Sanal O, Ersoy F, Yel L, et al. 1999. Impaired IgG antibody production to pheumococcal polysaccharides in patients with ataxia-telangeictasia. J. Clin. Immunol. 19:326–334.
12. Yuille MR, Colgnet LJ, Abraham SM, et al. 1998. ATM is usually rearranged in T-cell prolymphocytic leukemia. Oncogene 16:789–796.
13. Pan-Hammarstrom Q, Dai S, and Zhao Y, et al. 2003. ATM is not required in somatic hypermutation of VH, but is involved in the introduction of mutations in the switch u region. J. Immunol. 170:3707–3716.
14. Peterson RDA, Kelly WD, Good RA. 1964. Ataxia-telangiectasia: its association with a defective thymus, immunological-deficiency disease, and malignancy. Lancet 1:1189.
15. Amromin GD, Boder E, Teplitz R. 1979. Ataxia-telangiectasia with a 32 year survival. A clinicopathological report. J. Neuropath. Exp. Neurol. 38:621–643.

16. Gatti RA and Hall K: 1983.Ataxia-telangiectasia. Search for a central hypothesis. In: Chromosome Mutation and Neoplasia, German J, ed. Alan R. Liss, Inc., New York, pp. 23–41.

17. Lim D-S, Kirsch D, Canman CE, et al. 1998. ATM binds to beta-adaptin in cytoplasmic vesicles. Proc. Natl. Acad.Sci. USA 95:10,146–10,151.

18. Rivero-Carmena ME, Porras O, Pelaez B, Pacheco-Castro A, Gatti RA, Regueiro JR. 2000. Membrane and transmembrane signaling in Herpesvirus saimiri-translformed human CD4+ and CD8+ T cells is ATM-independent. Int. Immunol. 12:927–935.

19. Gatti RA and Good RA. l971. Occurrence of malignancy in immunodeficiency diseases. Cancer 28:89–98

20. Spector BD, Filipovich AH, Perry GS, Kersey JH. 1982. Epidemiology of cancer in ataxia-telangiectasia, in: Ataxia-Telangiectasia—Cellular and Molecular Link Between Cancer, Neuropathology and Immune Deficiency, Bridges BA and Harnden DG, eds., John Wiley: London, pp. 103–107.

21. Morrell D, Cromartie E, and Swift M. 1986. Mortality and cancer incidence in 263 patients with ataxia-telangiectasia. J. Natl. Cancer Inst. 77:89–92.

22. Taylor AMR, Metcalfe JA, Thick J, Mak Y-F. 1996. Leukemia and lymphoma in ataxia telangiectasia. Blood 87:423–438.

23. Su Y and Swift M. 2000. Mortality rates among carriers of ataxia-telangeictasia mutant alleles. Ann. Intern. Med. 133:770–778.

24. Chun HH, Castellvi-Bel S, Wang Z, et al. 2002. TCL-1, MTCP-1 and TML-1 gene expression profile in non-leukemic proliferations associated with ataxia-telangiectasia. Int. J. Cancer 97:726–731.

25. Barlow C, Hirotsune S, Paylor R, et al. 1996. Atm-deficient mice: a paradigm of ataxia telangiectasia. Cell 86:159–171.

26. Koike M, Takeuchi S Part S, et al. 1999. Overian cancer: loss of heterozygosity frequently occurs in the ATM gene, but structural alterations do not occur in this gene. Oncology 56:160–163.

27. Laake K Odegard A, Andersen TI, et al. 1997. Loss of heterozygosity at 11q23.1 in breast carcinomas: indication for involvement of a gene distal and close to ATM. Gene Chrom. Cancer 18:175–180.

28. Lu Y, Condie A, Bennett JD, Fry MJ, Yuille MR, Shipley J. 2001. Disruption of the ATM gene in breast cancer. Cancer Genet. Cytogenet. 126:97–101.

29. Carter SL, Negrini M, Baffa R, et al. 1994. Loss of heterozygosity at 11q22-q23 in breast cancer. Cancer Res. 54: 6270–6274.

30. Stilgenbauer S, Schaffner C, Litterst A, et al. 1997. Evidence for ATM as a tumor suppressor gene in T-prolymphocytic leukemia. Nat. Medicine 3:1155–1161.

31. Bullrich F, Tasio D, Kitada S, et al. 1999. ATM mutations in B-cell chronic lymphocytic leukemia. Cancer Res. 59:24–27.

32. Vorechovsky I, Luo L, Dyer MJS, et al. 1997. Clustering of missense mutations in the ataxia-telangiectasia gene in a sporadic T-cell leukaemia. Nat. Genet. 17:96–100.

33. Stankovic T, Weber P, Stewart G, et al. 1999. Inactivation of ataxia telangiectasia mutated gene in B-cell chronic lymphocytic leukaemia. Lancet 353:26–29.

34. Swift M, Reitnauer PJ, Morrell D, Chase CL. 1987. Breast and other cancers in families with ataxia-telangiectasia. N. Engl. J. Med. 316:1289–1294.

35. Swift A, Morrell D, Massey RB, Chase CL. 1991. Incidence of cancer in 161 families affected by ataxia-telangiectasia. N. Engl. J. Med. 325:1831–1836.

36. Easton DF. 1994. Cancer risks in A-T heterozygotes. Int. J. Radiat. Biol. 66:S177–S182.

37. Athma P, Rappaport R, Swift M. 1996. Molecular genotyping shows that ataxia-telangiectasia heterozygotes are predisposed to breast cancer. Cancer Genet. Cytogenet. 92:130–134.

38. Olsen JH, Hahnemann JM, Borresen-Dale A-L, et al. 2001. Cancer in patients with ataxia-telangiectasia and their relatives in the Nordic countries. J. Natl. Cancer Inst. 93:121–127.

39. Chen J, Birksholtz GC, Lindblom P, Rubio C, Lindblom A. 1998. The role of ataxia-telangiectasia heterozygotes in familial breast cancer. Cancer Res. 58:1376–1379.

40. Bay J-O, Grancho M, Pernin D, et al. 1998. No evidence for constitutional ATM mutation in breast/gastric cancer families. Int. J. Oncol. 12:1385–1390.

41. Vorechovsky I, Rasio D, Luo L, et al. 1996. The ATM gene and susecptibility to breast cancer: analysis of 38 breast tumors reveals no evidence for mutation. Canc Res. 56:2726–2732.

42. Stoppa-Lyonnet D, Soulier J, Lauge A, et al. 1998. ATM and breast cancer. Blood 91: 3920–3926.

43. FitzGerald MG, Bean JM, Hegde SR, et al. 1997. Heterozygous ATM mutations do not contribute to early onset of breast cancer. Nat. Genet. 15:307–310.

44. Broeks A, Floore AN, Urbanus JHM, et al. 2000. Classical ATM germline mutations contribute to breast cancer susceptibility. Amer. J. Hum. Genet. 66:494–500.

45. Chevenix-Trench G, Spurdle AB, Gatei M, et al. 2002. Dominant negative ATM mutations in breast cancer families. J. Nat. Cancer Inst. 94:205–215.

46. Thorstenson YR, Roxas A, Kroiss R, et al. 2003. Contributions of ATM mutations to familial breast and overian cancer. Cancer Res. 63:3325–3333.

47. Vorechovsky I, Luo L, Lindblom A, et al. 1996. ATM mutations in cancer families. Cancer Res. 56:4130–4133.

48. Gatti RA, Tward A, Concannon P. 1999. Cancer risk in ATM heterozygotes: a model of phenotypic and mechanistic differences between missense and truncating mutations. Mol. Genet. Metabol. 69:419–423.

49. Vorechovsky I, Luo L, Dyer MJS, et al. 1997. Clustering of missense mutations in the ataxia-telangiectasia gene in a sporadic T-cell leukaemia. Nature Genet. 17:96–100.

50. Bernstein JL, Teraoka S, Haile RW, et al. 2003. Designing and implementing quality control for multi-center screening of mutations in the ATM gene among women with breast cancer. Hum. Mut. 21: 542–550.

51. Scott SP, Bendix R, Chen P, Clark R, Dork T, Lavin MF. 2002. Missense mutations but not allelic variants alter the function of ATM by dominant interference in patients with breast cancer. Proc. Natl. Acad. Sci. USA 99:925–30.

52. Spring KF, Ahangari SP, Scott P, et al. 2002. Mice heterozygous for mutation in Atm, the gene involved in ataxia- telangiectasia, have heightened susceptibility to cancer. Nat. Genet. 32: 185–190.

53. Concannon P. 2002. ATM heterozygosity and cancer risk. Nat. Genet. 32:89–90.

54. Huo YK, Wang Z, Hong J-H, et al. 1994. Radiosensitivity of ataxia-telangiectasia, X-linked agammaglobulinemia and related syndromes. Cancer Res. 54: 2544–2547.

55. Sun X, Becker-Catania SG, Chun HH, et al. 2002. Early diagnosis of ataxia-telangiectasia using radiosensitivity testing. J. Pediat. 140:732–735.

56. McConville CM, Stankovic T, Byrd PJ, et al. 1996. AMR. Mutations associated with variant phenotypes in ataxia-telangiectasia. Am. J. Hum. Genet. 59:320–330.

57. Chun HH, Sun X, Nahas SA, et al. 2003. Improved diagnostic testing for ataxia-telangiectasia by immunoblotting of nuclear lysates for ATM protein expression and PI-3 kinase activity. Mol. Genet. Metab. In press.

58. Fukao T, Kaneko H, Birrell G, et al. 1999. ATM is upregulated during the mitogenic response in peripheral blood mononuclear cells. Blood 94:1998–2006.

59. Becker-Catania S, Chen G, Hwang M J, et al. 2000. Ataxia-telangiectasia: Phenotype/genotype studies of ATM protein expression, mutations, and radiosensitivity. Mol. Genet. Metab. 70:122–133.

60. Gilad S, Chessa L, Khosravi R, et al. 1998. Genotype-phenotype relationships in ataxia-telangiectasia and variants. Am. J. Hum. Genet. 62:551–561.

61. O'Driscoll M, Cerosaletti KM, Girard P-M, et al. 2001. DNA ligase IV mutations identified in patients exhibiting developal delay and immunodeficiency. Mol. Cell. 8:1175–1185.

62. Stewart GS, Maser RS, Stankovic T, et al. 1999. The DNA double-strand break repair gene hMRE11 is mutated in individuals with an ataxia-telangiectasia-like disorder. Cell 99:577–587.

63. Pitts SA, Kullar HS, Stankovic T, et al. 2001. HMRE11: genomic structure and a null mutation identified in a transcript protected from nonsese-mediated mRNA decay. Hum. Molec. Genet. 10:1155–1162.

64. Stankovic T, Kidd AMJ, Sutcliffe A, et al. 1998. ATM mutations and phenotypes in ataxia-telangiectasia families in the British Isles: expression of mutant ATM and the risk of leukemia, lymphoma, and breast cancer. Am. J. Hum. Genet. 62:334–345.

65. Stewart GS, Last JIK, Stakovic T, et al. 2001. Residual ataxia telanigiectasia mutated protein function in cells from A-T patients, with 5762ins137 and 7271T>G mutations, showing a less severe phenotype. J. Biol. Chem. 276:30103–30141.

66. Saviozzi S, Saluto A, Taylor AMR, et al. 2002. A late onset variant of ataxia-telangiectasia with a compound heterozygous genotype, A8030G/7481insA. J. Med. Genet. 39:57–61.

67. Shiloh Y. 2003. ATM and related protein kinases: safeguarding genome integrity. Nat. Rev. Cancer 3:155–168.

68. Bakkenist CJ and Kastan MB. 2003. DNA damage activates ATM through intermolecular autophosphorylation and dimer dissociation. Nature 421:499–506.

69. Savitsky K, Bar-Shira A, Gilad S, et al. 1995. A single ataxia-telangiectasia gene with a product similar to PI-3 kinase. Science 268:1749–1753.

70. Platzer M, Rotman G, Bauer D, Savitsky K, Shiloh Y, Rosenthal A. 1997. Ataxia-telangiectasia locus: analysis of 184 kb DNA provides evidence for mosaic genomic structure and complex transcriptional regulation of the ATM gene. Genome Res. 7:592–605.

71. Telatar M, Wang Z, Udar N, et al. 1996. Ataxia-telangiectasia: mutations in ATM cDNA detected by protein-truncation screening. Am. J. Hum. Genet. 59:40–44.

72. Concannon P and Gatti RA. 1997. Diversity of ATM gene mutations detected in patients with ataxia-telangiectasia. Hum. Mut. 10:100–107.

73. Telatar M, Teraoka S, Wang Z, et al. 1998. Ataxia-telangiectasia: identification and detection of founder-effect mutations in the ATM gene in ethnic populations. Am. J. Hum. Genet. 62:86–97.

74. Teraoka S, Telatar M, Becker-Catania S, et al. 1999. Splicing defects in the ataxia-telangiectasia gene, ATM: underlying mutations and phenotypic consequences. Am. J. Hum. Genet. 64: 1617–1631.

75. Orita M, Iwahana H, Kanazawa H, Hayashi K, Sekiya T. 1989. Detection of polymorphisms of human DNA by gel electrophoresis as single-strand conformation polymorphism. Proc. Natl. Acad. Sci. USA 86:2766–2770.

76. Castellvi-Bel S, Sheikhavandi S, Telatar M, et al. 1999. New mutations, polymorphisms, and rare variants in the ATM gene detected by a novel SSCP strategy. Hum. Mut. 14:156–162.

77. Campbell C, Mitui M, Eng L, Coutinho G, Thorstenson Y, Gatti RA. 2003. ATM mutations on distinct SNP and STR haplotypes in ataxia-telangiectasia patients of differing ethnicities reveal ancestral founder effects. Hum. Mut. 21:80–85.

78. Mitui M, Campbell C, Coutinho G, et al. 2003. Independent mutational events are rare in the ATM gene: haplotype prescreening enhances mutational detection rate. Hum. Mut. 22:43–50.

79. Buzin CH, Gatti RA, Nguyen VQ, et al. 2003. Comprehensive scanning of the ATM gene with DOVAM-S. Hum. Mut. 21:123–131.

80. Thorstenson YR, Shen P, Tusher VG, et al. 2001. Global analysis of ATM polymorphism reveals significant functional constrast. Am. J. Hum. Genet. 69:396–412.

81. Telatar M, Wang Z, Castellvi-Bel S, et al. 1998. A model for ATM heterozygote identification in a large population: Four founder-effect ATM mutations identify most of Costa Rican patients with ataxia Telangiectasia. Mol. Genet. Metab.64:36–43.

82. Coutinho G, Mitui M, Campbell C, et al. 2004. Five haplotypes account for fifty-five percent of ATM mutations in Brazilian patients with ataxia-telangiectasia: seven new mutations. Am. J. Med. Genet. In press.

Index